W9-BJH-627

Asthma

4th edition

Asthma

4th edition

Edited by

T.J.H. Clark MD BSc FRCP
Professor of Pulmonary Medicine, Imperial College,
London, UK

S. Godfrey MD PhD FRCP
Professor of Paediatrics and Director, Institute of
Pulmonology, Hadassah University Hospital, Jerusalem,
Israel

T.H. Lee MD FRCPath FRCP
National Asthma Campaign Professor, Department of
Respiratory Medicine and Allergy, GKT School of
Medicine, King's College, London, UK

N.C. Thomson MD FRCP
Professor of Respiratory Medicine, Department of
Respiratory Medicine, Western Infirmary, Glasgow, UK

A member of the Hodder Headline Group
LONDON

Co-published in the United States of America by
Oxford University Press Inc., New York

First published in Great Britain 2000 by
Arnold, a member of the Hodder Headline Group,
338 Euston Road, London NW1 3BH

http://www.arnoldpublishers.com

Co-published in the USA by
Oxford University Press Inc.,
198 Madison Avenue, New York, NY 10016
Oxford is a registered trademark of Oxford University Press

British Library Cataloguing in Publication Data
A catalogue record for this book is available from the British Library

Library of Congress Cataloguing-in-Publication Data
A catalog record for this book is available from the Library of Congress

ISBN 0 340 76123 7

1 2 3 4 5 6 7 8 9 10

Commissioning Editor: Joanna Koster
Production Editor: Lauren McAllister
Production Controller: Martin Kerans
Cover Design: Terry Griffiths

Typeset by Phoenix Photosetting, Chatham, Kent
Printed in Great Britain by St. Edmondsbury Press, Suffolk and bound by
Redwood Books, Wiltshire

What do you think about this book? Or any other Arnold title?
Please send your comments to feedback.arnold@hodder.co.uk

Contents

Contributors

Mrs G. Barnes
Director, National Asthma and Respiratory Training Centre, Warwick, UK

Professor P.J. Barnes
Department of Thoracic Medicine, National Heart and Lung Institute, Imperial College School of Medicine, London, UK

Professor E.R. Bleecker
Center for the Genetics of Asthma and Complex Diseases, University of Maryland, Baltimore, USA

Professor P.S. Burge
Consultant Physician, Birmingham Heartlands Hospital, Birmingham, UK

Professor P.G.J. Burney
Department of Public Health Sciences, Guy's Hospital, London, UK

Professor T.J.H. Clark
Pro Rector, Imperial College School of Medicine, National Heart and Lung Institute, London, UK

Professor G.J. Gibson
Department of Respiratory Medicine, Freeman Hospital, Newcastle upon Tyne, UK

Professor S. Godfrey
Director, Institute of Pulmonology, Hadassah University Hospital, Jerusalem, Israel

Dr C. Hawrylowicz
Department of Respiratory Medicine and Allergy, Guy's Hospital, London, UK

Professor S. Holgate
School of Medicine – Respiratory Cell and Molecular Biology Division, Southampton General Hospital, Southampton, UK

Professor P.K. Jeffery
Lung Pathology Unit, Imperial College School of Medicine and National Heart and Lung Institute, Royal Brompton Hospital, London, UK

G.H. Koppelman
Department of Pulmonary Rehabilitation, Beatrixoord Rehabilitation Centre, Haren, The Netherlands

Professor T.H. Lee
National Asthma Campaign Professor, Department of Respiratory Medicine and Allergy, GKT School of Medicine, King's College, London, UK

Dr W. McConnell
Southampton General Hospital, Southampton, UK

Dr G.G. Meijer
Department of Pulmonary Rehabilitation, Beatrixoord Rehabilitation Centre, Haren, The Netherlands

Dr S.P. Newman
Pharmaceutical Profiles Ltd, Ruddington, Nottingham, UK

Professor P.M. O'Byrne
Department of Medicine, McMasters University – Division of Respirology, Hamilton, Ontario, Canada

Dr M.R. Partridge
Consultant Physician, The Chest Clinic, Whipps Cross Hospital, London, UK

Professor D.S. Postma
Department of Pulmonary Diseases, University of Groningen, The Netherlands

Professor K.F. Rabe
Dept. of Pulmonology, Leiden University Medical Centre (LUMC), Leiden, The Netherlands

Dr D. Schmidt
Dept. of Pulmonology, Leiden University Medical Centre (LUMC), Leiden, The Netherlands

Professor A.E. Tattersfield
Division of Respiratory Medicine, City Hospital, Nottingham, UK

Professor N.C. Thomson
Department of Respiratory Medicine, Western Infirmary, Glasgow, UK

Professor J.O. Warner
School of Medicine – Allergy & Inflammation, Southampton General Hospital, Southampton, UK

Dr J. Warner
School of Medicine – Allergy & Inflammation, Southampton General Hospital, Southampton, UK

Professor A.J. Woolcock
Institute of Respiratory Medicine, Royal Prince Alfred Hospital, NSW, Australia

Preface to the fourth edition

Interest in asthma continues to grow apace and has an increasingly global dimension. This fourth edition reflects this need for timely reviews of asthma, a subject on which knowledge continues to accumulate. The third edition of *Asthma* appeared eight years ago and there have been some important advances since then. In planning for this fourth edition we have been very fortunate to recruit Professor Neil Thomson to join us as another editor as well as a number of new authors, all experts in their fields. As a result, the book has been substantially rewritten, both as chapters by the new authors but also thanks to extensive revisions to chapters written by our previous contributors.

We have continued the thrust of the last edition by assembling chapters which review the subject for practical clinicians and have further extended the list of supporting references, either by quoting more original articles or by giving a fuller list of further reading. Thus we hope this book will continue its original tradition of providing a comprehensive but readable synopsis of our understanding of asthma rather than being a reference textbook on the subject.

The need for this edition has been partly fuelled by the growing worldwide interest in the subject. Asthma management guidelines which had only just appeared in the last edition are now in widespread use. The Global Initiative for Asthma (GINA) has become well-established and has stimulated interest in many countries throughout the world while the British Thoracic Society guidelines provide clear and logical steps for the pharmacological management of asthma. These have in turn kindled further research in a range of communities which have added to our general knowledge. This stimulates a thirst for knowledge and a requirement for a broad-ranging review of the subject which is hopefully provided in this new edition.

As before, we recognize the reality of overlap between chapters and differences in style which stem from multi-author books. We hope this can be turned to good advantage as readers can continue to see slightly different approaches to the same subject which will enable them to form their own views.

Once again, we are deeply indebted to our contributors and to all those who have helped them produce their chapters. Our publishers have continued to be of great strength to us and we are delighted to have been able to achieve our target, thanks to their help, of getting this edition out in the millennium year.

We hope this new edition continues to provide useful contributions to our growing knowledge of asthma and will enable this better understanding to be reflected in improved treatment for our patients.

T.J.H. Clark
S. Godfrey
T.H. Lee
N.C. Thomson

2000

Preface to the third edition

It is less than a decade since the second edition was published but our understanding of asthma has grown immensely. Therefore in this third edition we have taken the opportunity largely to rewrite the book. Professor Godfrey and I felt it important to enlist some additional help and we were delighted when Professor Tak Lee agreed to join us. When the three of us planned this edition we realized that some new authors would be required and we were most fortunate in recruiting the new contributors as well as enlisting support from some of our original authors.

Since the first edition the book has gradually changed from being a review of the subject for clinicians to a collection of review articles which are more generously referenced. We have also included a greater proportion of chapters which examine the scientific origins of our knowledge about asthma and its treatment.

In the original edition the majority of chapters came from the Brompton Hospital and a consistent house style was achieved with relatively little overlap between chapters. In changing the format of this edition and by bringing in new authors there is greater overlap between some of the chapters. We have tried to minimize duplication as far as possible but some is inevitable and indeed much is desirable as the reader will be able to see more than one account of the subject, though written from a slightly different vantage point.

Occasionally the overlap between chapters is discordant and we recognize that this applies to some of our coverage of asthma treatment. Although the editors are committed to the more recent European, Canadian and Australasian guidelines concerning asthma treatment which involve the early use of anti-inflammatory therapy, we recognize that American practice differs somewhat, especially in the use of methylxanthines. We are therefore pleased that Dr Weinberger has produced an updated chapter on this subject. His advocacy of this treatment is in contrast to the advice given in other chapters but readers can come to their own conclusions as to what therapeutic mix is best for the individual patients. In this context the lack of uniformity of opinion is deliberate rather than accidental.

As usual this book owes almost everything to the contributors who have done all we have asked of them – to them we extend our gratitude. We are also grateful to our publishers for their help and in particular to Annalisa Page for both keeping us on our toes as well as always being there to help when we needed it.

We hope that this new edition will stimulate the better understanding of asthma that is required for its diagnosis and treatment.

T.J.H. Clark
S. Godfrey
T.H. Lee

1991

The definition of asthma: its relationship to other chronic obstructive lung diseases

WILLIAM D. McCONNELL AND STEPHEN T. HOLGATE

PREAMBLE

Asthma *circa* 1983 was a disease 'characterised by wide variations over short periods of time in resistance to flow in intrapulmonary airways' (Scadding, 1983).

Asthma *circa* 1998 was a:

chronic inflammatory disorder of the airways in which many cells play a role, in particular mast cells, eosinophils, and T lymphocytes. In susceptible individuals this inflammation causes recurrent episodes of wheezing, breathlessness, chest tightness, and cough particularly at night and/or in the early morning. These symptoms are usually associated with widespread but variable airflow limitation that is at least partly reversible either spontaneously or with treatment. The inflammation also causes an associated increase in airway responsiveness to a variety of stimuli (National Heart, Lung and Blood Institute, 1995).

A mere 12 years separates those two descriptions but they are clearly quite different. The more recent definition has introduced a further level of complexity. No longer is asthma a condition defined by a physiological, functional parameter. It now has a cellular and biochemical pathology underlying it. This change in definition encompasses the many advances that have been made in our understanding of asthma over the last 15 years but it is still far from the ideal definition that classifies patients into one group, with a common aetiology, pathology, clinical presentation, response to treatment and prognosis.

PURPOSE OF DISEASE DEFINITIONS

As has been illustrated above, any definition of a disease is dependent on the current state of clinical and scientific knowledge of the disease state. The specified common characteristic that exists in all individuals with a disease is known as the *defining characteristic* and any definition must encompass this characteristic as well as the other abnormalities that may be manifest (Campbell *et al.*, 1979). As our level of understanding of the disease processes deepens, the defining characteristic of the disease may change and patients that fell within the definition at one time may, advertently or inadvertently, fall outside it in due course. Therefore there exists a hierarchy in disease definition that reflects current understanding of the condition. As the level of knowledge increases, so we move closer to causation as the defining characteristic of a disease. Some conditions, such as chronic fatigue syndrome, have defining characteristics that are based purely on symptomatology, since little is known about the underlying pathophysiology or causative factors. Other conditions, such as peptic ulcer disease, can be defined according to pathogenetic characteristics that bring the definition closer to the aetiological factors responsible for the disease, such as the presence of *Helicobacter pylori*.

The main priority is for a definition to be useful to those individuals who are currently involved with the disease, so that it embraces those patients that share certain common characteristics. One of the most important groups that deals with the disease is clinicians, both general and specialist, who want to be able to communicate with colleagues and with patients about the aetiology, exacerbating factors, treatment options and the likely prognosis of the disease.

Another important group is basic scientists, investigating the pathophysiology of the condition. The range of investigations available to this group, such as tests of bronchial hyperresponsiveness, airway inflammation or allergy, is normally greater than those available to clinicians, and scientists are therefore able to characterize the patients in greater detail to ensure that they are dealing with a homogeneous sample.

Such investigations are usually not available to the epidemiologist, who often must study retrospectively populations of patients that may well not have been characterized according to modern standards. Epidemiological questionnaires enquiring merely about diagnosed asthma prove quite unreliable, because changes in the definition and nomenclature of a disease can change its apparent incidence quite considerably. Some have advocated that as asthma cannot be defined using criteria that are accessible to an epidemiologist, the most reliable way to study its epidemiology is to follow a large cohort and measure changes in the prevalence of certain well-defined end points, such as forced expiratory volume (FEV_1), presence of wheeze, cough and bronchial hyperresponsiveness (BHR) (Rijken *et al.*, 1991). Several questionnaires have been devised in an attempt to address this problem, with the emphasis on prospective cohort studies enquiring about current and past symptoms (O'Connor and Weiss, 1994). Questions enquiring about wheeze tend to be the most reliable marker of asthma (Jenkins *et al.*, 1996) but this only applies to certain age groups, since many infants develop wheeze during viral respiratory tract infections but do not subsequently develop asthma. Equally, in the older age groups, patients with chronic obstructive pulmonary disease (COPD) will frequently complain of wheezing. More recent epidemiological studies have combined symptom questionnaires with measures of BHR as an attempt to improve the sensitivity and specificity of the study (Toelle *et al.*, 1992) and to increase the objectivity of the measure taken. However, since BHR is neither a sensitive nor specific marker of asthma, it may not provide any additional level of accuracy (Jenkins *et al.*, 1996).

These sometimes complementary but often competing pressures on the agreed definition of a disease have led to prolonged and in-depth debates over the use of the word 'asthma'. In the absence of a full understanding of the conditions that we now group together as 'asthma', any definition will represent a compromise, albeit a temporary compromise.

DIAGNOSTIC CATEGORIES OF ASTHMA

In order to make a diagnosis of asthma, there is clearly no need for the clinician to attempt to confirm every feature of the asthma definition. This would not only be unnecessarily invasive and time-consuming for the patient, involving bronchial biopsies and challenge tests to assess airway hyperresponsiveness, it would also be prohibitively expensive. In most cases, the presence of a typical history in an individual with risk factors will strongly suggest the diagnosis, and the demonstration of variation in peak expiratory flow with time and treatment will confirm it. In general, a history of episodic breathlessness is given, associated with wheeze and cough, with intervening periods when they are relatively symptom-free. Clinical examination is generally unremarkable, except during exacerbations, though there may be evidence of associated diseases such as eczema. In some patients, however, with atypical presentations, there is a need for further investigations. Occasionally a history of cough alone is given. The condition may not display such a characteristically intermittent pattern and may present as chronic breathlessness. In some cases, the peak expiratory flow rate does not show the typical diurnal variation and the response to treatment is poor. These features may necessitate further confirmation of the diagnosis involving: skin-prick testing to assess allergy status; inhalational challenges with chemical (generally histamine or methacholine) or physical (exercise, hypertonic saline or cold air) stimuli to assess non-specific bronchial hyperresponsiveness; inhalational challenges to assess specific airway sensitivity to, for example, allergen; measurements of levels of exhaled nitric oxide, serum eosinophil cationic protein, urinary leukotriene E$_4$ or urinary glycosaminoglycans as indirect markers of airway inflammation; or induced sputum, bronchoalveolar lavage or bronchial biopsy measurements to look for evidence of the inflammatory and structural changes in the airway which are typical of asthma. As there is no 'gold standard' test for asthma, the eventual diagnosis in these more difficult patients may depend on a balance of probabilities and demonstration of the absence of any other pathology to explain the symptoms. In most cases in the United Kingdom, however, the diagnosis and management are carried out by a general practitioner on the basis of symptoms and a demonstration of variable intrapulmonary airflow limitation.

Traditionally, having arrived at the diagnosis of asthma, the patient is placed into one of three categories. Though these categories do still have some usefulness in the management of asthma patients, it is increasingly questioned whether pathogenetically there are substantial differences between the groups.

Category 1: extrinsic asthma

The term extrinsic refers to the observation that affected individuals show a hypersensitivity response to a range of external stimuli. This response is typically a type 1 immediate hypersensitivity reaction, involving the production of immunoglobulin E (IgE) to specific antigens that are present in the environment. These allergens can include proteins in the excreta of the house dust mite, *Dermatophagoides pteronyssinus* or *farinae*, various grass and tree pollens, household pets (cats, dogs) and, less commonly, certain proteins in food (e.g. cow's milk). Individuals tend to produce IgE to more than one antigen and are termed 'atopic'. Exposure to these allergens can produce a variety of clinical manifestations ranging from atopic dermatitis (eczema) and rhinitis (which may be seasonal if caused by pollen or perennial if caused by the house dust mite) to asthma or life-threatening anaphylaxis. The mechanism leading to these syndromes involves the allergen cross-linking high-affinity IgE receptors on the surface of mast cells, leading to degranulation of the cells and release of inflammatory mediators, including histamine, leukotrienes, enzymes and cytokines (Holgate *et al.*, 1986). These substances cause vasodilatation, leakage from blood vessels, recruitment of other inflammatory cells, contraction of bronchial smooth muscle and mucus hypersecretion. These processes lead to a variety of symptoms depending on the site affected (nasal mucosa, bronchi, skin, systemic circulation, etc.). Ongoing inflammation is caused by interaction of allergen with T lymphocytes, leading to further cytokine release and recruitment of inflammatory cells, particularly eosinophils. When this inflammatory process occurs in the airway wall, it leads to airway narrowing and the other characteristic feature of asthma, non-specific bronchial hyperresponsiveness (BHR).

A typical history may implicate a likely allergen with, for example, the presence of seasonal asthma symptoms or other allergic phenomena. Skin-prick testing, which involves the placing of dilute solutions of allergen on the skin and lightly piercing the epidermis, may confirm the identity of the allergen responsible by the development of a wheal-and-flare reaction in the skin within minutes. A RAST (radioallergoimmunosorbant test) of the serum may identify specific circulating IgE. Occasionally an inhalational allergen challenge is performed and the effect on lung function observed under carefully controlled conditions.

Less commonly, extrinsic asthma may be due to, or exacerbated by, the presence of IgG precipitating antibody to organic dusts such as from the fungus *Aspergillus*. After prior sensitization, exposure to the dust may cause a type 3 hypersensitivity reaction involving the deposition of immune complexes in the airways leading to wheeze and increased airflow obstruction after a delay of several hours. Extrinsic asthma may also result from exposure to a variety of organic or inorganic chemicals, such as diisocyanates and ethylene diamine, which may manifest itself as occupational asthma in the absence of IgE involvement.

Non-steroidal antiinflammatory agents, such as ibuprofen and aspirin, which inhibit the cyclooxygenase pathway of arachidonic acid metabolism, may exacerbate asthma, particularly in those individuals who have increased expression of the enzyme leukotriene C4 synthase in their mast cells and eosinophils (Cowburn *et al.*, 1998). Their disease is mediated largely by the leukotriene class of inflammatory mediators and therefore is a form of extrinsic asthma that is not immune-mediated. Such individuals, which account for 5–10% of asthmatics, typically present later in life with disease that responds poorly to corticosteroid therapy and is commonly associated with a history of nasal polyps.

Category 2: intrinsic asthma

Although an extrinsic cause for the asthma is often found, there is a significant number of individuals with airflow obstruction in whom there appears to be no antigenic or chemical factor causing the airway inflammation and who do not give a significant smoking history. These individuals are said to have 'intrinsic' or 'cryptogenic' asthma. This condition tends to present later in life than extrinsic asthma and may give a poorer response to bronchodilator medication. Prolonged courses of antiinflammatory drugs can often result in a substantial improvement in lung function but often there is some residual irreversible component to the airflow obstruction. Patients with intrinsic asthma may demonstrate a more rapid decline in pulmonary function than those with extrinsic disease (Ulrik *et al.*, 1992). In the presence of a smoking history, these patients may inadvertently be given the diagnosis of chronic obstructive pulmonary disease (COPD) caused by the smoking but further investigation may reveal a significant blood and sputum eosinophilia, typical of asthma. Histological examination of bronchial biopsies from these patients reveals changes more consistent with asthma than with COPD (Corrigan and Kay, 1990; Humbert *et al.*, 1996a,b; Humbert *et al.*, 1997; Ying *et al.*, 1997). Though there is a failure to identify an extrinsic cause for the asthma in these patients, it seems likely that the underlying pathogenetic processes are very similar to those of extrinsic asthma and it is tempting to speculate that these cases may represent the end-result of long-term, low-grade, untreated eosinophilic inflammation in the airways as a type 1 hypersensitivity reaction to some, at present, unknown allergen. Alternatively, there is some evidence to suggest that an atopic tendency declines with age (Burrows, 1995) and so negative skin-prick testing and low serum IgE levels in these older patients may fail to demonstrate a previous subclinical hypersensitivity to a common and well-known allergen.

Category 3: asthma associated with chronic obstructive pulmonary disease

The term 'chronic obstructive pulmonary disease' (COPD), and the related terms 'chronic bronchitis and emphysema', 'chronic airflow limitation', 'chronic obstructive airways disease' and 'non-specific chronic lung disease', have caused much controversy over the last 40 years. Pride *et al.* (1989) studied the use of terminology in these diseases and found much variation across the world, with Germany favouring the term 'chronic obstructive bronchitis', whilst the Netherlands employed 'chronic asthmatic bronchitis'. There was a tendency to prefer the older terms, such as 'chronic bronchitis' and 'emphysema' to the newer ones. Pride concluded that there was an unnecessary degree of redundancy in the terminology. The acronym COPD, which will be adopted for the remainder of this chapter, is generally used for a disease, usually in smokers or ex-smokers, in which there is progressive breathlessness and wheeze associated with airflow obstruction that shows little variation with time and poor reversibilty to bronchodilators or corticosteroids.

The typical COPD patient is quite dissimilar to the typical asthma patient and differentiation usually provides no difficulty to the clinician. Individuals with COPD are generally in their fifth decade or older, give a characteristic progressive history of breathlessness over several years, admit to a long smoking history and show abnormalities on clinical examination (cyanosis, hyperinflated chest, purse-lip breathing – signs which are generally only found in severe acute asthma attacks). Pulmonary function testing shows an obstructive defect with little reversibility with inhaled β_2-agonist and may demonstrate abnormalities consistent with emphysema (reduced gas transfer with a large residual volume suggesting air trapping). At similar levels of FEV_1, COPD patients tend to demonstrate greater hyperinflation of the lungs than do asthmatic subjects and have reduced gas transfer across the alveolar membrane (DLCO – transfer factor for carbone monoxide) whilst in asthma, gas transfer is normal or supernormal (Magnusson *et al.*, 1998). Difficulties arise, however, with the significant numbers of patients that have breathlessness, wheezing and airflow obstruction but show features compatible with both COPD and asthma. These will include the 'intrinsic asthmatic' with poorly reversible airflow obstruction and a moderate smoking history and the 'COPD patient' with evidence of emphysema but significant reversibility to their airflow obstruction. These difficulties are exacerbated by the problem of defining what degree of reversibility is 'significant'. In addition, since 10–15% of the UK population now have asthma and 30% smoke, and, of these, 20% will develop COPD, a significant number of patients will have both conditions.

These difficulties have remained for the last 40 years and the controversies have continued largely because of the lack of knowledge about the pathogenetic differences between COPD and asthma. Over the last 10 years, advances in our understanding of both asthma and COPD enable us to be more clear about the important features that distinguish these conditions, though we are still quite remote from a single defining characteristic. The remainder of this chapter will briefly discuss and compare our current knowledge of the pathogenesis of asthma and COPD and demonstrate how these processes lead to the clinical characteristics that define the two diseases. In this discussion, reference to the many other, less common conditions that can fall under the umbrella of 'obstructive lung disease' is omitted. These include bronchiectasis, bronchiolitis obliterans, diffuse panbronchiolitis and acute infective bronchiolitis. Most of these conditions have a distinct pathogenetic basis and can be distinguished and defined with relative ease.

REASONS TO DISTINGUISH ASTHMA AND COPD

For many clinicians in the past, the need to distinguish asthma from COPD has been of academic rather than practical interest, since the treatment of the two conditions seemed broadly similar – the use of bronchodilators for short-term relief of breathlessness and corticosteroids for prevention of breathless episodes. As our knowledge of the conditions has developed and the range of therapeutic options increased, a need has arisen to distinguish the two diseases. As stated in the British Thoracic Society (1997a) asthma management guidelines, 'whilst there is overlap between asthma and COPD related to smoking, they are different diseases with differing aetiologies, pathologies, natural histories and responses to treatment'.

The clarification of the diagnosis may allow more useful pursuit of the underlying cause of the disease, involving allergen avoidance, smoking cessation or genetic counselling (for example, in α1-antitrypsin deficiency). In addition, more accurate diagnostic labelling will more accurately predict a response to treatment. A common problem that is encountered is the dilemma faced when there is a poor response to a moderate dose of corticosteroid treatment. Is the treatment failure due to an inadequate dose, in which case the dose should be increased, or is it due to genuinely steroid-unresponsive disease (such as COPD), in which case the glucocorticoids should be stopped? Increasing knowledge of the side-effects of inhaled, as well as oral, corticosteroids and the high financial cost associated with these treatments, makes this an increasingly relevant point. Newer asthma treatments, such as the leukotriene receptor antagonists, will probably have no beneficial effect on smoking-related COPD but may produce dramatic improvements in the relatively steroid-unresponsive aspirin-sensitive asthma (Dahlen et al., 1993). Also, there are important differences in prognosis between asthma and COPD. Asthma has a low mortality and is associated with only a slightly increased rate of decline in lung function. COPD has a considerably higher mortality (Burrows et al., 1987) and continued smoking is associated with a progressive decline in lung function. There is some evidence that inhaled corticosteroids prevent the increased rate of loss of lung function in asthma (Haahtela et al., 1994) but that they have no effect in COPD (Pauwels et al., 1992). This prognostic difference may affect our advice to patients and, in addition, decisions concerning lung transplantation and mechanical ventilation may partly be dependent on the diagnostic label applied.

Accurate epidemiological evidence requires accurate diagnostic labels. Concerns have been expressed that part of the rapid increase in asthma prevalence is attributable to changes in diagnostic labelling, though further symptom-based studies have revealed this to be a relatively unimportant factor (Burney, 1993). Similarly, basic science and clinical research into these diseases requires accurate diagnosis, as errors will bias results. Finally, diagnostic mislabelling may have important implications for financial planning and resource allocation.

HISTORICAL BACKGROUND OF COPD

The CIBA symposium in 1959 attempted to define some of the processes involved in smoking-related airway disease. Prior to that there were two schools of thought. In the UK, chronic bronchitis was viewed as an inflammation of the airways caused by smoking and recurrent infection, leading to chronic sputum production ('smoker's cough'), progressive airflow obstruction and eventually to emphysema and respiratory failure. In the USA, a different view prevailed, regarding chronic bronchitis as a benign condition with most of the persistent airflow obstruction being due to emphysematous destruction of the lung parenchyma. Indeed, Fletcher and Peto (1977) demonstrated that chronic bronchitis was a benign condition and that the presence of 'smoker's cough' was not an early indication of subsequent progressive airflow limitation. It became clear that the patients diagnosed by the British as having chronic bronchitis were very similar to those given the diagnosis of emphysema by the US physicians and so the terms chronic obstructive lung disease (COLD), and subsequently COAD (*airway*) and COPD, were coined. Both the British and American theories regarded asthma as a separate entity.

The term chronic bronchitis was redefined by the CIBA symposium (1959) as 'chronic or recurrent excessive mucus secretion in the bronchial tree'. It therefore was a definition based on symptomatology and did not include any reference to the presence of airflow obstruction. Emphysema was defined pathologically as 'an increase beyond the normal in the size of air spaces distal to the terminal bronchiole either from dilatation or from destruction of their walls'. The elastic tissue of the alveolar walls normally keeps the small airways patent during expiration and provides elastic recoil for the lungs. Destruction of this tissue leads to airflow limitation, gas trapping and reduced gas transfer.

It was in the context of these various views that Orie and colleagues (1961) suggested the hypothesis that COPD and asthma were both different patterns of the same condition with common features of allergic hypersensitization, airway hyperresponsiveness and possibly eosinophilia. This has been termed the 'Dutch hypothesis' (Fletcher *et al.*, 1976) and, though its popularity has waxed and waned over the years, it has been difficult to find definitive evidence to confirm or refute it. Certainly COPD and asthmatic patients can exhibit many overlapping characteristics, including breathlessness, wheeze, peak expiratory flow rate variability, bronchial hyperresponsiveness and reversibility to bronchodilators and corticosteroids. There are now known to be important differences, however, in the pathogenesis of these conditions and in the mechanisms by which the common characteristics arise.

DEFINING CHARACTERISTICS OF ASTHMA IN COMPARISON TO COPD

Pathogenesis

Knowledge of the histopathology and pathogenesis of asthma and COPD has increased in the last 15 years largely as a result of the bronchoscopic evaluation of patients (Djukanovic *et al.*, 1990; Jeffery, 1998). Prior to this, most of the information regarding asthma was gleaned from post-mortem studies involving fatal acute severe asthma (Dunnill *et al.*, 1969) whilst the nature of chronic bronchitis, emphysema and COPD was elucidated from post-mortem studies and bronchial resections (lobectomies and pneumonectomies) in patients with pulmonary neoplasms. The realization that bronchoscopy could be performed safely in asthmatic and COPD patients allowed research into the airways during life, through the study both of bronchoalveolar lavage fluid (BALF), examining its cellular content, the markers of cellular activation and the levels of inflammatory mediators, and of endobronchial biopsies of large airways, assessing the distribution of the inflammatory and structural cells in the airway wall with particular emphasis on their activation status and their synthesis of inflammatory mediators, both at the protein and at the messenger RNA levels. In a few studies, transbronchial biopsies have been performed on patients, yielding information about the processes occurring in the smaller airways (Wenzel *et al.*, 1997).

These studies have shown that both asthma and COPD display inflammation of the airway wall associated with structural changes ('remodelling') but that the nature of these inflammatory and remodelling processes is different (Table 1.1). One of the major differences is in the site of the airflow obstruction in the two conditions, with airflow obstruction arising more from narrowing of the medium-sized airways in asthma, whilst in COPD it is preferentially expressed in the smaller airways (<3 mm diameter) (Hogg *et al.*, 1968).

INFLAMMATION

It has long been recognized that the sputum of asthmatic patients contains large numbers of eosinophils. This is also observed in biopsy specimens from the large airways of asthmatics and in bronchoalveolar lavage fluid (Djukanovic *et al.*, 1990). There are also increases in the metachromatic cells (mast cells and basophils) and in the lymphocyte population. Most notably, there seems to be a shift in the inflammatory cell phenotype away from the production of interleukin 2 (IL-2) and interferon gamma (IFN-γ) (a Th1 phenotype) towards

Table 1.1 *Comparison of pathological findings in COPD and asthma*

	COPD	Asthma
Airflow obstruction	Progressive deterioration of lung function (? reversible component)	Variable (± irreversible component)
Post-mortem	Excessive mucus (mucoid/ purulent), small airway disease, emphysema	Hyperinflation, airway plugs (exudate +mucus), no or little emphysema
Sputum	Macrophage, neutrophil (infective exacerbation)	Eosinophilia, metachromatic cells, Creola bodies
Surface epithelium	Fragility undetermined	Fragility/loss
Bronchiolar mucous cells	Metaplasia/hyperplasia	Mucous metaplasia is debated
Reticular basement membrane	Variable or normal	Homogeneously thickened and hyaline
Congestion/oedema	Variable/fibrotic	Present
Bronchial smooth muscle	Enlarged mass (small airways)	Enlarged mass (large airways)
Bronchial glands	Enlarged mass (increased acidic glycoprotein)	Enlarged mass (no change in mucin histochemistry)
Cellular infiltrate	Predominantly CD3, CD8, CD68, CD25, VLA-1 and HLA-DR +ve, mild eosinophilia (not degranulated?), mast cell increase	Predominantly CD3, CD4, CD25 (IL-2R) +ve, marked eosinophilia (EG2 +ve) (degranulated), mast cell increase (decrease in severe/fatal)
Cytokines (ISH)	GM-CSF protein ±IL-4 but not IL-5	IL-4 + IL-5 gene expression (Th2 profile)

Source: From Jeffery, 1998.

the production of interleukin 4 (IL-4), interleukin 5 (IL-5) and granulocyte-macrophage colony stimulating factor (GM-CSF) (a Th2 phenotype). This shift in cytokine production leads to an influx of other inflammatory cells, particularly the eosinophil. These cells all produce a variety of cytokines, growth factors and inflammatory mediators (histamine, leukotrienes, platelet activating factor) that activate other cells and enhance the inflammatory process.

The inflammatory process in COPD has proven a more elusive entity, partly because of the difficulties encountered in defining the various pathological processes that are encompassed by the term COPD. Chronic bronchitis is present in around 50% of smokers and does not contribute to airflow limitation. Until relatively recently, it was not clear whether inflammation played any part in chronic bronchitis or whether the mucus hypersecretion was solely due to mucous gland hypertrophy occurring as a response to cigarette smoke or particulate air pollution. Emphysema can cause airflow obstruction in the absence of any inflammatory process but it is likely that chronic inflammation in the small airways is at least partly responsible for emphysematous change in the lung parenchyma. Examination of the small airways does reveal an inflammatory process, referred to by Fletcher and Pride (1984) as a chronic obstructive bronchiolitis, which may well in its own right contribute significantly to the airflow limitation of COPD.

In recent years, bronchoscopic comparisons of patients with chronic bronchitis (without airflow obstruction), COPD and asthma with normals have demonstrated significant differences (Ollerenshaw and Woolcock, 1992; Lacoste et al., 1993; Saetta et al., 1993, 1994b; Di Stefano et al., 1996; O'Shaughnessy et al., 1997; Jeffery, 1998). The neutrophil is the commonest cell present in induced sputum and bronchoalveolar lavage fluid in normal non-smoking individuals but from patients with COPD these fluids demonstrate markedly elevated neutrophil and macrophage counts compared with asthmatics in whom airway neutrophilia is a much less prominent feature (Thompson et al., 1989; Ronchi et al., 1996) and biochemical markers of neutrophil activation are also markedly higher in COPD and chronic bronchitis than in asthma (Lacoste et al., 1993; Keating and Barnes, 1997). Patients with non-obstructed chronic bronchitis generally show less airway neutrophilia than those in whom obstruction is present (Lacoste et al., 1993) (Fig. 1.1), though this is not a consistent finding in all studies (Linden et al., 1993). However, severe chronic asthmatics on high doses of oral and inhaled corticosteroids tend to demonstrate high airway neutrophilia and low eosinophil counts (Wenzel et al., 1997) (Fig. 1.2). Whether this occurs as a result of the corticosteroid treatment or whether the neutrophils represent a corticosteroid-unresponsive component to the asthmatic inflammation is not known. Airway neutrophilia has also been demonstrated in asthmatics in sudden fatal asthma (Sur et al., 1993; Fahy et al., 1995) and during exacerbations (Turner et al., 1995). The neutrophils present in BALF from COPD patients may originate from the alveoli and respiratory bronchioles rather than from the larger airways, examination of which fails to show any significant neutrophil infiltrate.

On the other hand, airway eosinophilia is a less prominent feature of COPD, except during exacerbations (Saetta et al., 1994a). Even when eosinophils are present, markers of eosinophil activation (eosinophil cationic protein, ECP) are not elevated in BALF of COPD patients, in marked contrast to asthma where ECP is typically elevated (Lacoste et al., 1993), and the cytokine largely responsible for airway eosinophil recruitment and activation, IL-5, is only upregulated in asthmatic BALF and not during COPD exacerbations (Saetta et al., 1996). Examination of cytokine production by the airway cells in asthma and COPD also exposes significant differences. Whilst cells from asthmatic sputum produce increased levels of IL-5 and GM-CSF (which cause eosinophil recruitment), in COPD it is tumour necrosis factor alpha (TNF-α) and IL-8 with its neutrophil chemoattractant properties, that are over-produced (Hoshi et al., 1995; Keatings et al., 1996). In bronchial biopsies from COPD patients,

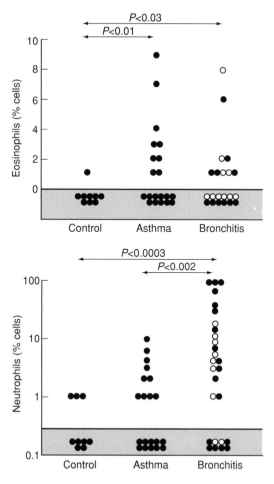

Figure 1.1 *Eosinophil and neutrophil content of BALF from normals, asthmatics, non-obstructed chronic bronchitics and COPD patients, demonstrating marked eosinophilia in asthma and predominant neutrophilia in chronic bronchitis, particularly when obstruction is present. Clear circles are non-obstructed (from Lacoste et al., 1993).*

the few eosinophils present normally contain granules, whereas in asthma they appear to be in an activated state and partially degranulated, having released inflammatory products stored in the cytoplasmic granules (Lacoste *et al.*, 1993). These differences are mimicked in the peripheral blood, where eosinophilia is significantly greater in asthmatics than in COPD or chronic bronchitis (Lacoste *et al.*, 1993). Keatings and Barnes (1997), by contrast, have studied induced sputum from COPD patients and found significantly elevated ECP concentrations compared to controls, which are comparable to those in asthma.

Endobronchial biopsies of large airways in normal non-smoking individuals show a predominantly lymphocytic infiltrate in the bronchial mucosa and submucosa, with relatively few granulocytes (neutrophils and eosinophils). Patients with COPD do not show a significant mucosal infiltrate of any granulocytes but instead reveal increased numbers of T lymphocytes (Ollerenshaw and Woolcock, 1992; Saetta *et al.*, 1993) and the numbers of T cells has been correlated with the presence of airflow obstruction (Di Stefano *et al.*, 1996) (Fig. 1.3). It is likely that the T cells exhibit different phenotypes in COPD from those in asthma, with excessive CD8+ T cells being present in endobronchial biopsies as airflow obstruction

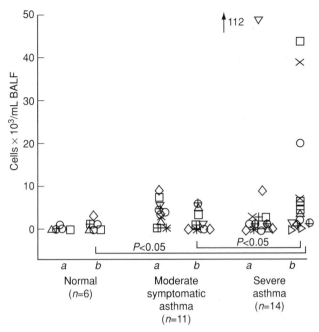

Figure 1.2 *Cellular content of BALF in non-asthmatics, moderate asthmatics and severe asthmatics, showing significant neutrophilia in severe asthmatics compared to moderates or normals (from Wenzel* et al., *1997). a, eosinophils; b, neutrophils.*

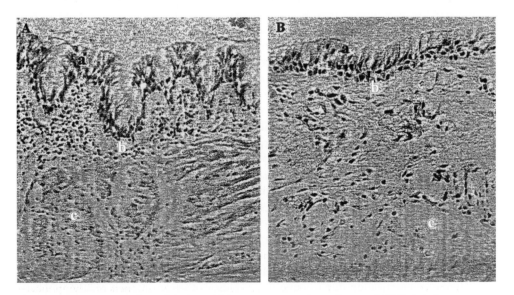

Figure 1.3 *Transverse sections of the bronchial mucosa contrasting asthma and COPD. A. Asthma demonstrating (a) epithelial disruption, (b) subepithelial fibrosis, (c) smooth muscle hypertrophy. B. COPD demonstrating (a) goblet cell hyperplasia, (b) normal subepithelial zone, (c) mucous gland hypertrophy (with grateful thanks to Dr John Wilson).*

increases in COPD (O'Shaughnessy *et al.*, 1997), in contrast to asthma in which the CD4+ cells predominate. A few studies have noted increased numbers of mast cells in the bronchial mucosa in COPD but this is not a universal finding (Lamb and Lumsden, 1982).

To what extent the inflammatory processes occurring in the small airways in COPD contribute to the airflow obstruction by thickening the airway wall internal to the smooth muscle layer is difficult to assess and probably varies from patient to patient, though several studies have correlated them (Cosio *et al.*, 1978; Cosio *et al.*, 1980; Mullen *et al.*, 1985; Bosken *et al.*, 1990; Linden *et al.*, 1993; Tiddens *et al.*, 1995). However it is likely that a significant contribution comes from the structural changes in the airway wall and alveoli.

AIRWAY REMODELLING

Characteristic structural changes are present in the walls of large airways of patients with any severity of asthma and even in asymptomatic atopic individuals (Roche *et al.*, 1989; Djukanovic *et al.*, 1992). It is likely that these changes, broadly termed airway remodelling, occur as a consequence of the chronic inflammatory processes and that they contribute to the asthma symptomatology (Redington and Howarth, 1997). Patchy shedding of the stratified ciliated epithelium has long been known to be a feature of asthma, with epithelial cells being commonly found in asthmatic sputum, but it can also be present in patients with non-asthmatic chronic cough (Boulet *et al.*, 1997). Post-mortem studies in fatal status asthmaticus frequently show areas of completely denuded epithelium, leaving only the basal cells. Under the epithelial basement membrane is the lamina reticularis which in asthmatics is thickened with layers of collagen. This subepithelial thickening is universal in asthma (Roche *et al.*, 1989) with the degree of thickening being correlated with the numbers of inflammatory cells and eosinophils in the epithelium (Chetta *et al.*, 1996). Outside the submucosa is the bronchial smooth muscle. In asthma this layer is markedly thickened due to hyperplasia and hypertrophy of the smooth muscle fibres. Other structural changes include increased airway wall vascularity and oedema (Li and Wilson, 1997). Several studies have employed the technique of high-resolution computed tomographic scanning to study these changes in wall thickness (Boulet *et al.*, 1995) and have shown that patients with increased asthma severity have greater airway wall thickening (Awadh *et al.*, 1998).

In COPD, the structural changes are quite different. Epithelial shedding is generally less marked than in asthma, with epithelial metaplasia being more prominent. In chronic bronchitis and in asthma, there is an increase in the large airway submucosal gland mass and in the number of epithelial goblet cells (Fig. 1.3) but in COPD this also occurs in the small airways (mucous metaplasia) and may contribute to airflow obstruction (Cosio *et al.*, 1980). The other structural changes in COPD are largely confined to the small airways (Ollerenshaw and Woolcock, 1992). The subepithelial fibrosis is present in COPD but the lamina reticularis is considerably less thickened than in asthma. Though there is a degree of smooth muscle hypertrophy in COPD, this is confined to the small airways, unlike in asthma where it is prominent in the larger bronchi but not in the smaller airways (Cosio *et al.*, 1980; Jeffery 1991).

The loss of alveolar attachments that is characteristic of the emphysematous component of COPD is not a feature of asthma. It is thought to result from a protease–antiprotease imbalance, possibly caused by the release of elastase due to neutrophilic inflammation and/or by antiprotease deactivation due to oxygen free-radicals that result from inhaling tobacco smoke (Gadek *et al.*, 1979; Cantin and Crystal, 1985; Saetta *et al.*, 1985; Linden *et al.*, 1993). This imbalance leads to proteolytic breakdown of lung tissue and so to the loss of elastic recoil that is characteristic of emphysema (Saetta *et al.*, 1985). Though cigarette smoke is by far the commonest cause of emphysema, there are occasional cases of emphysema in individuals who have never smoked and this is often due to deficiency of the antiprotease, α1-antitrypsin. In COPD, therefore, the airflow obstruction probably results from varying contributions from small airway inflammation, small airway remodelling and emphysema (Hale *et al.*, 1984).

Bronchial hyperresponsiveness

The tendency for the airways of asthmatic subjects to bronchoconstrict when exposed to various chemical and physical stimuli is known as bronchial hyperresponsiveness (BHR). Exposure to stimuli, such as allergen, which are specific for that individual produce a different effect, in that the non-specific stimuli generally cause a short-lived period of bronchoconstriction without inducing significant airway inflammation whilst antigenic stimuli cause more prolonged bronchoconstriction with an immediate response lasting for 1–2 hours followed by a late response at 4–8 hours, which is characterized by inflammatory cell recruitment to the airways. Various bronchoconstrictor stimuli can be used to measure the degree of BHR (Cockcroft *et al.*, 1977), including inhaled histamine or methacholine, inhaled hypertonic saline or distilled water, exercise or cold air. The chemical stimuli, histamine and methacholine, have the advantage of being simple to use and titrate, in order to give a measure of the concentration (PC_{20}) or dose (PD_{20}) required to produce a 20% fall in FEV_1. They are therefore the most widely used tests for clinical and scientific use. The physical stimuli are more difficult to titrate but probably mimic the day-to-day challenges on asthmatic airways more closely (Makker and Holgate, 1993). The response to exercise is a particularly physiological measure and is simple to use for epidemiological purposes but does not provide a numerical measure of the degree of BHR in an individual. Different stimuli give contrasting results as measures of BHR (Boulet *et al.*, 1987; Makker and Holgate, 1993), probably because each stimulus causes bronchoconstriction through different mechanisms, with the chemical stimuli causing smooth muscle contraction directly, whilst the physical stimuli may cause smooth muscle contraction indirectly through the release of mediators (histamine, leukotrienes, neuropeptides, etc.) from, for example, mast cells and nerve endings (Manning *et al.*, 1990). Thus different stimuli assess slightly different properties of the airways.

When normal individuals are challenged with a non-specific stimulus such as histamine there is usually a small degree of bronchoconstriction but the FEV_1 value forms a plateau before a 20% fall is achieved. In asthmatics, bronchoconstriction typically occurs at a much lower histamine concentration and there is no plateau, so that increasing the histamine dose further produces greater bronchoconstriction to a life-threatening degree (Sterk and Bell, 1991). BHR tends to be defined as a PC_{20} of less than 16 mg/mL, though some studies employ a different threshold concentration or a different percentage target fall in FEV_1, alterations which significantly affect the sensitivity and specificity of the test as a marker for asthma. Around 70% of patients with COPD also demonstrate BHR (Tashkin *et al.*, 1992), though usually at higher concentrations of agonist than in those with asthma (Fig. 1.4). There is, however, considerable overlap between the diseases, depending on the severity of disease and current treatment. The presence or absence of BHR cannot, therefore, be used alone as a defining characteristic that differentiates asthma from COPD. However, the relative responses to different bronchoconstrictor stimuli in COPD are notably different from asthma. Whilst COPD patients commonly demonstrate BHR to chemical stimuli, they rarely respond to physical stimuli (Arnup *et al.*, 1983; Ramsdale *et al.*, 1984) (Table 1.2), possibly because of the lesser role of primed mast cells in COPD. Also, the shape of the dose–response curve to chemical stimuli in COPD is different from asthma since COPD patients tend to demonstrate a plateau in their FEV_1 similar to normal individuals (Fig. 1.5).

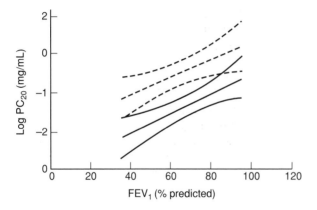

Figure 1.4 *Relationship between degree of airflow obstruction and BHR in asthma (solid lines) and COPD (broken lines). BHR increases as FEV$_1$ falls in both COPD and asthma, but at any level of FEV$_1$, BHR is greater in asthmatics (from Brand et al., 1991).*

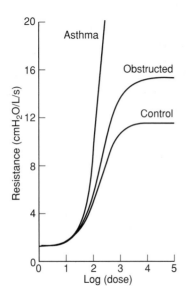

Figure 1.5 *Dose–response curves generated using a model of BHR, demonstrating how changes in the cross-sectional wall area can cause the dose–response curves typical of asthma and COPD (from Wiggs et al., 1992).*

Neither can the presence of BHR discriminate between asthmatics and normals because there are many individuals who exhibit BHR but report no asthma symptoms. The prevalence of BHR amongst children is around 20% but only half of these give a history suggestive of asthma (Sears *et al.*, 1986; Pattemore *et al.*, 1990). These individuals are commonly atopic, demonstrate greater variability in peak expiratory flow rate (PEFR) (Laprise and Boulet, 1997) and often have a family history of asthma (Lang *et al.*, 1987). Conversely, up to 50% of patients with asthma do not demonstrate BHR (Pattemore *et al.*, 1990), often because their disease is controlled with inhaled corticosteroids. Jones (1994) followed up children with asymptomatic BHR on exercise testing and found that 58% developed asthma in the subsequent 6 years, suggesting that they are at increased risk of developing asthma. A similar study in students with asymptomatic BHR showed a 45% incidence of asthma over 2 years (Zhong *et al.*, 1992). It seems likely that these individuals do not have a reduced perception of airway narrowing (Gibson *et al.*, 1995; Salome *et al.*, 1997), as has been suggested previously, but may have different factors contributing to their BHR. Pin *et al.* (1993) compared the eosinophil content of induced sputum in symptomatic and asymptomatic children with similar PC$_{20}$ values and

Table 1.2 *Airway responsiveness to different stimuli in patients with asthma and COPD (from Kerrebijn, 1989).*

Stimulus	Asthma (%)	COPD (%)
Methacholine (acetylcholine)	75	64
Histamine	82	36
Propranolol	67	21
Sulphur dioxide	95	30
Hyperventilation	96	11
Fog	30	81

found that it was lower in the asymptomatic individuals, whilst Power *et al.* (1993) studied asymptomatic adults with BHR and found no evidence of airway inflammation in bronchial biopsies compared to patients without BHR. Therefore, the nature of the BHR in these individuals may be different from that in asthmatics.

Even though BHR is present in a large proportion of COPD patients the mechanisms underlying it are probably different from those underlying BHR in asthma. There are multiple factors that contribute to BHR in asthma and COPD and the exact contributions of each factor are unknown.

EPITHELIAL FACTORS

The degree of epithelial loss has been correlated to BHR in asthma (Jeffery *et al.*, 1989). Epithelial damage may contribute to BHR through a variety of mechanisms (Saetta *et al.*, 1994b). There may be increased epithelial permeability, thus exposing afferent airway nerves and receptors to bronchoconstrictor and inflammatory stimuli. Greater plasma exudation through the epithelial barrier into the lumen may effectively alter the cross-sectional area of the lumen and change the surface tension properties of the airway. The epithelium also normally produces neutral endopeptidase which can inactivate bronchoconstrictor substances such as tachykinins. Epithelial loss may also reduce the responsiveness of the underlying smooth muscle to β_2-agonists.

CHRONIC INFLAMMATION

Since the inflammatory cells, particularly the mast cells and eosinophils, release many bronchoconstricting substances (leukotrienes, histamine), it is not surprising that the degree of BHR has been correlated to the inflammatory cell, particularly the eosinophil, content of the airway mucosa in asthma (Poulter *et al.*, 1990; Chetta *et al.*, 1996) (Fig. 1.6) and to the levels of the eosinophil activation marker (ECP) in BALF (Oddera *et al.*, 1996). BHR has also been correlated to the IL-5 expression in bronchial biopsies from atopic asthmatics (Ackerman *et al.*, 1994). However, a study by Makker *et al.* (1994) has failed to show an increase in the mast cell mediators (histamine, tryptase and prostaglandin D_2) following local airway challenge with hypertonic saline in asthmatic patients.

Allergen challenge in asthmatics causes airway inflammation and an increase in BHR. This temporal association implicates inflammation as a mediator of BHR. Similarly, treatment of asthmatic patients with antiinflammatory medication, such as inhaled corticosteroids, has profound effects on the inflammatory cell infiltrate in the airways and has a correspondingly profound effect on BHR (Cockcroft, 1988). Thus in most asthmatics the relationship between airway inflammation and BHR seems a causal one.

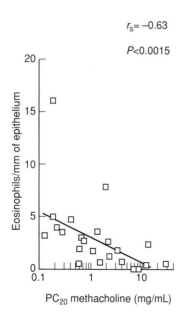

$r_s = -0.63$

$P < 0.0015$

Figure 1.6 *Relationship between eosinophil content of the epithelium and BHR in asthma. Correlation between intraepithelial eosinophils and PC$_{20}$ methacholine in 23 asthmatic patients (from Chetta et al., 1996). r$_s$ = Spearman rank correlation coefficient.*

AIRWAY REMODELLING

Models have been devised which demonstrate that BHR may result from normal smooth muscle shortening associated with thickening of the airway wall (Moreno *et al.*, 1986; Wiggs *et al.*, 1992). If the transverse cross-sectional area of the wall internal to the smooth muscle layer is increased, contraction of the smooth muscle to the same degree will produce a marked reduction in luminal diameter (Fig. 1.5). This increase in wall thickness will not necessarily impinge upon the lumen when the smooth muscle is relaxed and therefore there may not be a fall in baseline FEV$_1$. Several studies have been able to correlate airway wall thickness with BHR (Boulet *et al.*, 1995). Different features of the large airways in asthmatics may contribute to this wall thickening. Thickening of the subepithelial collagen layer has been correlated to airway hyperresponsiveness (Boulet *et al.*, 1997). Airway wall oedema, increased vascularity, increased bronchial smooth muscle mass and inflammatory cell infiltration may also play a role (Kuwano *et al.*, 1993). These changes are not present in the large airways in COPD but some may exist in the small airways (Bosken *et al.*, 1990).

Changes in airway wall structure external to the smooth muscle may also contribute to the BHR by uncoupling the lung's elastic forces from the smooth muscle, allowing it to shorten excessively (Macklem, 1991).

LOSS OF ALVEOLAR ATTACHMENTS

Seatta *et al.* (1985) correlated the degree of airway inflammation in the small airways of smokers having COPD with the loss of alveolar attachments which, in turn, is correlated with the loss of elastic recoil, increase in lung volumes and fall in FEV$_1$. The reduction in the forces holding the small airways patent will allow excessive contraction of the bronchial smooth muscle when a bronchoconstrictor stimulus is applied, thus contributing to the increased BHR found in patients with COPD. This emphysematous change is not a feature of asthma.

In asthma, the BHR is most closely correlated to the airway inflammation, whilst in COPD it is correlated with the baseline FEV$_1$ (Ramsdale *et al.*, 1984; Rijcken *et al.*, 1988; Tashkin *et al.*, 1992). However, in asthmatics exhibiting a degree of fixed airflow obstruction, the BHR is more related to the baseline FEV$_1$ (Ryan *et al.*, 1982) and to the airway wall thickness (Boulet *et al.*, 1995) (Fig. 1.5). It may be, therefore, that the irreversible airway remodelling processes that occur in COPD and in certain asthmatics lead both to progressive fall in FEV$_1$ and to increased BHR, whilst in asthmatics with completely reversible airflow obstruction, the BHR is caused by inflammation. Whether the BHR in smokers and asthmatics causes the progressive fall in FEV$_1$ or whether the BHR occurs as a result of the fixed airflow obstruction is a much debated and still unresolved subject (van Schayck *et al.*, 1994; Saetta *et al.*, 1994a), though it is likely that both theories may apply since BHR is a manifestation of so many properties of the airway.

Variability in airflow obstruction

Variation in the degree of airflow obstruction as assessed by measurement of the peak expiratory flow (PEF) is characteristic of asthma but, once again, cannot be used as a single defining characteristic because, like BHR, there is considerable overlap wi⁺h the normal population and with individuals having COPD (Brand *et al.*, 1991). This variation may, over relatively short periods of time, be associated with exacerbations of asthma or may occur in a diurnal pattern, with a marked reduction in PEF occurring in the morning (Fig. 1.7). This cyclical PEF variation in asthma is an exaggeration of the normal slight variations that occur in non-asthmatic individuals. It is impossible to set a threshold degree of PEF variability that defines asthma as subjects with well controlled asthma will exhibit stable PEFs whilst some patients with COPD may demonstrate exaggerated variability. Altering the threshold will change the sensitivity of the test at the expense of its specificity. Any dichotomy on the basis of PEF variability is therefore arbitrary.

It seems likely that diurnal PEF variability is caused by similar factors that determine BHR, since most studies find significant correlations between BHR and PEF variability both at a population level and at an individual level (Higgins *et al.*, 1992; Boezen *et al.*, 1996; Brand *et al.*, 1997) (Fig. 1.8) and many individuals exhibiting asymptomatic BHR will also demonstrate significant PEF variability (Gibson *et al.*, 1995). The correlation between BHR and PEF

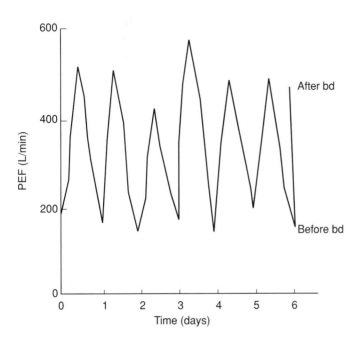

Figure 1.7 *Typical chart of peak expiratory flow (PEF) from a patient with uncontrolled asthma, demonstrating diurnal and between-day variation in PEF and the response of a low morning PEF to bronchodilator (from National Heart, Lung and Blood Institute, 1995). bd, bronchodilator.*

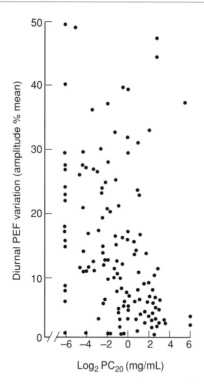

Figure 1.8 *Relationship between BHR and diurnal PEF variability in asthma (from Kerstjens* et al., *1994).*

variability is less strong in patients with COPD (Brand *et al.*, 1991). The correlation in asthma, however, is not exact and the two indices are therefore assessing similar but not identical properties of the airway (Boezen *et al.*, 1996). Like BHR, PEF variability responds to antiinflammatory treatment in asthma (Kerstjens *et al.*, 1994), and in clinical practice PEF variability is commonly used as a marker of disease severity and an early sign of deterioration in asthma control. However, Saetta *et al.* (1989) reported a case of fatal asthma in a patient demonstrating severe BHR but stable PEFs.

The correlation between PEF variability and BHR also depends on the method by which BHR is assessed and the way in which PEF variability is calculated. A variety of measures of PEF variability have been suggested, including the amplitude of variation expressed as a percentage of the mean, or the standard deviation of the PEF over a period of time, or the lowest PEF as a percentage of the highest. The latter is the simplest to measure and may be most clinically relevant (Brand *et al.*, 1997).

Reversibility

The characteristic that is used most commonly in clinical practice to differentiate asthma from COPD is the high degree of reversibility in airflow obstruction to bronchodilator or antiinflammatory medication that is present in asthma (Fig. 1.9). Different guidelines do not agree on the threshold of reversibility that is considered significant. The British Thoracic Society (1997b) Guidelines for the Management of COPD suggest that an increase in FEV_1 of 200 mL and 15% of the baseline value should be considered significant, whilst the American Thoracic Society (1991) recommends a 200 mL and 12% increase over baseline. However,

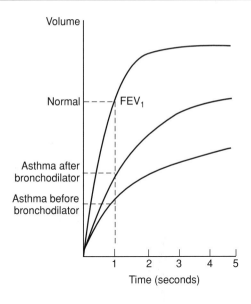

Figure 1.9 *Spirometric tracing demonstrating the reversibility of asthma to bronchodilators (from National Heart, Lung and Blood Institute, 1995).*

having assessed reversibility, it is still legitimate to refer to patients as having 'COPD with significant reversibility' or 'asthma with a large irreversible component', since reversibility is not the single defining characteristic of asthma. To add to the difficulties, as with PEF variability, reversibility can be expressed in several ways. Even though the guidelines tend to recommend measuring the change in the FEV_1 expressed as a percentage of the initial value, change in FEV_1 as a percentage of the predicted value discriminates asthma from COPD more reliably, as the former measure exaggerates the degree of reversibility in patients with lower baseline FEV_1 values (Brand *et al.*, 1992, Dompeling *et al.*, 1992). In addition, reversibility to β_2 agonist bronchodilators, such as salbutamol, does not predict reversibility to corticosteroids, though there is a reasonably strong correlation (Nisar *et al.*, 1990; Kerstjens *et al.*, 1993), and there is considerable within-subject variability in bronchodilator response in asthma and COPD (Kerstjens *et al.*, 1993).

Nagai *et al.* (1995) performed a post-mortem study examining the factors that determine the degree of reversibility to bronchodilators in patients with COPD. Greater reversibility was positively associated with bronchial inflammation, and particularly the degree of eosinophilic inflammation. Reduced reversibility and more severe airflow obstruction were associated with more severe emphysematous change. Interestingly, a positive correlation was found between bronchiolar fibrosis and the degree of reversibility to bronchodilator.

A proportion of COPD patients will demonstrate reversibility to a short course of oral corticosteroids. Such a course of corticosteroids is therefore recommended by COPD management guidelines (British Thoracic Society, 1997a). The factors that determine reversibility to corticosteroids are similar to those that determine reversibility to bronchodilators. Chanez *et al.* (1997) treated a group of COPD patients showing no response to bronchodilators with 2 weeks of oral prednisolone. Half of the patients showed a greater than 12% improvement in their FEV_1 and this steroid-responsive group had significantly higher indices of eosinophilic inflammation in their BALF (Fig. 1.10). Kerstjens *et al.* (1992) studied the factors that influenced responsiveness to inhaled corticosteroids over two-and-a-half years in a mixed group of patients with obstructive airways disease. They found that benefits were particularly marked in those patients who were non-smokers, had allergies, were under 40 years of age and had greater BHR, i.e. had asthmatic features.

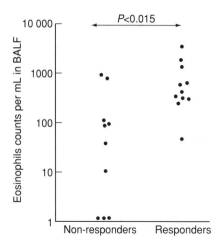

Figure 1.10 *Eosinophil counts in BALF of COPD patients divided into two groups on the basis of their reversibility to corticosteroids (from Chanez et al., 1997).*

In COPD, short courses of inhaled corticosteroids for up to 3 months at high doses tend to show slight improvements in lung function but lower doses have little benefit (van Schayck *et al.*, 1996). There is no effect on BHR (Dompeling *et al.*, 1993) and Keatings *et al.* (1997) demonstrated no effect of oral or inhaled corticosteroids on the neutrophilic or eosinophilic inflammation, or the IL-8 and TNF-α levels, in the sputum of patients with COPD. The effects on symptoms are also correspondingly marginal, with a small reduction in the number of exacerbations in the long term, and in the number of days requiring oral corticosteroids during an exacerbation. This is in contrast to asthma where all indices of disease activity (symptoms, FEV_1, peak flow variability, BHR, airway inflammation) show marked improvements with inhaled corticosteroids.

Symptomatology and natural history

The mechanisms by which the pathophysiological processes underlying the diseases result in the clinical manifestations of asthma and COPD are complex and embrace a multitude of contributing factors, including psychological, sociological and cultural influences. Therefore, although there are clearly relationships between the preceding characteristics (pathology, BHR, peak flow variability, reversibility) and symptomatology (Fig. 1.11), the correlation is by no means exact. For example, some authors have suggested that other measures of BHR may be more representative of symptoms than the traditionally used PC_{20}, such as the $PD_{15}FVC$ (dose of methacholine required to drop the forced vital capacity by 15%) (Sharma *et al.*, 1993).

The diagnosis of asthma is largely made on the symptomatology, which tends to be characteristic and is dictated by the pathophysiological processes underlying the condition. Given the rapid and large variations that occur in the level of airflow obstruction as a result of specific (i.e. allergen) and non-specific (exercise, cold air, etc.) stimuli that occur in asthma, it is not surprising that it tends to present relatively early during the disease process compared to COPD where the progression of airflow obstruction is more gradual. It is the non-specific BHR of asthma, which arises largely through eosinophilic inflammation and the subsequent remodelling of the airway wall, that is responsible for the marked variability in the disease symptomatology. In COPD, the neutrophilic inflammation tends to cause BHR not directly through release of bronchoconstrictor substances but indirectly through its effect on

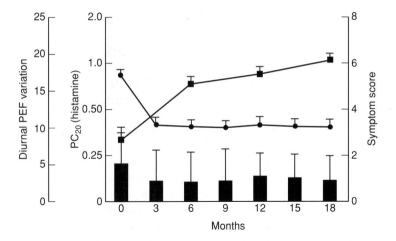

Figure 1.11 *Temporal relationship between diurnal PEF variation, BHR and symptoms following treatment with inhaled corticosteroids (from Kerstjens et al., 1994).* ■, PC_{20}; ● *diurnal PEF variation; bars – symptom score.*

structural changes within the walls of small airways and alveoli. Therefore, the BHR parallels the slow decline in FEV_1 that is characteristic of COPD. Thus, even though the symptoms described by COPD and asthma patients are similar (wheeze, cough, shortness of breath), the *pattern* of the symptomatology is quite different. The response of the symptoms to treatment mimics the responses of the other markers of disease activity, such as BHR, PEF variability and airway inflammation, as summarized in Fig. 1.12.

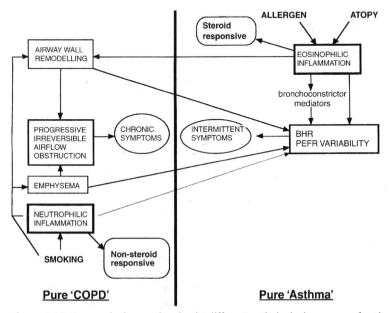

Figure 1.12 *Proposed schema whereby the different pathological processes of asthma and COPD result in similar symptomatology and clinical characteristics. The division of into 'pure asthma' and 'pure COPD' is artificial since most individuals will display features of both.*

Asthma is a difficult diagnosis to make before the age of 6 years because there is a high incidence of wheeze amongst infants and the majority of these children do not subsequently develop asthma. Martinez *et al.* (1995) demonstrated that a third of children under 3 years of age have a history of wheeze associated with lower respiratory tract infections (mostly viral) and that 60% of these had stopped wheezing by the age of 6. A risk factor for this transient wheezing is maternal smoking and it is thought that these infants may have congenitally small airways which become less prone to produce wheeze as the lungs develop. However, the risk factors for continuing to wheeze and developing asthma are atopy (eczema, rhinitis, raised serum IgE level at 9 months), maternal asthma and maternal smoking. Therefore there seems to be an inherited tendency for the persistence of wheeze leading to clinical asthma.

As childhood and adolescence progress there is a tendency for asthma symptoms to improve and remit. However, the more severe the asthma, the lower the probability of remission (Oswald *et al.*, 1997). Examination of the individuals in symptomatic remission commonly reveals some latent evidence of asthma, with persisting non-specific BHR (Martin *et al.*, 1980). Indeed, around a third of young adults in remission will subsequently develop symptomatic asthma within 7 years (Kelly *et al.*, 1987).

Once into adulthood, there is a relatively low incidence of remission. A recent study has confirmed previous reports of an accelerated rate of decline in lung function (FEV_1) amongst asthmatics of 38 mL per year, compared with about 22 mL in a normal adult (Finucane *et al.*, 1985; Peat *et al.*, 1987; Ulrik *et al.*, 1992; Lange *et al.*, 1998) (Fig. 1.13). This is manifest as an irreversible component to the airflow obstruction, irrespective of their smoking history. The longer the duration and the greater the severity of asthma, the greater is the fall in FEV_1 below the predicted value (Brown *et al.*, 1984; Hudon *et al.*, 1997) (Fig. 1.14). In asthma, the rate of decline in FEV_1 has also been correlated with increased BHR and with increased reversibility, in 'intrinsic' asthmatics, suggesting that more extreme, ongoing airway inflammation is associated with greater wall remodelling (Vollmer *et al.*, 1985; Ulrik *et al.*, 1992). Fletcher *et al.* (1976) coined the phrase 'the horse-racing effect' for the observation that the rate of decline in lung function was related to its absolute level. Thus, those asthmatics with most severe airflow obstruction had the greatest rate of loss of lung function. Ulrik *et al.* (1992) found that the horse-racing effect was confined to extrinsic asthmatics and was not present in intrinsic asthma, though the rate of decline depended on age in both types of disease.

Individuals with COPD generally present with largely fixed airflow obstruction after their fifth decade. The rate of decline in lung function in COPD of around 60–80 mL per year is markedly greater than in non-smokers (Fletcher and Peto, 1977) but if they discontinue

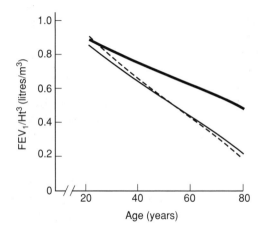

Figure 1.13 *Accelerated rate of decline in lung function amongst asthmatics (from Peat et al., 1987). Thick line, normal people; thin line, asthmatics; dashed line, asthmatic smokers.*

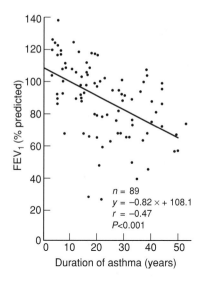

Figure 1.14 *Relationship between duration of asthma and pulmonary function (from Brown* et al.*, 1984).*

smoking the rate of decline returns to that of a non-smoker of that age (Fig. 1.15). In COPD, the rate of decline in lung function depends largely on the amount smoked but may also be related to the BHR (Xu *et al.*, 1997). The morbidity and mortality of the obstructive lung diseases are related to the level of the FEV_1 and to its rate of decline (Burrows *et al.*, 1987). Thus the prognosis of asthma is notably better than that of COPD (Fig. 1.16).

Reversibility to corticosteroids in the short term does not necessarily imply that they will prevent the progressive decline in lung function that occurs in asthmatics and smokers with COPD. Several longitudinal studies have investigated the effects of early or late introduction of inhaled corticosteroids on the course of asthma and found a beneficial slowing of the rate of decline of lung function by corticosteroids (Haahtela *et al.*, 1994; Overbeek *et al.*, 1996), suggesting that the irreversible airflow obstruction may occur as a result of long-term

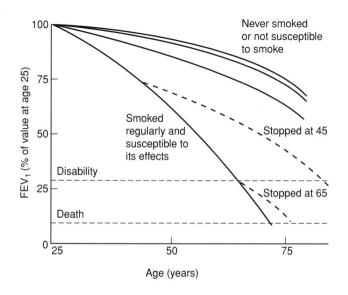

Figure 1.15 *The increased decline in lung function with time in smokers susceptible to COPD. Smoking cessation leads to reversion of the rate of decline to normal (from Fletcher and Peto, 1977).*

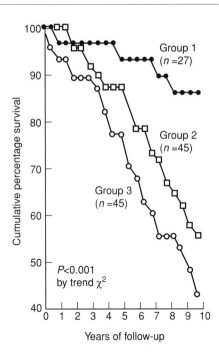

Figure 1.16 *Comparison of the 10-year survival in three groups of patients with obstructive airways disease. Group 1 constitutes those patients who had asthmatic features (non-smokers, atopic) whilst group 3 displayed features more suggestive of COPD (non-atopic smokers). Group 2 were those patients who could not be clearly classified into groups 1 or 3 (from Burrows* et al.*, 1987).*

uncontrolled airway inflammation leading to the fixed structural changes to the airways (Redington and Howarth, 1997; Hudon *et al.*, 1997; Backman *et al.*, 1997). Many have postulated that inhaled corticosteroids should be used very early in the disease course to prevent this decline, even in mild asthma. However, Oswald *et al.* (1997), in a 28-year longitudinal study of 286 children, found that those with mild asthma at age 7 did not subsequently have impaired airway function at age 35.

Studies of corticosteroids in smokers with COPD have been less conclusive with some studies showing long-term benefit and others not. Postma *et al.* (1985, 1988) demonstrated some reduction in this rate of decline with oral corticosteroids, but these studies may well have included some asthmatic patients. The recently released results of the large EUROSCOP (Pauwels *et al.*, 1992) study have failed to show any benefit of inhaled corticosteroids in smokers with mild-to-moderate COPD after the first 3 months. Thus either inflammation plays no part in the decline in lung function in COPD or the inflammation contributes to the decline but is itself little affected by corticosteroids. There is no doubt therefore that the most important intervention to slow the loss of FEV_1 in COPD is to stop smoking.

CONCLUSIONS

Having discussed the defining characteristics of asthma, it is possible to understand how the modern definition from the NHLBI/WHO workshop mentioned at the beginning of this chapter has been formulated. Clearly, research is needed to elucidate further the pathogenetic mechanisms underlying COPD and asthma but even at this stage we are able to distinguish clear differences between the two conditions. Woolcock and King (1995) attempted to clarify these differences by classifying the adult asthma phenotype into five categories as shown in Fig. 1.17, according to whether they demonstrated some of the defining characteristics of typical asthma, i.e. symptoms, pathology, atopy and airway hyperresponsiveness. It is clear

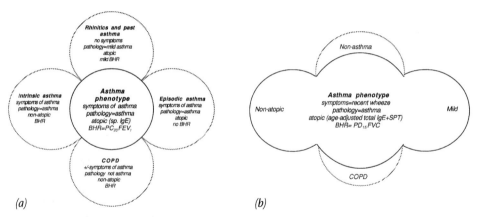

Figure 1.17 *(a) Variations on the asthma phenotype. (b) Redefining the asthma phenotype slightly enables all those with the symptoms and pathology of asthma to become included in the definition, whilst excluding asymptomatic atopics and COPD patients (from Woolcock and King, 1995).*

that there is considerable potential for the misclassification of individuals on the basis of one characteristic alone. The authors propose that the replacing of PC_{20} with $PD_{15}FVC$ (provocative dose producing a 15% fall in vital capacity) (Sharma *et al.*, 1993) as a measure of BHR and the use of age-adjusted measurement of total IgE can lead to the inclusion of more subjects with intrinsic and intermittent asthma within the central asthma diagnosis without including subjects with COPD or allergic rhinitis. However, it is difficult to envisage, using the current knowledge or technology, how a clear definition of asthma can be obtained. There is a need for a simple 'gold standard' test to distinguish COPD from asthma. It is unlikely, but still possible, that such a test may be based on tests of pulmonary function or radiological techniques. It is more likely that a cellular or biochemical parameter from blood, sputum or even urine will provide a sensitive and specific marker for asthma. Until that time, however, the debate over the definition of asthma will continue.

REFERENCES

Ackerman V, Marini M, Vittori E, *et al.* (1994) Detection of cytokines and their cell sources in bronchial biopsy specimens from asthmatic patients. Relationship to atopic status, symptoms and level of airway responsiveness. *Chest*, **105**, 687–96.

American Thoracic Society. (1991) Lung function testing: selection of reference values and interpretative strategies. *Am Rev Respir Dis*, **144**, 1202–18.

Arnup ME, Mendella LA, Anthonisen NR. (1983) Effects of cold air hyperpnoea in patients with chronic obstructive lung disease. *Am Rev Respir Dis*, **128**, 236–9.

Awadh N, Muller NL, Park CS, *et al.* (1998) Airway wall thickness in patients with near fatal asthma and control groups: assessment with high resolution computed tomographic scanning. *Thorax*, **53**, 248–53.

Backman KS, Greenberger PA, Patterson R. (1997) Airways obstruction in patients with long-term asthma consistent with 'irreversible asthma'. *Chest*, **112**, 1234–40.

Boezen HM, Postma DS, Schouten JP, *et al.* (1996) PEF variability, bronchial responsiveness and their relation to allergy markers in a random population (20–70 yr). *Am J Respir Crit Care Med*, **154**, 30–5.

Bosken CH, Wiggs BR, Pare PD, *et al.* (1990) Small airway dimensions in smokers with obstruction to airflow. *Am Rev Respir Dis*, **142**, 563–70.

Boulet L-P, Belanger M, Carrier G. (1995) Airway responsiveness and bronchial-wall thickness in asthma with or without fixed airflow obstruction. *Am J Respir Crit Care Med*, **152**, 865–71.

Boulet L-P, Laviolette M, Turcotte H, *et al*. (1997) Bronchial subepithelial fibrosis correlates with airway responsiveness to methacholine. *Chest*, **112**, 45–52.

Boulet LP, Legirs C, Thibault L. (1987) Comparative bronchial responses to hyperosmolar saline and methacholine in asthma. *Thorax*, **42**, 953–8.

Brand PLP, Duiverman EJ, Postma DS, *et al*. (1997) Peak flow variation in childhood asthma: relationship to symptoms, atopy, airways obstruction and hyperresponsiveness. *Eur Respir J*, **10**, 1242–47.

Brand PLP, Postma DS, Kerstjens HA, *et al*. (1991) Relationship of airway hyperresponsiveness to respiratory symptoms and diurnal PEFR variation in patients with obstructive lung disease. *Am Rev Respir Dis*, **143**, 916–21.

Brand PLP, Quanjer PH, Postma DS, *et al*. (1992) Interpretation of bronchodilator response in patients with obstructive airways disease. *Thorax*, **47**, 429–36.

British Thoracic Society. (1997a) The British guidelines on asthma management. *Thorax*, **52**(Suppl. 1), S2–S21.

British Thoracic Society. (1997b) BTS Guidelines for the management of chronic obstructive pulmonary disease. *Thorax*, **52**(Suppl. 5), S2–S28.

Brown PJ, Greville HW, Finucane KE. (1984) Asthma and irreversible airflow obstruction. *Thorax*, **39**, 131–6.

Burney PGJ. (1993) Epidemiology. In: *Asthma*, 3rd edn. Clark TJH, Godfrey S, Lee TH, eds. London: Chapman and Hall, pp. 254–308.

Burrows B. (1995) Allergy and the development of asthma and bronchial hyperresponsiveness. *Clin Exp Allergy*, **25**, 15–16.

Burrows B, Bloom JW, Traver GA, *et al*. (1987) The course and prognosis of different forms of chronic airways obstruction in a sample from the general population. *N Engl J Med*, **317**, 1309–14.

Campbell EJM, Scadding JG, Roberts RS. (1979) The concept of disease. *BMJ*, **2**, 757–62.

Cantin A, Crystal RG. (1985) Oxidants, antioxidants and the pathogenesis of emphysema. *Eur J Respir Dis*, **139**, 7–17.

Chanez P, Vignola AM, O'Shaugnessy T, *et al*. (1997) Corticosteroid reversibility in COPD is related to features of asthma. *Am J Respir Crit Care Med*, **155**, 1529–34.

Chetta A, Foresi A, Del Donno M, *et al*. (1996) Bronchial responsiveness to distilled water and methacholine and its relationship to inflammation and remodeling of the airways in asthma. *Am J Respir Crit Care Med*, **153**, 910–17.

Ciba Guest Symposium. (1959) Terminology, definitions and classifications of chronic pulmonary emphysema and related conditions. *Thorax*, **14**, 286–99.

Cockcroft DW. (1988) Modulation of airway hyperresponsiveness. *Ann Allergy*, **60**, 465–71.

Cockcroft DW, Killian DN, Mellon JJA, *et al*. (1977) Bronchial reactivity to inhaled histamine: a method and clinical survey. *Clin Allergy*, **7**, 235–43.

Corrigan CJ, Kay AB. (1990) CD4 T-lymphocyte activation in acute severe asthma. Relationship to disease severity and atopic status. *Am Rev Respir Dis*, **141**, 970.

Cosio MG, Ghezzo H, Hogg JC, *et al*. (1978) The relations between structural changes in small airways and pulmonary function test. *N Engl J Med*, **298**, 1277–81.

Cosio MG, Hale KA, Niewoehner DE. (1980) Morphologic and morphometric effects of prolonged cigarette smoking on the small airways. *Am Rev Respir Dis*, **122**, 265–71.

Cowburn AS, Sladek K, Soja J, *et al*. (1998) Overexpression of leukotriene C4 synthase in bronchial biopsies from patients with aspirin-intolerant asthma. *J Clin Invest*, **101**, 834–46.

Dahlen B, Kumlin M, Margolskee DJ, *et al*. (1993) The leukotriene receptor antagonist MK0679 blocks airway obstruction induced by inhaled lysine aspirin in aspirin-sensitive asthmatics. *Eur Respir J*, **6**, 1018–26.

Di Stefano A, Turato G, Maestrelli P, *et al*. (1996) Airflow limitation in chronic bronchitis is associated with T-lymphocyte and macrophage infiltration of the bronchial mucosa. *Am J Respir Crit Care Med*, **153**, 629–32.

Djukanovic R, Lai CK, Wilson JW, *et al*. (1992) Bronchial mucosal manifestations of atopy: a comparison of markers of inflammation between atopic asthmatics, atopic non-asthmatics and healthy controls. *Eur Respir J*, **5**, 538–44.

Djukanovic R, Roche WR, Wilson JW, *et al*. (1990) Mucosal inflammation in asthma. *Am Rev Respir Dis*, **142**, 434–57.

Dompeling E, van Schayck CP, Molema J, *et al*. (1992) A comparison of six different ways of expressing the bronchodilating response in asthma and COPD; reproducibility and dependence of prebronchodilator FEV_1. *Eur Respir J*, **5**, 975–81.

Dompeling E, van Schayck CP, van Grunsven PM, *et al*. (1993) Slowing the deterioration of asthma and chronic obstructive pulmonary disease observed during bronchodilator therapy by adding inhaled corticosteroids. *Ann Intern Med*, **118**, 770–8.

Dunnill MS, Massarella GR, Anderson JA. (1969) A comparison of the quantitative anatomy of the bronchi in normal subjects, in status asthmaticus, in chronic bronchitis and in emphysema. *Thorax*, **24**, 176–9.

Fahy JV, Kim KW, Boushey HA. (1995) Prominent neutrophilic inflammation in sputum from patients with asthma exacerbation. *J Allergy Clin Immunol*, **95**, 843–52.

Finucane KE, Greville HW, Brown PJE. (1985) Irreversible airflow obstruction: evolution in asthma. *Med J Aust*, **142**, 602–4.

Fletcher C, Peto R. (1977) The natural history of chronic airflow obstruction. *BMJ*, **1**(6077), 1645–8.

Fletcher CM, Peto R, Tinder CM, *et al*. (1976) *The natural history of chronic bronchitis and emphysema*. Oxford: Oxford University Press.

Fletcher CM, Pride NB. (1984) Definitions of emphysema, chronic bronchitis, asthma, and airflow obstruction: 25 years on from the Ciba symposium. *Thorax*, **39**, 81–5.

Gadek JE, Fells GA, Crystal RG. (1979) Cigarette smoking induces functional antiprotease deficiency in the lower respiratory tract of humans. *Science*, **206**, 1315–16.

Gibson PG, Mattoli S, Sears MR, *et al*. (1995) Increased peak flow variability in children with asymptomatic hyperresponsiveness. *Eur Respir J*, **8**, 1731–5.

Haahtela T, Jarvinen M, Kava T, *et al*. (1994) Effects of reducing or discontinuing inhaled budesonide in patients with mild asthma. *N Engl J Med*, **331**, 700–5.

Hale KA, Ewing SL, Gosnell BA, *et al*. (1984) Lung disease in long-term cigarette smokers with and without chronic airflow obstruction. *Am Rev Respir Dis*, **130**, 718–21.

Higgins BG, Britton JR, Chinn S, *et al*. (1992) Comparison of bronchial reactivity and peak expiratory flow variability measurements for epidemiologic studies. *Am Rev Respir Dis*, **145**, 588–93.

Hogg TC, Macklem PT, Thurlbeck NM. (1968) The site and nature of airway obstruction in chronic obstructive lung disease. *N Engl J Med*, **278**, 1355–60.

Holgate ST, Hardy C, Robinson C, *et al*. (1986) The mast cell as a primary effector cell in the pathogenesis of asthma. *J Allergy Clin Immunol*, **77**, 274–82.

Hoshi H, Ohno I, Honma M, *et al*. (1995) IL-5, IL-8 and GM-CSF immunostaining of sputum cells in bronchial asthma and chronic bronchitis. *Clin Exp Allergy*, **25**, 720–8.

Hudon C, Turcotte H, Laviolette M, *et al*. (1997) Characteristics of bronchial asthma with incomplete reversibility of airflow obstruction. *Ann All Asth Immunol*, **78**, 195–202.

Humbert M, Durham SR, Ying S, *et al*. (1996a) IL-4 and IL-5 mRNA and protein in bronchial biopsies from atopic and non-atopic asthmatics: evidence against 'intrinsic' asthma being a distinct immunopathological entity. *Am J Respir Crit Care Med*, **154**, 1497–504.

Humbert M, Grant JA, Taborda-Barata L, *et al*. (1996b) High-affinity IgE receptor (Fc epsilon RI)-bearing cells in bronchial biopsies from atopic and non-atopic asthma. *Am J Respir Crit Care Med*, **153**, 1931–7.

Humbert M, Ying S, Corrigan CJ, *et al*. (1997) Bronchial mucosal expression of the genes encoding chemokines RANTES and MCP-3 in symptomatic atopic and non-atopic asthmatics: relationship to the eosinophil-active cytokines interleukin (IL)-5, granulocyte macrophage-colony-stimulating factor, and IL-3. *Am J Respir Cell Mol Biol*, **16**, 1–8.

Jeffery PK. (1991) Morphology of the airway wall in asthma and in chronic obstructive pulmonary disease. *Am Rev Respir Dis*, **143**, 1152–8.

Jeffery PK. (1998) Structural and inflammatory changes in COPD: a comparison with asthma. *Thorax*, **53**, 129–36.

Jeffery PK, Wardlaw A, Nelson FC, *et al.* (1989) Bronchial biopsies in asthma: an ultrastructural quantification study and correlation with hyperreactivity. *Am Rev Respir Dis*, **140**, 1745–53.

Jenkins MA, Clarke JR, Carlin JB, *et al.* (1996) Validation of questionnaire and bronchial hyperresponsiveness against respiratory physician assessment in the diagnosis of asthma. *Int J Epidemiol*, **25**, 609–16.

Jones A. (1994) Asymptomatic bronchial hyperreactivity and the development of asthma and other respiratory tract illnesses in children. *Thorax*, **49**, 757–61.

Keatings VM, Barnes PJ. (1997) Granulocyte activation markers in induced sputum: comparison between chronic obstructive pulmonary disease, asthma and normal subjects. *Am J Respir Crit Care Med*, **155**, 449–53.

Keatings VM, Collins PD, Scott DM, *et al.* (1996) Differences in interleukin-8 and tumour necrosis factor-α in induced sputum from patients with chronic obstructive pulmonary disease and asthma. *Am J Respir Crit Care Med*, **153**, 530–4.

Keatings VM, Jatakanon A, Worsdell YM, *et al.* (1997) Effects of inhaled and oral glucocorticoids on inflammatory indices in asthma and COPD. *Am J Respir Crit Care Med*, **155**, 542–8.

Kelly WJW, Hudson I, Phelan PD, *et al.* (1987) Childhood asthma in adult life: a further study at 28 years of age. *BMJ*, **294**, 1059–62.

Kerrebijn KF. (1989) Clinical presentation. In: Holgate ST, ed. *The role of the inflammatory process in airway hyperresponsiveness*. Oxford: Blackwell Scientific Publications, 1–15.

Kerstjens HAM, Brand PLP, de Jong PM, *et al.* (1994) Influence of treatment on peak expiratory flow and its relation to airway hyperresponsiveness and symptoms. *Thorax*, **49**, 1109–15.

Kerstjens HAM, Brand PLP, Hughes MD, *et al.* (1992) A comparison of bronchodilator therapy with or without inhaled corticosteroid therapy for obstructive airway disease. *N Engl J Med*, **327**, 1413–19.

Kerstjens HAM, Brand PLP, Quanjer PH, *et al.* (1993) Variability of bronchodilator response and effects of inhaled corticosteroid treatment in obstructive airways disease. *Thorax*, **48**, 722–9.

Kuwano K, Bosken CH, Pare PD, *et al.* (1993) Small airways dimensions in asthma and in chronic obstructive pulmonary disease. *Am Rev Respir Dis*, **148**, 1220–5.

Lacoste J-Y, Bousquet J, Chanez P, *et al.* (1993) Eosinophilic and neutrophilic inflammation in asthma, chronic bronchitis and chronic obstructive pulmonary disease. *J Allergy Clin Immunol*, **92**, 537–48.

Lamb D, Lumsden A. (1982) Intra-epithelial mast cells in human airway epithelium: evidence for smoking-induced change in their frequency. *Thorax*, **37**, 334–42.

Lang DM, Hopp RJ, Bewtra AK, *et al.* (1987) Distribution of methacholine inhalation challenge responses in a selected adult population. *J Allergy Clin Immunol*, **79**, 533–40.

Lange P, Parner J, Vestbo J, *et al.* (1998) A 15 year follow-up study of ventilatory function in adults with asthma. *N Engl J Med*, **339**, 1194–200.

Laprise C, Boulet L-P. (1997) Asymptomatic airway hyperresponsiveness: a three year follow-up. *Am J Respir Crit Care Med*, **156**, 403–9.

Li X, Wilson JW. (1997) Increased vascularity of the bronchial mucosa in mild asthma. *Am J Respir Crit Care Med*, **156**, 229–33.

Linden M, Rasmussen JB, Piitulainen E, *et al.* (1993) Airway inflammation in smokers with nonobstructive and obstructive chronic bronchitis. *Am Rev Respir Dis*, **148**, 1226–32.

Macklem PT. (1991) Factors determining bronchial smooth muscle shortening. *Am Rev Respir Dis*, **143**, S47–S48.

Magnusson H, Richter K, Taube C. (1998) Are chronic obstructive pulmonary disease (COPD) and asthma different diseases? *Clin Exp Allergy*, **28**, 187–94.

Makker HK, Holgate ST. (1993) Relation of the hypertonic saline responsiveness of the airways to exercise induced asthma symptom severity and to histamine or methacholine reactivity. *Thorax*, **48**, 142–7.

Makker HK, Walls AF, Goulding D, *et al*. (1994) Airway effects of local allergen challenge with hypertonic saline in exercise-induced asthma. *Am J Respir Crit Care Med*, **149**, 1012–19.

Manning PJ, Watson RM, Margolskee DJ. (1990) Inhibition of exercise-induced bronchoconstriction by MK-571, a potent leukotriene D4-receptor antagonist. *N Engl J Med*, **323**, 1736–9.

Martin AJ, Landau LI, Phelan PD. (1980) Lung function in young adults who had asthma in childhood. *Am Rev Respir Dis*, **122**, 609–16.

Martinez FD, Wright AL, Taussig LM, *et al*. (1995) Asthma and wheezing in the first six years of life. *N Engl J Med*, **332**, 133–8.

Moreno RH, Hogg JC, Pare PD. (1986) Mechanics of airway narrowing. *Am Rev Respir Dis*, **133**, 1171.

Mullen JB, Wright JL, Wiggs BR, *et al*. (1985) Reassessment of inflammation of airways in chronic bronchitis. *BMJ (Clin Res Ed)*, **291**, 1235–9.

Nagai A, Thurlbeck WM, Konno K. (1995) Responsiveness and variability of airflow obstruction in chronic obstructive pulmonary disease. *Am J Respir Crit Care Med*, **151**, 635–9.

National Heart, Lung and Blood Institute. (1995) Global initiative for asthma. *Global strategy for asthma management and prevention*. NHLI/WHO Workshop Report.

Nisar M, Walshaw M, Pearson MG, *et al*. (1990) Assessment of reversibility of airway obstruction in patients with chronic obstructive airways disease. *Thorax*, **45**, 190–4.

O'Connor GT, Weiss ST. (1994) Clinical and symptom measures. *Am J Respir Crit Care Med*, **149**, S21–S28.

O'Shaughnessy TC, Ansari TW, Barnes NC, *et al*. (1997) Inflammation in bronchial biopsies of subjects with chronic bronchitis: inverse relationship of CD8+ T-lymphocytes with FEV_1. *Am J Respir Crit Care Med*, **155**, 852–7.

Oddera S, Silvestri M, Balbo A, *et al*. (1996) Airway eosinophilic inflammation, epithelial damage and bronchial hyperresponsiveness in patients with mild-moderate stable asthma. *Allergy*, **51**, 100–7.

Ollerenshaw SL, Woolcock AJ. (1992) Characteristics of the inflammation in biopsies from large airways of subjects with asthma and subjects with chronic airflow limitation. *Am Rev Respir Dis*, **145**, 922–7.

Orie NGM, Sluiter HJ, de Vries K, *et al*. (1961). The host factor in bronchitis. In: Orie NGM, Sluiyer HJ, eds. Assen, Netherlands: Royal van Gorcum, 43–59.

Oswald H, Phelan PD, Lanigan A, *et al*. (1997) Childhood asthma and lung function in mid-adult life. *Pediatr Pulmonol*, **23**, 14–20.

Overbeek SE, Kerstjens HAM, Bogaard JM, *et al*. (1996) Is delayed introduction of inhaled corticosteroids harmful in patients with obstructive airways disease (asthma and COPD)? *Chest*, **110**, 34–41.

Pattemore PK, Asher MI, Harrison AC, *et al*. (1990) The interrelationship among bronchial hyperresponsiveness, the diagnosis of asthma and asthma symptoms. *Am Rev Respir Dis*, **142**, 549–54.

Pauwels R, Lofdahl CG, Pride NB, *et al*. (1992) European Respiratory Society study on chronic obstructive pulmonary disease (EUROSCOP): hypothesis and design. *Eur Respir J*, **5**, 1254–61.

Peat JK, Woolcock AJ, Cullen K. (1987) Rate of decline of lung function in subjects with asthma. *Eur J Respir Dis*, **70**, 171–9.

Pin I, Radford S, Kolendowicz R, *et al*. (1993) Airway inflammation in symptomatic and asymptomatic children with methacholine hyperresponsiveness. *Eur Respir J*, **6**, 1249–56.

Postma DS, Peters I, Steenhuis EJ, *et al*. (1988) Moderately severe chronic airflow obstruction: can corticosteroids slow down obstruction? *Eur Respir J*, **1**, 22–6.

Postma DS, Steenhuis EJ, van der Weele LT, *et al*. (1985) Severe chronic airflow obstruction: can corticosteroids slow down progression? *Eur J Respir Dis*, **67**, 56–64.

Poulter LW, Power C, Burke C. (1990) The relationship between bronchial immunopathology and hyperresponsiveness in asthma. *Eur Respir J*, **3**, 792–9.

Power C, Sreenan S, Hurson B, *et al*. (1993) Distribution of immunocompetent cells in the bronchial walls of clinically healthy subjects showing bronchial hyperresponsiveness. *Thorax*, **48**, 1125–9.

Pride NB, Vermeire P, Allegra L. (1989) Diagnostic labels applied to model case histories of chronic airflow obstruction. Responses to a questionnaire in 11 North American and Western European countries. *Eur Respir J*, **2**, 702–9.

Ramsdale EH, Morris MM, Roberts KS, *et al*. (1984) Bronchial responsiveness to methacholine in chronic bronchitis: relationship to airflow obstruction and cold air responsiveness. *Thorax*, **39**, 912–18.

Redington AE, Howarth PH. (1997) Airway wall remodelling in asthma. *Thorax*, **52**, 310–12.

Rijcken B, Schouten JP, Weiss ST, *et al*. (1988) The relationship between airway responsiveness to histamine and pulmonary function level in a random population sample. *Am Rev Respir Dis*, **137**, 826–32.

Rijcken B, Schouten JP, Rosner B, *et al*. (1991) Is it useful to distinguish between asthma and COPD in respiratory epidemiology? *Am Rev Respir Dis*, **143**, 1456–7.

Roche WR, Williams JH, Beasley R, *et al*. (1989) Subepithelial fibrosis in the bronchi of asthmatics. *Lancet*, **1**, 520–4.

Ronchi MC, Piragino C, Rosi E, *et al*. (1996) Role of sputum differential cell count in detecting airway inflammation in patients with chronic bronchial asthma or COPD. *Thorax*, **51**, 1000–4.

Ryan G, Latimer KM, Dolovich J, *et al*. (1982) Bronchial responsiveness to histamine: relationship to diurnal variation of peak flow rate, improvement after bronchodilator and airway calibre. *Thorax*, **37**, 423–9.

Saetta M, Di Stefano A, Maestrelli P, *et al*. (1993) Activated T-lymphocytes and macrophages in bronchial mucosa of subjects with chronic bronchitis. *Am Rev Respir Dis*, **147**, 301–6.

Saetta M, Di Stefano A, Maestrelli P. (1994a) Airway eosinophilia in chronic bronchitis during exacerbations. *Am J Respir Crit Care Med*, **150**, 1646–52.

Saetta M, Di Stefano A, Maestrelli P, *et al*. (1996) Airway eosinophilia and expression of interleukin-5 protein in asthma and in exacerbations of chronic bronchitis. *Clin Exp Allergy*, **26**, 766–74.

Seatta M, Finkelstein R, Cosio MG. (1994b) Morphological and cellular basis for airflow limitation in smokers. *Eur Respir J*, **7**, 1505–15.

Saetta M, Ghezzo H, Kim WD, *et al*. (1985) Loss of alveolar attachments in smokers. A morphometric correlate of lung function impairment. *Am Rev Respir Dis*, **132**, 894–900.

Saetta M, Thiene G, Crescioli S, *et al*. (1989) Fatal asthma in a young patient with severe bronchial hyperresponsiveness but stable peak flow records. *Eur Respir J*, **2**, 1008–12.

Salome CM, Xuan W, Gray EJ, *et al*. (1997) Perception of airway narrowing in a general population sample. *Eur Respir J*, **10**, 1052–8.

Scadding JG. (1983) Definition and clinical categories of asthma. In: *Asthma*, 2nd Edn. Clark TJH, Godfrey S, eds. London: Chapman and Hall, 1–11.

Sears MR, Jones PR, Holdaway MD, *et al*. (1986) Prevalence of bronchial reactivity to inhaled methacholine in New Zealand children. *Thorax*, **41**, 283–9.

Sharma A, Gibbons WJ, Menzies R, *et al*. (1993) Relationship between falls in vital capacity during bronchoprovocation testing (BPT) and the clinical expression of asthma. *Am Rev Respir Dis*, **147**, A258.

Sterk PJ, Bel EH. (1991) The shape of the dose–response curve to inhaled bronchoconstrictor agents in asthma and COPD. *Am Rev Respir Dis*, **143**, 1433–7.

Sur S, Crotty TB, Kephart GM, *et al*. (1993) Sudden-onset fatal asthma. A distinct entity with few eosinophils and relatively more neutrophils in the airway submucosa? *Am Rev Respir Dis*, **148**, 713–19.

Tashkin DP, Altose MD, Bleecker ER, *et al*. (1992) The Lung Health Study: airway responsiveness to inhaled methacholine in smokers with mild to moderate airflow limitation. *Am Rev Respir Dis*, **145**, 301–10.

Thompson AB, Daughton D, Robbins GA, *et al*. (1989) Intraluminal airway inflammation in chronic bronchitis. Characterization and correlation with clinical parameters. *Am Rev Respir Dis*, **140**, 1527–37.

Tiddens HAWM, Pare PD, Hogg JC, *et al.* (1995) Cartilaginous airway dimensions and airflow obstruction in human lungs. *Am J Respir Crit Care Med*, **152**, 260–6.

Toelle BG, Peat JK, Salome CM, *et al.* (1992) Toward a definition of asthma for epidemiology. *Am Rev Respir Dis*, **146**, 633–7.

Turner MO, Hussack P, Sears MR, *et al.* (1995) Exacerbations of asthma without sputum eosinophilia. *Thorax*, **50**, 1057–61.

Ulrik CS, Backer V, Dirksen A. (1992) A 10 year follow-up of 180 adults with bronchial asthma: factors important for the decline in lung function. *Thorax*, **47**, 14–18.

van Schayck CP, Dompeling E, Molema J, *et al.* (1994) Does bronchial hyperresponsiveness precede or follow airway obstruction in asthma or COPD? *Neth J Med*, **45**, 145–53.

van Schayck CP, van Grunsven PM, Dekhuijzen PN, *et al.* (1996) Do patients with COPD benefit from treatment with inhaled corticosteroids? *Eur Respir J*, **9**, 1969–72.

Vollmer WM, Johnson LR, Buist AS. (1985) Relationship of response to a bronchodilator and decline in forced expiratory volume in one second in population studies. *Am Rev Respir Dis*, **132**, 1186–93.

Wenzel SE, Szefler SJ, Leung DYM, *et al.* (1997) Bronchoscopic evaluation of severe asthma: persistent inflammation associated with high dose glucocorticoids. *Am J Respir Crit Care Med*, **156**, 747–43.

Wiggs BR, Bosken C, Pare PD, *et al.* (1992) A model of airway narrowing in asthma and in chronic obstructive pulmonary disease. *Am Rev Respir Dis*, **145**, 1251–8.

Woolcock AJ, King G. (1995) Is there a specific phenotype for asthma? *Clin Exp Allergy*, **25**, 3–7.

Xu X, Rijcken B, Schouten JP, *et al.* (1997) Airways responsiveness and the development and remission of chronic respiratory symptoms in adults. *Lancet*, **350**, 1431–4.

Ying S, Humbert M, Barkens J, *et al.* (1997) Expression of IL-4 and IL-5 mRNA and protein by CD4+ and CD8+ T cells, eosinophils, and mast cells in bronchial biopsies obtained from atopic and nonatopic (intrinsic) asthmatics. *J Immunol*, **158**, 3539–44.

Zhong NS, Chen RC, Yang MO, *et al.* (1992) Is asymptomatic bronchial hyperresponsiveness an indication of potential asthma? A 2 year follow-up of young students with bronchial hyperresponsiveness. *Chest*, **102**, 1104–9.

2

Lung function and bronchial hyperresponsiveness: physiological aspects

G.J. GIBSON

The functional features characteristically associated with asthma are variable airway narrowing and unusual sensitivity of the airways to non-specific stimuli (bronchial hyperresponsiveness, BHR). In the great majority of patients with asthma both features are present. Occasionally, however, patients with otherwise typical asthma and variable airway obstruction have no demonstrable BHR. On the other hand, BHR without asthma also occurs in other situations such as following viral respiratory tract infections.

AIRWAY FUNCTION

Determinants of airway size in health

The bronchial tree is a complex branching system which extends from the trachea to the alveoli. With successive generations, individual airways narrow towards the lung periphery, but a marked increase in the total number of airways at each division implies that the overall cross-sectional area increases progressively. In healthy subjects the narrowest section, and hence the main site of resistance to breathing, is centrally in the trachea, larynx and upper airway.

The size of an individual airway depends on several factors including its relaxed, unstressed, dimensions, its elastic properties (which determine its susceptibility to compressing and distending forces) and the tone of the smooth muscle in its wall. The pressure distending the intrathoracic airways is closely related to the recoil pressure of the lungs – hence in emphysema, where lung recoil is diminished, the airways are narrowed. Since lung recoil pressure increases with lung volume, airway dimensions increase progressively over the vital capacity (VC) range from residual volume (RV) to total lung capacity (TLC).

During tidal inspiration the transmural pressure is slightly greater than during breath-holding and conversely during expiration rather less; consequently airway resistance is less when measured during inspiration than on expiration. During forceful expiration, as occurs with commonly used tests such as peak expiratory flow (PEF) and forced expiratory volume in one second (FEV_1), transmural pressures are greatly increased and the intrathoracic airways are compressed, resulting in the wheezing audible even in normal subjects during forced expiration.

In healthy individuals smooth muscle tone varies from time-to-time, dependent on activity of the autonomic nervous system, particularly the vagus nerve. Pre-ganglionic fibres in the vagus innervate efferent ganglia in the airway wall and post-ganglionic fibres release acetylcholine which stimulates muscarinic receptors on bronchial smooth muscle, causing it to contract. The effect of vagal tone is demonstrable, even in normal subjects, by the bronchodilatation that follows inhalation of an anticholinergic agent such as ipratropium bromide. The role of the sympathetic nervous system in normal control of bronchial tone is less clear. The sympathetic nerve supply to human airway smooth muscle is sparse even though β-adrenoceptors are plentiful (Barnes, 1986). They probably respond mainly to circulating catecholamines rather than to neural stimulation. Again, bronchodilatation is readily demonstrable in normal subjects by inhalation of a β-sympathomimetic agent such as salbutamol. Most studies have suggested that, at rest, β-blocking drugs have no effect on airway tone in normal subjects, suggesting no significant resting sympathetic or bronchial β-receptor activity. The non-adrenergic, non-cholinergic (NANC) autonomic system may also play a role in control of bronchial smooth muscle tone. Inhibitory NANC (i.e. bronchodilator) nerve fibres innervate human airways and it is likely that their bronchodilator effect is mediated by release of nitric oxide (Belvisi et al., 1992). Other factors involved in control of airway smooth muscle tone include the locally prevailing tensions of carbon dioxide and oxygen, which have an important role in regulating local ventilation and blood flow.

Vagal activity is increased by stimulation of irritant receptors, particularly in the upper airway and larynx. Relevant stimuli include inhaled particulates and noxious gases. Their consequences are exaggerated in asthma, a facet of bronchial hyperresponsiveness, the mechanisms and manifestations of which are discussed below.

Methods of assessment

AIRWAY RESISTANCE AND CONDUCTANCE

Direct estimation of airway resistance requires measurement of airflow together with the pressure difference along the airway, i.e. between mouth and alveoli. The former is readily obtained using a pneumotachograph or by electrical differentiation of volume expired. More difficult is measurement of alveolar pressure. The usual laboratory method is whole body plethysmography (DuBois et al., 1956). This allows simultaneous estimation of thoracic gas volume, so that the measurements can be related to each other as specific airway conductance (sG_{AW}) which is the reciprocal of airway resistance divided by lung volume. This index aims to take account of the inevitable variation of airway resistance with the lung volume at which it is measured (Fig. 2.1). Strictly, however, sG_{AW} is completely independent of volume only if the relation between airway conductance (G_{AW}) and volume passes through the origin. In practice

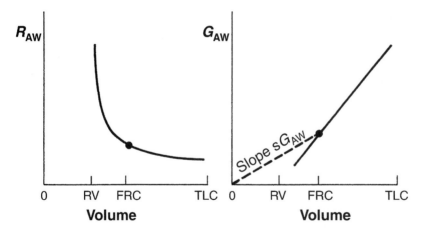

Figure 2.1 *Schematic diagram of variation of airway resistance (left) and conductance (right) with lung volume in a normal subject. Note that R$_{AW}$ increases considerably at volumes below functional residual capacity (FRC) and that its relation to volume is approximately hyperbolic. Hence its reciprocal, airway conductance, shows a linear relation to volume. Specific conductance (sG$_{AW}$) does not completely remove the effects of lung volume as the G$_{AW}$–volume plot does not usually pass through the origin. RV, residual volume; TLC, total lung capacity.*

this is not the case so that sG_{AW} tends to be greater at higher lung volumes (Fig. 2.1). Plethysmographic measurements are usually made during gentle panting efforts in order to minimize transmural pressures across the airways and hence to allow evaluation of airway calibre in its unstressed state. Panting also minimizes changes in the temperature and humidity of the respired gas, as well as producing abduction of the vocal cords, so that the contribution of laryngeal resistance (an appreciable proportion of total airway resistance in normal subjects) is minimized.

Two other methods for estimation of airway resistance in clinical practice use either forced oscillation or transient interruption of airflow. Both are applied during tidal breathing and hence have the theoretical advantage of directly estimating the load to breathing under more natural conditions than either panting or forced expiration. With forced oscillation sinusoidal oscillations of flow from a loudspeaker are superimposed on the normal tidal flow and by computerized analysis of the flow and the resulting change in pressure at the mouth the resistance of the total respiratory system can be derived (van Noord *et al.*, 1991). Resistance measured by forced oscillation tends to be slightly higher than with other techniques because it includes small contributions from lung tissue and chest wall resistance. With the interruptor method, airflow is transiently and repeatedly interrupted by a valve which closes the airway. The pressure on the mouth side of the valve immediately following closure is taken as the alveolar pressure which was generating the flow immediately before closure (Bates *et al.*, 1988). Both these techniques are relatively easily applied, they require little or no co-operation from the patient and, unlike the body plethysmograph, the equipment can be made portable. However, both involve theoretical assumptions that may be less valid in patients with airway obstruction, as estimation of representative alveolar pressure is then less reliable. All the measurements discussed above are generally less reproducible than the commonly applied indices based on forced expiration.

FORCED EXPIRATORY TESTS

All the measurements of airway resistance described in the previous section are performed with low pressures and flows and consequently they assess the dimensions of the airways in a relatively unstressed state. During quiet breathing the pressure surrounding the intrathoracic airways is more negative than the pressure within the airway and there is no tendency for the airway to be compressed. During forceful expiration, however, very positive pressures are generated, not only in the alveoli driving airflow, but also in the pleural space surrounding the larger intrathoracic airways. As air is forcibly expired, the pressure within the bronchial tree falls progressively from alveoli to mouth, so that at some points along the airways ('equal pressure points', EPP), the pressure outside becomes equal to that within. At all points downstream (i.e. on the mouth side of EPP) the intrathoracic airway is subject to a net compressing force. With further increases in effort, the degree of compression increases such that the resulting flow becomes independent of the effort applied. This phenomenon occurs particularly at lower lung volumes, while at high lung volumes close to full inflation expiratory flow is more effort-dependent. Hence PEF (which is developed very early during forced expiration) is more dependent on effort than FEV_1 which integrates maximum expiratory flow over a large range of lung volumes (more than 75% of the vital capacity in a normal subject).

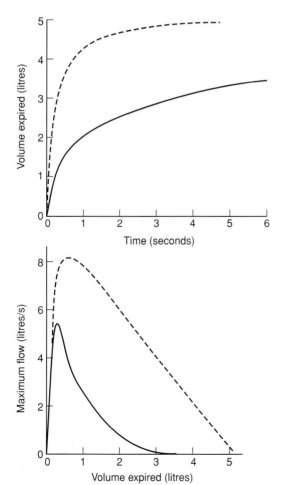

Figure 2.2 *Schematic diagram of spirogram (volume vs. time) and maximum expiratory flow volume curves in a normal subject (broken line) and a patient with airway obstruction due to asthma (solid line).*

The hallmark of generalized airway narrowing (from whatever cause) is reduction of the rate of forced expiration. This can be visualized in various ways, most commonly as volume expired against time (the conventional forced expiratory spirogram) or as instantaneous maximum expiratory flow plotted against volume expired (maximum expiratory flow volume, MEFV curve) (Fig. 2.2). Diffuse airway narrowing, as in asthma, causes a reduction in the ratio of FEV_1/forced vital capacity (FVC), while the contour of the MEFV curve is changed with a diminished peak and increasingly pronounced concavity (convexity to the volume axis). The proportionate reduction in maximum expiratory flow is greater the lower the lung volume and PEF (although diminished in symptomatic asthma) is affected less markedly. Measurements of maximum flow at lower lung volumes have theoretical advantages for detection of mild airway narrowing but in practice the normal inter-individual variation is so large that isolated measurements are rarely useful. Measurements at small lung volumes are of most value when sequential values are obtained in an individual. During forced expiration to smaller lung volumes there is progressive dynamic narrowing and probable closure of intrathoracic airways. As airway obstruction worsens, eventually the FVC is truncated by either airway closure or inability of the subject to sustain the prolonged effort necessary to continue expiration through increasingly narrow airways. In practice, in most symptomatic patients with airway obstruction the FVC is less than normal (but note that the reduction in FEV_1 is proportionately greater, so that the ratio FEV_1/FVC is also reduced).

The volume displayed on MEFV curves can be recorded in one of two ways – either as volume expired (the more usual), or as change in thoracic gas volume. The latter is measured with the subject seated within a body plethysmograph, using the plethysmographic signal as the index of change in thoracic volume. In this latter case volume change is due not only to bulk flow of gas out of the lungs, but also to compression of thoracic gas consequent on the high alveolar pressure (Boyle's law). Consequently the shapes of the two curves differ (Fig. 2.3). The difference between the two types of curve is exaggerated in the presence of

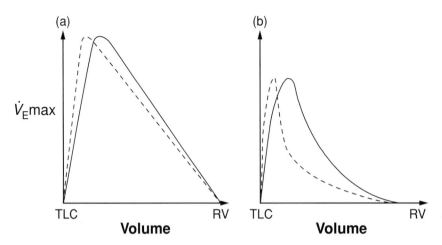

Figure 2.3 *Schematic diagram of MEFV curves plotted using two different volume signals in (a) a normal person and (b) a patient with airway obstruction caused by asthma. The broken line represents the curve obtained using volume expired and the solid line using change in thoracic gas volume. The normal person shows little difference but there is a marked difference in the patient with asthma owing to a greater effect of compression of thoracic gas during forced expiration. $\dot{V}_E max$, maximum expiratory flow. Abbreviations: see Fig. 2.1.*

significant airway obstruction because of the greater volume of intrathoracic gas (pulmonary hyperinflation).

One criticism of tests of forced expiration of particular relevance to asthma is that the manoeuvre itself, and in particular the preceding full inspiration, may alter the calibre of the airways. In normal subjects deep inspiration characteristically increases maximal expiratory flow at a specific lung volume, while in asthma more variable results have been described (see below). The effect of deep inspiration can be avoided by recording a partial expiratory flow volume (PEFV) curve, with the forced expiration started from a volume less than full inflation, usually from near the normal end-tidal inspiratory volume (Fig. 2.4). PEFV curves are particularly useful for visualizing the effect of a bronchodilator drug in normal subjects (Barnes *et al.*, 1981), as full inflation leads to diminution of bronchomotor tone – which limits the size of the effect on MEFV curves (or FEV_1). The relationship between MEFV and PEFV curves can be quantitated as the M/P ratio, i.e. the ratio of maximum expiratory flow at a particular lung volume taken from maximal and partial curves respectively.

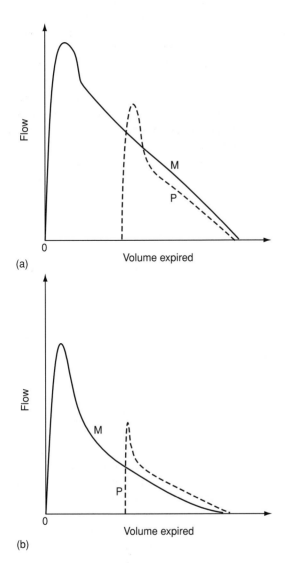

(a)

(b)

Figure 2.4 *Schematic maximum (M, solid line) and partial (P, broken line) flow volume curves in (a) a normal person and (b) a patient with asthma. In the healthy person the flow obtained from the maximum curve at a given lung volume exceeds that from the partial curve, i.e. deep inspiration has resulted in bronchodilatation (M/P > 1). By contrast, in the patient with asthma M/P < 1.*

The choice of test of airway function for evaluating and following patients with asthma depends on both theoretical and practical considerations. At first sight, airway resistance during tidal breathing would seem the most appropriate as, in principle, it ought to be the most closely related to the physiological situation. However all the techniques available for its measurement have practical and/or theoretical disadvantages. As conventionally measured, airway resistance is dominated, especially in normal subjects, by the calibre of the central airways but this does not necessarily apply in patients with airway obstruction. Once the resistance of the more peripheral airways increases sufficiently to produce symptoms, a measurable increase in total airway resistance will be found. Consequently, in asthma R_{AW} and sG_{AW} should not be regarded as dependent solely (or even mainly) on the calibre of the larger airways. FEV_1, also, is not very sensitive to early changes in small airways but the anticipated greater sensitivity of maximum expiratory flow at small lung volumes and other 'small airway tests' is usually outweighed by their greater variability.

Measurements of airway resistance and maximum flow generally give similar qualitative information in patients with airway obstruction. Since, however, they depend on different factors, there is no reason *a priori* why their quantitative relation should be close. One common situation where sequential measurements of airway function are required is in assessing the effects of bronchodilator drugs. In patients with established airway obstruction either sG_{AW} or forced expiratory tests are appropriate, but the changes in each are not necessarily related in a linear fashion. Consequently, any attempt to equate differential proportional changes with relative effects of a drug on 'large' or 'small' airways is likely to be unsound. Maximum expiratory flow at small lung volumes often shows the biggest proportional effects, but changes in FVC and absolute thoracic gas volume need to be taken into account for valid interpretation of changes in flow. In practice, despite its theoretical disadvantage, FEV_1 remains the most useful index for assessing the response to treatment. PEF has the further advantage of portability and easy availability in the domiciliary setting. However, single values of PEF give less specific information than spirometric indices and PEF is intrinsically more effort-dependent than FEV_1.

Airway function in asthma

The defining characteristic of asthma is *variability* of airway narrowing. Sometimes this variability is equated with 'reversibility' but evidence of persisting airway narrowing, however subtle, in many patients with asthma in apparent remission implies that reversibility is frequently incomplete. The time frame of variation of airway function is itself extremely variable. Some patients are prone to dramatic changes, with FEV_1 declining from relative normality to as little as 10–15% of normal over a few hours, others showing characteristic diurnal variation with persistently low values in the early morning and yet others with apparently 'fixed' airway obstruction with little apparent change over months or years and characteristic variation uncovered only after several days' treatment with corticosteroids.

As in normal subjects, both anticholinergic and β-sympathomimetic agents reduce bronchomotor tone and produce bronchodilatation. Unlike the situation in normal subjects, however, β-receptor blockade (e.g. with propranolol) frequently provokes broncho-constriction, suggesting resting activity of not only the cholinergic, but also the adrenergic system. The mechanism of this difference from normal is unclear. Plasma levels of adrenaline are similar to normal, even in acute severe asthma (Ind *et al.*, 1985).

The narrowing of the airways in asthma is widespread, including both small and large airways and even the extrathoracic airway and glottis. Experimental measurements of peripheral airway resistance during fibreoptic bronchoscopy have shown marked increases, even in patients with mild asymptomatic asthma who have normal values of FEV_1 and sG_{aw} (Wagner *et al.*, 1990). Several factors contribute to the airway narrowing. In addition to smooth muscle contraction, these include thickening of components of the airway wall including the epithelium and subepithelial layers (so called 'remodelling') (James *et al.*, 1989). An inverse relation between subepithelial thickening and FEV_1 in asthma has been shown by bronchial biopsy studies (Chetta *et al.*, 1997). Even if lesser degrees of airway wall thickening have little effect on baseline function, they amplify the effect of smooth muscle contraction so that marked increases in airway resistance occur with a relatively minor degree of shortening of smooth muscle (Wiggs *et al.*, 1992) (Fig. 2.5). Inflammatory changes and oedema, together with increased secretions, also contribute, especially during exacerbations.

During an asthma attack there is widespread airway narrowing and an increased tendency for airways to close completely. This results in increases in residual volume (RV) and functional residual capacity (FRC). Consequently, tidal breathing occurs at a greater absolute lung volume, an adaptive mechanism which may help to maintain airway patency due to the greater lung recoil pressure at higher volumes.

The effect of deep inspiration on airway function in asthma is more variable than in healthy subjects. In normal subjects in whom bronchoconstriction has been induced, e.g. by inhaling methacholine, deep inspiration reduces bronchomotor tone and consistently reduces airway resistance (increases sG_{AW}) and increases forced expiratory flow (M/P > 1). However, with methacholine-induced bronchoconstriction in asthmatic subjects, reduction in airway resistance following deep inspiration is less consistent and may be absent (Fish *et al.*, 1981). Furthermore, in spontaneously occurring asthma, the effect of deep inspiration is often to produce further bronchoconstriction, demonstrable as M/P ratio < 1. The M/P ratio tends to fall (i.e. greater bronchoconstriction post deep inspiration) as FEV_1 falls (Lim *et al.*, 1987). These

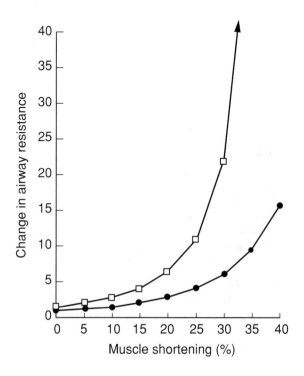

Figure 2.5 *Theoretical effect of increased airway wall thickness in asthma on the change in airway resistance with a given degree of shortening of airway smooth muscle in asthmatic and non-asthmatic airways. The baseline resistance of the non-asthmatic airway is set at 1.0. Although airway wall thickening in asthma has only a small effect on relaxed diameter, it greatly enhances the increase in resistance associated with smooth muscle shortening (from James* et al., *1989).* □, *asthma;* ●, *non-asthma.*

divergent findings emphasize that induced and spontaneous airway narrowing in asthma may have important functional differences. In particular, chemically induced bronchoconstriction may be a poor model for inflammatory narrowing of the smaller airways in spontaneous asthma.

BRONCHIAL HYPERRESPONSIVENESS

Bronchial hyperresponsiveness (BHR) in asthma is characterized by exaggerated airway constrictor responses to a variety of non-specific stimuli, usually when inhaled (Table 2.1). Thus, BHR is demonstrable following inhalation of chemical agents which mimic the effects of the parasympathetic nervous system (methacholine), substances that are released naturally from mast cells (histamine and other putative mediators of the asthmatic response), cold, dry air, otherwise inert hypertonic or hypotonic solutions and atmospheric pollutants. The precise mechanism(s) responsible for BHR is not established but its aetiology may be multifactorial and may vary depending on the particular stimulus concerned.

Pharmacological agents such as methacholine act directly on specific receptors on airway smooth muscle, whereas indirect stimuli such as hypertonic saline are thought to act by activation of cellular and/or neurogenic pathways. Inhaled hypertonic saline induces release of mediators such as histamine and also may activate nerve endings and irritant receptors by changes in local osmolality (Makker and Holgate, 1993). Enhanced vagal reflex mechanisms may be relevant to the temporary hyperresponsiveness demonstrable in normal subjects after viral respiratory tract infections. In this situation mucosal damage may allow greater access of inhalants to afferent nerve fibres, stimulating greater bronchoconstriction.

The wide variety of potential stimuli (Table 2.1) and their different modes of action suggest that the fundamental mechanism(s) of BHR are more likely due to the response of the asthmatic airway rather than to unusual sensitivity of the receptors which are stimulated. However, the response is not related simply to the bronchial smooth muscle. Indeed, there is no apparent correlation between in-vivo airway responsiveness and in-vitro smooth muscle responsiveness (Armour et al., 1984). Nevertheless, an increased amount of smooth muscle and/or an abnormality in its contractility may well interact with other factors to account for BHR in asthma. Other structural elements of the airway wall as well as its overall thickness are likely to be relevant (Fig. 2.5). Thus, for example, greater bronchial responsiveness is seen with increased subepithelial layer thickness on bronchial biopsy (Chetta et al., 1997) and with greater bronchial wall thickness as measured by CT scanning (Boulet et al., 1995).

Table 2.1 *Stimuli to which asthmatic airways show hyperresponsiveness.*

Type	Examples
Parasympathomimetic agents	Methacholine, pilocarpine
β-receptor antagonists	Propranolol
Mediators	Histamine, prostaglandins (PGF$_2$ α), leukotrienes (LTC$_4$, LTD$_4$, LTE$_4$), serotonin, adenosine, platelet activating factor, neuropeptides (substance P, neurokinin A)
Osmotic/physical	Hypotonic saline / fog, hypertonic saline, airway cooling/drying, exercise
Air pollutants	Sulphur dioxide, ozone, particulates

Another important factor determining the extent of bronchial narrowing is the load opposing smooth muscle shortening. This includes both the stiffness of the airway wall itself and the recoil of the surrounding lung parenchyma. Either a reduction in the load opposing muscle shortening or an increase in airway wall thickness could produce excessive airway narrowing without any need to invoke a change in properties of airway smooth muscle. Some, but not all, studies have shown relations between the presence of inflammatory cells in bronchial lavage or biopsy and increased airway responsiveness (Haley and Drazen, 1998), but the suggestion that BHR directly reflects 'airway inflammation' is an oversimplification. It has been proposed that hyperresponsiveness is due to a failure of deep inspiration to stretch airway smooth muscle (Skloot et al., 1995). This, in turn, might result from inflammation and oedema of the airway wall inhibiting the normal relaxation of smooth muscle associated with stretching during deep inspiration. However, the difference in responsiveness of asthmatic and normal airways is not limited to measurements requiring a preceding deep inspiration, and therefore asthmatic hyperresponsiveness cannot be due entirely to this mechanism (Burns and Gibson, 1998).

In experimental and clinical studies of bronchial responsiveness, the cholinergic agent methacholine is the most widely used provoking stimulus. Increasing concentrations or doses are administered by inhalation with their effect monitored using either tests of forced expiration or specific airway conductance. The most commonly used index of response is the provoking concentration (PC_{20}) or dose (PD_{20}) causing a reduction in FEV_1 of 20%. The degree of BHR in an asthmatic individual tends to increase when asthma is more troublesome (Josephs et al., 1989), even if there is little change in prechallenge airway function. Greater BHR is also associated with greater spontaneous variability of airway function, e.g. greater diurnal variation of PEF (Brand et al., 1991). Non-specific BHR also increases following exposure to specific allergens to which the subject is sensitive. This has been shown with natural exposure, e.g. during the pollen season in pollen-sensitive individuals (Boulet et al., 1983) and also following specific challenge, both single exposures (Cockcroft and Murdock, 1987) and repeated low-dose exposure (Ihre and Zetterstrom, 1993). The degree of BHR is generally greater in asthma than in chronic obstructive pulmonary disease (COPD), although there is some overlap (Brand et al., 1991). Unlike the situation in COPD, where there is a relation between BHR (PC_{20}) and baseline airway calibre, no such relation is found in asthma (Twentyman et al., 1993) and many patients with virtually normal prechallenge function show BHR.

In most clinical studies bronchial responsiveness has been assessed in terms of the concentration or dose of challenge agent which produces a specified change in respiratory function. Clearly, however, this is a considerable simplification of the response. In most normal subjects the full dose–response curve of FEV_1 to inhaled histamine is sigmoid with an apparent plateau at high concentrations (Woolcock et al., 1984; Moore et al., 1996) (Fig. 2.6). By contrast, some patients with asthma fail to show such a plateau response as the dose of histamine is increased, suggesting that they lack a mechanism present in healthy subjects that serves to limit airway narrowing. The possible implication of this type of response for deteriorating airway function in spontaneous asthma is obvious. The nature of the protective mechanism in healthy subjects and the cause of its reduced effectiveness in some patients with asthma remain uncertain. A maximal plateau response implies limitation of smooth muscle shortening despite increasing stimulation, i.e. the muscle is activated sufficiently to produce the maximal tension of which it is capable against the load on which it is acting. Again, it is likely that thickening of the airway walls is relevant to the abnormal response in asthma: attention has been drawn particularly to the possible role of peribronchial inflammation and oedema. This may effectively 'uncouple' intrapulmonary airways from the supporting effect of the surrounding lung parenchyma, which normally prevents excessive narrowing (Macklem, 1996).

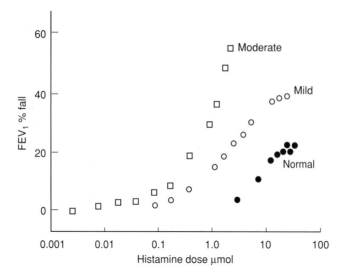

Figure 2.6 *Dose–response curves of FEV₁ to histamine challenge in a normal person and two patients with asthma. Both asthmatics show hyperresponsiveness compared to the normal but the patient with mild asthma and the healthy person show a plateau response at high histamine doses whereas the patient with more severe asthma shows no plateau despite a fall in FEV₁ >50% (redrawn from Woolcock et al., 1984).*

The level of maximal bronchoconstriction is related only weakly to the degree of hyperresponsiveness as assessed by PD_{20}, suggesting that the mechanisms underlying the plateau response and conventional BHR may be different. A decrease in load on the airway smooth muscle resulting from peribronchial oedema would result in progressive closure of small airways during challenge. It has therefore been suggested that a large reduction in FVC during challenge may indicate absence of a plateau response and a tendency to excessive bronchoconstriction (Gibbons *et al.*, 1996).

PULMONARY AND CHEST WALL MECHANICS

In radiographic surveys of patients with asthma, overinflation is frequently noted even without severe airway obstruction. Both radiographic and functional evidence of hyperinflation are much more likely if the onset of disease was in childhood (Merkus *et al.*, 1993). Changes during the acute attack have been more controversial. They were first recognized as progressive reduction in TLC over several days during recovery from acute asthma. Although doubt was subsequently cast on some of the plethysmographic measurements made during acute asthma, short-term changes have been supported by estimates using the inert gas technique and by careful radiographic studies. The time-scale over which such changes occur remains unclear, but is probably days rather than hours or minutes. The fall in TLC during recovery from spontaneous asthma is not closely related to the increase in FEV₁ (Blackie *et al.*, 1990). The TLC does not change consistently when airway narrowing is produced acutely during bronchial challenge (Lougheed *et al.*, 1993).

The mechanism by which TLC increases in asthma is not clear. Detailed analysis of the static pressure volume curve of the lungs using the exponential curve fitting method (which is independent of absolute lung volume) shows only a slight increase in lung distensibility (Colebatch *et al.*, 1979) and the static lung compliance over the tidal volume range is effectively normal. As with other causes of airway obstruction, residual volume is consistently increased. In asthma this is likely to reflect progressive airway closure as expiration continues due to a combination of increased bronchial smooth muscle tone, mucous obstruction, oedema and inflammation of the airway wall.

In normal individuals, FRC (i.e. lung volume at end-tidal expiration) is very close to the relaxation volume of the respiratory system, i.e. that volume at which lung and chest wall recoil are equal and opposite. In patients with asthma, changes in the elastic properties of the lungs and chest wall lead to an increase in this relaxation volume (static hyperinflation). In addition there is a variable degree of further 'dynamic hyperinflation' reflected by an increase in end-expiratory volume above the relaxation volume. In general, with increasing airway resistance and greater flow limitation, expiration towards the relaxation volume becomes increasingly prolonged, so that the next inspiration begins before this volume is reached. This results in an extra load on the inspiratory muscles in that they have to overcome a 'threshold' load related to the elastic recoil of the respiratory system before inspiratory flow can commence. Furthermore, this occurs in the face of worsening mechanical advantage of the inspiratory muscles due to the greater lung volume. Dynamic hyperinflation has been demonstrated during methacholine-induced asthma (Pellegrino *et al.*, 1993) and doubtless contributes to the distress of spontaneously occurring acute asthma. Dynamic hyperinflation is an adaptive response and its development correlates with the presence of dynamic compression of the airways during tidal breathing (Pellegrino *et al.*, 1993). Although beneficial in maintaining airway patency, the increased effort associated with breathing at higher lung volumes contributes to breathlessness (Lougheed *et al.*, 1993). Persistent tonic inspiratory muscle activity during expiration has been demonstrated with induced asthma (Muller *et al.*, 1981), but whether this occurs also in spontaneous asthma is not clear. The constraints imposed by severe airway obstruction are such that during tidal breathing both end-expiratory and end-inspiratory volumes rise. Another adaptive strategy that allows normal ventilation to be maintained is an increase in the frequency of breathing. Each of these imposes significant loads on the inspiratory muscles at the same time as their capacity is diminished secondary to the hyperinflation.

Static respiratory muscle function is generally well preserved in asthma. Hyperinflation itself results in some reduction in maximum inspiratory pressure at the elevated FRC, but in most patients even during acute attacks, this is usually well preserved. Respiratory muscle fatigue is very likely to occur in severe asthma but evidence in stable patients suggests that, if anything, fatigue is less easily demonstrable than in normal subjects (McKenzie and Gandevia, 1986).

In some patients reductions in maximum respiratory pressures related to chronic steroid treatment are seen (Decramer and Koenrad, 1992). Long-term steroid use may impair inspiratory muscle endurance to a greater extent than strength (Perez *et al.*, 1996). Such patients may also be unduly susceptible to further muscle weakness associated with use of neuromuscular blocking agents if assisted ventilation is required (Leatherman *et al.*, 1996).

PULMONARY GAS EXCHANGE

The distribution of pulmonary ventilation and perfusion in asthma is often markedly abnormal, even in patients with only mild airway obstruction. This maldistribution of ventilation and/or perfusion is demonstrable using simple tests of uneven ventilation, with radioisotope scans and with detailed studies of matching of ventilation and perfusion at a microscopic level. Delayed nitrogen washout from the lungs while breathing pure oxygen is demonstrable, even when standard tests of airway function are within the normal range (McFadden and Lyons, 1968a). Similarly, studies of regional distribution of ventilation using inhaled isotopes often show much more marked abnormalities than might be expected from the degree of airway obstruction (Sovijarvi *et al.*, 1982). Perfusion lung scans performed at the same time usually show a similar pattern of defects secondary to the local reduction in ventilation with apparently good matching on a regional basis. The reduced perfusion may result from either local pulmonary vasoconstriction secondary to hypoxia or passive obstruction of pulmonary vessels due to locally increased alveolar pressure consequent on airway narrowing. This may be seen as a useful compensatory mechanism, but appreciable mismatching remains at a microscopic level, resulting in the blood gas abnormalities described below.

More detailed study of the matching of alveolar ventilation to perfusion at a microscopic level is possible with the multiple inert gas elimination technique (MIGET). With this method the elimination by the lungs of an infused solution of six inert gases chosen to have a wide range of solubility in blood is measured. The pattern of elimination of the gases in the expired air depends on the distribution of ventilation/perfusion ($\dot{V}/\dot{Q}$) ratios and mathematical processing allows construction of this distribution in the form of a histogram relating $\dot{V}/\dot{Q}$ values to either blood flow or ventilation (Fig. 2.7). Alternatively, the range of maldistribution can be expressed as the logarithm of the standard deviation (log SD) of perfusion or ventilation values. Using MIGET, an increased dispersion of $\dot{V}/\dot{Q}$ ratios is demonstrable even in mild, asymptomatic asthma (Rodriguez-Roisin and Roca, 1994). In some subjects with stable asthma, a further population of alveoli is seen with a low $\dot{V}/\dot{Q}$ ratio (Wagner *et al.*, 1978). This corresponds to the pathological finding of mucus plugging of peripheral airways which has been demonstrated at autopsy, even in some subjects with only mild asthma. It is likely that alveoli beyond such occluded airways continue to receive slow collateral ventilation, consequently avoiding atelectasis. Nevertheless, reductions in PaO_2 in adults are usually only mild unless asthma is severe. Important factors which act to limit the reduction of PaO_2 include increases in total ventilation and in cardiac output, both common findings in asthma. The effect of the increased cardiac output is the maintenance of a relatively high mixed venous PO_2, which itself reduces the tendency for PaO_2 to fall. In mild asthma, therefore, the net effect on arterial blood gases is a relatively normal PaO_2, but often a reduced $PaCO_2$ due to the increased ventilation.

As airway narrowing worsens, the pattern of $\dot{V}/\dot{Q}$ matching becomes more abnormal, with an increase in the population of alveoli with low $\dot{V}/\dot{Q}$, i.e. retaining perfusion but poorly ventilated. Even in acute severe asthma, marked atelectasis is uncommon, corresponding to the usual absence of alveoli with $\dot{V}/\dot{Q} = 0$ (i.e. shunt). A shunt may, however, develop in patients with life-threatening asthma requiring assisted ventilation with high inspired oxygen concentrations (Ballester *et al.*, 1989).

Because of the increased ventilation and consequently reduced $PaCO_2$ the alveolar-arterial oxygen difference ($P(A–a)O_2$) is a more sensitive index of abnormal gas exchange than the PaO_2 alone. This is demonstrated in a recent analysis of six different studies using the MIGET technique in patients with asthma of all severities, from mild asymptomatic to acute life-threatening (Wagner *et al.*, 1996) (Fig. 2.8). Clearly as $\dot{V}/\dot{Q}$ mismatching increases and as the dispersion of perfusion to different lung units widens, gas exchange worsens. Even though in subjects with milder asthma (studies A, B, C in Fig. 2.8) PaO_2 was virtually normal; in all there was elevation of $P(A–a)O_2$.

During recovery from acute severe asthma, improvement in gas exchange characteristically

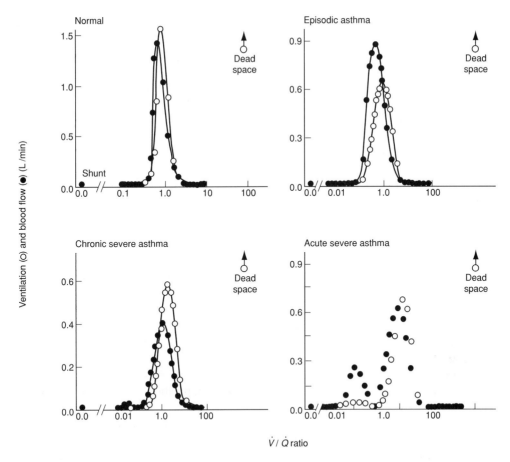

Figure 2.7 *Patterns of distribution of ventilation (○) and blood flow (●) plotted against V̇/Q̇ ratio using the MIGET technique in a normal person and three patients with asthma. In the healthy person the distributions are narrowly unimodal, while in the asthmatic patients the distributions are broader with populations of alveoli with very low V̇/Q̇ ratios in those with severe asthma (redrawn from Rodriguez-Roisin and Roca, 1994).*

lags behind improvement in airway function. If hypercapnia is present it is usually corrected rapidly, but maldistribution of perfusion and consequent hypoxaemia may persist for up to two weeks (Wagner *et al.*, 1996).

Several studies have shown that bronchodilator drugs, as well as improving airway function, can have effects on perfusion which potentially may be adverse. The worsening of hypoxaemia following a bronchodilator has been noted over many years and emphasizes the dichotomy that may occur between between airway and gas exchange function in asthma. This potentially adverse effect occurs particularly with β-sympathomimetic stimulants administered intravenously; a possible mechanism is via a reduction in pulmonary vascular tone and consequent reduction in hypoxic vasoconstriction, which normally acts as a compensatory mechanism for locally deficient ventilation. In practice, however, patients in whom this occurs will be receiving treatment with supplementary oxygen and its clinical significance is doubtful.

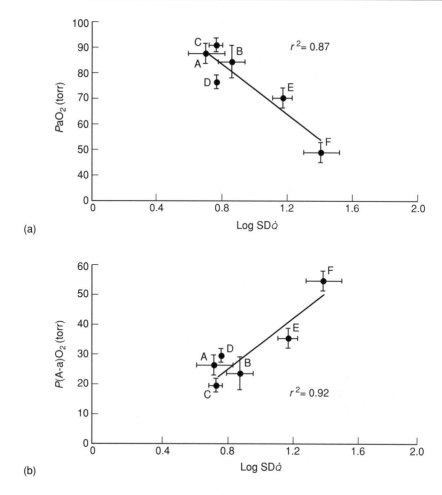

Figure 2.8 *Relations of arterial PO$_2$ and alveolar–arterial oxygen pressure difference (P(A–a)O$_2$) to the distribution of perfusion (log SD$_Q$) in six studies of asthma of increasing severity from A to F. In the three groups with milder asthma (A,B,C) PaO$_2$ is normal even though P(A–a)O$_2$ is increased. As the maldistribution of perfusion increases, P(A–a)O$_2$ increases and PaO$_2$ falls (redrawn from Wagner et al., 1996).*

CARBON MONOXIDE TRANSFER FACTOR

In most non-smoking patients with asthma, transfer of carbon monoxide measured by the standard single breath method is normal, or slightly greater than normal (Collard *et al.*, 1994). If elevated, it may fall towards normal values as airway narrowing improves with treatment (Keens *et al.*, 1979). The precise cause is not clear; suggested mechanisms include a mild increase in pulmonary arterial pressure leading to more even gravitational distribution of blood flow and blood volume, or an increased pulmonary capillary blood volume consequent on the more negative intrathoracic pressure required to overcome increased airway resistance. The former hypothesis is supported by the finding that carbon monoxide transfer factor (T$_L$CO) increases in normal subjects at altitude (presumably due to the associated increase in pulmonary artery pressure) and by scan data showing increased perfusion of the upper zones in some subjects with mild asthma (Collard *et al.*, 1994). On the other hand, the possible role of greater negative intrathoracic pressure is supported by an increase in T_LCO in normal subjects when breathing through an artificial resistance. The transfer coefficient for carbon monoxide (kCO) is more consistently elevated, partly because this index measures the rate of uptake of carbon monoxide in the better ventilated and perfused alveoli.

VENTILATORY CONTROL AND ACID–BASE STATUS

As with other conditions associated with increased airway resistance, the ventilatory response to CO_2 is likely to be impaired due to the abnormal respiratory mechanics, in particular the increased load on the inspiratory muscles and their reduced capacity in the presence of hyperinflation. This impaired response contrasts with the obviously increased ventilatory drive associated with an acute asthmatic attack. If the ventilatory response is expressed in terms of pressure output (mouth occlusion pressure) a truer picture is obtained and increased responses to CO_2 are demonstrable (Zackon *et al.*, 1976).

The main cause of hypercapnia in severe asthma is mechanical, and in particular a very adverse load/capacity relationship which ultimately compromises alveolar ventilation. However, other factors may contribute. For example, it has been shown (Rebuck and Read, 1971) in asthmatic subjects studied after recovery from a severe attack that those who developed hypercapnia during the acute attack did not show the anticipated improvement in ventilatory response to CO_2 in remission. It is also noteworthy that patients who develop hypercapnia during one severe attack are likely to develop it again in a subsequent episode (Mountain and Sahn, 1988). It therefore appears likely that in addition to the mechanical situation, constitutional sensitivity to CO_2 may influence whether or not CO_2 retention is likely during an acute attack. Psychological factors may also be interwoven, as an association has been reported between reduced chemosensitivity and impaired perception of a respiratory load (Gibson, 1995).

Because in most patients with acute severe asthma the drive to breathe is clearly increased, it is often assumed that, unlike patients with COPD, they are not at risk of hypercapnia when given oxygen to breathe. However, the mechanism of increasing hypercapnia during oxygen breathing is not simply depression of overall ventilation, and alterations in $\dot{V}/\dot{Q}$ relationships are also relevant. Patients with acute severe asthma and hypercapnia are at risk of further elevation of $PaCO_2$ if uncontrolled oxygen is given (Wasserfallen *et al.*, 1990).

The most common acid–base disturbance in asthma, even during severe episodes, is a respiratory alkalosis (Mountain *et al.*, 1990). If the $PaCO_2$ rises above normal, this is superseded by a respiratory acidosis. A metabolic acidosis has generally been regarded as unusual in acute severe asthma, but in one large detailed study a metabolic acidosis accompanied respiratory acidosis in more than half the cases with hypercapnia. These patients had had very severe hypoxaemia and also showed an increased 'anion gap', presumably due to accumulation of lactate by anaerobic metabolism (Mountain *et al.*, 1990). In another large study of acute severe asthma, only 8.5% of patients were classified as rapid onset, i.e. < 6 hours duration but, when compared with the remaining patients, they were much more likely to have hypercapnia and a respiratory acidosis on admission (Kolbe *et al.*, 1998).

RESPIRATORY FUNCTION AT NIGHT

Worsening of asthma during sleep and nocturnal or early morning waking due to airway obstruction are characteristic symptoms. The precise mechanism(s) involved are not clear, but several factors are likely to be involved. To some extent, nocturnal bronchoconstriction is an exaggeration of the normal diurnal pattern of airway function. In addition the sleeping state is accompanied by an abnormal increase in airway resistance in asthmatic subjects (Ballard *et al.*, 1989). Airway resistance is highest and the increase is maintained for the longest periods in stages 3 and 4 of non-REM sleep (slow wave sleep) (Bellia *et al.*, 1989). The effect of sleep stage has been attributed to lower sensitivity to a resistive load in deep slow wave sleep.

Detailed study of small groups of healthy and asthmatic subjects sleeping in a horizontal body plethysmograph showed a greater reduction in FRC during non-rapid eye movement (REM) sleep in the latter group (Fig. 2.9). The reduction was associated with less tonic activity of the inspiratory muscles than in the waking state (Ballard *et al.*, 1993). Although both reduction in FRC and increased airway resistance may predispose to hypoxaemia, in practice patients with well-controlled asthma show little oxygen desaturation during sleep (Neagley *et al.*, 1986).

Possible contributors to airway narrowing during sleep in asthma include exposure to house dust mite antigens, a greater tendency to mucus obstruction due to less effective mucociliary clearance and circadian rhythms in bronchial responsiveness and generation of mediators. The largest fall in peak flow coincides with the nadir of plasma adrenaline and follows the nadir in plasma cortisol by about three hours, but concentration profiles of these

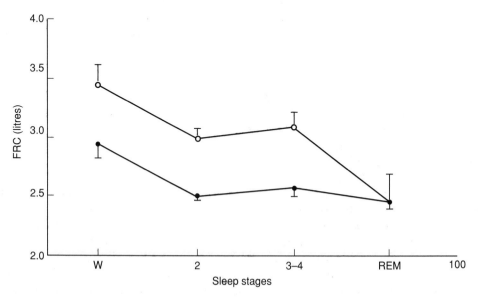

Figure 2.9 *Effect of sleep on functional residual capacity (FRC) in asthmatic (○) compared to normal (●) subjects. W, awake; 2, 3 and 4, stage 2, 3 and 4 non-rapid eye movement sleep; REM, rapid eye movement sleep. Note the marked reduction in FRC in asthmatic patients during REM sleep (redrawn from Ballard* et al., *1990). Error bars: SEM.*

hormones are similar in asthmatic and normal people. Asthmatics have, however, been shown to have an abnormal rise in plasma histamine coinciding with the early morning fall in peak flow (Barnes *et al.*, 1980).

Sleep itself is more frequently disrupted by transient arousal in patients with asthma than in healthy subjects (Montplaisir *et al.*, 1982). In some this may lead to impaired performance during the day (Fitzpatrick *et al.*, 1991).

CLINICAL APPLICATION OF LUNG FUNCTION TESTS

Recognition of asthma

In most situations, tests of respiratory function give rather non-specific information and their diagnostic role is essentially one of pattern recognition. Since, however, the definition of asthma is in terms of variable airway narrowing, functional tests have a greater diagnostic role in asthma than in many other conditions. Although the functional pattern of airway obstruction is not specific, its variation over minutes (bronchodilator response or bronchial challenge), hours (diurnal variation) or days is usually diagnostic. The marked diurnal variation of airway function so characteristic of asthma (Fig. 2.10) is essentially an exaggeration of the normal diurnal variability. The distribution of PEF variability in the population is unimodal with no clear cut separation between asthmatic and non-asthmatic subjects (Higgins *et al.*, 1989). The amplitude of diurnal PEF variation is most commonly defined as maximum–minimum expressed as a percentage of the mean daily value. In one study mean values for asthmatic and non-asthmatic individuals were 13.3 and 8.5% respectively (Higgins *et al.*, 1989). Others have found average values in asthma between 14 and 17%.

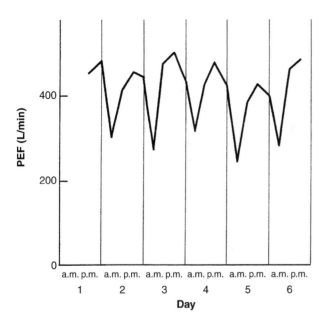

Figure 2.10 *Peak expiratory flow (PEF) recorded four times daily in an asthmatic patient showing the characteristic variability and morning dip.*

Differential diagnosis

The most common diagnostic problems arise in relation to the distinction between asthma and COPD. While this is clear in many patients, in others uncertainty remains even after detailed investigation. Not infrequently, both asthma and smoking-induced COPD co-exist in the same patient. The distinction is to some degree semantic, in that many patients with otherwise classical asthma have chronic persisting airway obstruction which may be severe even after maximal treatment (see below) and no universal consensus exists on whether the term 'COPD' should include these patients as well as the larger group in whom smoking is clearly the cause.

Most patients with smoking-related COPD have some degree of emphysema, in which case the functional distinction from asthma becomes more clear. In particular, patients with emphysema tend to have more markedly increased total lung capacity and greater reductions in lung elastic recoil. In practice, the most useful functional descriminators are often the T_LCO and kCO, which are usually both reduced with widespread emphysema, while in asthma they are well preserved.

In an acutely breathless patient the distinction between bronchial asthma and left ventricular failure (LVF) ('cardiac asthma') can be difficult, particularly in the elderly. Simple tests of respiratory function can be applied in most patients and may be helpful in differential diagnosis, as LVF is associated with only mild or moderate impairment of peak flow and FEV_1 (McNamara and Cionni, 1992).

Another situation which can cause diagnostic confusion occurs in patients with localized narrowing of the central airway, caused, for example, by benign tracheal stenosis or tumour. This gives a different functional pattern, that of extrathoracic airway obstruction in which, in general, maximum inspiratory flows are more reduced than maximum expiratory flows and PEF is more reduced than FEV_1. Of most value is examination of the full maximum expiratory and inspiratory flow volume curves (Miller and Hyatt, 1973). Inspiratory stridor which sometimes can be confused with asthma is also seen in patients with functional obstruction of the upper airway due to inspiratory laryngeal narrowing (Christopher et al., 1983). This syndrome, which is characteristically found in young women, may also be recognizable with use of maximum flow volume curves. Another type of functional wheezing results from forceful tidal breathing at volumes below FRC; in these individuals maximum flow volume curves are characteristically normal (Rodenstein et al., 1983).

Bronchodilator responses

In assessment of the response to bronchodilator, FEV_1 is most commonly used, but, as with spontaneous variability of airway function, no absolute 'cut-off' value distinguishes asthma from not asthma. Although arbitrary percentage increases in FEV_1 (e.g. 15% or 20%) are sometimes used to diagnose or exclude asthma, they can be misleading. Certainly a large increase (e.g. > 0.5 L) is effectively diagnostic but more commonly, a smaller increase is suggestive and a repeat on a second occasion may be supportive. In severe asthma very little increase may be found, but on the other hand a 20% increase when the FEV_1 is only 0.5 L is often seen in non-asthmatic chronic airway obstruction. For this reason, if a specific level of bronchodilator responsiveness is desired for diagnostic purposes, it is preferable to use both a minimum percentage and minimum absolute increase. In some patients with moderate or severe chronic, and apparently largely irreversible, airway obstruction, the characteristic variability of asthma only comes to light after treatment with corticosteroids.

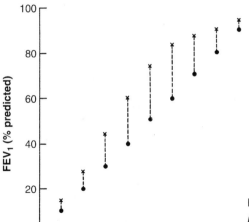

Figure 2.11 *Schematic relation of acute effect of inhaled bronchodilator to the pretreatment FEV₁ in asthma of varying severity.*

The magnitude of a bronchodilator response inevitably depends on the severity of pre-existing airway obstruction. This is illustrated schematically in Fig. 2.11. In general, the largest responses are seen in the mid-range of airway function. When airway narrowing is very severe, bronchodilators may be relatively ineffective, while at the other extreme, when airway function is close to normal, smaller responses may result from a 'ceiling effect'. None the less, even with relatively normal FEV_1, the improvement after bronchodilator in patients with asthma tends to be greater than in the non-asthmatic population (Lorber *et al.*, 1978).

Not infrequently following a bronchodilator a greater proportional increase is seen in forced or relaxed vital capacity than in FEV_1 with the result that the FEV_1/FVC or FEV_1/VC ratio actually falls. The improved vital capacity probably results from dilatation of smaller airways. Airway resistance and specific airway conductance measured by plethysmography may give a larger signal, particularly when assessing bronchodilators in patients with mild airway obstruction or normal people. Changes in maximum flow volume curves following bronchodilators are complicated by the increase in FVC and the only valid comparison is at a given percentage of the *prebronchodilator* FVC, which (as TLC does not change following bronchodilation) represents a comparable absolute lung volume.

Bronchial challenge tests

The clinical role of bronchial challenge testing is somewhat controversial and use of such tests varies considerably between countries. Testing for sensitivity to specific allergens is a specialized procedure which is rarely performed, apart from investigation of possible occupational sensitizers. More widely used is assessment of BHR to non-specific stimuli, most commonly histamine or methacholine. Methacholine has the advantage that larger doses can be given without the development of uncomfortable side-effects such as headache. Asthmatic patients are considerably more sensitive than normals to both agents. Theoretical considerations suggest that the response is likely to be influenced by prechallenge airway calibre with greater responses seen as airway narrowing progresses. Although dependence on baseline function is clearly demonstrable in patients with non-asthmatic COPD, this has little or no influence on the response in asthma (Twentyman *et al.*, 1993). In clinical testing of patients with more severe airway obstruction, however, challenge tests are usually precluded on the grounds of safety.

The most commonly used index of responsiveness is $PC_{20} FEV_1$ or $PD_{20} FEV_1$. In population studies such indices are dependent on lung size, with apparently greater responsiveness in smaller individuals (Peat *et al.*, 1996). In clinical practice, however, they usually suffice to distinguish most asthmatics from normals. The level of responsiveness correlates with severity as assessed by current symptoms or treatment requirements. Other indices of response have theoretical advantages, particularly those which avoid deep inspiration (see above), but it is not clear whether these theoretical advantages are of clinical relevance.

The severity of BHR may be relevant to the course and outcome of acute severe asthma. For example, it has been shown that patients requiring ventilatory support during an acute attack have greater BHR in remission than those not requiring assisted ventilation (Pouw *et al.*, 1990). Also, the resolution of BHR following acute severe asthma is relatively slow and continues for a period, even after FEV_1 has reached a stable value (Whyte *et al.*, 1993), possibly reflecting the gradual therapeutic effect of corticosteroids on airway inflammation. In stable asthma, similarly, the effect of an inhaled steroid on BHR is gradual over several weeks, with the benefit reversing only one week after cessation of treatment (Vathenen *et al.*, 1991).

In practice, the clinical situation in which tests of non-specific hyperreactivity are most useful is in the patient with suspected asthma, perhaps with atypical symptoms such as predominant cough, and with relatively normal function. With established airway obstruction, there are group differences between patients with asthma and COPD but in an individual the discriminatory power of a conventional inhalation challenge with methacholine or histamine is doubtful.

Routine monitoring of asthma

Current British guidelines (British Thoracic Society, 1997) for assessment and management of asthma are based on peak flow values and, surprisingly, make no mention of FEV_1. In this respect, they are at variance with international guidelines (National Heart, Blood and Lung Institute, 1991) which emphasize the complementary roles of the two types of measurement (Table 2.2). In principle, PEF is more effort-dependent but in practice most patients are able to deliver reproducible values. Clearly peak flow meters have the great advantage of economy and portability. Spirometry has traditionally been confined to hospitals but several small portable devices are now available, although they remain much more expensive than peak flow meters. Accuracy and reproducibility of FEV_1 is generally better than PEF. In general the two measurements correlate with each other but often not closely (Giannini *et al.*, 1997). Moreover, a given percentage change in one index should not be assumed to equate with the same proportional change in the other (Gautrin *et al.*, 1994).

The accuracy of portable peak flow meters has been assessed in several recent studies with somewhat disconcerting results. The commonly used 'mini-Wright' meter has been most widely studied but inaccuracies also affect other devices. The main problem is the non-linear response of these instruments to accurately measured increments of flow. Using the standard (linear) scales on the instruments, they tend to over-read in the mid-range with an error that may be as much as 80 L/min at values around 300 L/min (Miller *et al.*, 1992; Jackson, 1995). This non-linearity can affect the interpretation of changes within an individual patient, particularly if this is expressed in percentage terms to allow comparison over different ranges of values. For example, a meter over-reading in the mid-range will exaggerate diurnal variation in peak flow when values are between 100–300 L/min. Such inaccuracy could have important implications for therapy if management plans are based

Table 2.2 *Comparison of utility of peak expiratory flow (PEF) and spirometric measurements.*

	PEF	Spirometry (FEV$_1$, FVC)
Cost	Cheap	Expensive
Portability	Good	Poor but improving
Technical performance	Modest	Good
Dependence on effort	Considerable	Much less
Diagnostic specificity	Modest	Good
Assessment of severity of airway obstruction	Fair	Accurate

on threshold values of variation of peak flow (Miles *et al.*, 1996). The errors could be corrected by using an accurate non-linear scale. Moves are being made to agree appropriate national and international standards for calibration and accuracy, but at the time of writing this has not been achieved.

Airway function, severity and symptoms of asthma

Unlike the situation in COPD where severity of disease is clearly related to the level of airway function, the term 'severity' in asthma is used in various senses, including: (a) extent of variability of airway function (usually PEF); (b) severity of persistent airway narrowing (as in COPD), and (c) in relation to treatment requirements. Correlations between current airway function, its lability and symptoms are crude. Breathlessness is related not only to the severity of airway narrowing as judged by FEV$_1$ or PEF but also, importantly, to the severity of hyperinflation (Lougheed *et al.*, 1993).

Rubinfeld and Pain (1976) showed that when asthmatic subjects were asked to grade the severity of chest tightness during methacholine-induced bronchoconstriction, there was considerable variation in perception and the correlation between symptoms and objective assessment was only weak. Importantly, 15% of the patients in this study were found to be 'poor perceivers'. It has also been shown that the perception of severity of airway obstruction in spontaneous asthma is less good in patients who have had near fatal attacks and some evidence suggests that perception of bronchoconstriction is blunted when BHR is more pronounced (Ruffin *et al.*, 1991), factors which might have important implications for the outcome of acute severe asthma.

Natural history of asthma and 'fixed' airway narrowing

Cross-sectional studies of adults with a history of asthma show that spirometric measurements are on average less than predicted (Godden *et al.*, 1994; Strachan *et al.*, 1996). Some longitudinal studies, usually in smaller groups of patients, have also shown that those with asthma have a more rapid decline in FEV$_1$ with age than do controls (Peat *et al.*, 1987). The degree of functional impairment is related to both the duration and severity of previous asthma (Brown *et al.*, 1984), with lower FEV$_1$ in those with earlier age of onset and in whom symptoms persisted throughout childhood and adolescence (Strachan *et al.*, 1996; Oswald *et al.*, 1997). Normally, spirometric measurements increase markedly with age and overall growth, but in children with persistent wheezing the rate of increase of FEV$_1$ is less than normal (Gold *et al.*, 1994).

When studied in their thirties, most subjects with a history of childhood asthma have normal or virtually normal function if they have been symptom-free in recent years but more sensitive tests of airway function may show subtle abnormalities not detectable by conventional spirometry and many such individuals retain BHR to non-specific stimuli (Godden *et al.*, 1994). While remission, or apparent remission, of childhood asthma is common, this is much less frequent in young adults, but a minority of those with mild disease may achieve normal function or lose BHR over a period of several years (Panhuysen *et al.*, 1997). On the other hand, the recurrence in middle life of asthma and more marked airway obstruction in those who have apparently 'outgrown' childhood asthma is common.

In a hospital-based population of patients with asthma, a large proportion have persistent airway narrowing of varying severity, with incomplete or often only marginal reversibility to treatment. Such patients may be described as having 'irreversible' or 'fixed' airway obstruction

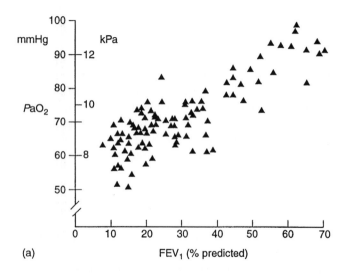

(a)

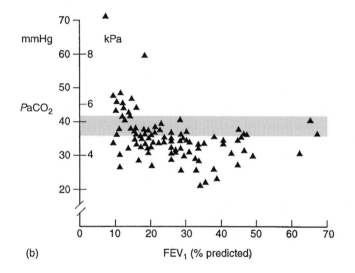

(b)

Figure 2.12 *Correlations of (a) PaO$_2$ and (b) PaCO$_2$ to FEV$_1$ in patients breathing room air on admission to hospital with asthma of varying severity (from McFadden and Lyons, 1968b).*

and their functional features merge with those of COPD. Sometimes marked persistent reduction of FEV_1 is seen even in lifelong non-smokers with a clear history of otherwise typical chronic asthma. A specific example of chronic and often largely 'fixed' airway obstruction in asthma occurs in patients with co-existent allergic bronchopulmonary aspergillosis who generally show less reversibility than is seen in typical asthma (Malo *et al.*, 1977).

Acute severe asthma

Correlations between gas exchange disturbance and tests of airway function in asthma are not close but across the broad range of patients admitted to hospital with acute asthma of varying severity there are clear trends (Fig. 2.12). As asthma worsens, the alveolar–arterial oxygen tension difference widens but PaO_2 is usually well preserved until airway obstruction is severe. The classic study of McFadden and Lyons (1968b), and general experience, show that PaO_2 < 8 kPa (60 mmHg) and/or any rise in $PaCO_2$ are likely only with very severe airway obstruction (FEV_1 < 20% predicted, *see* Fig. 2.12). Such values are, therefore, correctly regarded as ominous signs in acute asthma. Since $PaCO_2$ is less than normal in most patients with acute asthma, even a normal value should be regarded with concern as it may herald rapid deterioration. Although hypercapnia in acute asthma is often regarded as unusual, one large series showed it to be present on presentation in as many as 61 of 229 episodes. In the majority of these, however, hypercapnia responded rapidly to emergency treatment so that only in five episodes was assisted ventilation subsequently required (Mountain and Sahn, 1988). While inspired oxygen requires less strict control than in patients with COPD, a reasonable compromise in acute severe asthma is to use 35% oxygen via a venturi mask, which has been shown to be both safe and adequate (Ford and Rothwell, 1989).

REFERENCES

Armour CL, Lazar NM, Schellenberg RR, *et al.* (1984) A comparison of in-vivo and in-vitro human airway reactivity to histamine. *Am Rev Respir Dis*, **129**, 907–10.

Ballard RD, Clover CW, White DP. (1993) Influence of non-REM sleep on inspiratory activity and lung volume in asthmatic patients. *Am Rev Respir Dis*, **147**, 880–6.

Ballard RD, Irvin CG, Martin R, Pak J, Pandey R, White DP. (1990) Influence of sleep on lung volume in asthmatic patients and normal subjects. *J Appl Physiol*, **68**, 2034–41.

Ballard RD, Saathoff MC, Patel DK, Kelly PL, Martin RJ. (1989) Effect of sleep on nocturnal bronchoconstriction and ventilatory patterns in asthmatics. *J Appl Physiol*, **67**, 243–9.

Ballester E, Reyes A, Roca J, Guitart R, Wagner PD, Rodriguez-Roisin R. (1989) Ventilation–perfusion mismatching in acute severe asthma: effects of salbutamol and 100% oxygen. *Thorax*, **44**, 258–67.

Barnes PJ. (1986) Neural control of human airways in health and disease. *Am Rev Respir Dis*, **134**, 1289–314.

Barnes PJ, Fitzgerald G, Brown M, Dollery C. (1980) Nocturnal asthma and changes in circulating epinephrine, histamine and cortisol. *New Engl J Med*, **303**, 263–7.

Barnes PJ, Gribbin HR, Osmanliev D, Pride NB. (1981) Partial flow-volume curves to measure bronchodilator dose–response curves in normal humans. *J Appl Physiol*, **50**, 1193–7.

Bates JHT, Baconnier P, Milic Emili J. (1988) A theoretical analysis of the interruptor technique for measuring respiratory mechanics. *J Appl Physiol*, **64**, 2204–14.

Bellia V, Cuttitta G, Insalaco G, Visconti A, Bonsignore G. (1989) Relationship of nocturnal bronchoconstriction to sleep stages. *Am Rev Respir Dis*, **140**, 363–7.

Belvisi MG, Stretton CD, Barnes PJ. (1992) Nitric oxide is the endogenous neurotransmitter of bronchodilator nerves in human airways. *Eur J Pharmacol*, **210**, 221–2.

Blackie SP, Al-Majed S, Staples CA, Hilliam C, Pare PD. (1990) Changes in total lung capacity during acute spontaneous asthma. *Am Rev Respir Dis*, **142**, 79–83.

Boulet LP, Belanger M, Carrier G. (1995) Airway responsiveness and bronchial wall thickness in asthma with or without fixed airflow obstruction. *Am J Respir Crit Care Med*, **152**, 865–71.

Boulet LP, Cartier A, Thomson NC, *et al.* (1983) Asthma and increases in non-allergic bronchial responsiveness from seasonal pollen exposure. *J Allergy Clin Immunol*, **71**, 399–406.

Brand PLP, Postma DS, Kerstejns HAM, *et al.* (1991) Relationship of airway hyperresponsiveness to respiratory symptoms and diurnal peak flow variation in patients with obstructive lung disease. *Am Rev Respir Dis*, **143**, 916–21.

British Thoracic Society. (1997) The British guidelines on asthma management. *Thorax*, **52**, Suppl. 1.

Brown PJ, Greville HW, Finucane K. (1984) Asthma and irreversible airflow obstruction. *Thorax*, **39**, 131–6.

Burns GP, Gibson GJ. (1998) Airway hyperresponsiveness in asthma: not just a problem of smooth muscle relaxation with inspiration. *Am J Respir Crit Care Med*, **158**, 1–4.

Chetta A, Foresi A, DelDonno M, Bertorelli G, Pesci A, Olivieri D. (1997) Airway remodelling is a distinctive feature of asthma and is related to severity of disease. *Chest*, **111**, 852–7.

Christopher KL, Wood RP, Eckert RC, Blager FB, Raney RA, Souhrada JF. (1983) Vocal cord dysfunction presenting as asthma. *New Engl J Med*, **308**, 1566–70.

Colebatch HJH, Greaves IA, Ng CKY. (1979) Pulmonary mechanics in diagnosis. In: DeKock MA, Nadel JA, Lewis CM, eds. *Mechanisms of airways obstruction in human respiratory disease*. Capetown: Balkema, 25–47.

Cockcroft DW, Murdock KY. (1987) Changes in bronchial responsiveness to histamine at intervals after bronchial challenge. *Thorax*, **42**, 302–8.

Collard P, Njinou B, Nejadnik B, Keyeux A, Frans A. (1994) Single breath diffusing capacity for carbon monoxide in stable asthma. *Chest*, **105**, 1426–9.

Decramer M, Koenrad SJ. (1992) Corticosteroid-induced myopathy involving respiratory muscles in patients with chronic obstructive pulmonary disease or asthma. *Am Rev Respir Dis*, **146**, 800–2.

DuBois AB, Botelho SY, Comroe JH. (1956) A new method for measuring airway resistance in man using a body plethysmograph. *J Clin Invest*, **35**, 327–32.

Fish JE, Ankin MG, Kelly JF, Peterman VI. (1981) Regulation of bronchomotor tone by lung inflation in asthmatic and nonasthmatic subjects. *J Appl Physiol*, **50**, 1079–86.

Fitzpatrick MF, Engleman H, Whyte KF, Deary IJ, Shapiro CM, Douglas NJ. (1991) Morbidity in nocturnal asthma: sleep quality and daytime cognitive performance. *Thorax*, **48**, 100–2.

Ford DJ, Rothwell RPG. (1989) 'Safe oxygen' in acute asthma: prospective trial using 35% Ventimask prior to admission. *Respir Med*, **83**, 189–94.

Gautrin D, D'Aquino LC, Gagnon G, Malo JL, Cartier D. (1994) Comparison between peak expiratory flow rates and FEV, in the monitoring of asthmatic subjects at an out patient clinic. *Chest*, **106**, 1419–26.

Giannini D, Paggiaro PL, Moscato G, *et al.* (1997) Comparison between peak expiratory flow and forced expiratory volume in one second during bronchoconstriction induced by different stimuli. *J Asthma*, **34**, 105–11.

Gibbons WJ, Sharma A, Lougheed D, Macklem PT. (1996) Detection of excessive bronchoconstriction in asthma. *Am J Respir Crit Care Med*, **153**, 582–9.

Gibson GJ. (1995) Perception, personality and respiratory control in life-threatening asthma. *Thorax*, **50**, Suppl 1, S2–S4.

Gold DR, Wypij D, Wang X, *et al.* (1994) Gender- and race-specific effects of asthma and wheeze on level and growth of lung function in children in six US cities. *Am J Respir Crit Care Med*, **149**, 1198–208.

Godden DJ, Ross S, Abdalla M, *et al.* (1994) Outcome of wheeze in childhood: symptoms and pulmonary function 25 years later. *Am J Respir Crit Care Med*, **149**, 106–12.

Haley KJ, Drazen JM. (1998) Inflammation and airway function in asthma. *Am J Respir Crit Care Med*, **157**, 1–3.

Higgins BG, Britton JR, Chinn S, *et al.* (1989) The distribution of peak expiratory flow variability in a population sample. *Am Rev Respir Dis*, **140**, 1368–72.

Ihre E, Zetterstrom O. (1993) Increase in non-specific bronchial responsiveness after repeated inhalation of low doses of allergen. *Clin Exp Allergy*, **23**, 298–305.

Ind PW, Causon RC, Brown MJ, Barnes PJ. (1985) Circulating catecholamines in acute asthma. *BMJ*, **290**, 267–79.

Jackson AC. (1995) Accuracy, reproducibility and variability of portable peak flow meters. *Chest*, **107**, 648–51.

James AL, Pare PD, Hogg JC. (1989) The mechanics of airway narrowing in asthma. *Am Rev Respir Dis*, **139**, 242–6.

Josephs LK, Gregg I, Mullee MA, *et al.* (1989) Nonspecific bronchial reactivity and its relationship to the clinical expression of asthma. A longitudinal study. *Am Rev Respir Dis*, **140**, 350–7.

Keens TG, Mansell A, Krastins IRB, *et al.* (1979) Evaluation of the single breath diffusing capacity in asthma and cystic fibrosis. *Chest*, **76**, 41–4.

Kolbe J, Fergusson W, Garrett J. (1998) Rapid onset asthma: a severe but uncommon manifestation. *Thorax*, **53**, 241–7.

Leatherman JW, Fluegel WL, David WS, Davies SF, Iber C. (1996) Muscle weakness in mechanically ventilated patients with severe asthma. *Am J Respir Crit Care Med*, **153**, 1686–90.

Lim TK, Pride NB, Ingram RH Jr. (1987) Effects of volume history during spontaneous and acutely induced airflow obstruction in asthma. *Am Rev Respir Dis*, **135**, 591–6.

Lorber DB, Kattenborn W, Burrows B. (1978) Responses to isoproterenol in a general population sample. *Am Rev Respir Dis*, **118**, 855–61.

Lougheed MD, Lam M, Forkert L, Webb KA, O'Donnell DE. (1993) Breathlessness during acute bronchoconstriction in asthma: pathophysiologic mechanisms. *Am Rev Respir Dis*, **148**, 1452–9.

Macklem PT. (1996) A theoretical analysis of the effect of airway smooth muscle load on airway narrowing. *Am J Respir Crit Care Med*, **153**, 83–9.

Makker HK, Holgate ST. (1993) The contribution of neurogenic reflexes to hypertonic saline-induced broncho-constriction in asthma. *J Allergy Clin Immunol*, **92**, 82–8.

Malo JL, Inouye T, Hawkins R. *et al.* (1977) Studies in chronic allergic bronchopulmonary aspergillosis. *Thorax*, **32**, 275–80.

McFadden, ER, Lyons HA (1968a) Airway resistance and uneven ventilation in bronchial asthma. *J Appl Physiol*, **25**, 365–70.

McFadden ER, Lyons HA. (1968b) Arterial blood gas tension in asthma. *New Engl J Med*, **278**, 1027–32.

McKenzie DK, Gandevia SC. (1986) Strength and endurance of inspiratory, expiratory and limb muscles in asthma. *Am Rev Respir Dis*, **134**, 999–1004.

McNamara RM, Cionni DJ. (1992) Utility of the peak expiratory flow rate in the differentiation of acute dyspnoea: cardiac vs. pulmonary origin. *Chest*, **101**, 129–32.

Merkus PJFM, van Essen-Zandvliet EEM, Kouwenberg JM, *et al.* (1993) Large lungs after childhood asthma: a case control study. *Am Rev Respir Dis*, **148**, 1484–9.

Miles JF, Tunnicliffe, W, Cayton RM, Ayres JG, Miller MR. (1996) Potential effects of correction of inaccuracies of the Mini-Wright peak expiratory flow meter in the use of an asthma self management plan. *Thorax*, **51**, 403–6.

Miller MR, Dickinson SA, Hutchings DJ. (1992) The accuracy of portable peak flow meters. *Thorax*, **47**, 904–9.

Miller RD, Hyatt RE. (1973) Evaluation of obstructing lesions of the trachea and larynx by flow–volume curves. *Am Rev Respir Dis*, **108**, 476–81.

Moore BJ, Hilliam CC, Verbrugt LM, Wiggs BR, Vedal S, Pare PD. (1996) Shape and position of the complete dose–response curve for inhaled methacholine in normal subjects. *Am J Respir Crit Care Med*, **154**, 642–8.

Mountain RD, Heffner JE, Brackett NC, Sahn SA. (1990) Acid–base disturbance in acute asthma. Chest, **98**, 651–5.

Mountain RD, Sahn SA. (1988) Clinical features and outcome in patients with acute asthma presenting with hypercapnia. *Am Rev Respir Dis*, **138**, 535–9.

Montplaisir, J, Walsh, J, Malo JL. (1982) Nocturnal asthma: features of attacks, sleep and breathing patterns. *Am Rev Respir Dis*, **125**, 18–22.

Muller, N, Bryan AC, Zamel N. (1981) Tonic inspiratory muscle activity as a cause of hyperinflation in asthma. *J Appl Physiol*, **50**, 279–82.

National Heart, Lung and Blood Institute. (1991) Expert panel report: guidelines for the diagnosis and management of asthma. US Department of Health and Human Services, Bethesda, MD. NIGH, Publication no. **91–3042**.

Neagley SR, White DP, Zwillich CW. (1986) Breathing during sleep in stable asthmatic subjects: influence of inhaled bronchodilators. *Chest*, **90**, 334–7.

Oswald, H, Phelan PD, Lanigan A, *et al.* (1997) Childhood asthma and lung function mid-adult life. *Pediat Pulmonol*, **23**, 14–20.

Panhuysen CIM, Vonk JM, Koeter GH, *et al.* (1997) Adult patients may outgrow their asthma: a 25-year follow-up study. *Am J Respir Crit Care Med*, **155**, 1267–72.

Peat JK, Salome CM, Xuan W. (1996) On adjusting measurements of airway responsiveness for lung size and airway calibre. *Am J Respir Crit Care Med*, **154**, 870–5.

Peat JK, Woolcock AJ, Cullen K. (1987) Rate of decline of lung function in subjects with asthma. *Eur J Respir Dis*, **70**, 171–9.

Pellegrino R, Violante B, Nava S, Rampulla C, Brusasco V, Rodarte JR. (1993) Expiratory airflow limitation and hyperinflation during methacholine-induced bronchoconstriction. *J Appl Physiol*, **75**, 1720–7.

Perez T, Becquart L-A, Stach B, Wallaert B, Tonnel A-B. (1996) Inspiratory muscle strength and endurance in steroid-dependent asthma. *Am J Respir Crit Care Med*, **153**, 610–15.

Pouw EM, Koeter GH, de Monchy JGR, Homan AJ, Sluiter HJ. (1990) Clinical assessment after a life-threatening attack of asthma: the role of bronchial hyperreactivity. *Eur Respir J*, **3**, 861–6.

Rebuck AS, Read J. (1971) Patterns of ventilatory response to carbon dioxide during recovery from severe asthma. *Clin Sci*, **41**, 13–21.

Rodenstein DO, Francis, C, Stanescu DC. (1983) Emotional laryngeal wheezing: a new syndrome. *Am Rev Respir Dis*, **127**, 354–6.

Rodriguez-Roisin R, Roca J. (1994) Bronchial asthma. *Thorax*, **49**, 1027–33.

Rubinfeld AR, Pain MCF. (1976) Perception of asthma. *Lancet*, **i**, 882–4.

Ruffin RE, Latimer KM, Schemburi DA. (1991) Longitudinal study of near fatal asthma. *Chest*, **99**, 77–83.

Skloot G, Permutt S, Togias A. (1995) Airway hyperresponsiveness in asthma: a problem of limited smooth-muscle relaxation with inspiration. *J Clin Invest*, **96**, 2393–403.

Sovijarvi ARA, Poyhonen L, Kellomaki L, Muittari A. (1982) Effects of acute and long-term bronchodilator treatment on regional lung function in asthma assessed by krypton-81m and technetium-99m-labelled macroaggregates. *Thorax*, **37**, 516–20.

Strachan DP, Griffiths JM, Johnston IDA, Anderson HR. (1996) Ventilatory function in British adults after asthma or wheezing illness at ages 0–35. *Am J Respir Crit Care Med*, **154**, 1629–35.

Twentyman OP, Hood SV, Holgate ST. (1993) Does baseline airway calibre affect measurements of airway responsiveness to histamine? *J Appl Physiol*, **74**, 3034–9.

van Noord JA, Clement J, van de Woestijne KP, Demedts M. (1991) Total respiratory resistance in patients with asthma, chronic bronchitis and emphysema. *Am Rev Respir Dis*, **143**, 922–7.

Vathenen AS, Knox AJ, Wisniewski A, Tattersfield AE. (1991) The course of change in bronchial reactivity with an inhaled corticosteroid in asthma. *Am Rev Respir Dis*, **143**, 1317–21.

Wagner PD, Dantzker DR, Iacovoni VE, Tomlin WC, West JB. (1978) Ventilation–perfusion inequality in asymptomatic asthma. *Am Rev Respir Dis*, **118**, 511–24.

Wagner PD, Hedenstierna, G, Rodriguez-Roisin R. (1996) Gas exchange, expiratory flow obstruction and the clinical spectrum of asthma. *Eur Respir J*, **9**, 1278–82.

Wagner EM, Liu MC, Wienmann GG, Permutt, S, Bleecker ER. (1990) Peripheral lung resistance in normal and asthmatic subjects. *Am Rev Respir Dis*, **141**, 584–8.

Wasserfallen J-B, Schaller M-D, Feihl F, Perret CH. (1990) Sudden asphyxic asthma: a distinct entity? *Am Rev Respir Dis*, **142**, 108–11.

Wiggs BR, Bosken C, Pare PD, James A, Hogg JC. (1992) A model of airway narrowing in asthma and in chronic obstructive pulmonary disease. *Am Rev Respir Dis*, **145**, 1251–8.

Whyte MKB, Choudry NB, Ind PW. (1993) Bronchial hyperresponsiveness in patients recovering from acute severe asthma. *Respir Med*, **87**, 29–35.

Woolcock AJ, Salome CM, Yan K. (1984) The shape of dose–response curve to histamine in asthmatics and normal subjects. *Am Rev Respir Dis*, **130**, 71–5.

Zackon H, Despas PJ, Anthonisen N. (1976) Occlusion pressure responses in asthma and chronic obstructive pulmonary disease. *Am Rev Respir Dis*, **114**, 917–27.

3

Exercise and environmentally-induced asthma

S. GODFREY

INTRODUCTION

Exercise-induced asthma (EIA) has been a subject of interest to physicians for at least 300 years since Sir John Floyer, himself an asthmatic, clearly described the adverse effects of physical exercise on his asthma (Floyer, 1698). He wrote that 'all Violent Exercise makes the Asthmatic to breathe short' and then went on to relate how different types of exercise had differing potentials for causing trouble in the asthmatic. It now seems likely, but not certain, that he was not correct about the relative effects of different types of exercise unless they were of unequal intensity. However, he did suggest that the mechanism of EIA was related to 'putting the Spirits to a great Expansion' or making the 'Blood boyl' and perhaps the modern counterpart of this idea is the suggestion that EIA is primarily a vascular phenomenon (McFadden, 1990). Very little was known about the mechanisms underlying EIA for many years but it was known that a similar brief attack of asthma could also be provoked in a susceptible person by deep breathing, or even by laughing or crying.

The similarity between asthma induced by exercise and that induced by hyperventilation (hyperventilation-induced asthma, HIA) led to the suggestion first discussed seriously by Herxheimer (1946) that EIA was probably caused by the hyperventilation of exercise. Scientific investigation of this subject began with the remarkable pioneering observations by R. S. Jones and his colleagues in Liverpool (Jones et al., 1962, 1963; Jones, 1966; Jones and Jones, 1966). These studies clearly showed EIA to be a normal feature of childhood (and young adult) asthma and related the pattern of EIA to clinical severity. In another important study, McNeill et al. (1966) described the diminution of response to further exercise after an attack of EIA – a refractory period. Asthma which resembles that provoked by exercise or hyperventilation can also be provoked in the laboratory by the inhalation of non-isotonic fogs (osmotically-induced asthma, OIA) but this type of environmentally-induced asthma is unlikely to occur naturally although, as will be discussed later, climatic condition can profoundly affect the severity of EIA or HIA. Over the past 50 years there has been a great deal of interest in the subject of EIA which provides such an accessible, elegant and safe model of asthma for investigators interested in the pathophysiology of this disease.

Exercise continues to be problematic for many asthmatics, especially the younger, more active patients despite advances in treatment, and a recent quality of life survey of adolescents suggested that there was mild-to-moderate quality of life impairment due to exercise amongst the asthmatics in the population (Gibson *et al.*, 1995). In this study, knowledge about asthma was low not only amongst the normal children but also amongst their teachers and the asthmatics themselves; in particular, specific knowledge about the prevention and treatment of EIA was poor. EIA which prevents a child or adolescent from participating in normal sports or an adult from earning a livelihood that involves physical exertion is clearly a problem of clinical significance, apart from the light which EIA and other forms of environmentally-triggered asthma may shed on the pathophysiology of asthma itself.

PATTERN OF LUNG FUNCTION CHANGES IN EIA AND HIA

The changes in lung function which occur in response to about six minutes of reasonably hard exercise are quite characteristic and are illustrated in Fig. 3.1. During most of the actual period of exercise lung function changes little or may even improve somewhat. Towards the end of the exercise period lung function may begin to deteriorate and in some patients this fall can be quite marked, even during the exercise. The major fall in lung function normally occurs from 5 to 10 minutes after stopping the exercise after which lung function normally returns

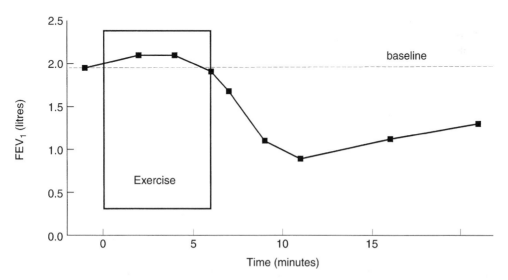

Figure 3.1   *Typical pattern of exercise-induced asthma in a child. Note that during exercise there is a minor improvement in lung function and the exercise-induced asthma only becomes fully manifest after stopping.*

spontaneously to baseline over 30 to 45 minutes. The recovery from EIA appears to be slower in older children compared with younger children which differs from the response to histamine bronchial provocation in which the recovery time is not age related (Hofstra *et al.*, 1995).

The pattern of change in lung function is independent of the parameter used to measure the change although the proportional change varies from parameter to parameter. Most studies have utilized the forced expired volume in one second (FEV_1) to document the changes but very similar results are obtained using even the simple measurement of peak expiratory flow (PEF). Asthma induced by steady-state hyperventilation for a similar time closely resembles EIA as far as the changes in lung function are concerned (Fig. 3.2).

Various indices have been used to quantitate the severity of environmentally-induced asthma. As far as steady-state exercise or hyperventilation challenges are concerned, most express the results as the percentage fall in lung function from the pre-challenge baseline:

$$\% \text{ fall in } FEV_1 = \frac{\text{baseline } FEV_1 - \text{post-exercise } FEV_1}{\text{baseline } FEV_1} \times 100$$

and there is little or nothing to be gained from more complicated indices. There is a problem if a drug that alters baseline lung function is given before the challenge and is to be compared with a placebo challenge or with a previous challenge. Under these conditions careful consideration must be given as to whether to use the predrug or pre-exercise lung function as the baseline value. When progressive challenges are used, as is common practice with hyperventilation and osmotic challenges, then the results are often expressed as the 'dose' of hyperventilation or non-isotonic solution inhaled that causes a 20% fall in FEV_1 – exactly analogous to the PC_{20} and PD_{20} indices used in methacholine or histamine inhalation challenges.

A number of studies have shown that early in exercise there is a small but generally significant bronchodilatation, and the onset of bronchoconstriction depends to some degree

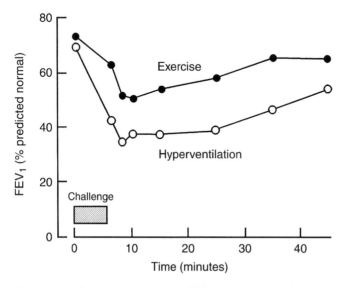

Figure 3.2 *The response to 6 minutes of steady-state exercise and voluntary isocapnic hyperventilation of similar intensity to that occurring during exercise in an asthmatic patient. The pattern of change in lung function is quite similar for the two challenges, although in this instance the change was more marked after hyperventilation.*

on the duration of the exercise. Early on in the modern investigation of EIA, Jones *et al.* (1962) noted that when children with asthma ran hard for just 1–2 minutes their lung function on stopping had actually improved but if they ran hard for 8–12 minutes they developed asthma on stopping. Measurements of pulmonary resistance during exercise by Stirling *et al.* (1983), and more recently by Suman *et al.* (1995), have shown a fall in resistance for the first 2 minutes which lasted for the whole 12 minutes of exercise in the former study but was not significant by the end of exercise in the latter. Not only is there some bronchodilatation, at least at the beginning of exercise, but there is also a marked reduction in the sensitivity to inhaled histamine or methacholine during exercise both in normal people and asthmatic patients (Stirling *et al.*, 1983; Freedman *et al.*, 1988; Inman *et al.*, 1990) which resulted in a more than tenfold protection from the effects of methacholine in the study by Inman *et al.* (1990). In both asthmatics and normals similar protection from histamine or methacholine bronchoconstriction was found when the individuals hyperventilated instead of exercised (Stirling *et al.*, 1983; Freedman *et al.*, 1988). These observations led the investigators to conclude that the bronchodilatation and inhibition of chemical bronchoconstriction was unrelated to the metabolic effects of exercise. Freedman (1992), reviewing the evidence that exercise can be a bronchodilator, suggested that the effect is the result of the deeper breathing during exercise (or hyperventilation) and that this operates through differences in the hysteresis of the airways and lung parenchyma.

There are considerable similarities in the time-course of the changes in lung function in exercise- or hyperventilation-induced asthma when compared with the early response to allergen inhalation. All are rapid in onset, pass-off over some 30 minutes, are largely prevented by prior administration of sodium cromoglycate and are easily prevented or reversed by the inhalation of a β_2-agonist. In many patients the early response to antigen inhalation is followed after some 6–8 hours by a second fall in lung function, the so-called late response, which is now believed to be due to an allergic inflammatory reaction in the airways. Given the similarity of EIA and the early response to allergen challenge it has been puzzling that late phase responses are uncommon after EIA occurring in between 10 and 38% of patients in carefully controlled studies (Boulet *et al.*, 1987; Speelberg *et al.*, 1989; Verhoeff *et al.*, 1990; Koh *et al.*, 1994). In the study of Speelberg *et al.* (1989), of the 86 patients challenged by exercise 27 developed an early response only, 7 a late response only, and 26 had a dual early and late phase response. Other investigators have not, however, obtained such definite results or even denied the existence of a late phase reaction (McFadden, 1987; Rubinstein *et al.*, 1987; Zawadski *et al.*, 1988), suggesting that the changes are just due to the random variation of lung function (McFadden, 1987; Zawadski *et al.*, 1988). On the whole, the bulk of evidence seems to support the existence of a late phase reaction in a small proportion of asthmatics, possibly those with greater responsiveness (Lee and O'Hickey, 1989; Crimi *et al.*, 1992). The lack of a late phase reaction in most patients after EIA is also compatible with the lack of evidence of an inflammatory response to exercise as shown by bronchoalveolar lavage (Jajour and Calhoun, 1992), although it is possible that this may occur in those who do indeed develop a late reaction after EIA.

Both challenges appear to operate through pathways involving a number of steps and are not simply the result of direct action on bronchial smooth muscle as would appear to be the case with methacholine or histamine challenges.

FACTORS AFFECTING THE SEVERITY OF THE RESPONSE

Both EIA and HIA have been used in population studies of bronchial reactivity, in attempts to define asthma, in the evaluation of the pathophysiology of asthma and in the evaluation of drugs used to treat asthma (Silverman *et al.*, 1973; Deal *et al.*, 1980; O'Byrne *et al.*, 1982; Weiss *et al.*, 1984). However, there are a number of important factors which influence the magnitude of the response.

Type of exercise

Sir John Floyer (1698) believed that different types of exercise affected the severity of EIA 'the most agreeable Exercise is Riding; the greatest are Sawing'. Patients and their physicians are aware that there are differences in the susceptibility to EIA with different types of exercise, although in many cases this is explained by differences in intensity, duration or pattern of exercise. Thus arm exercise is normally less intense than leg exercise and team sports such as soccer often involve intermittent exercise. However, in early controlled studies investigators found differences in EIA related to the type of exercise even if it was of identical intensity, duration and pattern. More specifically, EIA was noted to be minimal with swimming compared with running under normal conditions (Fitch and Morton, 1971; Godfrey *et al.*, 1973). This was very puzzling but, as so often happens, this enigma was to lead to some very important advances in our understanding of both EIA and the physiology of respiration in general. As discussed later, most of the difference between swimming and running depends on the fact that the air breathed during swimming is humid and this reduces the severity of EIA. Even so, when we arranged for children to swim breathing dry air they developed more EIA than when swimming while breathing humid air from the pool surface as expected but they still developed significantly less EIA than they did after running while breathing dry air (Bar-Yishay *et al.*, 1982). This suggests that there may be some effect of the type of exercise on the severity of EIA after all.

Severity and duration of the stimulus

The severity of the asthma that follows a period of exercise or hyperventilation depends upon the severity of the exercise and its duration (Silverman and Anderson, 1972). The results of a series of exercise tests of different severities and different durations in a group of asthmatic children are shown in Fig. 3.3. From this it can be seen that the severity of the post-exertional EIA increases with increasing work load up to a certain level after which the response reaches a plateau. In these studies each level of exercise or duration was performed once only on different occasions in random order. They were not tests of progressively increasing severity or duration. The level of exercise corresponding to this plateau is approximately two-thirds of the maximum working capacity of the patient which corresponds to a heart rate of about 170–180/min in children and somewhat less in adults. With a given severity of exercise, the post-exertional EIA increases with the duration of the exercise up to about 6–8 minutes after which it reaches a plateau or even becomes less severe. These studies also showed what asthmatics often claim, namely that they can sometimes 'run through' their asthma and get less trouble after a long run compared with a shorter run.

   A treadmill test is a particularly useful type of exercise challenge since the work performed depends on body weight and hence at a given setting, such as 3 m.p.h. (5 k.p.h.) and a 10% slope, all patients will be working at a similar relative level. Others have essentially confirmed these findings (Eggleston and Guerrant, 1976) and recommend a test consisting of 5 minutes continuous treadmill exercise adjusting slope and speed to produce a heart rate of 90% of the predicted maximal heart rate for the age and sex of the patient. In view of the plateau effects seen in Fig. 3.3 it is probably unnecessary to be overly exact about the work rate and time as long as they are close to the values producing the plateau. With isocapnic hyperventilation

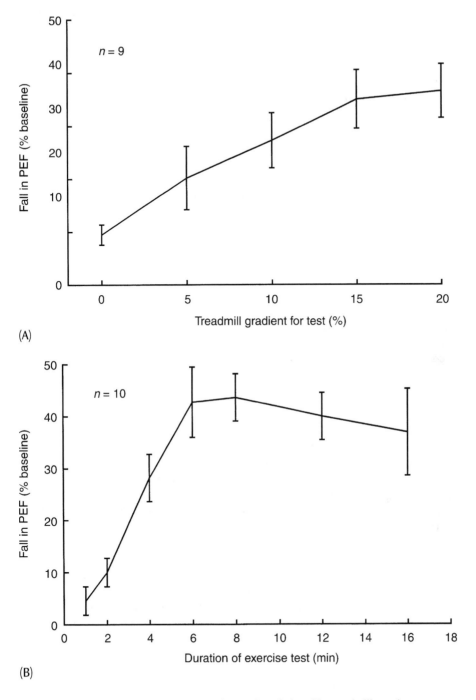

Figure 3.3 *(A) Effect of gradient (work rate) on asthma induced by treadmill running at a constant speed for 6 minutes. Each point represents the mean of tests in nine children who performed each gradient on a different occasion. (B) The effect of the duration of exercise on asthma induced by treadmill running at constant speed and gradient. Each point represents the mean of tests in 10 children who performed each duration on a different occasion. PEF, peak expiratory flow. (Redrawn from the data of Silverman and Anderson, 1972.)*

there is also increasingly severe HIA following more intense hyperventilation (Deal *et al.*, 1979) but there do not appear to be any studies relating to the duration of hyperventilation analogous to those with exercise.

While dose–response curves have been used to evaluate hyperventilation and osmotically-induced asthma, this has not been particularly helpful as far as exercise is concerned even though exercise physiologists have traditionally been interested in progressively increasing levels of exercise to the maximum the patient can tolerate. Such challenges have not been very effective in provoking EIA either because of the prolonged duration of exercise in some tests or because the patient has been allowed to rest between relatively short stages of a stepwise test. More recently, Inbar *et al.* (1992) undertook a formal comparison of continuously progressive and steady-state treadmill exercise lasting 6-8 minutes in which the total metabolic load and ventilation were the same in each type of protocol. The severity of the EIA after exercise was the same for both types of challenge even though the minute ventilation was much higher in the latter portion of the progressive exercise test. It is possible that their patients reached the plateau level of EIA in both types of protocol and could not develop more EIA in the progressive challenge even though the stimulus at the end of the progressive challenge was greater.

Pattern of exercise and refractoriness

It has been known for a long time that prior exercise reduces the response to a subsequent challenge and that asthmatics can become refractory to exercise challenges repeated over a short period (McNeill *et al.*, 1966; James *et al.*, 1976). This prior exercise may take the form of brief warming-up periods (Schnall and Landau, 1980) or a single, more prolonged, exercise period (Edmunds *et al.*, 1978; Reiff *et al.*, 1989). The appearance of relative refractoriness to a subsequent exercise challenge following an initial period of exercise is shown in Fig. 3.4. We undertook a formal study of this aspect of EIA by having a group of nine children exercise twice on a treadmill with varying lengths of time between the two equally intense exercise challenges (Edmunds *et al.*, 1978). We found that the refractoriness shown in the second of the pair of tests depended upon the time between the challenges and that the half-life of the effect was about 45 minutes, so that after about 2–3 hours the children were again fully responsive to an exercise challenge. Because of this phenomenon of refractoriness to EIA, the severity of EIA at any given time will be affected by the amount of exercise that the subject has recently undertaken. This helps explain why not all exercise encountered in everyday life, especially if it is intermittent, is prone to cause EIA even if the exercise is apparently intense. This is the case with many team games in which the participants run, slow down, run again and so on, effectively inducing a state of refractoriness. The situation with respect to HIA and OIA is less well defined. There is no doubt that refractoriness is seen in some patients following HIA and OIA (Bar-Yishay *et al.*, 1983a; Soto *et al.*, 1985; Belcher *et al.*, 1987), and indeed refractoriness to both HIA and osmotically-induced asthma can cross-react with that to EIA (Bar-Yishay *et al.*, 1983b; Belcher *et al.*, 1987).

In our original studies of refractoriness to EIA we noticed a very curious phenomenon – the exercise which induced the refractoriness in a subsequent challenge did not itself need to provoke EIA (Ben-Dov *et al.*, 1982). In this study we noted refractoriness to a second exercise challenge in subjects breathing cold, dry air following a previous exercise challenge breathing warm, humid air which itself did not provoke asthma for reasons discussed below (Fig. 3.5). In fact, such an observation can be deduced from an earlier study by Henriksen *et al.* (1981) and was repeated with exactly the same results by Wilson *et al.* (1990). Originally it was thought that refractoriness to exercise was due to the liberation of chemical mediators in the

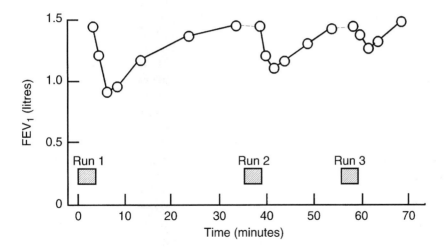

Figure 3.4   *Refractoriness to exercise-induced asthma demonstrated by a decreasing amount of asthma following each of a series of equally severe running tests. The second and third runs were begun once the FEV₁ had returned to baseline following the previous challenge.*

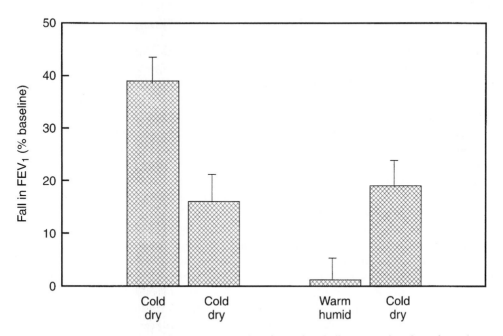

Figure 3.5   *Response of 12 children to two pairs of exercise challenges, each pair performed on a different day. In one pair (left) the children breathed cold dry air for both challenges and were refractory to the second challenge undertaken 30 minutes later. In the other pair (right) they breathed warm humid air for the first challenge and did not develop EIA. In the second challenge of this pair undertaken 30 minutes later they breathed cold dry air but their response showed them to be refractory even though they had not developed asthma after the first warm humid challenge. (Redrawn from the data of Ben-Dov et al., 1982.)*

first attack that were used up and took time to be re-synthesized, but these observations suggested that neither bronchospasm nor the presumed mediator release and depletion of stores are necessary for the development of refractoriness to EIA. Direct measurements of at least one mediator (neutrophil chemotactic factor) did not show any reduction in release when the patient was refractory to a challenge with inhaled hypertonic saline EIA (Belcher *et al.*, 1988). This phenomenon of refractoriness without preceding asthma is quite compatible with the studies of O'Byrne and others (O'Byrne and Jones, 1986; Manning *et al.*, 1993; Melillo *et al.*, 1994; Wilson *et al.*, 1994), which suggested it was not due to the using up of stored mediators but rather to the release of inhibitory prostaglandins by the first exercise challenge.

Climatic conditions during the challenge

In a number of important studies it has been noted that the severity of EIA or HIA is greatly influenced by the climate of the air breathed (Weinstein *et al.*, 1976; Bar-Or *et al.*, 1977; Chen and Horton, 1977). Breathing warm, humid air virtually abolishes EIA while breathing cold, dry air increases its intensity. Indeed, a study from Sweden (Larsson *et al.*, 1993) found an incidence of asthma with bronchial hyperreactivity of no less than 56% in cross-country skiers. Voluntary hyperventilation or the hyperventilation associated with exercise leads to drying and cooling of the airway mucosa as the water evaporates from the surface and this cooling is accentuated if the dry air is also cold. For a given level of ventilation similar losses of heat and water occur whether the challenge is exercise or isocapnic hyperventilation, provided they are carried out under identical climatic conditions. The cooling was first demonstrated by recording temperature change in the oesophagus (Deal *et al.*, 1979) and later by direct recording within the airways (McFadden *et al.*, 1982, 1985).

Cooling, or more probably drying, of the airways explains the differences in the severity of EIA induced by swimming, in which the patient breathes relatively humid air, and running, in which under normal laboratory conditions the air is relatively dry. Realizing the fundamental importance of this phenomenon in the pathogenesis of EIA, Anderson (1984) and her colleagues began to investigate the possibility that it was the changes in osmolarity of the fluid lining the airways that was the triggering event in EIA. They had previously shown that asthma closely resembling EIA could be provoked by inhaling fogs of hypotonic or hypertonic salt solutions (Schoeffel *et al.*, 1981). Careful inspection of the earlier data relating the severity of induced asthma to the temperature of the air breathed showed that there could be very wide fluctuations of temperature with relatively little difference in the severity of the asthma provided the water loss was similar (Anderson *et al.*, 1989).

Argyros *et al.* (1993) studied the response to isocapnic hyperventilation of air at different temperatures but with identical heat contents that induced different amounts of water loss. They found increasing amount of HIA related to the increasing water loss despite *increasing* inspired air temperatures. There has been some argument as to where the evaporation takes place within the airway and whether or not the volume of fluid available could prevent any significant change in osmolarity (Anderson, 1984; Gilbert *et al.*, 1987; Anderson *et al.*, 1989). However, Anderson and her colleagues (1989) have produced compelling evidence to suggest that drying of the mucosa would take place over the most relevant generations of airways. Animal experiments involving the perfusion and ventilation of isolated lung lobes with gases and blood of different temperatures lend some support to the concept that the climatic effect operates primarily through water exchange (Freed *et al.*, 1987). In these studies, cooling of the lobe by ventilation increased resistance but not cooling by perfusion with cool blood. If both were cooled then resistance did not increase because there was no loss of water from the (cool) blood to the (cool) gas. In this latter situation the lung was, of course, cold and the resistance should have increased had cooling been the important stimulus.

Allergenic environment and air pollution

It has been known for some time that non-specific bronchial reactivity to histamine can be markedly increased for several days or weeks following a specific bronchial provocation challenge with allergen (Cockcroft *et al.*, 1977). Equally, removal of an individual from an environment in which exposure to sensitizing allergens has occurred reduces non-specific reactivity to histamine (Platts-Mills *et al.*, 1982). To see if this also applied to exercise we undertook exercise challenges in asthmatic children on the day before and during the week after a specific allergen bronchial provocation test (Mussaffi *et al.*, 1986). There was a clear-cut increase in the response to the same level of exercise with the fall in FEV$_1$ almost doubling. This was true whether or not there were both early and late reactions to the allergen but, as has been documented before, histamine responsiveness in our study only increased in those children with both early and late reactions. From these observations it is to be expected that the severity of EIA will vary from time to time, even for the same severity of stimulus and climatic conditions, depending upon the recent exposure of the patient to relevant allergens. In a recent study of asthmatic children who had spent a month in the relatively allergen-free alpine town of Davos, Switzerland, Benckhuijsen *et al.* (1996) showed a modest but significant decrease in the severity of EIA using a standard challenge. Air pollution, simulated in the laboratory by adding small amounts of sulphur dioxide to the air, has also been shown to considerably enhance EIA (Roger *et al.*, 1985), further complicating the prediction of the severity of EIA under conditions of natural exposure.

The clinical severity of the asthma

It would be expected that the clinical severity of asthma would influence the severity of EIA or HIA obtained with a standard challenge but hard data to support this idea are difficult to find. In the original studies of EIA in children by Jones (1966) he related response to exercise to severity of asthma. He categorized his patients according to what we would now term bronchial hyperreactivity but this included taking note of both the post-exercise bronchoconstriction and the bronchodilatation after inhaling a bronchodilator. Although this appeared to distinguish between mild and moderate asthmatics his most severe patients were indistinguishable on this basis from the mild and moderate groups. In a new analysis of the severity of EIA in 272 mild, moderate and severe young asthmatics defined according to accepted management guidelines, we found that the mean fall in FEV$_1$ was 15.8%, 22.8% and 21.1% respectively, and the only significant difference was between the mild group and the other asthmatic groups (Godfrey *et al.*, 1999). Sly (1970) studied asthmatic children and found a correlation between the severity of EIA, age and the number of days of wheeze in the previous year but not with the time since the last episode of wheezing. On the other hand, Silverman (1973) found no significant correlations between the severity of EIA and the number of days of illness in the preceding 3 months or 12 months, the symptoms recorded in a diary over the previous day, week or month or the mean of twice-daily PEF recording over the preceding month. More modern data on the relationship between the severity of asthma and EIA are notable by their absence and it seems likely that exercise is a poor tool for distinguishing between asthmatics of different clinical severity. This is hardly surprising, as even if EIA were more severe in patients with more severe asthma they are likely to be receiving treatment which reduces the response.

Medications

It has been known for a long time that the most effective method of preventing or reversing EIA is the simple administration of a selective β_2-agonist. Improvements have also been made in the β_2-agonist drugs over the years and a new generation of long-acting inhaled drugs has been developed which inhibit EIA for substantially longer than the older β_2-agonists (Henriksen et al., 1992; Kemp et al., 1994). This means that if the patient has used a short-acting β_2-agonist within about 4 hours or a long-acting β_2-agonist within about 12 hours of exercise the severity of the resultant EIA is likely to be reduced considerably. Some care is needed because it has also been shown that tolerance may develop to the protective effect of salmeterol against EIA over a period of 1 month (Simons et al., 1997). Other drugs that have been shown to prevent or reduce EIA if given before exercise include the specific anti-histamine drug terfenadine (Wiebicke et al., 1988; Finnerty and Holgate, 1990) and the cromones, sodium cromoglycate and nedocromil sodium (Shaw and Kay, 1985; Henriksen, 1988; de Benedictis et al., 1995). Sodium cromoglycate is not a bronchodilator and its exact mechanism of action is disputed but it is interesting that it only inhibits EIA if given before exercise but not if given at the end of the exercise but before the onset of the EIA (Silverman and Andrea, 1972). Drugs that inhibit the release or binding of potential mediators of EIA have been studied and some have been shown to be effective in preventing EIA. Leukotriene antagonists have been shown to reduce EIA significantly (Makker et al., 1993; Meltzer et al., 1996; Reiss et al., 1997; van Schoor et al., 1997). The inhalation of prostaglandin E_2 is effective in inhibiting EIA and had no effect on methacholine hyperreactivity (Melillo et al., 1994). There are also a number of other agents that inhibit EIA to varying degrees but for which there is no obvious pharmacological explanation of their mode of action. The diuretic frusemide blocks both EIA and OIA when given by inhalation (Bianco et al., 1988; Moscato et al., 1991) but although it is tempting to link this to osmotic changes in the airway lining fluid other similar diuretics do not have this effect. Inhaled heparin which was without any effect on blood coagulation reduced EIA even more than sodium cromoglycate in the study of Ahmed et al. (1993). The mode of action and the significance of the effects of frusemide and heparin remain to be determined.

There has long been an argument as to whether or not corticosteroids affect EIA. For many years it was generally believed that corticosteroids did not affect EIA, which was similar to the lack of effect of corticosteroids in preventing the early response to the inhalation of allergen. From more recent studies it now appears that inhaled corticosteroids can reduce the response to both exercise and pharmacological agents (Henriksen, 1985; Vathenen et al., 1991). It may be that the efficacy of inhaled steroids is drug-specific and depends on both the dose and duration of treatment. A single (1000 µg) dose of budesonide was unable to inhibit EIA in the study of Venge et al. (1990), while 4 weeks of the same daily dose produced a significant reduction. Pedersen and Hansen (1995) carried out a dose–response study of the effect of inhaled budesonide on asthmatic children with moderate and severe asthma, each dose being given for 4 weeks. They found that 100 µg/day was effective in controlling symptoms and no further clinical benefit was seen with higher doses. However, they found a considerable dose–response effect on the inhibition of EIA with 100 µg/day reducing the fall in FEV_1 to 26% compared with 55% before treatment and 400 µg/day reducing the fall in FEV_1 to 10% (Fig. 3.6). There is now little doubt that EIA is likely to be reduced significantly if the patient is taking a moderate or high dose of an inhaled corticosteroid on a regular basis.

PATHOGENESIS OF EIA, HIA AND OIA

The pathophysiological processes underlying exercise, hyperventilation and osmotically-triggered asthma have excited considerable interest and stimulated much controversy over a

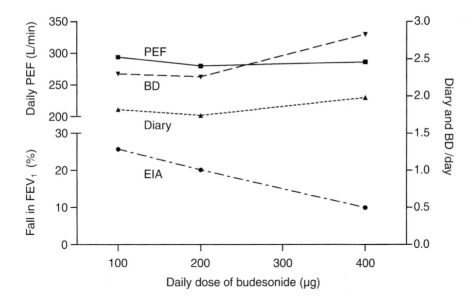

Figure 3.6 *Dose–response curves for diary scores, use of supplementary bronchodilators (BD), mean of twice daily peak expiratory flow (PEF) and exercise-induced asthma (EIA) in 19 asthmatic children treated with inhaled budesonide. Each dose of drug was taken for 4 weeks. There was no dose-related effect on the clinical parameters but the severity of EIA was reduced in a dose–response fashion. (Redrawn from the data of Pedersen and Hansen, 1995.)*

number of years. When trying to decide among the various hypotheses it is worth recalling that Popper (1968) clearly pointed out that in science it is impossible to prove a theory to be correct but if observations are not compatible with the theory then it can be shown to be inadequate. Like any other physiological phenomenon, EIA, HIA and OIA can be considered as events which require a receptor site for the triggering stimulus, an intermediate pathway and an effector mechanism. Although there is much similarity between EIA and HIA the bland assumption that they are identical may lead to erroneous conclusions because haemodynamic changes are present during exercise in addition to the hyperventilation common to both types of challenge.

The trigger mechanism

From what has been described above it is almost certain that a change in the osmolarity of the lining fluid of the larger central airways resulting from the need to warm and humidify inspired air is the major triggering event in EIA and probably in HIA. OIA, which does not occur under natural conditions, is used in the laboratory to attempt to mimic the trigger which is presumed to occur with EIA or HIA. To what extent the nature of the exercise itself or the pattern of breathing independent of the total metabolic or ventilatory changes contribute to the stimulus is as yet uncertain, although such effects are likely to be of minor importance compared with the osmotic stimulus. The role of temperature changes in the airway independent of the water loss and osmotic stimulus is still a subject of controversy and future research may provide further insights into airway receptor physiology. We have no evidence at present about the nature of the presumed osmoreceptor and whether this is neural, chemical or mechanical.

The cooling and drying hypothesis cannot entirely account for the triggering of EIA and HIA. Were they the only factors involved, then neither exercise nor hyperventilation should be able to provoke an attack of asthma under conditions in which cooling and drying of the airway are prevented. Normally when patients breath warm, humid air at body temperature and humidity they develop little if any EIA. However, there is the occasional patient who does develop EIA under these conditions (Ben-Dov *et al.*, 1982). In the study of Anderson and her colleagues (1982) 14 out of 24 patients developed a greater than 10% fall (mean 20%) in FEV_1 after exercising while breathing air conditioned to body temperature and humidity. Continuing this line of thought, if heat and water loss from the airways are held constant, then the severity of EIA should be constant whatever the severity of the exercise. To study this idea we exercised a group of children at two levels of exercise while the amount of heat and water loss from the airways was kept constant by varying the conditions of the inspired air (Noviski *et al.*, 1987). Thus during the lesser work load they breathed cooler, dry air while at the harder work load they breathed warmer, more humid air. There was almost twice as much asthma after the harder exercise challenge as compared with the lighter challenge even though the heat and water losses were virtually identical. This apparent paradox may be explained by the observations that the inhalation of hypotonic solutions also provokes asthma (Schoeffel *et al.*, 1981) and it has been shown that HIA is least when air equilibrated to body conditions is breathed but increases under conditions in which water (and heat) is either removed or added to the airway (Aitken and Marini, 1985). During hyperventilation or exercise under normal climatic conditions some water and heat is lost from the airway and preventing this by breathing warm humid air could result in a hypotonic stimulus in some patients. Keeping the heat and water loss constant but varying the exercise or hyperventilation load could also mean that the drying affected different generations of airway as the flow profiles of ventilation changed. Thus both EIA breathing air equilibrated to body conditions and different quantities of EIA for the same heat and water loss but different exercise levels are still compatible with the trigger being a change in osmolarity in the airways.

The intermediary pathway

Whatever the exact nature of the trigger, the intermediary pathway leading from the receptor site to the airways which narrow could be humoral, neural or a combination of these mechanisms. A direct neural reflex originating in the airway and terminating in the bronchial smooth muscle seems an unlikely mechanism given the relatively slow onset of EIA or HIA and the even slower return to baseline. The possibility that chemical mediators are involved in the intermediary pathway seems more likely, although much of the evidence in favour is highly circumstantial. Thus sodium cromoglycate, which certainly prevents mediator release *in vitro*, prevents EIA if given before exercise but not if given immediately afterwards (Silverman and Andrea, 1972). Neutrophil chemotactic factor, a mast cell-derived mediator, has been found to rise in the blood during EIA (Lee *et al.*, 1982). A potent H_1 histamine antagonist, terfenadine, has been shown to markedly reduce the severity of EIA, HIA and OIA (Wiebecke *et al.*, 1988; Finney *et al.*, 1990). EIA has also been shown to be reduced by treatment with an inhibitor of leukotriene D_4 (Manning *et al.*, 1990; Finnerty *et al.*, 1992; Makker *et al.*, 1993; Reiss *et al.*, 1997) and HIA by an inhibitor of 5-lipoxygenase (Israel *et al.*, 1990). In animals, HIA is reduced by pretreatment with capsaicin which reduces the availability of ecosinoids (Ray *et al.*, 1989). The fact that Broide *et al.* (1990) failed to detect significant elevations of mast cell-derived histamine or tryptase in bronchoalveolar lavages from subjects with EIA could easily be explained by the increased pulmonary blood flow during exercise simply washing the mediators out of the lungs.

As already noted, one of the characteristic features of EIA is that the subject becomes relatively refractory to a subsequent challenge for some time after the initial attack. Originally, this refractoriness which was seen after EIA and sometimes after HIA and OIA was thought to be due to the depletion of the presumed stores of mediators that were liberated by the trigger and caused bronchospasm. It was assumed that time was required to resynthesize these stores and the observed half-life of the recovery of responsiveness to EIA of about 45 minutes (Edmunds et al., 1978) would fit well with a metabolic function. Refractoriness does not seem to reside in end-organ hyporesponsiveness because subjects remain responsive to histamine after developing EIA (Hamielic et al., 1988; Zawadski et al., 1988). However, bronchial reactivity is not entirely without influence on refractoriness, because O'Hickey et al. (1989) showed that the more reactive the patient to methacholine the less was the refractoriness to hypertonic saline. The fact that there is also some degree of cross-refractoriness between EIA and HIA (Bar-Yishay et al., 1983b) and between EIA and OIA (Belcher et al., 1987) supports the concept that similar mediator mechanisms are involved in all three types of asthma.

The appearance of refractoriness does not require that the initial exercise challenge provoke an attack of asthma although his phenomenon of refractoriness without preceding asthma could not be demonstrated with hyperventilation (Bar-Yishay et al., 1983a) which suggests that EIA and HIA are not completely identical. The mystery surrounding refractoriness was considerably clarified by a series of studies which showed that the prostaglandin inhibitor, indomethacin, could prevent the appearance of refractoriness to EIA and OIA but not to HIA (O'Byrne and Jones, 1986; Mattoli et al., 1987; Margolski et al., 1988). This suggested that refractoriness, at least to exercise and hyperosmolar challenges, was due to the release of an inhibitory prostaglandin whose effect persisted for 30 to 60 minutes or so after the initial challenge and whose release did not require that the initial challenge cause an attack of asthma. A direct approach was used by Melillo et al. (1994) who showed that inhaled prostaglandin E$_2$ (PGE$_2$) caused substantial protection from EIA when the exercise was performed 30 minutes after the inhalation. As PGE$_2$ had no effect on bronchial reactivity to methacholine, they reasoned that the effect of PGE$_2$ in EIA was not a direct effect on the bronchial smooth muscle. Cross-refractoriness between asthma induced by exercise and the leukotriene (LTD$_4$) has been investigated by Manning et al. (1993) with or without the blocking of prostaglandin synthetase by flurbiprofen. The inhibition of prostaglandin synthetase had no effect on the initial challenges by either exercise or LTD$_4$ but substantially reduced the refractoriness that was seen in control studies with the repetition of either type of challenge. Of particular interest in this study was that cross-refractoriness was seen with exercise rendering the patients less responsive to LTD$_4$ and vice versa. In this situation prostaglandin synthetase inhibition also reduced the cross-refractoriness so that the authors concluded that EIA was at least in part due to the release of LTD$_4$ and that this in turn released inhibitory prostaglandins which rendered the individual refractory to a subsequent exercise challenge.

On balance, it now seems almost certain that all forms of challenge that cause changes in the osmolarity of the fluid lining the airways result in the release of mediators in the lungs. Moreover, it seems that the intermediary pathway involves the release of rapidly acting bronchoconstricting mediators amongst which are LTD$_4$ and slowly reacting, bronchodilating prostaglandins.

The effector mechanism

The most straightforward concept of the effector mechanism of EIA, HIA or OIA is that the airways obstruction is simply due to bronchospasm because it is rapid in onset and recovery, and is prevented or rapidly reversed by the inhalation of a β_2-agonist. An alternative hypothesis for the mechanism of the airways obstruction of EIA and HIA has been proposed by McFadden and his colleagues (1986) which attributes the obstruction to reactive hyperaemia of the bronchial epithelium. They suggested that the airways cool during exercise or hyperventilation and rewarm once the exercise or hyperventilation stops. The rewarming of these cooled airways caused reactive hyperaemia and obstructed the airflow. In support of their hypothesis they reported greater airways obstruction when the rewarming was increased by breathing warm, humid air at the end of the challenge. It must be pointed out that other investigators have not confirmed that the rate of rewarming affects the degree of obstruction (Smith *et al.*, 1989; Smith and Anderson, 1990). If cooling and subsequent vasodilatation on rewarming are the effector mechanisms of EIA and HIA it is difficult to understand why the severity of post-exertional asthma should be directly related to the duration of exercise for durations at least up to 6–8 minutes (Eggleston and Guerrant, 1976) since airway cooling reaches a low plateau level after about 2–3 minutes of exercise (Gilbert *et al.*, 1987, 1991). In any case, this hypothesis seems unlikely because many asthmatics develop moderate or even marked airways obstruction towards the end of the exercise period while their airways are still cold. Anderson and Daviskas (1992) have reviewed the possible role of the airway microvasculature in EIA and conclude that reactive hyperaemia is most unlikely to be the mechanism whereby the airways are narrowed and if anything the evidence suggests an increase in airway blood flow during cooling. However, a recent study by Ichinose *et al.* (1996) could suggest an interesting 'compromise' for these alternative effector hypotheses. They found that a specific antagonist of the neurokinin-1 receptor shortens the duration but not the severity of EIA and as this agent may well act by reducing vascular engorgement and permeability they consider that the initial fall in lung function in EIA is due to bronchospasm while the speed of recovery depends upon vascular events.

A model of the pathophysiology of EIA

On the basis of the established facts a possible model of the pathophysiology of EIA has been developed as illustrated in Fig. 3.7. Physical exercise is seen as having four major effects on the asthmatic person:

- it causes hyperventilation with consequent cooling and drying of the bronchial mucosa and in turn liberates bronchoconstricting mediators such as LTD_4
- it may have a direct (intrinsic) trigger effect – which would explain residual differences between different types of exercise or different exercise protocols
- it increases sympathetic drive or reduces bronchial tone which generally prevents much change in lung function during the exercise
- it releases an inhibitory prostaglandin possibly via LTD_4 which results in refractoriness to a subsequent exercise challenge.

The cooling and drying of the airways is dependent upon the climatic conditions of the inspired air. During exercise the patient is relatively (though not always completely) protected either by an increased sympathetic drive or alternatively by a reduction in bronchial tone which has also been found with isocapnic hyperventilation. This short-term protection stops as soon as the exercise ends allowing the bronchospasm to become manifest. Another type of protection is built up more slowly by the release of an inhibitory prostaglandin and which probably accounts for the refractory period after EIA and possibly for that following HIA. The effect of the released mediator on the airways also depends upon the basic level of bronchial reactivity which, in turn, depends upon such factors as the level of allergenic stimulation,

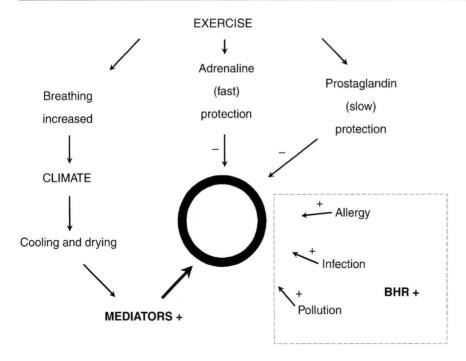

Figure 3.7 *Model of pathways involved in EIA. Exercise is believed to trigger EIA by increasing ventilation which, influenced by climatic conditions, produces cooling and drying of the airways. The type of exercise may have some independent influence on the severity of the EIA. As a result of the stimulus, mediators are liberated from storage in mast cells and possibly other cells which act on the airway causing bronchospasm. The response of the airway depends on its reactivity which is influenced by environmental factors including the level of allergic stimulation, recent viral infection and pollution. During exercise this effect is opposed by increased sympathomimetic drive (short protection) so that in most subjects (but not all) lung function changes little until exercise ceases and the sympathomimetic drive is turned off. In addition, exercise releases protective mediators such as prostaglandins which cause refractoriness to subsequent exercise (slow protection).*

recent viral infections and air pollution. This model emphasizes the following points about EIA:

- EIA and HIA are inherently variable because of the many factors which interact to produce the bronchoconstriction.
- The severity of the response on any one occasion is largely unpredictable as not all the variables can be quantified.
- When using exercise or hyperventilation as a challenge in the same person on different occasions or in different persons, it is vital to standardize the stimulus, environmental and allergenic factors as far as possible.

EIA, HIA AND BRONCHIAL HYPERREACTIVITY

While bronchial hyperreactivity (BHR) is thought to be the fundamental physiological manifestation of the airway inflammation that characterizes asthma, it has also been known for some time that bronchial hyperreactivity occurs in other diseases. In an earlier review

(Anderson *et al.*, 1975) it was noted that increased fluctuations in lung function in response to exercise could be found in persons other than those with active asthma, for example in close relatives of asthmatic children, formerly wheezy infants and their close relatives, and in children with cystic fibrosis. However, it was only patients with active asthma who developed the post-exercise fall in lung function characteristic of EIA, and in others with bronchial reactivity the main change was bronchodilatation during the exercise. More recently, Phillips *et al.* (1998) showed that children with obstructive lung disease due to primary ciliary dyskinesia usually developed bronchodilatation after exercise and bronchoconstriction occurred in only 3 out of the 12 studied. These observations suggested that there might be important differences in the pathophysiology of bronchial hyperreactivity in the individual with active asthma as compared to those with other pulmonary diseases.

We have recently compared the non-specific bronchial reactivity to exercise, the inhalation of methacholine and the inhalation of adenosine 5′-monophosphate (AMP) in children with asthma and other paediatric chronic obstructive lung diseases (Avital *et al.*, 1995). As shown in Fig. 3.8 the asthmatic children were responsive to all three challenges but the children with other lung diseases were only responsive to methacholine. There was close agreement between the responsiveness to exercise and AMP in the asthmatics. Since AMP is a potent liberator of mediators from mast cells (Cushley and Holgate, 1985; Driver *et al.*, 1991; Polosa and Holgate, 1997) this supports the concept that bronchial reactivity in asthma involves a chemical intermediary pathway which is a feature of the disease and not found in other types of chronic lung diseases with end-organ hyperresponsiveness. A very similar result was obtained by Carlsen *et al.* (1998) who compared responsiveness to exercise and methacholine in children with asthma and children with other types of paediatric chronic obstructive lung diseases. They found no difference in responsiveness to methacholine but the EIA was three times as severe in the asthmatic children compared with those having other diseases. Studies in adults comparing responsiveness to hyperventilation, methacholine or AMP in patients with asthma or chronic obstructive pulmonary disease (COPD) have yielded similar results. Thus Ramsdale *et al.* (1984, 1985) found that 19 out of 27 COPD patients responded abnormally to a methacholine challenge but only 3 responded to hyperventilation with cold air while 26 out

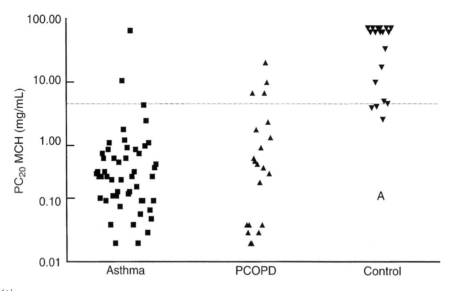

(A)

Figure 3.8

of 27 asthmatics responded to cold air hyperventilation as well as to methacholine. Oosterhoff *et al.* (1993) showed that both asthmatic and COPD patients were responsive to methacholine when compared with controls but the former were also far more responsive to AMP, especially when compared with non-smoking COPD patients.

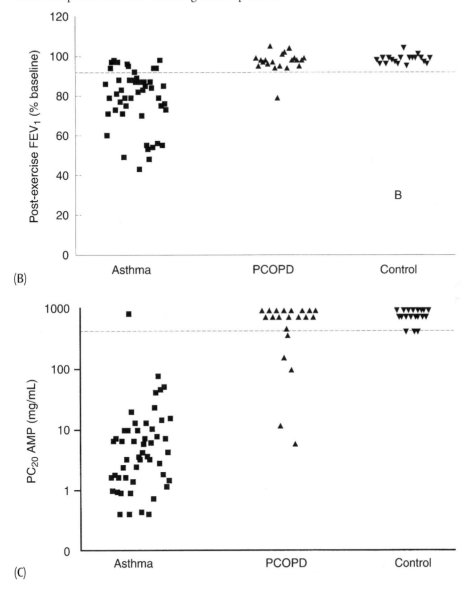

(B)

(C)

Figure 3.8 cont.   *Response of children with asthma, other chronic lung diseases (PCOPD) and children without organic lung disease (Control) to bronchial provocation by (A) methacholine (MCH) inhalation, (B) exercise and (C) adenosine (AMP) inhalation. The results are expressed in terms of the concentration of methacholine or adenosine causing a 20% fall in FEV_1 (PC_{20}) and the post-exercise fall in FEV_1. The horizontal dashed line represents the lower limit of normal as determined by 2 SD below the log mean PC_{20} of the normal group for the inhalation challenges and 2 SD below the mean exercise-induced fall in FEV_1 for the exercise challenge. Most patients with asthma and/or PCOPD responded abnormally to methacholine. While most asthmatics also responded abnormally to both exercise and AMP, very few of the PCOPD patients responded to these two challenges. (Redrawn from the data of Avital et al., 1995.)*

It is also apparent from some studies that the pattern of reactivity in asthmatics may change as their disease changes. Thus we found (Balfour-Lyn *et al.*, 1980) that while EIA persisted in asthmatic children, even while their clinical condition showed signs of improving, once they had become totally free of symptoms for at least 6 months their exercise-induced bronchial reactivity returned to normal. Martin *et al.* (1980) showed a dissociation between reactivity to exercise and to non-specific pharmacological agents in children who grew out of their asthma. In their study the children who were in complete remission often retained their responsiveness to histamine but no longer reacted to exercise. This may mean that pharmacological agents merely demonstrate end-organ responsiveness while exercise invokes a whole physiological pathway that is only found in patients with active asthma.

EPIDEMIOLOGY OF EIA AND HIA

Exercise, hyperventilation and to some extent non-isotonic fogs have been used in attempts to define asthma epidemiologically by studying the responses of populations of normal and asthmatic people. An exercise challenge is one method of demonstrating bronchial reactivity and could theoretically be used as an aid to the diagnosis of asthma provided the limits of the response of the normal population are established. In many studies purely arbitrary levels of response such as a fall in FEV_1 of 10 or 15% have been accepted as the upper limit of normal with no statistical justification. Owing to the different methods used to induce asthma by hyperventilation and non-isotonic fogs there is relatively little useful epidemiological information to date using these techniques and most of the literature relates to asthma induced by exercise.

Response of normal subjects to exercise

There have been a number of studies of exercise-induced bronchial hyperreactivity in populations of totally healthy people who have never had asthma and in some cases they were also unrelated to asthmatics. The upper limit of the fall in lung function in normal people undertaking an exercise challenge in earlier studies (Burr *et al.*, 1974; Anderson *et al.*, 1975) was found to be about 9–10%, this being the mean plus 2 SD of the fall in peak expiratory flow (PEF). At that time there were no good data using other indices of lung function nor studies which took account of the influence of climate and other factors discussed above on the severity of EIA. More recently there have been studies using standardized exercise challenges which examined large randomly selected populations of children and adolescents who had never had any symptoms of lung disease (Backer *et al.*, 1991; Riedler *et al.*, 1994; Haby *et al.*, 1995). From the combined results of these studies we calculated that the mean fall in FEV_1 after 6 minutes of hard running in a moderate climate was 5.3% with a weighted standard deviation of 5.6% (Godfrey *et al.*, 1999) giving a mean plus 2 SD of 16.4%. There is a particular problem with surveys of bronchial reactivity to exercise which have attempted to examine total populations in that they inevitably include asthmatics who, in our experience comprise some 10% of the male population up to age 17 years (Auerbach *et al.*, 1993) and in other studies even twice or more this incidence (Ninan and Russell, 1992; Peat *et al.*, 1994). These asthmatics would increase the overall range of response to exercise and probably account for the variation in the reported upper limit of 'normal' fall in FEV_1. The situation with hyperventilation is not so well studied but it has been suggested that a fall in FEV_1 greater than 9% strongly suggests the diagnosis of asthma using a steady-state type of hyperventilation challenge when the individual exceeds a ventilation of about 25 times baseline FEV_1 breathing cold, dry air (Weiss *et al.*, 1984).

Incidence of EIA in asthmatics

As far as the incidence of EIA in asthmatics is concerned, it is clear that this is influenced by the adequacy of the exercise challenge, by the severity of the asthma in the population being studied and by the factors discussed above which influence the response of the asthmatic to exercise. In our recent analysis (Godfrey *et al.*, 1999) of 232 children and young adults with asthma of varying degrees of severity the mean fall in FEV_1 was 18.8% with a wide SD of 14.8%. Because of this variability in response as well as the variability in the normal population the proportion of asthmatics attending a specialized clinic with an abnormal exercise challenge would be expected to be relatively low and the predictive value of the test relatively poor (see below). Random testing of asthmatics in the community might be expected to yield even fewer positive results because there will be many more very mild asthmatics amongst them although in our study the differences between the mild, moderate and severe groups of asthmatics were very small.

Sensitivity and specificity of exercise tests for asthma

The sensitivity and specificity of exercise testing in asthma has been addressed in a number of studies but it must be pointed out that the results are influenced by the choice of the population and the choice of the cut-off point for accepting the test as positive. When attempting to answer the question as to the value of exercise testing for diagnosing asthma in epidemiological studies, it is essential to study a randomly selected population and to use a meaningful cut-off based on a statistical analysis of the responses of normal and asthmatic populations. We undertook such an analysis of the response to exercise and inhalation challenges for children and young adults (Godfrey *et al.*, 1999) using data on normals collected from the literature (Backer *et al.*, 1991; Riedler *et al.*, 1994; Haby *et al.*, 1995). From the three studies of exercise in normal children there were a total of 978 results to compare with our own studies of 232 asthmatics. Using a graphical computer program normal distribution curves for the normal and asthmatic children were produced (Fig. 3.9) assuming that the total number of asthmatics (the area under the curve for asthmatics) was 10% of the total population. The result shows the range of responses of asthmatics to be wide (as indicated by the relatively large SD) but nevertheless there was a good separation between the asthmatic and the normal children at approximately a 10% fall in FEV_1 with most of the normal children having less than a 10% fall in FEV_1 and most of the asthmatic children having a greater than 10% fall.

For any given value of a fall in FEV_1 it is possibly to calculate the proportion of asthmatic children with a positive response (i.e. sensitivity) and the proportion of normal children with a negative response (i.e. specificity) using a table of the area of the tail in the normal distribution for a given SD ('Z-score' table). The optimal balanced value where sensitivity and specificity of a fall in FEV_1 for separating asthmatic from normal children are equal can be calculated or read from the graph. For our study (Godfrey *et al.*, 1999) the optimal balanced value of a fall in FEV_1 was 8.95% with a sensitivity and specificity of 74.7%. Choosing a higher cut-off point for a fall in FEV_1 of say 15% would yield a specificity of 96% but a sensitivity of only 60%. On the other hand choosing a lower cut-off point for a fall in

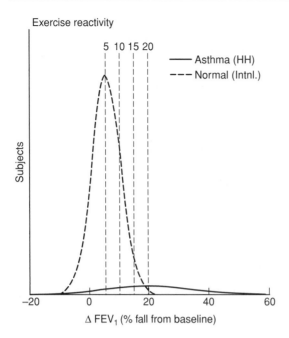

Figure 3.9 *Theoretical population distribution of bronchial reactivity to exercise expressed as the fall in FEV$_1$ (DFEV$_1$) based on data for normal children from studies in the literature (Intnl) and in asthmatics from studies at Hadassah University Hospital (HH). The area under the curve represents the total size of the population and this has been drawn as 90% of the total for the normal children and 10% for the asthmatics. The vertical dotted lines indicate cut-off points at various values of ΔFEV$_1$. (From Godfrey et al., 1998.)*

FEV$_1$ of say 5% would yield a sensitivity of 82.5% but a specificity of only 48.0%. For comparison the optimal balanced value of the cut-off cumulative dose of methacholine or histamine causing a 20% fall in FEV$_1$ in an inhalation challenge was 5.5 μmol with a sensitivity and specificity of 90.7%. However, the balanced optimal cut-off is only the best estimate when the variability of the data in the two populations is similar as was the case with inhalation challenges. For exercise a better estimate is obtained when the sum of sensitivity and specificity is greatest and in our study (Godfrey *et al.*, 1999) this occurred at a fall in FEV$_1$ of 13% with a sensitivity of 62.8% and a specificity of 94.2%. Thus a fall in FEV$_1$ of 13% or more is very specific for diagnosing asthma but the test has a relatively low sensitivity.

Although a bronchial challenge by the inhalation of methacholine or histamine is more sensitive than an exercise challenge, and quite specific when comparing known asthmatics with known normal people, bronchial hyperreactivity to methacholine or histamine is commonly found in other types of chronic obstructive lung disease in adults and children. Such non-asthmatic patients rarely, if ever, respond abnormally to exercise, hyperventilation or the inhalation of adenosine 5'-monophosphate (AMP). In a comparison of these challenges for distinguishing asthma from COPD we found that sensitivity and specificity of a methacholine challenge was only 50% compared with 85% for exercise and 90% AMP (Avital *et al.*, 1995). Interestingly, Carlsen *et al.* (1998) found a very similar result for sensitivity and specificity of exercise compared with methacholine (72%) for distinguishing asthma from COPD in children.

Reproducibility of EIA

From what has been discussed above it is clear that the severity of EIA in any one person depends on a number of variables, some of which are difficult to control, so that the reproducibility of the challenge is likely to be low. In their original study of free-range running in asthmatic children followed over a year, Silverman and Anderson (1972) found an individual coefficient of variation of the fall in PEF of 21% for challenges repeated at weekly intervals compared with 53% for those repeated at monthly intervals. Similar results for the coefficient of variation using FEV_1 as the test of lung function were found by Eggleston and Guerrant (1976). More recently Haby et al. (1995) measured repeatability (95% CI within which difference between result and 'true' value should lie) to two exercise challenges within 3 days in a total population study of 8–11-year-old children and found this range to be + 12% for this shorter interval. Using a rather different approach in which they determined the proportion of a total population of children who had a positive exercise test at monthly intervals over a year, Powell et al. (1996) obtained a coefficient of variation of 24.6% for patients with a 15% fall in FEV_1.

LIVING WITH EIA

Apart from the hyperventilation associated with laughing or crying in some young children, hyperventilation or osmotic challenges are unlikely to occur in normal everyday life. On the other hand, exercise commonly causes trouble in the everyday life of asthmatics. The typical sufferer from EIA is the adolescent or young adult who actively engages in competitive sports, especially medium distance track running, although even gymnastics or dancing can be very troublesome if the exercise is fairly continuous. Younger children may be troubled by EIA when they run about and get very excited during play and older people when they have to climb several flights of stairs. The only physical activity unlikely to cause EIA is swimming. In warm humid climates EIA is less likely to cause problems for the asthmatic person while in temperate or cold climates most continuous strenuous exercise other than swimming is likely to cause some problems unless the patient is receiving appropriate medication. In the past it was common for doctors to advise parents against allowing their children to partake in sports which provoked EIA and even when not so advised the children were often kept out of sports either because they became ill or because the teacher would not allow them to take part. Because of the commonly held belief that asthma was 'all in the mind', children who missed games because of EIA were often considered to be malingerers of varying degrees.

A number of studies of physical fitness have been undertaken in children with asthma and these have generally shown that asthmatic children have a modest reduction in cardiopulmonary performance compared with control children (Clark and Cochrane, 1988; Fink et al., 1993). Of particular interest was the study of Fink et al. (1993) who measured physical performance in 11–12-year-old asthmatic and non-asthmatic children who were physically active in comparison with those who were not. Their young asthmatic children were either sedentary, inactive (no participation in sports) or active (participation in sports) and their control groups of non-asthmatics were either inactive or active to a similar degree. They found no significant differences between the asthmatics and controls as far as the groups who were inactive and active were concerned but the performance of the sedentary asthmatics was significantly reduced for all parameters compared with the other asthmatic groups and the controls. The tests were performed after the inhalation of salbutamol and the resting FEV_1 was above 95% of predicted in all the asthmatic groups so that the poor performance of the habitually sedentary asthmatics was not due to bronchospasm. In a study of children in South Africa, Terblanche and Stewart (1990) found that all but the most severely asthmatic participated in sports as much as their healthy peers. The implications of these studies are that asthmatic children who are allowed to be physically active perform similarly to non-asthmatics but if the child is forced to be sedentary for whatever reason then physical fitness is likely to be reduced.

There are many examples of asthmatics who compete successfully in sports and may reach world class champion status. In the 1988 Olympic Games there were 67 members of the 597-strong USA team who had EIA and these asthmatics won between them no less than 41 medals, including 15 gold and 21 silver in a variety of sports including endurance running events (Pierson and Voy, 1988). This could only have been possible through the use of appropriate and approved medication for sportsmen and women, including short-acting β_2-agonists, ipratropium bromide, sodium cromoglycate and inhaled corticosteroids (Harries, 1994). On a more modest level Silvers *et al.* (1994) found no problems with asthmatic children who participated in cross-country skiing provided they took appropriate medication. Surveys of teachers in both the UK and France showed that the large majority were aware that exercise could be problematic for the asthmatic child but the teachers had little if any knowledge about how to enable the child to take part in games or what to do if the child became sick (Menardo-Mazeran *et al.*, 1990; Brookes and Jones, 1992). Even some asthmatics are unaware either that they have asthma or that exercise can cause them problems. Rupp *et al.* (1992) conducted a survey of 1241 middle and high school athletes and after excluding the known asthmatics and those without any relevant symptoms they found that an exercise test provoked EIA in no less than 29% of those not previously diagnosed as asthmatics who either had suspicious symptoms or abnormal resting lung function.

MANAGEMENT OF EIA

From what has already been discussed, asthma as provoked by exercise depends on many factors including the type of exercise, the pattern of exercise, the climate and any medications being used. The conditions most likely to be associated with EIA are summarized in Table 3.1.

Many of these considerations also apply to HIA and OIA. If it is practical (and desirable) for the asthmatic person to adopt a pattern of exercise unlikely to be associated with EIA then the problem may be avoided but this should not be at the cost of preventing the patient from participating in activities which he or she considers to be normal.

Table 3.1 *Conditions most likely and least likely to facilitate EIA.*

Most likely to facilitate EIA	Least likely to facilitate EIA
Continuous exercise: about 6–8 min	Intermittent exercise / team games
Hard exercise: heart rate > 160 (children)	Light exercise: heart rate < 140 (children)
Running	Swimming
Dry or cold climate	Humid climate
In allergy season (if atopic)	Out of allergy season (if atopic)
Air pollution – especially SO_2	Clean air
No medication	Correct medication – mainly β_2-agonists
	High dose inhaled corticosteroids

Medications

If it is impractical to avoid precipitating EIA then it can be treated by the use of appropriate medications. Without doubt the inhaled β_2-agonists are the most effective agents at preventing EIA or reversing it if lung function has already fallen. Two puffs of a short-acting β_2-agonist taken correctly a few minutes before starting to exercise will almost completely prevent the appearance of EIA in most asthmatics and the effect will persist for 2–3 hours. The newer long-acting β_2-agonists have a similar protective effect which may last for up to 12 hours. For the asthmatic who expects to be undertaking physical activity which he or she knows from experience is likely to provoke EIA and which is likely to continue over several hours, a long-acting β_2-agonist would probably be more appropriate than a short-acting agent.

Good control of asthma is also likely to reduce but not totally prevent the appearance of EIA and for patients with frequent or perennial symptoms appropriate corticosteroid prophylaxis is indicated although this is rarely likely to be justified if the patient only suffers from asthma related to exercise. As discussed earlier, other agents including cromones, leukotriene antagonists, methyl xanthines, and some antihistamines can also reduce EIA but they are generally less effective than the β_2-agonists and are not recommended solely for the management of EIA.

Physical training

Because sedentary asthmatics are generally unfit and because of the adverse psychological effects of being excluded from games as well as the inherent belief that physical exercise can somehow 'develop the lungs' a number of investigators have explored the use of physical training for asthmatics. Properly controlled studies have demonstrated that asthmatics who undergo physical training can improve their fitness, as measured by maximum oxygen uptake, to a similar degree as non-asthmatics who undergo similar training (Bundgaard, 1982; Cochrane and Clark, 1990). Whether this improved fitness can reduce the likelihood of developing EIA is not a simple issue because improved physical fitness results in decreased minute ventilation for a given level of oxygen consumption, and as the trigger for EIA is probably related to the level of ventilation, one might expect less EIA after training for a similar exercise stress. A small reduction in EIA of this type at a given level of exercise has been obtained by training in some studies (Svenonius et al., 1983; Haas et al., 1987). Others have found improvements in lung function and asthma control after general fitness training but it is difficult to ensure adequate controls in such studies and to separate the effects, if any, of training from those of better supervision of the asthma. Several investigators have failed to find any change in bronchial reactivity after physical training (Cochrane and Clark, 1990; Robinson et al., 1992) which casts some doubt on the ability of general exercise training to improve the asthma. However, Weiner et al. (1992) using inspiratory muscle training or sham training in a control group did show an improvement in muscle strength, asthma symptoms and lower drug consumption in the treated group. Physical training can restore normal levels of physical fitness to the asthmatic although it is uncertain whether it makes a significant reduction in the severity of the bronchial hyperreactivity which is the basis of the disease. Training undoubtedly improves the sense of well-being of the patient and provides important psychological support.

Alternative medicine

Some patients or parents of asthmatic children believe or are led to believe that various types of alternative or complementary medicine are useful in the treatment of asthma, usually when they have been inadequately managed by conventional means. Few controlled studies of these treatments have been undertaken with respect to EIA but a small reduction has been obtained with hypnosis (Ben Zvi *et al.*, 1982). Controlled studies with acupuncture in EIA have yielded conflicting results (Fung *et al.*, 1986; Morton *et al.*, 1993) and there appear to be no controlled studies of homeopathy or other forms of alternative medicine. In short, these treatments are of dubious value and incomparably inferior to an inhaled β_2-agonist in managing EIA.

CONCLUSION

Exercise-induced asthma (EIA) is a common problem in most young asthmatics who partake in sports and in many other asthmatics even with everyday exertion. The trigger for EIA and for hyperventilation-induced asthma (HIA) or osmotically-induced asthma (OIA) which mimic it, appears to be the drying of the respiratory mucosa. Hence exercise performed breathing warm, humid air is less likely to trigger an attack than exercising while breathing cold, dry air. The intermediary pathway almost certainly involves chemical mediators which result in bronchospasm but also involves the release of inhibitory prostaglandins which render the asthmatic refractory to a subsequent attack of EIA. The severity of EIA also depends on the overall level of bronchial hyperreactivity and therefore varies in relation to other factors, such as allergic stimulation, which alter bronchial reactivity. EIA and HIA can be prevented or reversed by bronchodilator medications, especially β_2-agonists, but can also be partly prevented by sodium cromoglycate and by antagonists of the mediators involved in the intermediary pathway. Corticosteroids by inhalation also reduce the severity of EIA but relatively large doses are required. Asthmatics who habitually refrain from normal physical activity lack the normal cardiorespiratory fitness of physically active asthmatics and normal people but physical training can restore normal levels of fitness. It is uncertain whether physical training actually improves asthma control or reduces the severity of EIA.

REFERENCES

Ahmed T, Garrigo J, Danta I. (1993) Preventing bronchoconstriction in exercise-induced asthma with inhaled heparin. *N Engl J Med*, **329**, 90–5.

Aitken ML, Marini JJ. (1985) Effect of heat delivery and extraction on airway conductance in normal and in asthmatic subjects. *Am Rev Respir Dis*, **13**, 357–61.

Anderson SD. (1984) Is there a unifying hypothesis for exercise induced asthma. *J Allergy Clin Immunol*, **73**, 660–5.

Anderson SD, Daviskas E, Smith CM. (1989) Exercise-induced asthma: a difference in opinion regarding the stimulus. *Allergy Proc*, **10**, 215–26.

Anderson SD, Daviskas E. (1992) The airway microvasculature and exercise induced asthma. *Thorax*, **47**, 748–52.

Anderson SD, Schoeffel RE, Follet R, Perry CP, Daviskas E, Kendall M. (1982) Sensitivity to heat and water loss at rest and during exercise in asthmatic patients. *Eur J Respir Dis*, **63**, 459–571.

Anderson SD, Silverman M, Konig P, Godfrey S. (1975) Exercise-induced asthma. *Br J Dis Chest*, **69**, 1–39.

Argyros GJ, Phillips YY, Rayburn DB, Rosenthal RR, Jaeger JJ. (1993) Water loss without heat flux in exercise-induced bronchospasm. *Am Rev Respir Dis*, **147**, 1419–24.

Auerbach I, Springer C, Godfrey S. (1993) Total population survey of the frequency and severity of asthma in 17 year old boys in an urban area in Israel. *Thorax*, **48**, 139–41.

Avital A, Springer C, Bar-Yishay E, Godfrey S. (1995) Adenosine, methacholine and exercise challenges in children with asthma or paediatric COPD. *Thorax*, **50**, 511–16.

Backer V, Dirksen A, Bach-Mortensen N, Hansen KK, Laursen EM, Wendelboe D. (1991) The distribution of bronchial responsiveness to histamine and exercise in 527 children and adolescents. *J Allergy Clin Immunol*, **88**, 68–76.

Balfour-Lynn L, Tooley M, Godfrey S. (1980) A study comparing the relationship of exercise induced asthma to clinical asthma in childhood. *Arch Dis Child*, **56**, 450–4.

Bar-Or O, Neuman I, Dotan R. (1977) Effects of dry and humid climates on exercise-induced asthma in children and adolescents. *J Allergy Clin Immunol*, **60**, 163–8.

Bar-Yishay E, Gur I, Inbar O, Neuman I, Dlin RA, Godfrey S. (1982) Differences between running and swimming as stimuli for exercise induced asthma. *Eur J Applied Physiol*, **48**, 387–97.

Bar-Yishay E, Ben-Dov I, Godfrey S. (1983a) Refractory period following hyperventilation-induced asthma. *Am Rev Respir Dis*, **127**, 572–4.

Bar-Yishay E, Gur I, Ben-Dov I and Godfrey S. (1983b) Refractory period following induced asthma: contributions of exercise and isocapnic hyperventilation. *Thorax*, **38**, 849–53.

Belcher NG, Murdoch RD, Dalton N, *et al.* (1988) A comparison of mediator and catecholamine release between exercise- and hypertonic saline-induced asthma. *Am Rev Respir Dis*, **137**, 1026–32

Belcher NG, Rees PJ, Clark TJH, Lee TH. (1987) A comparison of the refractory periods induced by hypertonic airway challenge and exercise in bronchial asthma. *Am Rev Respir Dis*, **135**, 822–5.

Ben-Dov I, Bar-Yishay E, Godfrey S. (1982a) Refractory period following exercise induced asthma unexplained by respiratory heat loss. *Am Rev Respir Dis*, **125**, 530–4.

Ben-Dov I, Bar-Yishay E, Godfrey S. (1982b) Exercise induced asthma without respiratory heat loss. *Thorax*, **37**, 630–1.

Ben Zvi Z, Spohn WA, Young SH, Kattan M. (1982) Hypnosis for exercise-induced asthma. *Am Rev Respir Dis*, **125**, 392–5.

Benckhuijsen J, van den Bos J-W, van Velzen E, de Bruin R, Aalbers R. (1996) Differences in the effect of allergen avoidance on bronchial hyperresponsiveness as measured by methacholine, adenosine 5′-monophosphate, and exercise in asthmatic children. *Pediatr Pulmonol*, **22**, 147–53.

Bianco S, Vaghi A, Robuschi M, Pasargiklian M. (1988) Prevention of exercise-induced bronchoconstriction by inhaled furosemide. *Lancet*, **2**, 252–5.

Boulet L-P, Legris C, Turcotte H, Hebert J. (1987) Prevalence and characteristics of late asthmatic responses to exercise. *J Allergy Clin Immunol*, **80**, 655–62.

Broide DH, Eisman S, Ramsdell JW, Ferguson P, Schwartz LB, Wasserman SI. (1990) Airway levels of mast cell-derived mediators in exercise-induced asthma. *Am Rev Respir Dis*, **141**, 563–8.

Brookes J, Jones K. (1992) Schoolteachers' perceptions and knowledge of asthma in primary schoolchildren. *Br J Gen Pract*, **42**, 504–7.

Bundgaard A. (1982) Effect of physical training on peak oxygen consumption rate and exercise-induced asthma in adult asthmatics. *Scand J Clin Lab Invest*, **42**, 9–13.

Burr ML, Eldridge BA, Borysiewicz LK. (1974) Peak expiratory flow rates before and after exercise in school children. *Arch Dis Child*, **49**, 923–6.

Carlsen K-H, Engh G, Mork M, Schroder E. (1998) Cold air inhalation and exercise-induced bronchoconstriction in relationship to methacholine bronchial responsiveness: different patterns in asthmatic children and children with other chronic lung diseases. *Respir Med*, **92**, 308–15.

Chen WY, Horton DJ. (1977) Heat and water loss from the airways and exercise induced asthma. *Respiration*, **34**, 305–13.

Clark CJ, Cochrane LM. (1988) Assessment of work performance in asthma for determination of cardiorespiratory fitness and training capacity. *Thorax*, **43**, 745–9.

Cochrane LM, Clark CJ. (1990) Benefits and problems of a physical training programme for asthmatic patients. *Thorax*, **45**, 345–51.

Cockcroft DW, Ruffin RE, Dolovich J, Hargreave FE. (1977) Allergen induced increase in non-allergic bronchial reactivity. *Clin Allergy*, **7**, 503–13.

Crimi E, Balbo A, Milanese M, Miadonna A, Rossi GA, Brusasco V. (1992) Airway inflammation and occurrence of delayed bronchoconstriction in exercise-induced asthma. *Am Rev Respir Dis*, **146**, 507–12.

Cushley MJ, Holgate ST. (1985) Adenosine-induced bronchoconstriction in asthma: role of mast cell-mediator release. *J Allergy Clin Immunol*,**75**, 272–8.

de Benedictis FM, Tuteri G, Pazzelli P, Bertotto A, Bruni L, Vaccaro R. (1995) Cromolyn versus nedocromil: duration of action in exercise-induced asthma in children. *J Allergy Clin Immunol*, **96**, 510–24.

Deal EC, McFadden ER Jr, Ingram RH, Jaeger JJ. (1979a) Hyperpnea and heat flux: initial reaction sequence in exercise-induced asthma. *J Appl Physiol*, **46**, 476–83.

Deal EC, McFadden ER Jr, Ingram RH, Jaeger JJ. (1979b) Esophageal temperature during exercise in asthmatic and non-asthmatic subjects. *J Appl Physiol*, **46**, 484–90.

Deal EC, McFadden ER Jr, Ingram RH, Breslin FJ, Jaeger JJ. (1980) Airway responsiveness to cold air and hyperpnea in normal subjects and in those with hay fever and asthma. *Am Rev Respir Dis*, **121**, 621–8.

Driver AG, Kukoly CA, Metzger WJ, Mustafa SJ. (1991) Bronchial challenge with adenosine causes the release of serum neutrophil chemotactic factor in asthma. *Am Rev Respir Dis*, **143**, 1002–7.

Edmunds AT, Tooley M, Godfrey S. (1978) The refractory period after exercise induced asthma, its duration and relation to severity of exercise. *Amer Rev Respir Dis*, **117**, 247–54.

Eggleston PA, Guerrant JL. (1976) A standardised method of evaluating exercise-induced asthma. *J Allergy Clin Immunol*, **58**, 414–25.

Fink G, Kaye C, Blau H, Spitzer SA. (1993) Assessment of exercise capacity in asthmatic children with various degrees of activity. *Pediatr Pulmonol*, **15**, 41–3.

Finnerty JP, Holgate ST. (1990) Evidence for the roles of histamine and prostaglandins as mediators in exercise-induced asthma: the inhibitory effect of terfenadine and flurbiprofen alone and in combination. *Eur Respir J*, **3**, 540–5.

Finnerty JP, Wood-Baker R, Thomson H, Holgate ST. (1992) Role of leukotrienes in exercise-induced asthma. Inhibitory effect of ICI 204219, a potent leukotriene D4-receptor antagonist. *Am Rev Respir Dis*, **145**, 746–9.

Finney MJB, Anderson SD, Black JL. (1990) Terfenadine modifies airway narrowing induced by the inhalation of nonisotonic aerosols in subjects with asthma. *Am Rev Respir Dis*, **141**, 1151–7.

Fitch KD, Morton AR. (1971) Specificity of exercise-induced asthma. *BMJ*, **4**, 577–81.

Floyer J, Sir. (1698) *A treatise of the asthma*. London: R Wilkin and W Innis.

Freed AN, Kelly LJ, Menkes HA. (1987) Airflow-induced bronchospasm. Imbalance between airway cooling and airway drying. *Am Rev Respir Dis*, **136**, 595–9.

Freedman S, Lane R, Gillett MK, Guz A. (1988) Abolition of methacholine induced bronchoconstriction by the hyperventilation of exercise or volition. *Thorax*, **43**, 631–6.

Freedman S. (1992) Exercise as a bronchodilator. *Clin Sci*, **83**, 383–9.

Fung KP, Chow OK, So SY. (1986) Attenuation of exercise-induced asthma by acupuncture. *Lancet*, **2**, 1419–22.

Gibson PG, Henry RL, Vimpani GV, Halliday J. (1995) Asthma knowledge, attitudes, and quality of life in adolescents. *Arch Dis Child*,**73**, 321–6.

Gilbert IA, Fouke JM, McFadden ER Jr. (1987) Heat and water flux in the intrathoracic airways and exercise-induced asthma. *J Appl Physiol*, **63**, 1681–91.

Gilbert IA, Regnard J, Lenner KA, Nelson JA, McFadden ER. (1991) Intrathoracic airstream temperatures during acute expansions of thoracic blood volume. *Clin Sci*, **81**, 655–61.

Godfrey S, Silverman M, Anderson S. (1973) Problems of interpreting exercise induced asthma. *J Allergy Clin Immunol*, **52**, 199–209.

Godfrey S, Springer C, Bar-Yishay E, Avital A. (1999) Cut-off points defining normal and asthmatic bronchial reactivity to exercise and inhalation challenges in children and young adults. *Eur Respir J*, **14**, 559–68.

Haas F, Pasierski S, Levine N, *et al.* (1987) Effect of aerobic training on forced expiratory airflow in exercising asthmatic humans. *J Appl Physiol*, **63**, 1230–5.

Haby MM, Peat JK, Mellis CM, Anderson SD, Woolcock AJ. (1995) An exercise challenge for epidemiological studies of childhood asthma: validity and repeatability. *Eur Respir J*, **8**, 729–36.

Hamielec CM, Manning PJ, O'Byrne PM. (1988) Exercise refractoriness after histamine inhalation in asthmatic subjects. *Am Rev Respir Dis*, **138**, 794–8.

Harries M. (1994) Pulmonary limitations to performance in sport. *BMJ*, **309**, 113–15.

Henriksen JM. (1985) Effect of inhalation of corticosteroids on exercise induced asthma: randomised double blind crossover study of budesonide in asthmatic children. *BMJ*, **291**, 248–9.

Henriksen JM. (1988) Effect of nedocromil sodium on exercise-induced broncho-constriction in children. *Allergy*, **43**, 449–53.

Henriksen JM, Agertoft L, Pedersen S. (1992) Protective effect and duration of action of inhaled formoterol and salbutamol on exercise-induced asthma in children. *J Allergy Clin Immunol*, **89**, 1176–82.

Henriksen JM, Dahl R, Lundquist GR. (1981) Influence of relative humidity and repeated exercise on exercise-induced bronchoconstriction. *Allergy*, **36**, 463–70.

Herxheimer H. (1946) Hyperventilation asthma. *Lancet*, **1**, 83–7.

Hofstra WB, Sterk PJ, Neijens HJ, Kouwenberg JM, Duiverman EJ. (1995) Prolonged recovery from exercise-induced asthma with increasing age in childhood. *Pediatr Pulmonol*, **20**, 177–83.

Ichinose M, Miura M, Yamauchi H, Kegeyama N, Tomaki M, Oyake T, Ohuchi Y, Hida W, Miki H, Tamura G, Shirato K. (1996) A neurokinin 1-receptor antagonist improves exercise-induced airway narrowing in asthmatic patients. *Am J Respir Crit Care Med*, **153**, 936–41.

Inbar O, Rotstein A, Neuman I, Dlin R. (1992) Comparison of maximal and submaximal exercise protocols in the provocation of exercise-induced asthma in drug-controlled asthmatics. *Clin J Sports Med*, **2**, 98–104.

Inman MD, Watson RM, Killian KJ, O'Byrne PM. (1990) Methacholine airway responsiveness decreases during exercise in asthmatic subjects. *Am Rev Respir Dis*, **141**, 1414–17.

Israel E, Dermarkarian R, Rosenberg M, *et al.* (1990) The effects of a 5-lipoxygenase inhibitor on asthma induced by cold, dry air. *N Engl J Med*, **323**, 1740–4.

James L, Faciane J, Sly RM. (1976) Effect of treadmill exercise on asthmatic children. *J Allergy Clin Immunol*, **57**, 408–16.

Jarjour NN, Calhoun WJ. (1992) Exercise-induced asthma is not associated with mast cell activation or airway inflammation. *J Allergy Clin Immunol*, **89**, 60–8.

Jones RHT, Jones RS (1966) Ventilation capacity in young adults with a history of asthma in childhood. *BMJ*, **2**, 976–8.

Jones RS, Buston MH, Wharton MJ. (1962) The effect of exercise on ventilatory function in the child with asthma. *Br J Dis Chest*, **56**, 78–86.

Jones RS, Wharton MJ, Buston MH. (1963) The place of physical exercise and bronchodilator drugs in the assessment of the asthmatic child. *Arch Dis Child*, **38**, 539–45.

Jones RS. (1966) Assessment of respiratory function in the asthmatic child. *BMJ*, **2**, 972–5.

Kemp JP, Dockhorn RJ, Busse WW, Bleecker ER, Van-As A. (1994) Prolonged effect of inhaled salmeterol against exercise-induced bronchospasm. *Am J Respir Crit Care Med*, **150**, 1612–15.

Koh YY, Lim HS, Min KU. (1994) Airway responsiveness to allergen is increased 24 hours after exercise challenge. *J Allergy Clin Immunol*, **94**, 507–16.

Larsson K, Ohlson P, Larsson L, Malmberg P, Rydstrom PO, Ulriksen H. (1993) High prevalence of asthma in cross-country skiers. *BMJ*, **307**, 1326–9.

Lee TH, Brown MJ, Nagy L, Causon R, Walport MJ, Kay AB. (1982) Exercise induced release of histamine and neutrophil chemotactic factor in atopic asthmatics. *J Allergy Clin Immunol*, **70**, 73–81.

Lee TH, O'Hickey SP. (1989) Exercise-induced asthma and late phase reactions. *Eur Respir J*, **2**, 195–7.

Makker HK, Lau LC, Thomson HW, Binks SM, Holgate ST. (1993) The protective effect of inhaled leukotriene D4 receptor antagonist ICI 204219 against exercise-induced asthma. *Am Rev Respir Dis*, **147**, 1413–18.

Manning PJ, Watson RM, Margolskee DJ, Williams VC, Schwartz JI, O'Byrne PM. (1990) Inhibition of exercise-induced bronchoconstriction by MK-571, a potent leukotriene D4-receptor antagonist. *N Engl J Med*, **323**, 1736–9.

Manning PJ, Watson RM, O'Byrne PM. (1993) Exercise-induced refractoriness in asthmatic subjects involves leukotriene and prostaglandin interdependent mechanisms. *Am Rev Respir Dis*, **148**, 950–4.

Margolski DJ, Bigby BG, Boushey HA. (1988) Indomethacin blocks airway tolerance to repetitive exercise but not to eucapnic hyperpnea in asthmatic subjects. *Am Rev Respir Dis*, **137**, 842–6.

Martin AJ, Landau LI, Phelan PD. (1980) Lung function in young adults who had asthma in childhood. *Am Rev Respir Dis*, **122**, 609–16.

Mattoli S, Foresi A, Corbo GM, Valente S, Ciappi G. (1987) The effect of indomethacin on the refractory period occurring after the inhalation of ultrasonically nebulised distilled water. *J Allergy Clin Immunol*, **79**, 678–83.

McFadden ER. (1987) Exercise and asthma. *N Engl J Med*, **317**, 502–4.

McFadden ER. (1990) Hypothesis: exercise-induced asthma as a vascular phenomenon. *Lancet*, **335**, 880–3.

McFadden ER Jr, Denison DM, Waller JF, Assoufi B, Peacock A. (1982) Direct recordings of the temperatures in the tracheobronchial tree in normal man. *J Clin Invest*, **69**, 700–5.

McFadden ER, Lenner KAM, Strohl KP. (1986) Postexertional airway rewarming and thermally induced asthma. New insights into pathophysiology and possible pathogenesis. *J Clin Invest*, **78**, 18–25.

McFadden ER, Pichurko BM, Bowman HF, *et al*. (1985) Thermal mapping of the airways in humans. *J Appl Physiol*, **58**, 564–70.

McNeill RS, Nairn JR, Millar JS, Ingram CG. (1966) Exercise induced asthma. *Q J Med*, **35**, 55–67.

Melillo E, Woolley KL, Manning PJ, Watson RM, O'Byrne PM. (1994) Effect of inhaled PGE_2 on exercise-induced bronchoconstriction in asthmatic subjects. *Am J Respir Crit Care Med*, **149**, 1138–41.

Meltzer SS, Hasday JD, Cohn J, Bleecker ER. (1996) Inhibition of exercise-induced bronchospasm by Zileuton: a 5-lipoxygenase inhibitor. *Am J Respir Crit Care Med*, **153**, 931–5.

Menardo-Mazeran G, Michel FB, Menardo JL. (1990) L'enfant asthmatique et le sport au college: enquete aupres des professeur d'education physique et sportive. *Rev Mal Respir*, **7**, 45–9.

Morton AR, Fazio SM, Miller D. (1993) Efficacy of laser-acupuncture in the prevention of exercise-induced asthma. *Ann Allergy*, **70**, 295–8.

Moscato G, DellaBianca A, Falagiani P, Mistrello G, Rossi G, Rampulla C. (1991) Inhaled furosemide prevents both the bronchoconstriction and the increase in neutrophil chemotactic activity induced by ultrasonic 'fog' of distilled water in asthmatics. *Am Rev Respir Dis*, **143**, 561–6.

Mussaffi H, Springer C, Godfrey S. (1986) Increased bronchial responsiveness to exercise and histamine after allergen challenge in asthmatic children. *J Allergy Clin Immunol*, **77**, 48–52.

Ninan TK, Russell G. (1992) Respiratory symptoms and atopy in Aberdeen schoolchildren: evidence from two surveys 25 years apart. *BMJ*, **304**, 873–7.

Noviski N, Bar-Yishay E, Gur I, Godfrey S. (1987) Exercise intensity determines and climatic conditions modify the severity of exercise induced asthma. *Am Rev Respir Dis*, **136**, 592–4.

O'Byrne PM, Jones GM. (1986) The effect of indomethecin on exercise-induced bronchoconstriction and refractoriness after exercise. *Am Rev Respir Dis*, **134**, 69–72.

O'Byrne PM, Ryan G, Morris M, *et al*. (1982) Asthma induced by cold air and its relation to nonspecific bronchial responsiveness to methacholine. *Am Rev Respir Dis*, **125**, 281–5.

O'Hickey SP, Arm JP, Rees PJ, Lee TH. (1989) Airway responsiveness to methacholine after inhalation of nebulized hypertonic saline in bronchial asthma. *J Allergy Clin Immunol*, **83**, 472–6.

Oosterhoff Y, DeJong JW, Jansen MAM, Koeter GH, Postma DS. (1993) Airway responsiveness to adenosine 5'-monophosphate in chronic obstructive pulmonary disease is determined by smoking. *Am Rev Respir Dis*, **147**, 553–8.

Peat JK, van den Berg RH, Green WF, Mellis CM, Leeder SR, Woolcock AJ. (1994) Changing prevalence of asthma in Australian children. *BMJ*, **308**, 1591–6.

Pedersen S, Hansen OR. (1995) Budesonide treatment of moderate and severe asthma in children: a dose-response study. *J Allergy Clin Immunol*, **95**, 29–33.

Phillips GE, Thomas S, Heather S, Bush A. (1998) Airway response of children with primary ciliary dyskinesia to exercise and β_2-agonist challenge. *Eur Respir J*, **11**, 1389–91.

Pierson WE, Voy RO. (1988) Exercise-induced bronchospasm in the XXIII summer Olympic games. *N Engl Reg Allergy Proc*, **9**, 209–13.

Platts-Mills TAE, Tovey UR, Mitchell EB, Moszoro H, Nock P, Wilkins SR. (1982) Reduction of bronchial hyperreactivity during prolonged allergen avoidance. *Lancet*, **2**, 675–8.

Polosa R, Holgate ST. (1997) Adenosine bronchoprovocation: a promising marker of allergic inflammation in asthma? *Thorax*, **52**, 919–23.

Popper KR. (1968) *Conjectures and refutations*. New York: Harper and Row.

Powell CVE, White RD, Primhak RA. (1996) Longitudinal study of free running exercise challenge: reproducibility. *Arch Dis Child*, **74**, 108–14.

Ramsdale EH, Morris MM, Roberts RS, Hargreave FE. (1984) Bronchial responsiveness to methacholine in chronic bronchitis; relationship to airflow obstruction and cold air responsiveness. *Thorax*, **39**, 912–18.

Ramsdale EH, Roberts RS, Morris MM, Hargreave FE. (1985) Differences in responsiveness to hyperventilation and methacholine in asthma and chronic bronchitis. *Thorax*, **40**, 422–6.

Ray DW, Hernandez C, Leff AR, Drazen JM, Solway J. (1989) Tachykinins mediate bronchoconstriction elicited by isocapnic hyperpnea in guinea pigs. *J Appl Physiol*, **66**, 1108–12.

Reiff DB, Choudry NB, Pride NB, Ind PW. (1989) The effect of prolonged submaximal warm-up exercise on exercise-induced asthma. *Am Rev Respir Dis*, **139**, 479–84.

Reiss TF, Hill JB, Harman E, *et al*. (1997) Increased urinary excretion of LTE4 after exercise and attenuation of exercise-induced bronchospasm by montelukast, a cysteinyl leukotriene receptor antagonist. *Thorax*, **52**, 1030–5.

Riedler J, Reade T, Dalton M, Holst D, Robertson C. (1994) Hypertonic saline challenge in an epidemiologic survey of asthma in children. *Am J Respir Crit Care Med*, **150**, 1632–9.

Robinson DM, Egglestone DM, Hill PM, Rea HH, Richards GN, Robinson SM. (1992) Effects of a physical conditioning programme on asthmatic patients. *NZ Med J*, **105**, 253–6.

Roger LJ, Kehrl HR, Hazucha M, Horstman DH. (1985) Bronchoconstriction in asthmatics exposed to sulphur dioxide during repeated exercise. *J Appl Physiol*, **59**, 784–91.

Rubinstein I, Levison H, Slutsky AS, *et al*. (1987) Immediate and delayed bronchoconstriction after exercise in patients with asthma. *N Engl J Med*, **317**, 482–5.

Rupp NT, Guill MF, Brudno S. (1992) Unrecognized exercise-induced bronchospasm in adolescent athletes. *Am J Dis Child*, **146**, 941–4.

Schnall RP, Landau LI. (1980) The protective effects of short sprints in exercise induced asthma. *Thorax*, **35**, 828–32.

Schoeffel RE, Anderson SD, Altounyan RE. (1981) Bronchial hyperreactivity in response to inhalation of ultrasonically nebulised solutions of distilled water and saline. *BMJ*, **283**, 1285–7.

Shaw RJ, Kay AB. (1985) Nedocromil, a mucosal and connective tissue mast cell stabilizer, inhibits exercise-induced asthma in adults. *Br J Dis Chest*, **79**, 385–9.

Silverman M, Anderson SD. (1972) Standardization of exercise tests in asthmatic children. *Arch Dis Child*, **47**, 882–9.

Silverman M, Andrea T. (1972) Time course of effect of disodium cromoglycate on exercise-induced asthma. *Arch Dis Child*, **47**, 419–22.

Silverman M, Konig P, Godfrey S. (1973) Use of serial exercise tests to assess the efficacy and duration of action of drugs for asthma. *Thorax*, **28**, 574–8.

Silverman M. (1973) Exercise studies in asthmatic children. MD Thesis, University of Cambridge.

Silvers W, Morrison M, Wiener M. (1994) Asthma ski day: cold air sports safe with peak flow monitoring. *Ann Allergy*, **73**, 105–8.

Simons FER, Gerstner TV, Cheang MS. (1997) Tolerance to the bronchoprotective effect of salmetarol in adolescents with exercise-induced asthma using concurrent inhaled glucocorticoid treatment. *Pediatrics*, **99**, 655–9.

Sly RM. (1970) Exercise related changes in airway obstruction: frequency and clinical correlates in asthmatic children. *Ann Allergy*, **28**, 1–16.

Smith CM, Anderson SD, Walsh S, McElrea MS. (1989) An investigation of the effects of heat and water exchange in the recovery period after exercise in children with asthma. *Am Rev Respir Dis*, **140**, 598–605.

Smith CM, Anderson SD. (1990) The effects of heat and water exchange in the recovery period after exercise in children with asthma. Letter. *Am Rev Respir Dis*, **141**, 802–3.

Soto ME, Schnall R, Landau LI. (1985) Refractoriness to bronchoconstriction following hyperventilation with cold dry air. *Pediatr Pulmonol*, **1**, 80–4.

Speelberg B, van den Berg NJ, Oosthoek CHA, Verhoeff NPLG, van den Brink WTJ. (1989) Immediate and late asthmatic responses induced by exercise in patients with reversible airflow limitation. *Eur Respir J*, **2**, 402–8.

Stirling DR, Cotton DJ, Graham BL, Hodgson WC, Cockroft DW, Dosman JA. (1983) Characteristics of airway tone during exercise in patients with asthma. *J Appl Physiol*, **54**, 934–42.

Suman OE, Babcock MA, Pegelow DF, Jarjour NN, Reddan WG. (1995) Airway obstruction during exercise in asthma. *Am J Respir Crit Care Med*, **152**, 24–31.

Svenonius E, Kautto R, Arborelius M. (1983) Improvement after training of children with exercise-induced asthma. *Acta Paediatr Scand*, **72**, 23–30.

Terblanche E, Stewart RI. (1990) The influence of exercise-induced bronchoconstriction on participation in organized sport. *S Afr Med J*, **78**, 741–3.

van Schoor J, Joos GF, Kips JC, Drajesk JF, Carpentier PJ, Pauwels RA. (1997) The effect of ABT-761, a novel 5-lipoxygenase inhibitor, on exercise- and adenosine-induced bronchoconstriction in asthmatic subjects. *Am J Respir Crit Care Med*, **155**, 875–80.

Vathenen AS, Knox AJ, Wisniewski A, Tattersfield AE. (1991) Effect of inhaled budesonide on bronchial reactivity to histamine, exercise, and eucapnic dry air hyperventilation in patients with asthma. *Thorax*, **46**, 811–16.

Venge P, Henriksen J, Dahl R, Hakansson L. (1990) Exercise-induced asthma and the generation of neutrophil chemotactic activity. *J Allergy Clin Immunol*, **85**, 498–504.

Verhoeff NPLG, Speelberg B, van Den Berg NJ, Oosthoek CHA, Stijnen T. (1990) Real and pseudo late asthmatic reactions after submaximal exercise challenge in patients with bronchial asthma. *Chest*, **98**, 1194–9.

Weiner P, Azgad Y, Ganam R, Weiner M. (1992) Inspiratory muscle training in patients with bronchial asthma. *Chest*, **102**, 1357–61.

Weinstein RE, Anderson JA, Kvale P, Sweet LC. (1976) Effects of humidification exercise-induced asthma (EIA). *J Allergy Clin Immunol*, **57**, 250–1.

Weiss ST, Tager IB, Weiss JW, Munoz A, Speizer FE, Ingram RH. (1984) Airway responsiveness in a population sample of adults and children. *Am Rev Respir Dis*, **129**, 898–902.

Wiebicke W, Poynter A, Montgomery M, Chernick V, Pasterkamp H. (1988) Effect of terfenadine on the response to exercise and cold air in asthma. *Pediatr Pulmonol*, **4**, 225–9.

Wilson BA, Bar-Or O, Seed LG. (1990) Effects of humid air breathing during arm or treadmill exercise on exercise-induced bronchoconstriction and refractoriness. *Am Rev Respir Dis*, **142**, 349–52.

Wilson BA, Bar-Or O, O'Byrne PM. (1994) The effects of indomethacin on refractoriness following exercise both with and without a bronchoconstrictor response. *Eur Respir J*, **7**, 2174–8.

Zawadski DK, Lenner KA, McFadden ER. (1988) Effect of exercise on nonspecific airway reactivity in asthmatics. *J Appl Physiol*, **64**, 812–16.

Zawadski DK, Lenner KA, McFadden ER. (1988) Re-examination of the late asthmatic response to exercise. *Am Rev Respir Dis*, **137**, 837–41.

4

Bronchial challenge by pharmacological agents

P.M. O'BYRNE

INTRODUCTION

Inhalation challenges with pharmacological agents that are airway constrictor agonists, such as histamine or methacholine, are widely used in both clinical and research laboratories to measure airway responsiveness. This is because airway hyperresponsiveness has been identified as an important feature in patients with current, symptomatic asthma, and indeed has been included in the defining characteristics of asthma (Sheffer *et al.*, 1995).

Airway responsiveness is a term which describes the ability of the airways to narrow after exposure to constrictor agonists. Thus, airway hyperresponsiveness is an increased ability to develop this response. Airway hyperresponsiveness consists both of an increased sensitivity of the airways to constrictor agonists, as indicated by a smaller concentration of a constrictor agonist needed to initiate the bronchoconstrictor response (Hargreave *et al.*, 1981), a steeper slope of the dose–response, as well as a greater maximal response to the agonist (Woolcock *et al.*, 1984) (Fig. 4.1).

There has been extensive research interest in airway hyperresponsiveness over the past 30 years. In populations of asthmatic patients, the severity of airway hyperresponsiveness correlates with the severity of asthma (Cockcroft *et al.*, 1977b) and with the amount of treatment needed to control symptoms (Juniper *et al.*, 1981). Studies in this area have examined a variety of methods of measuring airway responsiveness, the clinical significance and the effects of anti-asthma medications on these measurements, and the pathophysiology and pathogenesis of airway hyperresponsiveness in asthmatic patients. As a result of this

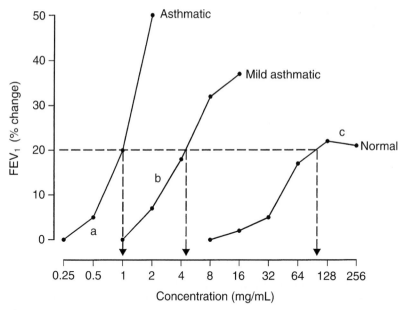

Figure 4.1 *Dose–response curves obtained in a normal person and asthmatic patients with increasing severity of airway hyperresponsiveness, by inhaling increasing concentrations of a constrictor agonist. In normals and mild asthmatics, (a) a threshold response (sensitivity), (b) a slope of the dose–response (reactivity), and (c) a maximal response (plateau) can be obtained. In most patients with current asthma, a plateau response cannot be obtained. For clinical purposes, the response is usually measured as the percentage change in FEV_1 from baseline and is expressed as the provocation concentration (PC) of the agonist causing a 20% fall in FEV_1 (PC_{20}).*

research, the methods of its measurement have been standardized, and are widely accepted. The commonly used methods of measuring airway responsiveness have been carefully characterized and compared to each other (Ryan *et al.*, 1981a). These will be fully described in this chapter, together with the methods of measuring the responses and expressing the results.

Other methods of measuring airway responsiveness to sensitizing stimuli, such as inhaled allergen (Cockcroft *et al.*, 1977b), occupational sensitizing agents (Chan-Yeung and Malo, 1995), or non-sensitizing naturally occurring stimuli, such as exercise (McFadden and Gilbert, 1994) or isocapnic hyperventilation (O'Byrne *et al.*, 1982), have also been described. Inhalation challenges with sensitizing stimuli are indicated in very specific circumstances. They are most commonly used in identifying occupational sensitizing agents. Chemical agonists, which are easier to administer and which have short-lived airway constrictor responses, should be used routinely to measure airway responsiveness.

HISTORICAL PERSPECTIVE

The initial observation that bronchoconstriction occurs more readily in asthmatics when compared to non-asthmatics after exposure to a constrictor agonist was made by Alexander and Paddock (1921), who demonstrated an 'asthmatic breathing' in asthmatics, but not normals, after subcutaneous administration of the cholinergic agonist pilocarpine. This observation was confirmed subsequently by Weiss *et al.* (1932), who reported that asthmatic patients, but not normals, developed bronchoconstriction, as measured by changes in the vital capacity, after being given intravenous histamine. Later Curry (1946), noted that this increased bronchoconstrictor response to histamine occurred with intramuscular, intravenous and nebulized histamine, again only in asthmatic patients. Tiffeneau and Beauvallet (1945) were the first to describe the use of acetylcholine inhalation tests to determine the degree of airway responsiveness in asthmatics.

It is now accepted that airway hyperresponsiveness is present in asthmatic people to many chemical or physical stimuli such as histamine (Juniper *et al.*, 1982); the cholinergic agonists acetylcholine (Simonssen, 1965), methacholine (Juniper *et al.*, 1978) and carbachol (Sotomayor *et al.*, 1984); the cysteinyl leukotrienes (LT) C_4, D_4 (Adelroth *et al.*, 1986b); prostaglandin (PG) D_2 (Hardy *et al.*, 1984) and $PGF_{2\alpha}$ (Thomson *et al.*, 1981); adenosine (Holgate *et al.*, 1984); as well as to physical stimuli such as exercise (McFadden and Gilbert, 1994), hyperventilation of cold, dry air (O'Byrne *et al.*, 1982), and both hypotonic and hypertonic solutions (Anderson *et al.*, 1983).

METHODS OF MEASURING AIRWAY RESPONSIVENESS

The two most widely used methods of measuring airway responsiveness use inhalation of an aerosolized pharmacological agonist, generated by a nebulizer, to provoke generally mild, short-lived airway constriction. In one method (Cockcroft *et al.*, 1977a), which is a modification of a method originally described by de Vries *et al.* (1962), aerosol is generated by a Wright nebulizer, delivered either to a face mask or a mouth piece, and inhaled by tidal breathing for 2 min. In the second method (Chai *et al.*, 1975), aerosol is generated by a DeVilbiss 646 nebulizer attached to a Rosenthal–French dosimeter, delivered to a mouthpiece and inhaled by five inspiratory capacity breaths. These two methods have been compared to each other, and with the appropriate standardization of features that influence the response, the two methods give very similar results and are of similar reproducibility (Ryan *et al.*, 1981).

A subsequently described method of measuring airway responsiveness by Yan *et al.* (1983) uses a hand-operated nebulizer, with the aerosol being generated by squeezing the bulb of the nebulizer. This removes the necessity of a source of compressed air. The potential advantages of this method are that it is portable and can be performed more quickly than the other methods. These reasons make it an attractive alternative for use in epidemiology studies where measurements of airway responsiveness are being made.

FACTORS THAT AFFECT INHALATION TESTS

The important technical factors of inhalation tests, that influence the response and must be standardized to accurately interpret results, are nebulizer output (Ryan *et al.*, 1981a), the particle size of the aerosol and the speed and volume of inspiration (Ryan *et al.*, 1981b), and the temperature of the solution. Nebulizer output varies between different types of nebulizers and even between different nebulizers of the same type. Therefore, each nebulizer needs to be calibrated before use. This is done by weighing the nebulizer before and after operation with compressed air at a constant pressure but with different flow rates to obtain the flow rate of compressed air which achieves the desired output. With the Wright nebulizer, an output of 0.13 mL/min is used. The particle size of the aerosol does not appear to be an important variable, once it is between 1.5–4.0 μm (Ryan *et al.*, 1981a). The volume and speed of inspiration is not an important variable if the tidal breathing method is used; however this may be more important in the method that uses inspiratory capacity breaths.

Bronchodilator medications must be avoided before the inhalation test, as these will antagonize the response to the constrictor aerosol. It is standard practice to withhold short-acting β_2-adrenoceptor agonists and anticholinergic agents for at least 8 h; short-acting xanthines for at least 24 h; long-acting xanthines, β_2-agonists and some antihistamines for at least 48–72 h; the longer acting antihistamines may influence the response to inhaled histamine for several weeks. Regular treatment with inhaled corticosteroids (Juniper et al., 1990) or nedocromil sodium (Bel et al., 1990) have been demonstrated to improve airway responsiveness in asthmatic patients. The effects of inhaled corticosteroids are slowly progressive over time and may persist for more than 3 months after they are discontinued in mild asthmatics (Juniper et al., 1991). For these reasons, inhaled or oral corticosteroids, cromolyn or nedocromil are continued without interruption during the inhalation test. However, it must be understood that the results obtained may be different (almost always improved) from a measurement made when the patient is not taking these medications.

In research studies, where the reproducibility of the inhalation test is an important consideration, other factors need to be considered. For example, inhalation of allergens (Cartier et al., 1982), atmospheric pollutants such as ozone (Golden et al., 1978) or recent viral respiratory infections (Empey et al., 1976), can cause airway hyperresponsiveness. The duration of this effect varies between stimuli and between individuals. Therefore, in research studies, inhalation tests are not performed within 6 weeks of exposure to these stimuli. However, in certain clinical situations, it may be important to perform inhalation tests both before and during exposure to an allergen or occupational sensitizing agent, to determine whether this exposure is important in causing symptoms. Inhalation of other stimuli known to cause bronchoconstriction, such as exercise or cold air, should be avoided before all inhalation tests. If all of the factors that can influence the response to inhaled bronchoconstrictor agonists are standardized, inhalation tests to measure airway responsiveness are very reproducible from day to day (Juniper et al., 1978).

CHOICE OF CONSTRICTOR AGONIST

Inhaled histamine or methacholine have been the most widely used constrictor agonists in clinical laboratories to measure airway responsiveness. Many other aerosol agonists have been used, as described above, however these have been mainly in research studies. Airway responsiveness to histamine correlates extremely well with airway responsiveness to methacholine (Juniper et al., 1978). There are, however, inherent disadvantages to inhaled histamine which makes inhaled methacholine a more useful agonist for many research studies. These disadvantages are the development of systemic side-effects, such as flushing, headache and tachycardia, when high concentrations (albeit concentrations not required in most asthmatic patients) are inhaled. These side-effects are generally not seen with even high concentrations of inhaled methacholine. Also, at high concentrations (>32 mg/mL) histamine precipitates out of solution. However, as all of these disadvantages exist only with high concentrations, histamine is as useful as methacholine for measuring airway responsiveness in clinical practice, where lower concentrations are used (Table 4.1).

A second potential problem with using histamine in research studies, is that tachyphylaxis (a decreased response to repeated stimulation) occurs following repeated challenges with inhaled histamine in mildly asthmatic people, when challenges are separated by up to 6 h (Manning et al., 1987). Tachyphylaxis does not occur to repeated challenges with inhaled

Table 4.1 *Inhalation tests with histamine or methacholine.*

Indications	Evaluation of symptoms suggestive of asthma (in patients with normal airway caliber)
	Evaluation of the presence of occupational asthma (together with other parameters)
	Evaluation of the severity of asthma (together with other parameters)
	Research studies in asthma
Contraindications	Severe airflow obstruction (FEV_1 <40% predicted or <1.5 L)
Factors enhancing response	Recent exposure to relevant inhaled allergens
	Recent exposure to relevant occupational agents
	Recent respiratory viral infections
	Exposure to atmospheric pollutants (ozone)
Factors reducing response	Avoidance of relevant allergens or occupational agents
	Bronchodilator drugs (β_2-adrenoceptor agonists, theophylline)
	Specific antagonists (antihistamines, anticholinergics)
	Regular treatment with corticosteroids
	Previous inhalation challenge with histamine (within 6 h)

acetylcholine in asthmatic patients (Manning and O'Byrne, 1988). These results suggest that histamine tachyphylaxis in asthmatics is specific to histamine stimulation and not due to bronchoconstriction *per se*. However, prior histamine inhalation reduces airway responsiveness to other bronchoconstrictor stimuli such as acetylcholine (Manning and O'Byrne, 1988) or exercise (Hamilec *et al.*, 1988). Therefore, repeated histamine inhalation tests should be separated by 1 day and histamine inhalation should not precede other inhalation challenges. Tachyphylaxis does not appear to occur to inhaled methacholine at the concentrations used in asthmatics (Stevens *et al.*, 1990), but does occur when higher concentrations are inhaled by non-asthmatic people (Beckett *et al.*, 1988).

Prolonged bronchoconstriction has been reported following methacholine inhalation challenge (Thomson *et al.*, 1983). This only occurs if very high concentrations of methacholine are used. Also, methacholine is unstable when diluted in phosphate-buffered saline; therefore normal saline must be used as the diluent. Other cholinergic agonists, such as acetylcholine (Simonssen, 1965) or carbachol (Sotomayor *et al.*, 1984) have been used to measure airway responsiveness in humans. A major disadvantage of acetylcholine is that it must be prepared freshly prior to the inhalation challenge and kept cool, to keep the solutions stable. Both histamine and methacholine are stable in solution for up to 3 months at the concentrations commonly used.

MEASUREMENT OF THE RESPONSE

Measurement of the response of the airways to an inhalation challenge can be obtained in a number of different ways. Mostly, the response is measured using non-invasive methods such as the forced expired volume in 1 second (FEV_1), airways resistance, maximum expiratory flow volume curves or total respiratory resistance. The FEV_1 is the most commonly used method of measuring response in clinical practice. However, other methods may have advantages in certain situations, depending on the objective of the test, and are used mostly in research studies.

The FEV_1 is the most popular test of pulmonary function, extensively used for detection of airflow limitation, for evaluating the effects of bronchodilators and in epidemiologic surveys. The main advantages of this test are that it is simple to perform, requires relatively less expensive equipment than other tests, and is very reproducible. The main disadvantages are that the FEV_1 requires a full inspiration, which may alter the measurement as described above. As with measurements of airways resistance, the FEV_1 is relatively insensitive to obstruction of the peripheral airways. Finally, although most of the flow expired in the first second of the forced vital capacity is effort independent, the initial part of the forced vital capacity is effort dependent, which may slightly affect the FEV_1.

The measurement of airways resistance using a whole body plethysmograph was introduced by DuBois *et al.* (1956). Airways resistance can be measured during either panting or resting breathing. As some of the agonists used may cause laryngeal narrowing, and panting partly overcomes this, it appears that measurement of airways resistance during panting is preferable. Airways resistance measured in the body plethysmograph includes the resistance of the central and peripheral airways. Because central airways resistance is the predominant component of total airways resistance, the measurement of airways resistance is not very sensitive to change in resistance of the smaller airways. In addition, as already described, some bronchoconstrictor agonists cause laryngeal constriction, therefore measurements of airways resistance may reflect laryngeal more than lower airway changes. The main advantage of measuring airways resistance is that the measurements can be obtained while avoiding a deep inspiration, which is known to alter airway smooth muscle tone in both normals and asthmatics during inhalation challenges. In normal people, a deep inspiration causes airway dilation, while in asthmatics the effect ranges from no effect, to airway dilation in some, to airway constriction in others. Since airways resistance varies with lung volume, it is important to relate changes in resistance to changes in lung volume. This can be done by calculating either specific airways resistance (sR_{AW}) or specific airways conductance (sG_{AW}). The sR_{AW} is obtained by multiplying airways resistance by the corresponding lung volume (usually close to functional residual capacity) at which the resistance is measured. The sG_{AW} is obtained by taking the reciprocal of the airways resistance, the airways conductance, and dividing it by the corresponding lung volume. Thus, during an inhalation challenge, with increasing severity of airways constriction, the sR_{AW} will increase while the sG_{AW} will decrease. The only advantage of one method over the other is that the scale of sR_{AW} tends to be bigger than sG_{AW}, therefore changes are easier to recognize. Measurements of airways resistance and functional residual capacity require a whole body plethsymograph, which is expensive to buy and relatively complex to use.

Maximum expiratory flow volume curves were first described by Hyatt *et al.* (1958). The flow volume curves can be obtained using either a variable volume whole body plethysmograph or a spirometer. The complete flow volume curves again require a full inspiration and are therefore affected by this manoeuvre in the same way as the FEV_1. The data from the flow volume curves are usually expressed as one or two flows measured at given volumes. When total lung capacity (TLC) is measured, the maximum flows are determined at a fixed percentage of TLC, usually 60 or 40%. If TLC is not measured, the flows are determined at a given percentage of vital capacity (VC), usually 50 or 25%. However, this has the disadvantage that VC falls as airway constriction occurs, and therefore the flows are not measured at the same lung volume during an inhalation challenge. To overcome this problem, considering that TLC does not change significantly during airway constriction, flows can be measured at a fixed distance from the beginning of the complete flow volume curve, even if TLC is not measured. In this way, flows are measured at the same lung volume during the inhalation challenge. The main advantage of maximum expiratory flow volume curves is that the flows in the last portion of the VC are determined by the geometry of the peripheral airways. Also, the equipment, if an electronic spirometer and an X–Y plotter are used, is relatively simple.

Bouhuys *et al.* (1969) demonstrated that, in the presence of induced airway constriction, flow volume curves following a partial inspiration had lower flows than after a complete inspiration. This difference between partial and complete curves has been attributed to airway dilation following lung inflation. Thus, partial flow volume curves, which avoid a deep inspiration, have the same advantages as measurements of airways resistance, with the additional advantage of reflecting the geometry of the peripheral airways. Therefore, measurements of sR_{AW} will reflect more the effect of a constrictor agonist on the more central airways, while partial flow volume curves will reflect more the effect on peripheral airways. Since the airway dilation following lung inflation depends on the degree of inflation, the partial flow volume curves should be started at a fixed lung volume. A standard method of performing partial flow volume curves has been described, in which the partial manoeuvre starts from the same lung volume using TLC as the reference volume (Zamel, 1984).

DuBois (1953) described a method of measuring total respiratory system resistance, $R(rs)$, by sinusoidally oscillating the system at its resonant frequency. The method was further modified so that $R(rs)$ was measured by oscillatory frequencies of 3 and 5 cycles/s. Takishima *et al.* (1981) have developed a fully automated method of aerosol delivery and continuous recording of $R(rs)$. The major advantage of this method is its simplicity, in that the patient just has to breath with resting tidal volume. However, $R(rs)$ measures the resistance of the total respiratory system, including the chest wall, and while it is a sensitive method of measuring the response, it is not specific regarding the different components of the respiratory system.

EXPRESSING THE RESULTS

Most recent studies in which airway responsiveness has been measured have plotted the changes in lung function against the log of the concentration of the agonist administered (Fig. 4.1). There are several ways of expressing the results from these semi-log dose–response curves. The most usual way is to determine the provocative concentration (PC) or provocative dose (PD) of the agonist which causes a predetermined change in lung function, usually a fixed percentage of baseline. If FEV_1 is the parameter used to assess lung function, a 20% fall from baseline is usually used and the results expressed as the PC_{20} FEV_1, i.e. the concentration of the agonist that causes a 20% fall in FEV_1 (Fig. 4.1). For sG_{AW}, a 35% reduction is usually used because of the greater variability of the measurement.

Other ways of expressing the results include applying a curve-fitting equation to the dose–response curve and obtaining various parameters from the equation. Woolcock *et al.* (1984) have described parameters related to the position, slope and plateau of the dose–response curve. They found differences in all parameters between normal and asthmatic people. Normals and mild asthmatics have a plateau response at higher concentrations of inhaled agonists. By contrast, more severe asthmatics do not demonstrate a plateau response, even with very severe degrees of airway constriction. The use of parameters such as these may be very useful in studies of mechanisms of airway responsiveness. However, for most clinical applications of measurements of airway responsiveness, the simpler method of expressing results, such as PC_{20} FEV_1 is the most useful.

SIGNIFICANCE OF AIRWAY HYPERRESPONSIVENESS

Airway hyperresponsiveness can be demonstrated in almost all patients with current symptomatic asthma (Cockcroft *et al.*, 1977a). Using the method described by Cockcroft *et al.*

(1977a), asthmatic individuals generally have a histamine or methacholine PC_{20} FEV_1 of less than 8 mg/mL. Most non-asthmatics will have a PC_{20} of greater 16 mg/mL. There is however some overlap, and defining an exact level of airway responsiveness, which would distinguish asthmatics from non-asthmatics, is not possible. This is because there appears to be a continuous distribution of non-specific airway responsiveness in the general population, with asthmatic people in one tail of this distribution (Cockcroft et al., 1983). In addition, even those with normal histamine or methacholine airway responsiveness can develop symptoms of asthma if exposed to specific stimuli to which they are sensitized, such as inhaled allergen or Toluene Diisocyanate (TDI) (Hargreave et al., 1984).

As has already been described, the severity of airway hyperresponsiveness generally correlates with the severity of asthma. The degree of airway hyperresponsiveness correlates with another important variable in asthma, that is variations in peak expiratory flow rates (Ryan et al., 1982) and with the improvement in FEV_1 after inhaled bronchodilator (Ryan et al., 1982). Lastly, the degree of airway constriction caused by exercise (Anderton et al., 1979) or hyperventilation of cold, dry air in asthmatic people, is related to the level of airway hyperresponsiveness (O'Byrne et al., 1982). As these stimuli are considered to act through release of endogenous mediators, it is likely that hyperresponsiveness of asthmatic airways to these released constrictor mediators plays a role in causing symptoms in asthmatic patients.

Airway hyperresponsiveness has been correlated to a number of markers of persisting airway inflammation in asthmatics. These include the number of eosinophils and mast cells in bronchoalveolar lavage fluid (Kirby, 1987), and the extent of deposition of collagen and other extracellular matrix proteins below the basement membrane in asthmatic airways (Jeffery, 1989). Airway hyperresponsiveness improves in most asthmatics when treated with inhaled corticosteroids over weeks to months in both children (van Essen-Zandvliet et al., 1992) and adults (Juniper et al., 1990). Taken together, these results suggest that persisting airway hyperresponsiveness in asthmatics is caused by inflammatory and structural changes in the airways.

Airway hyperresponsiveness to inhaled histamine or methacholine can also be demonstrated in patients with airflow obstruction apparently due to chronic bronchitis (Ramsdale et al., 1984). The degree of airflow obstruction, as indicated by the reduction on FEV_1 and FEV_1/VC ratio, correlates with the increase in airway responsiveness (Ramsdale et al., 1984). This suggests that, in patients with airflow obstruction, the airway hyperresponsiveness demonstrated is a result of reduced airway caliber. By contrast, many patients with airway hyperresponsiveness and asthma, have normal airway caliber at the time the inhalation challenge is being performed. This can, however, pose a problem in interpreting the result of an inhalation challenge with a constrictor agonist in a patient with significant airflow obstruction at the time of the study. Results from McClean et al. (1993) have demonstrated that the only parameter extracted from the methacholine dose–response curve that is not associated with baseline lung function is the dose–response threshold (defined as the concentration which produces a statistically significant change in FEV_1 or $\dot{V}40p$). Therefore, the threshold concentration may be a more specific measure of airway hyperresponssiveness than the PC_{20}; however, this independence of the dose–response threshold from the baseline lung function needs to be studied in populations of asthmatics.

The likelihood of identifying the presence of airway hyperresponsiveness in patients suspected of having asthma, based on history and physical examination, and in whom airway caliber is normal, is only slightly better than chance alone, even by physicians experienced in treating asthma (Adelroth et al., 1986a). Therefore, objective measurements of airway responsiveness are particularly useful in such patients with normal airway caliber, in whom a diagnosis of asthma is being considered. Another important application of measuring airway responsiveness is the diagnosis of occupational asthma (Vedal et al., 1988). Lastly, measurement of airway responsiveness has been suggested to be useful in determining the optimal treatment requirements of asthmatics, but this requires further study.

GENETICS OF AIRWAY HYPERRESPONSIVENESS

It has been recognized for many years that familial clustering exists for asthma, and more recently for airway hyperresponsiveness (Longo *et al.*, 1987; Hopp *et al.*, 1988). This could reflect a genetic predisposition for the development of asthma, a shared environmental risk(s), or most likely a combination of both. Efforts have also been made to examine the genetic basis of airway hyperresponsiveness. Studies of monozygotic and dizygotic twins have suggested that there is some genetic basis for the development of airway hyperresponsiveness, but that environmental factors are more important (Nieminen, 1991). Also measurements of airway hyperresponsiveness in young infants (mean age 4.5 weeks) have indicated that airway hyperresponsiveness can be present very early in life, and that a family history of asthma and parental smoking were risk factors for its development (Young *et al.*, 1991). More recently, reports of genetic linkage of airway hyperresponsiveness have been published. One study has identified genetic linkage between histamine airway hyperresponsiveness and several genetic markers on chromosome 5q, near a locus that regulates serum IgE levels (Postma *et al.*, 1995). Another study has identified linkage between a highly polymorphic marker of the B subunit of the high-affinity IgE receptor on chromosome 11q and methacholine airway hyper-responsiveness, even in patients with non-atopic asthma (van Herwerden *et al.*, 1995). Thus, a genetic basis for airway hyperresponsiveness seems very likely; however, the genetic linkage studies need to be confirmed by other investigators in different patient populations. One specific gene polymorphism (Glu 27) of the nine identified of the β_2-adrenoceptor has also been associated with increased methacholine airway hyperresponsiveness (Hall *et al.*, 1995), while another polymorphism (Gly 16) was associated with the presence of nocturnal asthma (Turki *et al.*, 1995).

CONCLUSIONS

Measurements of airway responsiveness to inhaled bronchoconstrictor mediators, histamine or methacholine can be useful in making a diagnosis of asthma, particularly in patients with symptoms consistent with asthma, who have no evidence of airflow obstruction. Histamine or methacholine inhalation tests can be performed quickly, safely and reproducibly by experienced technicians, once the factors known to influence the tests are appropriately controlled.

REFERENCES

Adelroth E, Hargreave FE, Ramsdale EH. (1986a) Do physicians need objective measurements to diagnose asthma? *Am Rev Respir Dis*, **134**, 704–7.
Adelroth E, Morris MM, Hargreave FE, O'Byrne PM. (1986b) Airway responsiveness to leukotrienes C4 and D4 and to methacholine in patients with asthma and normal controls. *N Engl J Med*, **315**, 480–4.
Alexander HL, Paddock R. (1921) Bronchial asthma: response to pilocarpine and epinephrine. *Arch Intern Med*, **27**, 184–91.

Anderson S, Schoeffel R, Finney M. (1983) Evaluation of ultrasonically nebulized solutions for provocative testing in patients with asthma. *Thorax*, **38**, 284–91.

Anderton RC, Cuff MT, Frith PA, *et al.* (1979) Bronchial responsiveness to inhaled histamine and exercise. *J Allergy Clin Immunol*, **63**, 315–20.

Beckett WS, McDonnell WF, Wong ND. (1988) Tolerance to methacholine inhalation challenge in nonasthmatic subjects. *Am Rev Respir Dis*, **137**, 1499–501.

Bel EH, Timmers MC, Hermans J, Dijkman JH, Sterk PJ. (1990) The long-term effect of nedocromil sodium and beclomethasone dipropionate on bronchial responsiveness to methacholine in nonatopic asthmatic subjects. *Am Rev Respir Dis*, **141**, 21–8.

Bouhuys A, Hunt VR, Kim BM, Zapletal A. (1969) Maximum expiratory flow rates in induced bronchoconstriction in man. *J Clin Invest*, **48**, 1159–68.

Cartier A, Thomson NC, Frith PA, Roberts R, Hargreave FE. (1982) Allergen-induced increase in bronchial responsiveness to histamine: relationship to the late asthmatic response and change in airway caliber. *J Allergy Clin Immunol*, **70**, 170–7.

Chai H, Farr RS, Froehlich LA, *et al.* (1975) Standardization of bronchial inhalation challenge procedures. *J Allergy Clin Immunol*, **56**, 323–7.

Chan-Yeung M, Malo JL. (1995) Occupational Asthma. *N Engl J Med*, **333**, 107–12.

Cockcroft DW, Berscheid BA, Murdock KY. (1983) Unimodal distribution of bronchial responsiveness to inhaled histamine in a random human population. *Chest*, **83**, 751–4.

Cockcroft DW, Killian DN, Mellon JJA, Hargreave FE. (1977a) Bronchial reactivity of inhaled histamine: a method and clinical survey. *Clin Allergy*, **7**, 235–43.

Cockcroft DW, Ruffin RE, Dolovich J, Hargreave FE. (1977b) Allergen-induced increase in non-allergic bronchial reactivity. *Clin Allergy*, **7**, 503–13.

Curry JJ. (1946) The action of histamine on the respiratory tract in normal and asthmatic subjects. *J Clin Invest*, **25**, 785–91.

De Vries K, Goei JT, Booy-Noord H, Orie NGM. (1962) Changes during 24 hours in the lung function and histamine hyperreactivity of the bronchial tree in asthmatic and chronic bronchitis patients. *Int Arch Allergy*, **20**, 93–99.

DuBois AB, Botelho SY, Comroe JH Jr. (1956) A new method for measuring airway resistance in man using a body plethysmograph: values in normal subjects and in patients with respiratory disease. *J Clin Invest*, **35**, 327–35.

DuBois AB. (1953) Resistance to breathing measured by driving the chest at 6 cps. *Fed Proc*, **12**, 35–6.

Empey DW, Laitinen LA, Jacobs L, Gold WM, Nadel JA. (1976) Mechanisms of bronchial hyperreactivity in normal subjects after upper respiratory tract infections. *Am Rev Respir Dis*, **113**, 131–9.

Golden JA, Nadel JA, Boushey HA. (1978) Bronchial hyperirritability in healthy subjects after exposure to ozone. *Am Rev Respir Dis*, **118**, 287–94.

Hall IP, Wheatley A, Wilding P, Liggett SB. (1995) Association of Glu 27 beta 2-adrenoceptor polymorphism with lower airway reactivity in asthmatic subjects. *Lancet*, **345**, 1213–14.

Hamilec CM, Manning PJ, O'Byrne PM. (1988) Exercise refractoriness post histamine bronchoconstriction in asthmatic subjects. *Am Rev Respir Dis*, **138**, 794–8.

Hardy CC, Robinson C, Tattersfield AE, Holgate ST. (1984) The bronchoconstrictor effect of inhaled prostaglandin D2 in normal and asthmatic men. *N Engl J Med*, **311**, 209–13.

Hargreave FE, Ramsdale EH, Pugsley SO. (1984) Occupational asthma without bronchial hyperresponsiveness. *Am Rev Respir Dis*, **130**, 513–15.

Hargreave FE, Ryan G, Thomson NC, *et al.* (1981) Bronchial responsiveness to histamine or methacholine in asthma: measurement and clinical significance. *J Allergy Clin Immunol*, **68**, 347–55.

Holgate ST, Mann JS, Cushley MJ. (1984) Adenosine as a bronchoconstrictor mediator in asthma and its antagonism by methylxanthines. *J Allergy Clin Immunol*, **74**, 302–6.

Hopp RJ, Bewtra AK, Biven R, Nair NM, Townley RG. (1988) Bronchial reactivity pattern in nonasthmatic parents of asthmatics. *Ann Allergy*, **61**, 184–6.

Hyatt RE, Schilder DP, Fry DL. (1958) Relationship between maximum expiratory flow and degree of lung inflation. *J Appl Physiol*, **13**, 331–6.

Jeffery PK, Wardlaw AJ, Nelson FC, Collins JV, Kay AB. (1989) Bronchial biopsies in asthma. An ultrastructural, quantitative study and correlation with hyperreactivity. *Am Rev Respir Dis*, **140**, 1745–53.

Juniper EF, Frith PA, Dunnett C, Cockcroft DW, Hargreave FE. (1978) Reproducibility and comparison of responses to inhaled histamine and methacholine. *Thorax*, **33**, 705–10.

Juniper EF, Frith PA, Hargreave FE. (1981) Airway responsiveness to histamine and methacholine: relationship to minimum treatment to control symptoms of asthma. *Thorax*, **36**, 575–9.

Juniper EF, Frith PA, Hargreave FE. (1982) Long term stability of bronchial responsiveness to histamine. *Thorax*, **37**, 288–91.

Juniper EF, Kline P, Vanzieleghem M, Hargreave F. (1991) Reduction of Budesonide after a year of increased use: a randomized controlled trial to evaluate whether improvements in airway responsiveness and clinical asthma are maintained. *J Allergy Clin Immunol*, **87**, 483–9.

Juniper EF, Kline PA, Vanzieleghem MA, Ramsdale EH, O'Byrne PM, Hargreave FE. (1990) Effect of long-term treatment with inhaled corticosteroids on airway hyperresponsiveness and clinical asthma in nonsteroid dependent asthmatics. *Am Rev Respir Dis*, **142**, 832–6.

Kirby JG, Hargreave FE, Gleich GJ, O'Byrne PM. (1987) Bronchoalveolar cell profiles of asthmatic and nonasthmatic subjects. *Am Rev Respir Dis*, **136**, 379–83.

Longo G, Strinati R, Poli F, Fumi F. (1987) Genetic factors in nonspecific bronchial hyperreactivity. An epidemiologic study. *Am J Dis Child*, **141**, 331–4.

McClean PA, van der Doelen J, Zamel N. (1993) Dose–response threshold is independent of baseline lung function. *Am Rev Respir Dis*, **147**, A830 (abstract).

McFadden ER, Gilbert IA. (1994) Exercise-induced asthma. *N Engl J Med*, **330**, 1362–7.

Manning PJ, Jones GL, O'Byrne PM. (1987) Tachyphylaxis to inhaled histamine in asthmatic subjects. *J Appl Physiol*, **63**, 1572–7.

Manning PJ, O'Byrne PM. (1988) Histamine bronchoconstriction reduces airway responsiveness in asthmatic subjects. *Am Rev Respir Dis*, **137**, 1323–5.

Nieminen MM, Kaprio J, Koskenvuo M. (1991) A population based study of bronchial asthma in adult twin pairs. *Chest*, **100**, 70–5.

O'Byrne PM, Ryan G, Morris M, *et al.* (1982) Asthma induced by cold air and its relation to nonspecific bronchial responsiveness to methacholine. *Am Rev Respir Dis*, **125**, 281–5.

Postma DS, Bleecker ER, Amelung PJ, *et al.* (1995) Genetic susceptibility to asthma: bronchial hyperresponsiveness coinherited with a major gene for atopy. *N Engl J Med*, **333**, 894–900.

Ramsdale EH, Morris MM, Roberts RS, Hargreave FE. (1984) Bronchial responsiveness to methacholine in chronic bronchitis: relationship to airflow obstruction and cold air responsiveness. *Thorax*, **39**, 912–18.

Ryan G, Dolovich MB, Obminski G, *et al.* (1981a) Standardization of inhalation provocation tests: influence of nebulizer output, particle size, and methods of inhalation. *J Allergy Clin Immunol*, **67**, 156–61.

Ryan G, Dolovich MB, Roberts RS, *et al.* (1981b) Standardization of inhalation provocation tests: two techniques of aerosol generation and inhalation compared. *Am Rev Respir Dis*, **123**, 195–9.

Ryan G, Latimer KM, Dolovich J, Hargreave FE. (1982) Bronchial responsiveness to histamine: relationship to diurnal variation of peak flow rate, improvement after bronchodilator, and airway caliber. *Thorax*, **37**, 423–9.

Sheffer AL, Bartal M, Bousquet J, Carrasco E, *et al.* (1995) Global strategy for asthma management and prevention. Bethesda, MD: National Institutes of Health. 95-3659, 70–114.

Simonssen BG. (1965) Clinical and physiological studies on chronic bronchitis. III. Bronchial reactivity to inhaled acetylcholine. *Acta Allergol*, **20**, 325–48.

Sotomayor H, Badier M, Vervloet D, Orehek J. (1984) Seasonal increase of carbachol airway responsiveness in patients allergic to grass pollen. *Am Rev Respir Dis*, **130**, 56–8.

Stevens WH, Manning PJ, O'Byrne PM. (1990) Tachyphylaxis to inhaled methacholine in normal but not asthmatic subjects. *J Appl Physiol*, **69**, 875–9.

Takishima T, Hida W, Sasaki H, Suzuki S, Sasaki T. (1981) Direct writing recorder of dose–response curves of airways to methacholine – clinical application. *Chest*, **80**, 600–6.

Thomson NC, O'Byrne PM, Hargreave FE. (1983) Prolonged asthmatic responses to inhaled methacholine. *J Allergy Clin Immunol*, **71**, 357–62.

Thomson NC, Roberts R, Bandouvakis J, Newball H, Hargreave FE. (1981) Comparison of bronchial responses to prostaglandin F2a and methacholine. *J Allergy Clin Immunol*, **68**, 392–8.

Tiffeneau R, Beauvallet. (1945) Epreuve de bronchoconstriction et de bronchodilatation par aerosols. *Bull Acad Med*, **129**, 165–8.

Turki J, Pak J, Green SA, Martin RJ, Liggett SB. (1995) Genetic polymorphisms of the beta 2-adrenergic receptor in nocturnal and nonnocturnal asthma. Evidence that Gly16 correlates with the nocturnal phenotype. *J Clin Invest*, **95**, 1635–41.

van Essen-Zandvliet EE, Hughes MD, Waalkens HJ, Duiverman EJ, Pocock SJ, Kerrebijn KF. (1992) Effect of 22 months of treatment with inhaled corticosteroids and/or beta2-agonists on lung function, airway responsiveness and symptoms in patients with asthma. *Am Rev Respir Dis*, **146**, 547–54.

van Herwerden L, Harrap SB, Wong ZYH, *et al*. (1995) Linkage of high-affinity IgE receptor gene with bronchial hyperreactivity, even in absence of atopy. *Lancet*, **346**, 1262–5.

Vedal S, Enarson DA, Chan H, Ochnio J, Tse KS, Chan-Yeung M. (1988) A longitudinal study of the occurrence of bronchial hyperresponsiveness in western red cedar workers. *Am Rev Respir Dis*, **137**, 651–5.

Weiss S, Robb GP, Ellis LB. (1932) The systemic effects of histamine in man. *Arch Intern Med*, **49**, 360–96.

Woolcock AJ, Salome CM, Yan K. (1984) The shape of the dose–response curve to histamine in asthmatic and normal subjects. *Am Rev Respir Dis*, **130**, 71–5.

Yan K, Salome CM, Woolcock AJ. (1983) Rapid method for measurement of bronchial responsiveness. *Thorax*, **38**, 760–5.

Young S, Le Souef PN, Geelhoed GC, Stick SM, Turner KJ, Landau LI. (1991) The influence of a family history of asthma and parental smoking on airway responsiveness in early infancy. *N Engl J Med*, **324**, 1168–73.

Zamel N. Partial flow–volume curves. (1984) *Bull Eur Physiopathol Respir*, **20**, 471–5.

5

The autonomic nervous system in asthma

DUNJA SCHMIDT AND KLAUS F. RABE

INTRODUCTION

The autonomic nervous system is involved in the control of airway function, including smooth muscle tone, epithelial cell function, mucus secretion, blood flow, microvascular permeability and inflammatory mediator release. Under normal circumstances, there is a balance between excitatory (bronchoconstricting) and inhibitory (bronchodilating) pathways, which regulate airway calibre. Conceivably, an imbalance between the counteracting components can lead to a decrease in airway lumen and severe airway obstruction as well as distinct pathological changes involved in asthma.

Bronchial asthma is characterized by reversible airway narrowing, which is associated with airway smooth muscle hypercontractility and airway inflammation, i.e. mucus hypersecretion, airway wall oedema, epithelial desquamation and infiltration of the airway wall by inflammatory cells. As all of these aspects can be modulated by the autonomic nervous system, it has been suggested that dysfunction of neural control might be a substantial component for the development and clinical presentation of asthma. This chapter will review the anatomy and physiology of the autonomic nervous system of the human airway and its possible role in the pathophysiology of bronchial asthma.

AUTONOMIC NERVOUS SYSTEM IN THE LUNG

The autonomic nervous system of the human lung comprises efferent pathways mediated through cholinergic, adrenergic and peptidergic mechanisms, as well as several types of afferent pathways. Airway calibre is regulated by a balance of excitatory, bronchoconstricting and inhibitory, bronchodilating mechanisms. These counteracting systems are – in the classical view – the cholinergic parasympathetic and the adrenergic sympathetic system, with its neurotransmitters acetylcholine and noradrenaline, respectively. While the parasympathetic nervous system is more important in the regulation of airway tone, i.e. the direct innervation of airways smooth muscle, the sympathetic nervous system is rather more important in the control of airways blood flow and glandular secretion, with little histological or functional evidence for a direct innervation of the human bronchial smooth muscle (Barnes, 1986b).

However, the autonomic neural control of the lung cannot be fully explained by the effects exerted by the cholinergic and adrenergic systems alone. Airway responses to nerve stimulation are still observed after adrenergic and cholinergic blockade (Richardson and Beland, 1976), and these responses, which are independent from the adrenergic and cholinergic pathways, are hence defined as non-adrenergic non-cholinergic (NANC) mechanisms. Depending on the stimulus, the NANC nervous system can elicit excitatory bronchoconstricting as well as inhibitory bronchodilating responses. Since the first neurotransmitters to be identified in the NANC system were peptides, it was initially named the peptidergic system to define it as a separate entity. Later it became clear that even small molecules such as nitric oxide (NO), carbon monoxide and hydroxyl radicals are functioning as important neurotransmitters of the NANC system, so that the term 'peptidergic' is strictly speaking no longer appropriate.

The majority of the afferent sensory nerves are non-myelinated C-fibres but they also comprise large numbers of fine myelinated fibres coming from lung irritant or rapidly adapting receptors. The sensory nerve fibres not only act as afferent pathways but are also believed to contain neurotransmitters of the NANC system which are released after activation and exhibit efferent functions (Barnes, 1986a; Spina and Page, 1996).

The efferent and afferent neural pathways form an intricate network with nerve fibres in direct anatomical contact but also functional and reflex mechanisms, including local axonal reflexes with antidromic stimulation of the nerves to accomplish an effective control of airway calibre and functions (Fig. 5.1).

Cholinergic system

The cholinergic nervous system is the predominant neural bronchoconstrictor pathway in the human lung. Efferent nerves run from the vagus nuclei in the brain stem through the vagus nerves towards small ganglia in the bronchial wall.

The neurotransmitter of the cholinergic system is acetylcholine, which acts in the airways preferentially on excitatory, muscarinic receptors. Until now five muscarinic cholinoceptor subtypes have been cloned of which four subtypes have been discriminated pharmacologically (Hulme et al., 1990). Of these only M_1 to M_3 are present in the human lung (Mak et al., 1992). The receptors that mediate bronchoconstriction, vasodilatation and mucus secretion belong to the M_3-cholinoceptor subtype (Barnes, 1993; Watson et al., 1995b). Those muscarinic receptors that are localized to nerves and parasympathetic ganglia in the airways are believed to belong to the M_1- and M_2-receptor subtypes (van Koppen et al., 1987). While the prejunctional M_1-receptor serves an autofacilitatory role – i.e. its activation causes an increase in neurotransmitter release from the nerve terminal – the prejunctional M_2-receptor has an autoinhibitory function, limiting acetycholine release after cholinergic stimulation (Minette and Barnes, 1988).

The functional involvement of the cholinergic system in the regulation of airway tone in humans under normal conditions is best illustrated by the observations that inhalation of the

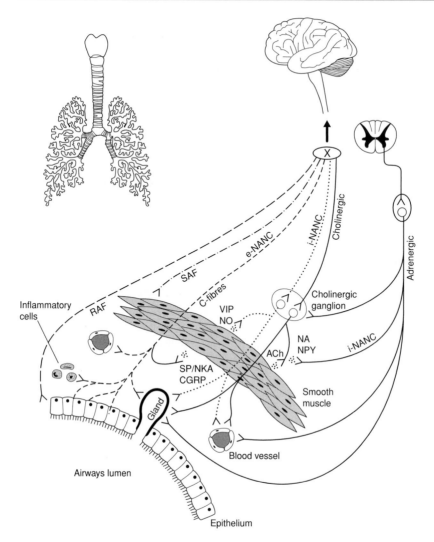

Figure 5.1 *Schematic representation of neural control of the airways, which comprises an adrenergic, cholinergic and non-adrenergic non-cholinergic (NANC) nervous system (Dupont, 1999). ACh, acetylcholine; SP, substance P; NKA, neurokinin A; NPY, neuropeptide Y; CGRP, calcitonin gene-related peptide; NA, noradrenaline; e-NANC, excitatory non-adrenergic non-cholinergic; i-NANC, inhibitory non-adrenergic non-cholinergic; SAF, slowly adapting fibres; RAF, rapidly adapting fibres; X, nervus vagus; NO, nitric oxide; VIP, vasoactive intestinal peptide.*

anticholinergic agent ipratropium bromide significantly increases specific airway conductance (sG_{AW}) in these individuals (Douglas *et al.*, 1979; MacNee *et al.*, 1982).

Adrenergic system

The sympathetic innervation of the human lung is relatively sparse in comparison to the parasympathetic nerve supply. Postganglionic adrenergic fibres enter the lung through the hilum and follow the cholinergic nerves into the peribronchial plexus to glands and blood vessels (Spencer and Leof, 1964; Richardson and Fergusson, 1979; Partanen *et al.*, 1982;

Sheppard *et al.*, 1983). The direct innervation of airways smooth muscle is almost absent. Sympathetic nerves are, however, also found in close anatomical relationship to cholinergic nerves (Daniel *et al.*, 1986) and ganglia (Richardson and Fergusson, 1979) suggesting mainly a neuromodulatory function for cholinergic neurotransmission.

In accordance with the above-mentioned histological studies, pharmacological evidence suggests only minor roles for sympathetic nerves and their neurotransmitter noradrenaline in the regulation of airway calibre in humans. Despite clear cardiovascular (side-) effects, neither circulating noradrenaline nor the α_1-selective adrenoceptor agonist phenylephrine exerts an effect on basal bronchial tone either in healthy or in asthmatic people (Larsson *et al.*, 1986). This comes as no surprise since noradrenaline, preferentially activates β_1- and α-adrenoceptors which are functionally not relevant for the regulation of bronchial tone, while its effect on β_2-adrenoceptors is insignificant.

However, the adrenergic system includes not only the sympathetic innervation but also the adrenal medulla which secrets adrenaline as a circulating hormone. Adrenaline, in contrast to noradrenaline, does activate β_2-adrenoceptors with a similar selectivity to α- and β_1-adrenoceptors. Obviously, the sparse sympathetic innervation of the human lung is out of proportion to the numerous β_2-adrenergic receptors found on smooth muscle cells, blood vessels, glands, epithelium and inflammatory cells (Carstairs *et al.*, 1985) which respond primarily to the circulating catecholamine produced primarily outside the lungs' innervation. Therefore, while the parasympathetic pathways represent anatomically the most abundant and important direct regulating system of airway functions, the physiological role and relevance of the numerous β_2-receptors have yet to be fully determined.

Peptidergic system

In addition to the 'classical' pathways, i.e. the cholinergic and adrenergic systems, the non-adrenergic non-cholinergic (NANC) nervous system also elicits excitatory broncho-constricting as well as inhibitory bronchodilating responses (Richardson and Beland, 1976; Richardson, 1981). Neurotransmitters of the NANC system are predominantly neuropeptides, but also small molecules such as NO. According to current knowledge, the NANC system does not consist of independent nerve fibres, as the neurotransmitters of the excitatory (e-)NANC system are predominantly localized to the endings of sensory nerve fibres, whereas the neurotransmitters of the inhibitory (i-)NANC system are mainly co-localized to acetylcholine and noradrenaline containing nerves.

e-NANC

Excitatory (e-)NANC contraction is believed to be mediated by antidromic stimulation of sensory nerve fibres from which substance P and other tachykinins such as neurokinin A (NKA), neurokinin B, neuropeptide K and calcitonin gene-related peptide (CGRP) are released. Histological and pharmacological studies have shown that e-NANC nerve fibres directly innervate bronchial smooth muscle, blood vessels and submucosal glands and form a diffuse network immediately beneath the epithelium with branches penetrating the epithelial layer (Barnes *et al.*, 1991a,b). Furthermore, a close interaction between the e-NANC and the cholinergic system seems likely because substance P and neurokinin A have been shown to release other neurotransmitters, including acetylcholine, from cholinergic nerves (Joos and Pauwels, 1990).

Although it was shown that tachykinins given directly to the lung by inhalation at high concentrations and in the presence of endopeptidase inhibitors are capable of producing bronchoconstriction and mimicking other symptoms of asthma, it is debated whether endogenous neuropeptides play a dominant role in the regulation of airway tone in healthy or asthmatic subjects (Cheung *et al.*, 1992, 1993).

i-NANC

The inhibitory (i)-NANC system is considered to be the most important bronchodilator pathway present in the human airways (Richardson and Beland, 1976; Richardson, 1981; Ichinose *et al.*, 1988; Lammers *et al.*, 1988). Neurotransmitters of the i-NANC system and/or their generating enzymes can be co-localized to parasympathetic (vasoactive intestinal peptide, NO) or sympathetic (neuropeptide Y) nerves.

Vasoactive intestinal peptide (VIP)-containing nerve fibres follow the vagus nerve and reach into the subepithelial layer. They are found around blood vessels, mucous glands and within smooth muscle bundles (Dey *et al.*, 1981). There is evidence that i-NANC transmitters are co-released with acetylcholine from parasympathetic nerves at the level of the airways smooth muscle. VIP and closely related peptides such as peptide histidine methionine (PHM) and pituitary adenylyl cyclase-activating peptide (PACAP) are believed to be the neurotransmitters within the i-NANC system (Palmer *et al.*, 1986a). Moreover, the VIP-containing neurones seem to be identical with cholinergic neurones in the upper airways; correspondingly, coexistence of VIP and acetylcholine in parasympathetic ganglia supplying the respiratory tract has been reported (Lundberg *et al.*, 1984a; Uddman and Sundler, 1987). The recent classification describes three receptor subtypes for VIP and PACAP: the PAC_1, $VPAC_1$ and $VPAC_2$ receptors (Harmar *et al.*, 1998), however, their role within the human lung has not been fully evaluated as yet.

Although there are large numbers of VIP-immunoreactive nerves in human airway smooth muscle (Laitinen *et al.*, 1985), and despite the bronchodilating effects of VIP (Saga and Said, 1984), the role of VIP as endogenous mediator of i-NANC responses appears to be questionable. This was suggested by the finding that phosphoramidon, a neutral endopeptidase inhibitor, significantly potentiated relaxations to low doses of VIP but at the same time did not have an effect on i-NANC responses in isolated human airways (Belvisi *et al.*, 1992a).

The lower respiratory tract in humans receives a relatively rich supply of PACAP-containing fibres (Luts *et al.*, 1993), which can be detected around smooth muscle, blood vessels and glands. In the respiratory tract the majority of the PACAP-containing fibres also contain VIP. It has been shown that PACAP is a potent dilator of human pulmonary arteries *in vitro*. However, in contrast to VIP-induced dilatation, the effect of PACAP was found to be endothelium-dependent (Cardell *et al.*, 1997), thereby suggesting an indirect action. Furthermore, in isolated bronchi obtained from primates, PACAP caused long-lasting smooth muscle relaxation (Yoshihara *et al.*, 1997). Until now there is no published information on the effect of PACAP in human airways.

During recent years evidence has accumulated that NO might be an important neurotransmitter of the i-NANC system (Belvisi *et al.*, 1992a, b). The enzyme, which is thought to be responsible for the NO production, is the neuronal nitric oxide synthase (nNOS), which may be activated by calcium entry upon nerve depolarization (Bredt *et al.*, 1990). Although human airways *in vitro* do not show basal release of NO this can be initiated upon stimulation of cholinergic nerves by electrical field stimulation (EFS) (Ward *et al.*, 1993).

Another neurotransmitter of the i-NANC system, neuropeptide Y (NPY), is often co-localized with noradrenaline at adrenergic nerve terminals of the airways (Bowden and Gibbins, 1992). Neuropeptide Y inhibits EFS-induced contractions in human bronchial smooth muscle (Fujiwara *et al.*, 1993) and causes contractions of airway vascular smooth muscle (Widdicombe, 1991).

Afferent nerves

The lung is densely innervated by sensory nerves (Widdicombe, 1976) which are involved in reflexes to protect the airways and maintain homeostasis under different ambient conditions. Those reflexes include coughing, changes in the rate and depth of breathing and further neuromodulatory functions which are achieved by altering the activity of the autonomic efferent system. Through the close linkage to and interaction with the efferent nerves, afferent pathways can modulate airway as well as vascular smooth muscle tone and mucus secretion.

Most of the studies that investigated the role of afferent nerves in the control of airway functions have been performed in animals and little information is available regarding the role of afferent nerve fibres in humans. Nevertheless, it appears that the majority of the sensory nerves in the lung are non-myelinated C-fibres, which not only act as afferent pathways but also are believed to contain neurotransmitters of the NANC system that can be released after activation and exhibit efferent functions. Activation of C-fibres by stimuli such as capsaicin and bradykinin causes rapid shallow breathing, preceded by apnoea, with hypotension, bradycardia, airway mucus secretion and vasodilatation, suggesting that all of these responses are part of a vagal reflex (Coleridge and Coleridge, 1984; Paintal, 1973).

Moreover, fine myelinated fibres can be identified, which originate from rapidly adapting irritant receptors as well as slowly adapting stretch receptors. Mechanical stimulation and the inhalation of irritants such as citric acid as well as non-iso-osmolal solutions activate rapidly adapting receptors that can cause coughing, alteration of breathing pattern, reflex mucus secretion and bronchoconstriction. Bronchodilation, on the other hand, may be achieved through activation of slowly adapting receptors after lung inflation.

Activation of extrapulmonary afferent pathways can modulate airway functions through interaction with the central nervous system and/or preganglionic parasympathetic fibres. While on the one hand reflex-induced bronchoconstriction can be observed in response to a variety of stimuli including hypoxia, hypercapnia and gastroesophageal reflux, bronchodilation, on the other hand, can result from hyperventilation and hypocapnia. For a more detailed review *see* Undem and Riccio, 1997; Karlsson *et al.*, 1988; Sant'Ambrogio, 1987.

PHYSIOLOGY: AUTONOMIC CONTROL OF AIRWAY FUNCTIONS

The airway calibre is predominantly determined by the mechanical balance of various forces that act upon the airways. These forces result from the tractions exerted by the lung parenchyma, airway walls and thoracic wall, as well as intrapleural and transmural pressures. The mechanical characteristics of these components depend on the structure and function or activation of cells, all of which can be modulated by neuronal and humoral mediators. The regulation and 'fine-tuning' of airway calibre is mainly determined by the bronchial tone through smooth muscle contraction or relaxation. In addition, the bronchial lumen can be affected by pulmonary blood flow, vascular permeability, cell infiltrations and airway secretions. Under normal conditions, contractile and relaxant factors maintain a sensitive balance in which the parasympathetic system appears to play the single most important role (Barnes, 1986b). The following paragraphs will give a condensed overview on the mechanisms by which the autonomic nervous system controls airway calibre through acting on bronchial and vascular smooth muscle as well as secretory cells (Table 5.1).

Table 5.1 *Regulation of airway calibre.*

Part of the autonomic nervous system	Neurotransmitter	Bronchial smooth muscle	Vascular smooth muscle	Mucus secretion	Net effect on airway calibre
Cholinergic	ACh	↑ contr.	→ dil.	↑ incr.	⎱ ⇒ decrease in airway calibre
e-NANC	SP, NKA	↑	→	↑	
Adrenergic	NA	–	←	↑	⎱ ⇒ increase in airway calibre
i-NANC	VIP	→	→	→	
	NO	→	→	←	
	NPY	→ (indir.)	←	→	

Abbreviations: e-NANC, excitatory non-adrenergic non-cholinergic; i-NANC, inhibitory non-adrenergic non-cholinergic; ACh, acetylcholine; SP, substance P; NKA, neurokinin A; NA, noradrenaline; VIP, vasoactive intestinal peptide; NPY, neuropeptide Y; contr., contraction; dil., dilatation; incr., increase; indir., indirect effect.

Autonomic innervation of airway smooth muscle

Throughout the bronchial tree, human airway smooth muscle is densely innervated by the parasympathetic system in which the cholinergic nerves represent the predominant excitatory bronchoconstricting pathway. Stimulation of the vagus nerve causes bronchoconstriction, which is inhibited by muscarinic receptor antagonists and potentiated by cholinesterase inhibitors (Nadel, 1980; Nadel and Barnes, 1984). The receptors, which mediate contraction of human airways smooth muscle, belong to the M_3-cholinoceptor subtype (Barnes, 1993; Watson *et al.*, 1995b).

Animal studies suggested a role of post-junctional M_2-receptors on airway smooth muscle cells in limiting β_2-adrenoceptor-mediated relaxation under conditions of cholinergic tone (Fernandes *et al.*, 1992; Watson and Eglen, 1994); in contrast, this M_2-receptor involvement could not be demonstrated in human airways (Watson *et al.*, 1995a).

NANC-mediated contractile responses are elicited through the release of tachykinins from sensory nerve fibre endings (see above, p. 107). Although these mediators can activate a variety of receptors (Barnes *et al.*, 1991a, b), there is evidence that tachykinin-induced contraction of human airways is mediated only by NK_2-receptors (Sheldrick *et al.*, 1995). However, there is no evidence, that under normal, i.e. non-asthmatic, conditions these pathways are likely to have important regulatory function in the control of bronchial tone (Cheung *et al.*, 1992).

Sympathetic nerves are found in close association with parasympathetic fibres and ganglia. However, the interaction of these two neural networks in airway smooth muscle is still poorly understood. The observations that the blockade of neuronal re-uptake of noradrenaline by cocaine is without effect on isolated bronchi and lung strips suggest that the sympathetic innervation plays only a minor functional role, if at all, in human airways smooth muscle (Ind *et al.*, 1983; Davis *et al.*, 1980; Zaagsma *et al.*, 1987). In accordance with these *in vitro* findings, neither noradrenaline nor infusion of selective α-adrenoceptor agonists produced significant effects *in vivo* (Larsson *et al.*, 1986), although α-adrenergic receptors have been found on airway smooth muscle. The adrenoceptors on airway smooth muscle are entirely of the β_2-receptor subtype (Carstairs *et al.*, 1985), which is consistent with the functional studies. However, it seems that under normal conditions the contribution of β_2-adrenoceptors to the regulation of airway tone is of minor importance.

Inhibitory NANC responses were first described in guinea pig airways, but in human airways also electrical field stimulation can lead to a propranolol-resistant (non-adrenergic), neurally-mediated relaxation of bronchial smooth muscle (Richardson and Beland, 1976; Davis *et al.*, 1980). However, in comparison to the pronounced i-NANC responses in guinea-pig airways, i-NANC responses in human tissue are rather small. Nevertheless, *in vitro* studies in humans suggest a possible involvement of the i-NANC system in the regulation of bronchial tone, while its *in vivo* function and relative importance are still to be determined.

It has been suggested that VIP is an important mediator of the i-NANC system given that it relaxes isolated strips of human bronchus, pulmonary artery and lung parenchyma (Saga and Said, 1984). Palmer *et al.* (1986a) showed that the VIP-induced bronchial relaxation *in vitro* is not altered by propranolol or indomethacine and suggested a direct effect of this peptide on airway smooth muscle. The same group failed to confirm a bronchodilating effect of infused VIP in normal subjects *in vivo* (Palmer *et al.*, 1986b), whereby the dosage was limited by cardiovascular side-effects. However, in asthmatic patients bronchodilation was observed after infusion of VIP (Morice and Sever, 1986). While inhalation of VIP had no significant bronchodilating effect and only a weak bronchoprotective effect (Barnes and Dixon, 1984) and the former was thought to be due to immediate metabolism of VIP by resident enzymes.

Although the above-mentioned studies showed small bronchodilating effects of VIP in human bronchi, it seems rather unlikely that it is the major mediator of i-NANC responses in airway smooth muscle, as was initially speculated. Belvisi *et al.* (1992a) showed that an increase in VIP concentrations – by inhibition of its degrading enzyme – significantly potentiated its relaxing effect, but did not alter i-NANC responses. Furthermore, they suggested that instead NO might be a more important mediator, as i-NANC responses are blocked by the NOS inhibitor L-NAME (Belvisi *et al.*, 1992a,b).

While NO and VIP are co-localized to cholinergic nerves, another potential mediator of i-NANC responses, NPY, is co-localized to adrenergic nerve endings. Interestingly, NPY inhibits cholinergic contractions induced by EFS in human isolated bronchi in a dose-dependent way, whereby this effect can be enhanced by phosphoramidon, an inhibitor of the enzyme neutral endopeptidase that degrades NPY. Since the same study showed that NPY neither affected resting tension nor the response to exogenously applied acetylcholine the authors suggested an indirect effect of NPY on airway smooth muscle by inhibiting the release of acetylcholine from nerve endings (Fujiwara *et al.*, 1993), most likely through presynaptic NPY_2 receptors (Gehlert, 1994).

Mediators of the NANC system are likely to modulate not only the cholinergic system, but there is also evidence that excitatory, bronchoconstricting as well as inhibitory, bronchodilating NANC responses interact with the adrenergic system. Activation of prejunctional β_2-adrenoceptors by salbutamol and aformoterol was shown to regulate the release of tachykinins from airway sensory nerves, causing a decrease in e-NANC contractile responses in guinea-pig airways (Verleden *et al.*, 1993). Since regulation of bronchial tone by the NANC system is more important in guinea-pig than in human airways, it is not surprising that similar data have not been obtained in human tissues so far. However, in isolated human airways the type 4 selective, cAMP-specific phosphodiesterase inhibitor rolipram enhanced i-NANC responses (Fernandes *et al.*, 1994), suggesting that also other drugs that cause an elevation of cAMP, such as β_2-adrenoceptor agonists, might be able to alter NANC responses in human airways.

Autonomic innervation of vascular smooth muscle

The autonomic innervation of airway vascular smooth muscle and its functional role in the regulation of pulmonary and/or bronchial blood flow are difficult to discuss on the basis of available data. Histological studies cannot clearly localize receptors to vascular smooth muscle cells and/or the endothelium and often do not differentiate between bronchial and pulmonary vasculature. The investigation of differentiation between pulmonary and bronchial blood flow in human beings under normal conditions, for obvious reasons, is rather difficult. Therefore, most of the functional data are limited to *in vivo* studies in animals, which cannot clearly distinguish between pulmonary or bronchial circulation, or *in vitro* findings in isolated human and animal pulmonary arteries.

According to animal studies, the vasculature is predominantly controlled by the adrenergic and peptidergic nervous system (Widdicombe, 1991). However, at present there is still no information regarding the innervation of airway vascular smooth muscle in humans. The only exception is the observation that no acetylcholinesterase-positive nerve fibres were found in connection with the blood vessels (Partanen *et al.*, 1982).

Despite the lack of cholinergic nerves distributed directly to the pulmonary vasculature, acetylcholine as well as VIP and PACAP have been shown to cause vasodilatation (Cardell *et al.*, 1997). However, the effects of both acetylcholine and PACAP were endothelium-dependent, in contrast to VIP-induced dilatation (Cardell *et al.*, 1997). These functional findings are in accordance with the demonstration of numerous VIP (Carstairs and Barnes, 1986b) but no muscarinic (Mak and Barnes, 1990) receptors on vascular smooth muscle, indicating an indirect action through the endothelium. The muscarinic receptors involved in the endothelium-dependent, acetylcholinesterase-induced vasodilatation of human pulmonary artery have been shown to be predominantly of the M_3 subtype (Barnes, 1993; Walch et al., 1999).

In accordance with the anatomically described sympathetic innervation of the vasculature, stimulation of these nerves leads to release of noradrenaline and neuropeptide Y, both of which can cause vasoconstriction (Widdicombe, 1991, 1998). Furthermore, the involvement of the adrenergic system in the regulation of pulmonary blood flow is supported by the observation that α-adrenoceptors mediate constriction of blood vessels in animals (Matran, 1991) while β-adrenergic agonists led to an increase in airway blood flow in humans (Onorato et al., 1994). However, neither α- nor β-receptor blockade significantly effected airway blood flow, at least under resting conditions (Baile et al., 1987).

Stimulation of the vagus nerve results in airway vasodilatation (Laitinen et al., 1987), which cannot completely be blocked by atropine; therefore it is likely to be caused by co-release of e-NANC neurotransmitters such as substance P (SP), CGRP and neurokinins A and B (Laitinen et al., 1987; Matran et al., 1989; Martling et al., 1989). Moreover, also mediators of the i-NANC system such as NO (Barnes, 1996) and VIP might contribute to this vasodilatation, whereas neuropeptide Y, as mentioned above, can cause vasoconstriction (Widdicombe, 1998).

In addition, airway vascular tone can be influenced by cardiac and chemoreceptor reflexes as well as by local axon reflexes through stimulation of sensory nerves in the airway mucosa (for review see Widdicombe, 1991). Until now, however, the role and relative importance of the components of the autonomic nervous system in the regulation of airway vascular tone has not been sufficiently clarified in humans under normal, physiological conditions.

Autonomic innervation of glands

Airway mucus is mainly derived from two sources, goblet and serous cells, which are localized to the surface epithelium and the sero-mucous glands in the subepithelial layer. Mucus-secreting cells of the epithelium are found predominantly in the proximal airways and less frequently in bronchioli with less than 1 mm in diameter (Cerkez et al., 1986a,b). The submucosal glands are mainly located to the proximal airways below the surface epithelium. In the proximal airways, where secretions can easily be coughed up, the volume of gland to epithelial secretion is 40:1 (Reid, 1954). In the more distal, non-cartilaginous airways goblet cells are more numerous than submucosal glands and secretions within the airway cannot be cleared as easily. Therefore, even small alterations in the amount or viscosity of goblet cell secretions are capable of exerting pronounced effects on airway calibre.

In contrast to the goblet cells, which lack cholinergic innervation (Partanen et al., 1982; Sheppard et al., 1983), the submucosal glands are predominantly innervated (Laitinen et al., 1985) and regulated (Baker et al., 1985) by cholinergic nerves, but also scarcely by adrenergic nerve fibres (Laitinen et al., 1985) as well as the NANC system (Baker et al., 1985). However, cholinergic receptors are found on both submucosal glands and epithelium. Therefore, it is not surprising, that mucus secretion can be altered by acetylcholine as well as the muscarinic receptor antagonist atropine. In vitro experiments not only support the notion that mucus secretion in human bronchus is predominantly regulated by cholinergic nerves but also that neither adrenergic nor NANC nerves have a direct action on bronchial secretory cells in humans (Sturgess and Reid, 1972; Pack et al., 1984; Baker et al., 1985).

Besides cholinergic innervation, there are also data available that demonstrated the presence of adrenergic and NANC nerves around glands (Pack and Richardson, 1984; Lundberg *et al.*, 1984b), the localization of β-adrenoceptors and SP receptors to glands (Carstairs and Barnes, 1986a; Carstairs *et al.*, 1985), and the stimulation of mucus secretion by α- as well as β-adrenoceptor agonists (Phipps *et al.*, 1982) and SP (Rogers *et al.*, 1989). In addition, stimulation of sensory nerves by capsaicin – with concomitant release of tachykinins – was shown to enhance mucus secretion in human airways *in vitro* (Rogers and Barnes, 1989). Furthermore, there is evidence that the i-NANC transmitter NO stimulates submucosal secretion (Nagaki *et al.*, 1995), whilst VIP inhibits baseline secretion from mucous and serous acini in human bronchi (Coles *et al.*, 1981); and in accordance with that, VIP-containing nerves as well as VIP receptors are found around submucosal glands (Laitinen *et al.*, 1985; Carstairs and Barnes, 1986b).

Unfortunately, there is only sparse information on the neuronal control of goblet cells in human airways, although this cell type may significantly contribute to the pathological changes observed in chronic airway diseases such as asthma (Aikawa *et al.*, 1992), where large amounts of highly viscous mucus are produced which then leads to airway plugging and eventually a fatal outcome of asthma attacks. So far the clinical relevance of the *in vitro* data obtained in animal and human airways is not clear (for review *see* Rogers and Dewar, 1990; Tavakoli *et al.*, 1997).

Autonomic innervation of the airway epithelium

The airway epithelium serves as a barrier between the external environment and the lung, protecting the airways from inhaled irritants. Its substantial role in defense and control mechanisms may be reflected by the fact that efferent pathways are scarce or even absent, whereas afferent pathways and receptors for transmitters that are released from the efferent nervous system are numerous. Therefore, epithelial damage and desquamation in connection with airway inflammation and diseases such as asthma can greatly affect its role in the regulation of airway function.

The sensory nerves (Widdicombe, 1976; Chanez *et al.*, 1998), which innervate the airway epithelium, can be involved in local neuronal as well as CNS-mediated reflexes such as cough, sneezing and alteration of the breathing pattern. Excitation of afferent receptors in the epithelium initiates reflexes via the vagus, thereby affecting bronchial and vascular smooth muscle tone as well as secretory cells.

Interestingly, the bronchial epithelium in human beings is not associated with acetylcholinesterase-positive nerve fibres (Partanen *et al.*, 1982) or muscarinic receptors (Mak and Barnes, 1990). However, extra-neuronal acetylcholine as well as its synthesizing enzyme have been detected in small amounts within human airway epithelial cells (Klapproth *et al.*, 1997), whereby the physiological role of this extra-neuronal acetylcholine has not been investigated yet.

Considering acetylcholine and VIP are frequently co-localized to cholinergic nerves, it is not surprising that VIP-positive nerve fibres do not occur in the bronchial epithelium (Laitinen *et al.*, 1985) but that VIP receptors have been found in high density (Carstairs and Barnes, 1986b). Similarly, high numbers of β_2-adrenoceptors (Carstairs *et al.*, 1985) as well as their mRNA (Hamid *et al.*, 1991) have been detected, although there is no indication for a sympathetic innervation of the epithelium (Pack and Richardson, 1984). The functional role of these numerous β_2-adrenoceptors on human airway epithelial cells has so far not been fully investigated.

PATHOPHYSIOLOGY: AUTONOMIC DYSFUNCTION IN ASTHMA

Reversible airway narrowing is a characteristic symptom of asthma, while bronchial smooth muscle hyperresponsiveness as well as airway inflammation can contribute to a decrease in airway calibre. Since the autonomic nervous system regulates bronchial and vascular smooth muscle tone as well as mucus secretion, and is involved in the modulation of epithelial cell function and inflammatory cell trafficking, it has been suggested that dysfunction of the neural control might be a substantial component for the development and clinical presentation of asthma.

However, histological studies failed to show a major difference in the distribution of autonomic nerve fibres between normal and asthmatic individuals but demonstrated, in addition to various aspects of airway inflammation, alterations in the morphology of bronchial smooth muscle including hypertrophy and hyperplasia (Ebina *et al.*, 1993). It still is a point of discussion as to what degree airway inflammation and changes in smooth muscle morphology might be involved in altered bronchial smooth muscle function which is clinically reflected in increased bronchial responsiveness to bronchospasmogenic stimuli (Sterk and Bel, 1989). So far, studies aiming to investigate the nature of bronchial hyperresponsiveness and addressing the interaction between inflammation and smooth muscle cells are inconclusive. However, there is increasing evidence that the smooth muscle itself plays an important role in the development of bronchial hyperresponsiveness (Solway and Fredberg, 1997; Schmidt and Rabe, 2000) and undergoes significant functional changes after sensitization and exposure to serum from asthmatic patients (Mitchell *et al.*, 1994, 1997).

Furthermore, recent reports describe that smooth muscle cells not only exhibit contractile but also secretory functions (Johnson and Knox, 1997). Similar to the changes in contractility, the secretory function also can be altered by exposure to serum from asthmatic patients and inflammatory cytokines (Hakonarson *et al.*, 1999). Therefore, looking at the interaction between smooth muscle and inflammatory cells, it has to be considered that smooth muscle itself is able to produce and secrete pro-inflammatory cytokines and chemotaxins (Johnson and Knox, 1997) and hence contributes to airway inflammation.

Although the pathophysiological basis of asthma can be thought of as a combination of altered bronchial smooth muscle function on one hand and airway inflammation on the other, it is not clear whether inflammatory processes cause the alterations of bronchial smooth muscle or, conversely, whether the alterations in smooth muscle secretory function support or even initiate airway inflammation.

All of this could affect parts of the autonomic nervous system and owing to their neuromodulatory function, even small changes in some of the neurotransmitters and receptors might cause an imbalance that substantially affects the overall control of airway calibre. From a clinical perspective, the functional significance of receptors and neurotransmitters associated with the autonomic nervous system in asthma is primarily underlined by the fact that β_2-adrenoceptor agonists and anticholinergics are among the most widespread used anti-asthmatic drugs.

Cholinergic nervous system and asthma

Several observations suggest that an increased activity of the cholinergic nervous system plays a key role in the pathophysiology of bronchial asthma. Because airway tone is primarily regulated by the parasympathetic nervous system, it has been speculated that dysfunction of this system might lead to obstructive airways diseases such as bronchial asthma. Importantly, clinical studies have demonstrated that anticholinergic drugs effectively reverse bronchospasm in patients with either stable or acute asthma (Ward *et al.*, 1981; Gross and Skordoin, 1984). Moreover, acetylcholine is capable of affecting mucus secretion as well as pulmonary blood flow, both of which could contribute to a decrease in airway calibre observed in asthma.

One hypothesis assumes that in asthma the prejunctional autoinhibitory M_2-cholinoceptor function is impaired, leading to bronchial obstruction through an increased and uncontrolled release of acetylcholine. Several different mechanisms for loss of neuronal M_2-receptor function have been suggested, including blockade by endogenous antagonists such as eosinophil major basic protein, decreased expression of M_2-receptors following infection with viruses or exposure to pro-inflammatory cytokines such as interferon-γ (Fryer *et al.*, 1999). This M_2-dysfunction concept is supported by the observation that activation of autoinhibitory M_2-cholinoceptors inhibited reflex bronchoconstriction in non-asthmatics but not in mildly asthmatic patients (Minette *et al.*, 1989) (Fig. 5.2). Similarly, it is likely that the alteration in autoinhibitory M_2-receptors also affects secretory cells and that these changes cause enhanced mucus production and mucus plugging of the airways. Hypersecretion of airway surface liquid – as a component of obstructive airway diseases – can lead to a reduction in airway calibre. Although it is unlikely that this change alone induces severe airway obstruction, it can add to other mechanisms and amplify their effects, particularly those of smooth muscle hypercontractility.

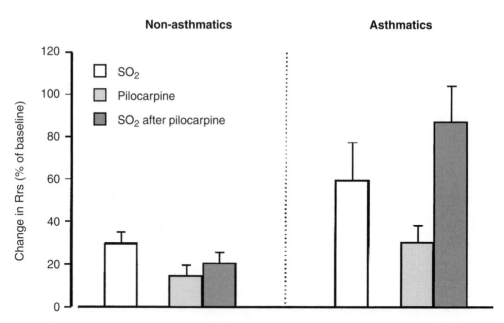

Figure 5.2 *Effect of the prejunctional M_2-muscarinic receptor agonist pilocarpine on sulphur dioxide (SO_2)-induced bronchoconstriction in non-asthmatic and asthmatic subjects (modified from Minette et al., 1989). Total respiratory resistance (Rrs) was measured in 7 non-asthmatics and 6 asthmatic patients. Airway responses to inhaled SO_2 without and after pretreatment with pilocarpine were determined and expressed as percentage of baseline values. Data shown are means ± SE. SO_2 significantly increased Rrs in the non-asthmatics and asthmatic patients (P < 0.01, for both groups). Although inhalation of pilocarpine significantly increased respiratory resistance (P < 0.05 in non-asthmatics and P < 0.01 in asthmatic patients) it also prevented SO_2-induced bronchoconstriction in the group of non-asthmatics, while a significant contractile response to SO_2 was still observed in the group of asthmatic patients (P < 0.01). Therefore, these results suggested an impaired autoinhibitory M_2-receptor function in patients with asthma.*

Adrenergic nervous system and asthma

Although the sympathetic innervation of the human lung plays only a minor role, the numerous β_2-adrenoceptors on airway smooth muscle indicate that the adrenergic system nevertheless is involved in the regulation of airway tone. This is underlined by the observation that in patients with bronchial asthma infusion of noradrenaline or phenylephrine (Larsson *et al.*, 1986) or tyramine (Ind *et al.*, 1983) – an indirect sympathomimetic agent releasing noradrenaline locally from sympathetic nerves – produced marked cardiovascular, but no bronchodilating effects. However, patients showed bronchodilation after intravenous administration of the β_2-adrenoceptor agonist salbutamol (Ind *et al.*, 1983).

Furthermore, after β-adrenoceptor blockade many asthmatic patients develop severe bronchoconstriction, whereas in normal people no significant effect on airway calibre can be observed (Zaid and Beall, 1966; Richardson and Sterling, 1969). The mechanism underlying β-adrenoceptor blockade-induced bronchoconstriction in asthmatic patients has not been identified yet. Based on the observation that in asthmatic patients propranolol-induced bronchoconstriction can be inhibited by anticholinergic pretreatment (Ind *et al.*, 1989), an indirect effect of these drugs has been postulated. On the one hand this observation might support an increased cholinergic input in patients with asthma, whereby the blockade of the subsequently upregulated adrenergic system would cause bronchoconstriction. On the other hand it led to the concept of a '*per se*' enhanced adrenergic stimulation in asthmatic patients, e.g. increased adrenaline plasma levels. However, despite widespread measurement of circulating plasma concentrations under various conditions (Warren *et al.*, 1982; Barnes *et al.*, 1982; Ind *et al.*, 1985; Dahlof *et al.*, 1988) the role and importance of adrenaline in the control of airway calibre in asthma remains uncertain.

So far, no significant differences in adrenaline and noradrenaline plasma levels have been found between normals and patients with or without exercise-induced asthma, neither under baseline conditions nor during or following exercise (Larsson *et al.*, 1982). Furthermore, adrenergic ganglion or neurone blockade as well as adrenalectomy have not been reported to result in bronchoconstriction or even in asthma. However, regardless of the limited knowledge on the function or dysfunction of β_2-adrenoceptors under normal as well as asthmatic conditions, β_2-adrenoceptor agonists belong to the most important as well as the most effective group of drugs used in the treatment of asthma.

Peptidergic, non-adrenergic non-cholinergic (NANC) nervous system and asthma

Under normal, physiological conditions the inhibitory NANC system of airways smooth muscle represents the only innervation in the human lung that has relevant bronchorelaxant function. Therefore, it is conceivable that a dysfunction of this system might lead to bronchospasm.

Previous reports suggested that the absence of VIP in the lungs of asthmatics might contribute to asthma pathogenesis and pathophysiology (Ollerenshaw *et al.*, 1989). More recent studies, however, demonstrated that the number of VIP immunoreactive nerves is not reduced in asthma, but that the number of NPY immunoreactive nerves is significantly decreased in these patients as compared to normals (Chanez *et al.*, 1998). Together with the *in vitro* finding that NPY can inhibit the release of acetylcholine (Fujiwara *et al.*, 1993), a reduction of nerves containing NPY would support the hypothesis of an increased cholinergic 'input' in asthma.

During recent years evidence has accumulated that NO might be an important neurotransmitter of the i-NANC system (Belvisi *et al.*, 1992a,b) and its role and function in asthma is still under intensive investigation and discussion (Barnes, 1996; Sanders, 1999). However, the relative importance of neuronally synthesized NO as a bronchodilator is not clear. Besides the report that human airways *in vitro* do not show basal release of NO but that its release can be initiated upon stimulation of cholinergic nerves by EFS (Ward *et al.*, 1993), there is only little published information.

Inhaled irritants as well as inflammatory mediators are believed to stimulate the e-NANC system leading to a release of neuropeptides such as SP, NKA, and CGRP (Barnes, 1991). These neuropeptides may induce so-called 'neurogenic inflammation' in the airways, which is characterized by increased vascular permeability, with subsequent plasma extravasation, and airway wall oedema, epithelial desquamation, mucus hypersecretion, and smooth muscle contraction as well as inflammatory cell infiltration (Barnes, 1991). The tachykinins can affect a number of inflammatory cells such as neutrophils, eosinophils, mast cells, dendritic cells, B and T lymphocytes, and may enhance chemotaxis, migration, cytokine production and mediator release, among other factors (Maggi, 1997). However, it has to be kept in mind that the whole concept of neurogenic inflammation has been developed in rodents, whereas in human airways there is only weak evidence for this pathomechanism (for review *see* Solway and Leff, 1991; Widdicombe, 1998).

Effects of isolated neuropeptides on airway function have been studied *in vitro*. However, the clinical implications of the findings are questionable, as under *in vivo* conditions neuropeptides are more likely to be co-released from nerve endings. Substance P, for example, primarily activates neurokinin (NK)-1 receptors (Barnes *et al.*, 1991a,b). There are reports that NK_1-receptor gene expression is increased in airways obtained from asthmatic patients compared with normal individuals (Peters *et al.*, 1992) and that SP immunoreactive nerves are more abundant in lung tissue from patients with asthma (Ollerenshaw *et al.*, 1991). However, although SP contracts isolated human bronchi *in vitro* in a dose-dependent manner (Lundberg *et al.*, 1983), it does not have an effect on lung function *in vivo* when inhaled by normals or asthmatic patients (Joos *et al.*, 1987).

Furthermore, inhalation studies have shown that NKA, an activator of NK_2-receptors, and bradykinin, which is believed to elicit release of tachykinins from sensory nerve endings, cause bronchoconstriction in patients with asthma, but not in normal individuals (Joos *et al.*, 1987; Polosa and Holgate, 1990). Despite this, however, neither NKA nor bradykinin-induced bronchoconstriction in asthmatic patients could be significantly attenuated by pretreatment with inhaled receptor antagonists that had NK_1- or NK_2-receptor selectivity (Joos *et al.*, 1996; Schmidt *et al.*, 1996). Although the potency of the antagonists may play a role, these observations suggest that released tachykinins elicit bronchoconstriction not through a single pathway. Besides NK-receptor activation, other mechanisms such as neurokinin-induced release of acetylcholine from cholinergic nerves (Joos and Pauwels, 1990), may be involved.

Apart from the involvement of sensory nerves in local reflexes – as a part of the e-NANC system – the role of afferent nerve excitation in asthma remains rather unclear. For example, stimulation of rapidly adapting receptors of the lung by citric acid induces cough, but does not cause significant bronchoconstriction, neither in asthmatic nor in normal individuals (Schmidt *et al.*, 1997; Lowry *et al.*, 1988). Probably, the afferent autonomic nervous system is more involved in sensation leading to cough and dyspnea, both of which are frequent symptoms that accompany bronchial asthma, rather than in direct bronchoconstricting mechanisms.

Initially the study of the excitatory and inhibitory NANC nervous system was focused on its regulation of bronchial tone. Meanwhile it has been noticed that NANC mediators not only have bronchoconstricting but also pro-inflammatory properties, and consequently the involvement of the NANC system in airway inflammation – as the second important component of bronchial asthma – has gained increasing interest.

The airway epithelial damage, which accompanies the asthmatic disease ultimately, causes exposure of C-fibre endings. This exposure can lead to increased sensitivity to inhaled irritants as well as to enhanced mediator release under baseline conditions. Conversely, it would be reasonable to assume that the release of neuropeptides can cause or at least enhance epithelial desquamation and shedding as observed in asthma. In response to the release of tachykinins, mucus secretion from submucosal glands and surface epithelial goblet cells could be stimulated. The importance of alterations in mucus secretion in asthma is underlined by several studies which found severe mucus plugging of peripheral airways in patients who died from asthma (Dunhill, 1960; Flora *et al.*, 1991; Shimura *et al.*, 1996; Carroll *et al.*, 1996). It has been suggested that hypertrophy and degranulation of goblet cells could be the cause of this airway plugging (Aikawa *et al.*, 1992; Shimura *et al.*, 1996).

Furthermore, activation of pulmonary C-fibre receptors by irritants and inflammatory mediators is known to produce powerful vasodilatation, mainly via sympathetic motor nerves. Besides vasodilatation and the concomitant increase in pulmonary blood flow, however, sensory neuropeptides might also lead to extravasation of plasma proteins and an increase in interstitial fluid volume, i.e. mucosal edema (Widdicombe, 1991). Thus, in addition to bronchoconstriction and mucus secretion, alterations within the pulmonary vascular system have to be taken into account as factors that contribute to the pathological changes observed in asthma.

In addition, neuropeptides might be involved in the increase in bronchial responsiveness which can be observed in asthma. In contrast to normals, patients with asthma can develop severe bronchoconstriction to inhaled stimuli, such as histamine, adenosine, cold air, exercise and others. The lack of correlation between the degrees of responsiveness against these stimuli suggests different bronchoconstricting pathways. Stimuli such as histamine, but also methacholine and leukotrienes, are considered direct challenges, since they exhibit their action through receptor stimulation, while indirect challenges, which are believed to be even more specific for asthma (Avital *et al.*, 1995), such as exercise tests and cold air inhalation, might involve reflex activation of cholinergic pathways through a release of neuropeptides from afferent nerve endings (Spina *et al.*, 1998). Therefore, an increase in the activity and/or sensitivity of these sensory nerves could contribute to the changes in airway hyperresponsiveness in asthma.

SUMMARY AND CONCLUDING REMARKS

The two most important systems in the regulation of airway calibre under normal conditions appear to be the bronchoconstricting cholinergic and the bronchorelaxing i-NANC system. Stimulation of cholinergic nerves can result in a decrease in airway lumen through bronchoconstriction, mucus hypersecretion and vasodilatation while the i-NANC system is capable of counteracting these effects. Under normal conditions, excitatory and inhibitory pathways are in balance to establish normal airway function and calibre, whereby this balance serves as a 'regulatory buffer' to enable the airways to interact with and respond to various (irritative) stimuli, without obvious alterations in airway functions.

One hypothesis suggests that an imbalance in the autonomic nervous system is involved in the pathophysiology of bronchial asthma, with a dominating cholinergic control and/or a diminished activity of the counteracting systems. So far, there is no clear evidence for alterations within the direct bronchodilating components, such as plasma adrenaline, β-adrenoceptor function, VIP and (neuronal) NO concentrations as well as in the number of

VIP- and NO-containing nerves. However, current data suggest that the imbalance might be related to an increased cholinergic input. Dysfunction of prejunctional muscarinic M_2-receptors (Minette *et al.*, 1989) as well as a decrease in the number of NPY immunoreactive nerves (Chanez *et al.*, 1998) have been observed in patients with asthma. Both alterations could lead to an increase in acetylcholine release through impaired negative feedback mechanisms at cholinergic nerve endings (Fig. 5.3).

The role of the NANC system, especially in the regulation of airway calibre in asthma, is far from being completely understood (Widdicombe, 1998). It has been hypothesized that activation of sensory nerve endings with subsequent release of neuropeptides is a major contributor to the inflammatory component in asthma, causing vasodilatation, increased vascular permeability and mucus production as well as inflammatory cell influx and activation. Nevertheless, the concept of 'neurogenic inflammation', which has been established in animal models, is not well supported in human airways.

Asthma is thought of as a combination of altered bronchial smooth muscle function – including altered sensitivity and contractility as well as hypertrophy and hyperplasia – together with airway inflammation. However, there is no evidence for how the autonomic nervous system could directly alter airway smooth muscle sensitivity and contractility. Bronchial hyperresponsiveness, which is characteristic of patients with asthma, is reflected not only in increased sensitivity of the bronchi to stimuli but also in increased maximal airway narrowing as compared to normal controls. This alteration can be observed *in vivo* (Woolcock

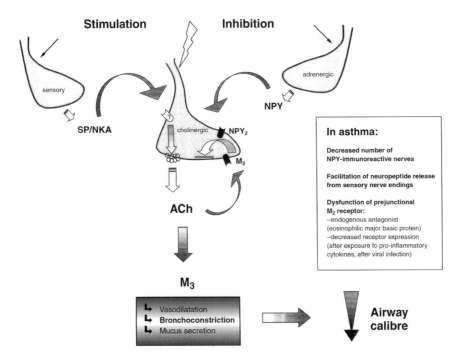

Figure 5.3 *Pathways within the autonomic nervous system which could contribute to an increased acetylcholine release from cholinergic nerves and, subsequently, to a decrease in airway calibre, which might be relevant in the pathophysiology of asthma. M_2, prejunctional, autoinhibitory muscarinic receptors, which upon stimulation inhibit acetylcholine release from cholinergic nerves; M_3, postjunctional receptors; NPY_2, prejunctional receptors for NPY; ⬦, nerve activation; ?, unknown mechanism; ⬐, inhibition of acetylcholine release. For other abbreviations, see Fig. 5.1.*

et al., 1984) as well as *ex vivo* and *in vitro*, after passive sensitization of isolated human airways (Schmidt *et al.*, 2000), and cannot be easily explained on the basis of changes in the autonomic nervous system.

Therefore, an alternative hypothesis suggests that alterations of smooth muscle cell itself are also involved in the pathogenesis of hyperresponsiveness and asthma (Schmidt and Rabe, 2000). Smooth muscle cells have been shown to be able to produce interleukins, growth factors and proinflammatory cytokines (Johnson and Knox, 1997), which could initiate, trigger and/or sustain inflammation and neuronal, facilitatory responses. Furthermore, it has been suggested that in relation to sensitization, smooth muscle cells alter their secretory function and receptor expression (Hakonarson *et al.*, 1999). Therefore, it might be speculated that the smooth muscle, in response to sensitization, would release interferon-γ (Hakonarson *et al.*, 1999), which could interact with the prejunctional M_2-receptor leading to an inhibition of its autoinhibitory function (Fryer *et al.*, 1999), and subsequently to an increased release of acetylcholine.

Despite the incomplete understanding of the role of the autonomic nervous system in asthma, current guidelines for the pharmacological treatment include substances, that interact with the autonomic nervous system, most importantly β_2-adrenoceptor agonists and muscarinic receptor antagonists. Neurokinin receptor antagonists, so far, do not play a major role in the treatment strategies and it can only be speculated that cromolyn sodium and related substances might be useful as inhibitors of mediator release from sensory nerve fibres. As a consequence, the combination of classical bronchospasmolytic drugs with those that have pronounced anti-inflammatory effects, such as corticosteroids, are currently considered as the best approach for the treatment of asthma.

Taking together, the autonomic nervous system is likely to have an important modulatory and regulatory function in the pathophysiology of asthma, but it is clearly not directly implicated in the cause of asthma. The imbalance within this system, however, appears to be a response to other factors causative for asthma, in an attempt to re-establish normal airway function.

REFERENCES

Aikawa T, Shimura S, Sasaki H, Ebina M, Takishima T. (1992) Marked goblet cell hyperplasia with mucus accumulation in the airways of patients who died of severe acute asthma attack. *Chest*, **101**, 916–21.

Avital A, Springer C, Bar-Yishay E, Godfrey S. (1995) Adenosine, methacholine, and exercise challenges in children with asthma or paediatric chronic obstructive pulmonary disease. *Thorax*, **50**, 511–16.

Baile EM, Osborne S, Pare PD. (1987) Effect of autonomic blockade on tracheobronchial blood flow. *J Appl Physiol*, **62**, 520–5.

Baker B, Peatfield AC, Richardson PS. (1985) Nervous control of mucin secretion into human bronchi. *J Physiol*, **365**, 297–305.

Barnes PJ. (1986a) Asthma as an axon reflex. *Lancet*, **1**, 242–5.

Barnes PJ. (1986b) Neural control of human airways in health and disease. *Am Rev Respir Dis*, **134**, 1289–314.

Barnes PJ. (1991) Neurogenic inflammation in airways. *Int Arch Allergy Appl Immunol*, **94**, 303–9.

Barnes PJ. (1993) Muscarinic receptor subtypes in airways. *Life Sci*, **52**, 521–8.

Barnes PJ. (1996) NO or no NO in asthma? *Thorax*, **51**, 218–20.

Barnes PJ, Baraniuk JN, Belvisi MG. (1991a) Neuropeptides in the respiratory tract. Part II. *Am Rev Respir Dis*, **144**, 1391–9.

Barnes PJ, Baraniuk JN, Belvisi MG. (1991b) Neuropeptides in the respiratory tract. Part I. *Am Rev Respir Dis*, **144**, 1187–98.

Barnes PJ, Dixon CM. (1984) The effect of inhaled vasoactive intestinal peptide on bronchial reactivity to histamine in humans. *Am Rev Respir Dis*, **130**, 162–6.

Barnes PJ, Ind PW, Brown MJ. (1982) Plasma histamine and catecholamines in stable asthmatic subjects. *Clin Sci*, **62**, 661–5.

Belvisi MG, Stretton CD, Miura M, *et al.* (1992a) Inhibitory NANC nerves in human tracheal smooth muscle: a quest for the neurotransmitter. *J Appl Physiol*, **73**, 2505–10.

Belvisi MG, Stretton CD, Yacoub MH, Barnes PJ. (1992b) Nitric oxide is the endogenous neurotransmitter of bronchodilator nerves in humans. *Eur J Pharmacol*, **210**, 221–2.

Bowden JJ, Gibbins IL. (1992) Colocalisation of neurotransmitters in autonomic neurones supplying the respiratory tract of various species, including humans. *Am Rev Respir Dis*, **145**, A259.

Bredt DS, Hwang PM, Snyder SH. (1990) Localisation of nitric oxide synthase indicating a neural role for nitric oxide. *Nature*, **347**, 768–70.

Cardell LO, Hjert O, Uddman R. (1997) The induction of nitric oxide-mediated relaxation of human isolated pulmonary arteries by PACAP. *Br J Pharmacol*, **120**, 1096–100.

Carroll N, Carello S, Cooke C, James A. (1996) Airway structure and inflammatory cells in fatal attacks of asthma. *Eur Respir J*, **9**, 709–15.

Carstairs JR, Barnes PJ. (1986a) Autoradiographic mapping of substance P receptors in lung. *Eur J Pharmacol*, **127**, 295–6.

Carstairs JR, Barnes PJ. (1986b) Visualization of vasoactive intestinal peptide receptors in human and guinea pig lung. *J Pharmacol Exp Ther*, **239**, 249–55.

Carstairs JR, Nimmo AJ, Barnes PJ. (1985) Autoradiographic visualization of beta-adrenoceptor subtypes in human lung. *Am Rev Respir Dis*, **132**, 541–7.

Cerkez V, Tos M, Mygind N. (1986a) Goblet-cell density in the human lung whole-mount study of the normal left lower lobe. *Anat Anz*, **162**, 205–213.

Cerkez V, Tos M, Mygind N. (1986b) Quantitative study of goblet cells in the upper lobe of the normal human lung. *Arch Otolaryngol Head Neck Surg*, **112**, 316–20.

Chanez P, Springall D, Vignola AM, *et al.* (1998) Bronchial mucosal immunoreactivity of sensory neuropeptides in severe airway diseases. *Am J Respir Crit Care Med*, **158**, 985–90.

Cheung D, Bel EH, den Hartigh J, Dijkman JH, Sterk PJ. (1992) The effect of an inhaled neutral endopeptidase inhibitor, thiorphan, on airway responses to neurokinin A in normal humans *in vivo*. *Am Rev Respir Dis*, **145**, 1275–80.

Cheung D, Timmers MC, Zwinderman AH, den Hartigh J, Dijkman JH, Sterk PJ. (1993) Neutral endopeptidase activity and airway hyperresponsiveness to neurokinin A in asthmatic subjects *in vivo*. *Am Rev Respir Dis*, **148**, 1467–73.

Coleridge JCG, Coleridge HMG. (1984) Afferent vagal C fibre innervation of the lungs and airways and its functional significance. *Rev Physiol Biochem Pharmacol*, **99**, 1–110.

Coles SJ, Said SI, Reid L. (1981) Inhibition by vasoactive intestinal peptide of glycoconjugate and lysozyme secretion by human airways *in vitro*. *Am Rev Respir Dis*, **124**, 531–6.

Dahlof C, Dahlof P, Lundberg JM, Strombom U. (1988) Elevated plasma concentration of neuropeptide Y and low level of circulating adrenaline in elderly asthmatics during rest and acute severe asthma. *Pulm Pharmacol*, **1**, 3–6.

Daniel EE, Kannan M, Davis C, Posey-Daniel V. (1986) Ultrastructural studies on the neuromuscular control of human tracheal and bronchial smooth muscle. *Respir Physiol*, **63**, 109–28.

Davis C, Connolly ME, Greenacre JK. (1980) Beta-adrenoceptors in human lung, bronchus and lymphocytes. *Br J Clin Pharmacol*, **10**, 425–32.

Dey RD, Shannon WA Jr, Said SI. (1981) Localization of VIP-immunoreactive nerves in airways and pulmonary vessels of dogs, cats and human subjects. *Cell Tissue Res*, **220**, 231–8.

Douglas NJ, Sudlow MF, Flenley DC. (1979) Effect of an inhaled atropinelike agent on normal airway function. *J Appl Physiol*, **46**, 256–66.

Dunhill MS. (1960) The pathology of asthma with special reference to changes in the bronchial mucosa. *J Clin Pathol*, **13**, 27–33.

Dupont L. (1999) Characterization of 5-HT receptors modulating airways smooth muscle contraction: an *in vitro* study. Catholic University Leuven, Belgie.

Ebina M, Takahashi T, Chiba T, Motomiya M. (1993) Cellular hypertrophy and hyperplasia of airway smooth muscles underlying bronchial asthma. A 3-D morphometric study. *Am Rev Respir Dis*, **148**, 720–6.

Fernandes LB, Ellis JL, Undem BJ. (1994) Potentiation of nonadrenergic noncholinergic relaxation of human isolated bronchus by selective inhibitors of phosphodiesterase isozymes. *Am J Respir Crit Care Med*, **150**, 1384–90.

Fernandes LB, Fryer AS, Hirshman CA. (1992) M_2-muscarinic receptors inhibit isoproterenol-induced relaxation of canine airway smooth muscle. *J Pharmacol Exp Ther*, **262**, 119–26.

Flora GS, Sharma AM, Sharma OP. (1991) Asthma mortality in a metropolitan county hospital, a 38-year study. *Allergy Proc*, **12**, 169–79.

Fryer AD, Adamko DJ, Yost BL, Jacoby DB. (1999) Effects of inflammatory cells on neuronal M_2 muscarinic receptor function in the lung. *Life Sci*, **64**, 449–55.

Fujiwara H, Kurihara N, Hirata K, Ohta K, Kanazawa H, Takeda T. (1993) Effect of neuropeptide Y on human bronchus and its modulation of neutral endopeptidase. *J Allergy Clin Immunol*, **92**, 89–94.

Gehlert DR. (1994) Subtypes of receptors for neuropeptide Y: implications for the targeting of therapeutics. *Life Sci*, **55**, 551–62.

Gross N, Skordoin M. (1984) Anticholinergic, antimuscarinic bronchodilators. *Am Rev Respir Dis*, **129**, 856–70.

Hakonarson H, Maskeri N, Carter C, Grunstein MM. (1999) Regulation of TH1- and TH2-type cytokine expression and action in atopic asthmatic sensitized airway smooth muscle. *J Clin Invest*, **103**, 1077–87.

Hamid QA, Mak JC, Sheppard MN, Corrin B, Venter JC, Barnes PJ. (1991) Localization of beta 2-adrenoceptor messenger RNA in human and rat lung using in-situ hybridization: correlation with receptor autoradiography. *Eur J Pharmacol*, **206**, 133–8.

Harmar AJ, Arimura A, Gozes I, *et al*. (1998) International Union of Pharmacology. XVIII. Nomenclature of receptors for vasoactive intestinal peptide and pituitary adenylate cyclase-activating polypeptide. *Pharmacol Rev*, **50**, 265–70.

Hulme EC, Birdsall JM, Buckley NJ. (1990) Muscarinic receptor subtypes. *Annu Rev Pharmacol Toxicol*, **30**, 633–73.

Ichinose M, Inoue H, Miura M, Takishima T. (1988) Non-adrenergic bronchodilation in normal subjects. *Am Rev Respir Dis*, **138**, 31–4.

Ind PW, Causon RC, Brown MJ, Barnes PJ. (1985) Circulating catecholamines in acute asthma. *Br Med J Clin Res Ed*, **290**, 267–9.

Ind PW, Dixon CMS, Fuller RW, Barnes PJ. (1989) Anticholinergic blockade of beta-blocker induced bronchoconstriction. *Am Rev Respir Dis*, **139**, 1390–4.

Ind PW, Scriven AJI, Dollery CT. (1983) Use of tyramine to probe pulmonary noradrenaline release in asthma. *Clin Sci Mol Med*, **65**, 9.

Johnson SR, Knox AJ. (1997) Synthetic functions of airway smooth muscle in asthma. *Trends Pharmacol Sci*, **18**, 288–92.

Joos GF, Pauwels RA, van der Straeten M. (1987) Effect of inhaled substance P and neurokinin A on the airways of normal and asthmatic subjects. *Thorax*, **42**, 779–83.

Joos GF, Pauwels RA. (1990) Mechanisms involved in neurokinin-induced bronchoconstriction. *Arch Int Pharmacodynamie Therapie*, **303**, 132–46.

Joos GF, Van Schoor J, Kips JC, Pauwels RA. (1996) The effect of inhaled FK224, a tachykinin NK-1 and NK-2 receptor antagonist, on neurokinin A-induced bronchoconstriction in asthmatics. *Am J Respir Crit Care Med*, **153**, 1781–4.

Karlsson JA, Sant'Ambrogio G, Widdicombe J. (1988) Afferent neural pathways in cough and reflex bronchoconstriction. *J Appl Physiol*, **65**, 1007–23.

Klapproth H, Reinheimer T, Metzen J, *et al.* (1997) Non-neuronal acetylcholine, a signalling molecule synthesized by surface cells of rat and man. *Naunyn Schmiedebergs Arch Pharmacol*, **355**, 515–23.

Laitinen A, Partanen M, Hervonen A, Pelto-Huikko M, Laitinen LA. (1985) VIP-like immunoreactive nerves in human respiratory tract. *Histochemistry*, **82**, 313–19.

Laitinen LA, Laitinen MV, Widdicombe JG. (1987) Parasympathetic nervous control of tracheal vascular resistance in the dog. *J Physiol*, **385**, 135–46.

Lammers JWJ, Minette P, McCusker MT, Chung KF, Barnes PJ. (1988) Non-adrenergic bronchodilator mechanisms in normal human subjects *in vivo*. *J Appl Physiol*, **64**, 1817–22.

Larsson K, Hjemdahl P, Martinsson A. (1982) Sympathoadrenal reactivity in exercise-induced asthma. *Chest*, **82**, 561–7.

Larsson K, Hjemdahl P, Martinsson A. (1986) Influence of circulating alpha-adrenoceptor agonists on lung function in patients with exercise-induced asthma and healthy subjects. *Thorax*, **41**, 552–8.

Lowry RH, Wood AM, Higenbottam TW. (1988) Effects of pH and osmolarity on aerosol-induced cough in normal volunteers. *Clin Sci*, **74**, 373–6.

Lundberg JM, Fahrenkrug J, Hokfelt T, *et al.* (1984a) Coexistence of peptide histidine isoleucine (PHI) and VIP in nerves regulating blood flow and bronchial smooth muscle tone in various mammals including man. *Peptides*, **5**, 593–606.

Lundberg JM, Hokfelt T, Martling CR, Saria A, Cuello C. (1984b) Substance P-immunoreactive sensory nerves in the lower respiratory tract of various mammals including man. *Cell Tissue Res*, **235**, 251–61.

Lundberg JM, Martling CR, Saria A. (1983) Substance P and capsaicin-induced contraction of human bronchi. *Acta Physiol Scand*, **119**, 49–53.

Luts A, Uddman R, Alm P, Basterra J, Sundler F. (1993) Peptide-containing nerve fibers in human airways: distribution and coexistence pattern. *Int Arch Allergy Immunol*, **101**, 52–60.

MacNee W, Douglas NJ, Sudlow MF. (1982) Effects of inhalation of beta-sympathomimetic and atropine-like drugs on airway calibre in normal subjects. *Clin Sci*, **63**, 137–43.

Maggi CA. (1997) The effects of tachykinins on inflammatory and immune cells. *Regul Pept*, **70**, 75–90.

Mak JC, Barnes PJ. (1990) Autoradiographic visualization of muscarinic receptor subtypes in human and guinea pig lung. *Am Rev Respir Dis*, **141**, 1559–68.

Mak JC.W, Baraniuk JN, Barnes PJ. (1992) Localization of muscarinic receptor subtype mRNAs in human lung. *Am J Respir Cell Mol Biol*, **7**, 344–8.

Martling CR, Matran R, Alving K, Lacroix JS, Lundberg JM. (1989) Vagal vasodilatory mechanisms in the pig bronchial circulation preferentially involves sensory nerves. *Neurosci Lett*, **96**, 306–11.

Matran R. (1991) Neural control of lower airway vasculature. Involvement of classical transmitters and neuropeptides. *Acta Physiol Scand Suppl*, **601**, 1–54.

Matran R, Alving K, Martling CR, Lacroix JS, Lundberg JM. (1989) Vagally mediated vasodilatation by motor and sensory nerves in the tracheal and bronchial circulation of the pig. *Acta Physiol Scand*, **135**, 29–37.

Minette P, Lammers JWJ, Dixon CMS, McCusker MT, Barnes PJ. (1989) A muscarinic agonist inhibits reflex bronchoconstriction in normal but not in asthmatic subjects. *J Appl Physiol*, **67**, 2461–5.

Minette PA, Barnes PJ. (1988) Prejunctional inhibitory muscarinic receptors on cholinergic nerves in human and guinea pig airways. *J Appl Physiol*, **64**, 2532–7.

Mitchell RW, Rabe KF, Magnussen H, Leff AR. (1997) Passive sensitization of human airways induces myogenic contractile responses *in vitro*. *J Appl Physiol*, **83**, 1276–81.

Mitchell RW, Rühlmann E, Magnussen H, Leff AR, Rabe KF. (1994) Passive sensitization of human bronchi augments smooth muscle shortening velocity and capacity. *Am J Physiol*, **267**, 218–22.

Morice AH, Sever PS. (1986) Vasoactive intestinal peptide as a bronchodilator in severe asthma. *Peptides*, **7**, 279–80.

Nadel JA. (1980) Autonomic regulation of airway smooth muscle. In: Nadel JA, ed. *Physiology and pharmacology of the airways*. New York: Dekker, 215–57.

Nadel JA, Barnes PJ. (1984) Autonomic regulation of the airways. *Ann Rev Med*, **35**, 451–67.

Nagaki M, Shimura MN, Irokawa T, Sasaki T, Shirato K. (1995) Nitric oxide regulation of glycoconjugate secretion from feline and human airways *in vitro*. *Respir Physiol*, **102**, 89–95.

Ollerenshaw S, Jarvis D, Woolcock A, Sullivan C, Scheibner T. (1989) Absence of immunoreactive vasoactive intestinal polypeptide in tissue from the lungs of patients with asthma. *N Engl J Med*, **320**, 1244–8.

Ollerenshaw SL, Jarvis DL, Sullivan CE, Woolcock AJ. (1991) Substance P immunoreactive nerves in airways from asthmatics and non-asthmatics. *Eur Respir J*, **4**, 673–82.

Onorato DJ, Demirozu MC, Breitenbucher A, Atkins ND, Chediak AD, Wanner A. (1994) Airway mucosal blood flow in humans. Response to adrenergic agonists. *Am J Respir Crit Care Med*, **149**, 1132–7.

Pack RJ, Richardson PS. (1984) The aminergic innervation of the human bronchus: a light and electron microscopic study. *J Anat*, **138**, 493–502.

Pack RJ, Williams IP, Phipps RJ, Richardson PS, Riche B. (1984) A preparation for the study of secretory function of the human bronchus *in vitro*. *Eur J Respir Dis*, **65**, 239–50.

Paintal AS. (1973) Vagal sensory receptors and their reflex effects. *Physiol Rev*, **53**, 159–227.

Palmer JB, Cuss FM, Barnes PJ. (1986a) VIP and PHM and their role in nonadrenergic inhibitory responses in isolated human airways. *J Appl Physiol*, **61**, 1322–8.

Palmer JB, Cuss FM, Warren JB, Blank M, Bloom SR, Barnes PJ. (1986b) Effect of infused vasoactive intestinal peptide on airway function in normal subjects. *Thorax*, **41**, 663–6.

Partanen M, Laitinen A, Hervonen A, Toivanen M, Laitinen LA. (1982) Catecholamine and acetylcholinesterase containing nerves in human lower respiratory tract. *Histochemistry*, **76**, 175–88.

Peters MJ, Adcock IM, Gelder CM, *et al*. (1992) NK$_1$ receptor gene expression is increased in asthmatic lung and reduced by corticosteroids. *Am Rev Respir Dis*, **145**, A835.

Phipps RJ, Williams IP, Richardson PS, Pell J, Pack RH, Wright N. (1982) Sympathomimetic drugs stimulate the output of secretory glycoprotein from human bronchi *in vitro*. *Clin Sci*, **63**, 23–8.

Polosa R, Holgate ST. (1990) Comparative airway response to inhalted bradykinin, kallidin and [des-Arg9]bradykinin in normal and asthmatic subjects. *Am Rev Respir Dis*, **142**, 1367–71.

Reid L. (1954) Pathology of chronic bronchitis. *Lancet*, **i**, 275–8.

Richardson J, Beland J. (1976) Nonadrenergic inhibitory nervous system in human airways. *J Appl Physiol*, **41**, 764–71.

Richardson J, Fergusson CC. (1979) Neuromuscular structure and function in the airways. *Fed Proc*, **38**, 202–8.

Richardson JB. (1981) Nonadrenergic inhibitory nervous system in human airways. *Lung*, **159**, 315–22.

Richardson PS, Sterling GM. (1969) Effects of beta adrenergic receptor blockade on airway conductance and lung volume in normal and asthmatic subjects. *BMJ*, **3**, 143–5.

Rogers DF, Aursudkij B, Barnes PJ. (1989) Effects of tachykinins on mucus secretion in human bronchi *in vitro*. *Eur J Pharmacol*, **174**, 283–6.

Rogers DF, Barnes PJ. (1989) Opioid inhibition of neurally mediated mucus secretion in human bronchi. *Lancet*, **1**, 930–2.

Rogers DF, Dewar A. (1990) Neural control of airway mucus secretion. *Biomed Pharmacother*, **44**, 447–53.

Saga T, Said SI. (1984) Vasoactive intestinal peptide relaxes isolated strips of human bronchus, pulmonary artery, and lung parenchyma. *Trans Assoc Am Physicians*, **97**, 304–10.

Sanders SP. (1999) Nitric oxide in asthma. Pathogenic, therapeutic, or diagnostic? *Am J Respir Cell Mol Biol*, **21**, 147–9.

Sant'Ambrogio G. (1987) Afferent nerves in reflex bronchoconstriction. *Bull Eur Physiopathol Respir*, **23**, 81S–88S.

Schmidt D, Jorres RA, Rabe KF, Magnussen H. (1996) Reproducibility of airway response to inhaled bradykinin and effect of the neurokinin receptor antagonist FK-224 in asthmatic subjects. *Eur J Clin Pharmacol*, **50**, 269–73.

Schmidt D, Jörres RA, Magnussen H. (1997) Citric acid-induced cough thresholds in normal subjects, patients with bronchial asthma, and smokers. *Eur J Med Res*, **2**, 384–8.

Schmidt D, Watson N, Ruehlmann E, Magnussen H, Rabe KF. (2000) Serum IgE levels predict human airway reactivity *in vitro*. *Clin Exp Allergy*, **30**, 233–41.

Schmidt D, Rabe KF. (2000) Immune mechanisms of smooth muscle hyperreactivity in asthma. *J Allergy Clin Immunol*, **105**, 673–82.

Sheldrick RLG, Rabe KF, Fischer A, Magnussen H, Coleman RA. (1995) Further evidence that tachykinin-induced contraction of human isolated bronchus is mediated only by NK$_2$-receptors. *Neuropeptides*, **29**, 281–92.

Sheppard MN, Kurian SS, Henzen-Logmans SC, *et al.* (1983) Neurone-specific enolase and S-100: new markers for delineating the innervation of the respiratory tract in man and other mammals. *Thorax*, **38**, 333–40.

Shimura S, Andoh Y, Haraguchi M, Shirato K. (1996) Continuity of airway goblet cells and intraluminal mucus in the airways of patients with bronchial asthma. *Eur Respir J*, **9**, 1395–401.

Solway J, Leff AR. (1991) Sensory neuropeptides and airway function. *J Appl Physiol*, 71, 2077–87.

Solway J, Fredberg JJ. (1997) Perhaps airway smooth muscle dysfunction contributes to asthmatic bronchial hyperresponsiveness after all. *Am J Respir Cell Mol Biol*, **17**, 144–6.

Spencer H, Leof D. (1964) The innervation of the human lung. *J Anat*, **98**, 599–609.

Spina D, Page CP. (1996) Airway sensory nerves in asthma – targets for therapy? *Pulm Pharmacol*, **9**, 1–18.

Spina D, Shah S, Harrison S. (1998) Modulation of sensory nerve function in the airways. *Trends Pharmacol Sci*, **19**, 460–6.

Sterk PJ, Bel EH. (1989) Bronchial hyperresponsiveness: the need for a distinction between hypersensitivity and excessive airway narrowing. *Eur Respir J*, **2**, 267–74.

Sturgess J, Reid L. (1972) An organ culture study of the effect of drugs on the secretory activity of the human bronchial submucosal gland. *Clin Sci*, **43**, 533–43.

Tavakoli S, Levine SJ, Shelhamer JH. (1997) Airway mucus secretion. In: Barnes PJ, Grunstein MM, Leff AR, Woolcock AJ, eds. *Asthma*, 1st edn. Philadelphia: Lippincott-Raven, 834–57.

Uddman R, Sundler F. (1987) Neuropeptides in the airways: a review. *Am Rev Respir Dis*, **136**, S3–S8.

Undem BJ, Riccio MM. (1997) Activation of airway afferent nerves. In: Barnes PJ, Grunstein MM, Leff AR, Woolcock AJ, eds. *Asthma*, 1st edn. Philadelphia: Lippincott-Raven, 843–57.

van Koppen CJ, Blankensteijn WM, Klaassen ARM, Rodrigues de Miranda F, Beld AJ, van Ginneken CAM. (1987) Autoradiographic visualization of muscarinic receptors in human bronchi. *J Pharmacol Exp Ther*, **244**, 760–4.

Verleden GM, Belvisi MG, Rabe KF, Miura M, Barnes PJ. (1993) Beta 2-adrenoceptor agonists inhibit NANC neural bronchoconstrictor responses *in vitro*. *J Appl Physiol*, **74**, 1195–9.

Walch L, Norel X, Leconte B, Gascard JP, Brink C. (1999) Cholinergic control of human and animal pulmonary vascular tone. *Therapie*, **54**, 99–102.

Ward JK, Belvisi MG, Fox AJ, *et al.* (1993) Modulation of cholinergic bronchoconstrictor responses by endogenous nitric oxide and vasoactive intestinal peptide in human airways *in vitro*. *J Clin Invest*, **92**, 736–42.

Ward M, Rentem P, Roderick Smith W, Davies D. (1981) Ipratropium bromide in acute asthma. *BMJ*, **282**, 598–600.

Warren JB, Keynes RJ, Brown MJ, Jenner DA, McNicol MW. (1982) Blunted sympathoadrenal response to exercise in asthmatic subjects. *Br J Dis Chest*, **76**, 147–50.

Watson N, Eglen RM. (1994) Effect of muscarinic M$_2$ and M$_3$ receptor stimulation and antagonism on responses to isoprenaline of guinea-pig trachea *in vitro*. *Br J Pharmacol*, **112**, 179–87.

Watson N, Magnussen H, Rabe KF. (1995a) Antagonism of β-adrenoceptor-mediated relaxations of human bronchial smooth muscle by carbachol. *Eur J Pharmacol*, **275**, 307–10.

Watson N, Magnussen H, Rabe KF. (1995b) Pharmacological characterization of the muscarinic receptor subtype mediating contraction of human peripheral airways. *J Pharmacol Exp Ther*, **274**, 1293–7.

Widdicombe JG. (1976) Modes of excitation of respiratory tract receptors. *Prog Brain Res*, **43**, 243–52.

Widdicombe JG. (1991) Neural control of airway vasculature and edema. *Am Rev Respir Dis*, **143**, S18–S21.

Widdicombe JG. (1998) Autonomic regulation. i-NANC/e-NANC. *Am J Respir Crit Care Med*, **158**, S171–S175.

Woolcock AJ, Salome CM, Yan K. (1984) The shape of the dose–response curve to histamine in asthmatic and normal subjects. *Am Rev Respir Dis*, **130**, 71–5.

Yoshihara S, Linden A, Kashimoto K, Nagano Y, Ichimura T, Nadel JA. (1997) Long lasting smooth muscle relaxation by a novel PACAP analogue in guinea-pig and primate airways *in vitro*. *Br J Pharmacol*, **121**, 1730–4.

Zaagsma J, van Amsterdam RGM, Brouwer F, Watson N, Magnussen H, Rabe KF. (1987) Adrenergic control of airway function. *Am Rev Respir Dis*, **136**, S45–S50.

Zaid G, Beall GN. (1966) Bronchial response to beta-adrenergic blockade. *N Engl J Med*, **275**, 580–4.

6

Inflammatory mediators and cytokines in asthma

TAK H. LEE AND CATHERINE M. HAWRYLOWICZ

INTRODUCTION

Many different inflammatory mediators have been implicated in the pathogenesis of asthma and bronchial hyperresponsiveness (BHR). Major advances have been made in the understanding of their biochemistry and biology. Sensitive assays for their identification have been introduced and, most importantly, specific antagonists have been developed. However, there is still uncertainty about the role of individual mediators in asthma and in their complex interactions.

Inflammatory mediators produce their effects by activation of specific cell surface receptors (Barnes, 1990), resulting in a complex cascade of signalling events (Nishizuka, 1992). These receptors are also proving to be of increasing interest for the development of novel therapeutic antagonists.

CELLULAR ORIGIN OF MEDIATORS

The release of mediators from mast cells has been assumed to play a central role in the pathogenesis of asthma. Thus, the action of mast cells and release of histamine, leukotrienes and prostaglandins may account for the immediate bronchial response to allergen, exercise, cold air and fog. Recent evidence, however, argues against the critical involvement of mast cells in BHR or in the continuing inflammation of asthmatic airways. Although disodium cromoglycate, which is clinically efficacious, was shown to stabilize rat mast cells, more potent mast cell stabilizers failed to show any clinically useful effect. Furthermore, β-adrenoceptor agonists, which are potent stabilizers of human mast cells, fail to inhibit late asthmatic responses following allergen challenge or to reduce BHR. By contrast, acute administration of corticosteroids has no mast cell stabilizing action and fails to inhibit the early response but is very effective in inhibiting the late response and in preventing the subsequent BHR.

Macrophages are present throughout the respiratory tract and may be activated by IgE-dependent mechanisms acting through both the high and low affinity receptors for IgE, FcεRI and FcεRII (Joseph et al., 1983; Maurer et al., 1994). However other stimuli including immune complexes, pro-inflammatory cytokines and T-cell interactions are also likely to be important. Increased numbers of MHC (major histocompatibility complex) class II positive, immature macrophages are observed in the pulmonary mucosa of asthmatic patients (Poston et al., 1992) and may contribute to the synthesis of pro-inflammatory mediators, tissue damage and the presentation of allergen to T lymphocytes resulting in increased lymphokine production. Macrophages are characterized by their capacity to synthesize large quantities of a broad array of mediators. Cells from asthmatic patients release increased amounts of mediators such as thromboxane, prostaglandins, leukotriene C_4 (LTC_4), platelet activating factor (PAF), chemokines and cytokines, including IL-1, IL-6, tumour necrosis factor (TNF) and granulocyte-macrophage colony stimulating factor (GM-CSF) which plays a central role in eosinophil survival and function and regulation of antigen presentation. Macrophages have the capacity to synthesize both pro- and antiinflammatory cytokines depending upon the nature of the stimulus and alveolar macrophages from asthmatic individuals reportedly synthesize decreased amounts of the deactivating cytokine interleukin (IL-)10 (Borish et al., 1996). Inhaled corticosteroids alter the balance of pro- and antiinflammatory cytokine expression, increasing IL-10 production by alveolar macrophages in asthma (John et al., 1998).

Eosinophil infiltration is a prominent feature of asthmatic airways. Allergen inhalation results in a marked increase in eosinophils in bronchoalveolar lavage (BAL) fluid at the time of the late reaction and there is a relationship between peripheral blood eosinophilia and BHR (Frigas and Gleich, 1986). Eosinophils release a variety of membrane-derived mediators, including LTC_4 and PAF, and granule-associated proteins such as major basic protein and eosinophil cationic protein, which are toxic to airway epithelium. Activated eosinophils in the airway lumen may thus lead to the epithelial damage that is characteristic of severe asthma. Eosinophils, and mast cells, have however also been shown to synthesize and store or secrete a number of cytokines, notably the Th2 cytokines IL-4 and IL-5 (Kay et al., 1997). Eosinophils also synthesize chemokines such as IL-8, MIP-1α (macrophage inflammatory problem), RANTES (regulated upon activation, normal T-cell expressed and secreted) and monocyte chemoattractant protein (MCP)-1 which are inhibited by glucocorticoids (reviewed by Weller, 1997).

While neutrophil infiltration of the airways is a feature of some animal models of asthma, the role of neutrophils in human asthma is less certain. However, high numbers of neutrophils and increased amounts of neutrophil chemoattractant, IL-8, have been described in acute severe asthma (Ondonez et al., 2000). In some animal models, neutrophil infiltration follows the development of increased responsiveness and neutrophil depletion does not affect the development of BHR.

T lymphocytes are also prominent in asthmatic airways. They may release a variety of lymphokines, which are important in perpetuating the allergic inflammatory response (Busse et al., 1995). Thus, IL-3 is important in differentiating mast cells, whereas GM-CSF, IL-3 and IL-5 may be important in maintaining eosinophil survival in the tissue and augmenting its pro-inflammatory function (Yamaguchi et al., 1988). IL-4 is critical for B-cell activation for synthesis of IgE production. IL-13 is a newly described T-cell-derived cytokine with similar functions to IL-4 that regulates B-cell, monocyte and endothelial cell functions. A significant increase in IL-13 mRNA and secreted protein was detected in BAL fluid from allergen, but not saline challenged patients with asthma (Huang *et al.*, 1995).

The pulmonary epithelium is increasingly recognized as an important source of pro-inflammatory cytokines in asthma. The increased expression of a number of cytokines in this tissue in asthma has been described and these include GM-CSF (Sousa *et al.*, 1993), monocyte chemoattractant protein (MCP)-1 (Sousa *et al.*, 1994), the eosinophil-specific chemo-attractant eotaxin (Ying *et al.*, 1997; Lamkhioued *et al.*, 1997), the T-cell chemoattractant IL-16, (Laberge *et al.*, 1997), the pro-inflammatory cytokine IL-1β and its natural antagonist, IL-1 receptor antagonist (IL-1ra). Most are inhibited following inhalation of glucocorticoids, although expression of the inhibitor molecule, IL-1ra, remains unaffected (Sousa *et al.*, 1997). Bronchial epithelial cells have recently been reported to express the high affinity receptor for IgE (Campbell *et al.*, 1998) and may therefore interact directly with inhaled allergens.

INFLAMMATORY MEDIATORS

The production of the different mediators that have been implicated in the pathogenesis of asthma can account for many of the pathological features of the disease. Thus, mediators such as histamine, chemotactic factors, prostaglandins and leukotrienes contract airway smooth muscle, increase microvascular leakage, increase mucus secretion and attract other inflammatory cells. Interactions among different inflammatory mediators might account for BHR. For instance, prostaglandin D_2 (PGD_2) potentiates the bronchoconstrictor response to histamine and cholinergic agonists in asthmatics (Fuller *et al.*, 1986). This effect is transient and is therefore unlikely to account for the sustained BHR found in asthmatic patients (Arm *et al.*, 1988a), whereas PAF causes a sustained increase in bronchial responsiveness in normal but not in asthmatic individuals (Cuss *et al.*, 1986). Recent studies involving both animals and humans are increasingly implicating a role not only for cytokines but also for members of the chemokine superfamily in cellular recruitment and activation in asthma.

Histamine

Histamine has been implicated in asthma since the finding that infusion of histamine intravenously mimics anaphylaxis in animals and was later shown to cause bronchoconstriction in asthmatic people. There is evidence for histamine release in asthmatic patients after experimental provocation, including exercise and allergen bronchial challenge, as indicated by elevated sputum, BAL fluid and plasma concentrations of histamine (Lee *et al.*, 1982a). However, interpretation of plasma histamine measurements is difficult and it has been suggested that most of the reported changes reflect release from circulating basophils, rather than from airway mast cells. Recent studies *in vitro* suggest that in addition histamine release is also induced by chemokines (Dahinden *et al.*, 1994).

Inhaled histamine causes bronchoconstriction *in vivo* and contraction of large and small human airways *in vitro* by activating H_1-receptors. In addition, histamine may stimulate irritant receptors in the airway epithelium, causing reflex bronchoconstriction. In human airways there is no evidence for the H_2-receptor-mediated bronchodilatation that has been reported in other species. H_2-receptors that inhibit further release of histamine have been described in human basophils, but not in pulmonary mast cells, and there is no evidence that H_2-receptor antagonists cause any worsening of asthma. Histamine also causes airway mucosal oedema and plasma extravasation by an H_1-mediated contraction of endothelial cells in postcapillary venules, thus increasing microvascular permeability. H_3-receptors, which inhibit cholinergic and non-cholinergic excitatory nerves in airways, have also been described

(Ichinose *et al.*, 1989). These receptors, which are very sensitive to histamine, inhibit neural bronchoconstriction and therefore may serve to limit the bronchoconstriction caused by histamine release.

Despite the fact that histamine is probably produced in asthmatic airways and has several effects on airway function that might contribute to the pathology of asthma, there is little evidence that antihistamines give significant improvement in clinical asthma.

Leukotrienes

Since the identity of slow-reacting substance of anaphylaxis (SRS-A) was shown to be a mixture of LTC_4, LTD_4 and LTE_4 there has been a substantial increase in the knowledge about the synthesis, release and biological effects of these potent mediators. Arachidonic acid (AA) released from membrane phospholipids during cell activation may be oxidatively metabolized by the enzymes of the lipoxygenase or cyclooxygenase pathways (Fig. 6.1) The 5-lipoxygenase

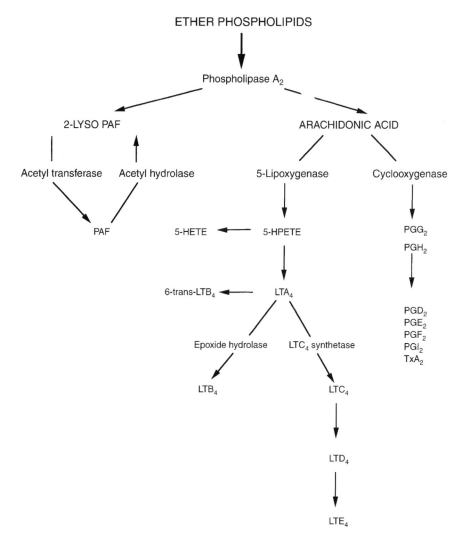

Figure 6.1 *The synthetic pathways for the synthesis of platelet activating factor (PAF-acether), leukotrienes (LT) and prostaglandins (PG). 5-HPETE, 5-hydroperoxyeicosatetraenoic acid; Tx, thromboxane.*

pathway generates 5-hydroperoxyeicosatetraenoic acid (5-HPETE) or is converted enzymatically to the unstable intermediate LTA_4, which is metabolized by an epoxide hydrolase to LTB_4, or by a glutathione-S-transferase, termed LTC_4 synthase, to LTC_4. The latter is cleaved by γ-glutamyl-transpeptidase to LTD_4, which is converted by a dipeptidase to LTE_4.

LTB_4 is a potent chemoattractant for neutrophils, while the sulphidopeptide leukotrienes (LTC_4, LTD_4 and LTE_4) are potent spasmogens for non-vascular smooth muscle and cause mucus secretion and capillary leak. The contribution of leukotrienes to the pathophysiology of bronchial asthma is suggested by their presence in the airways of asthmatic patients at rest and following allergen challenge, and by their potent bronchoconstrictor properties *in vitro* and *in vivo* (Samuelsson, 1983).

Functional studies with LTC_4 and LTD_4 indicate that there are probably discrete receptors for each of them, whereas LTE_4 may bind to the LTD_4 receptor. Recently, human and murine G-protein coupled receptors specific for LTB_4 have been characterized at the biological and molecular levels (Yokomizo *et al.*, 1997; Huang *et al.*, 1998). Sulphidopeptide leukotrienes are potent constrictors in human airways *in vitro* and *in vivo*, with an order of potency $LTD_4 > LTC_4 > LTE_4$, being more than 1000 times as potent as histamine on a molar basis and having a longer duration of action (Drazen and Austen, 1987). Animal studies also indicated that the SRS-A leukotrienes may have a greater effect on peripheral than on central airways (Drazen and Austen, 1987). In humans, SRS-A leukotrienes affect both central and peripheral airways. Leukotrienes stimulate mucus secretion in human airways *in vitro* and in guinea-pigs produce microvascular leakiness and airway oedema.

The sulphidopeptide leukotrienes are potent bronchoconstrictor agents when inhaled. They are approximately 100–1000-fold more potent than histamine. Although the airways of asthmatic individuals are hyperresponsive to the leukotrienes as to other bronchoconstrictor agonists, the responsiveness of asthmatics to these agonists demonstrates several unusual properties. While the airways of asthmatic patients are relatively less responsive to LTC_4 and LTD_4, compared with agents such as histamine or methacholine (Adelroth *et al.*, 1986), they demonstrate a marked and selective hyperresponsiveness to LTE_4 (Arm *et al.*, 1990), suggesting a possibly unique role for this mediator in the pathogenesis of airways hyperresponsiveness.

A clinical situation in which leukotrienes may play a role is in aspirin sensitivity (Arm *et al.*, 1989). A proportion of people with asthma are intolerant of aspirin. In these individuals ingestion of aspirin is followed within 1–2 hours by the onset of bronchospasm, which may be accompanied by rhinitis and/or urticaria. The majority of subjects with aspirin-induced asthma (AIA) may be desensitized to aspirin by the administration of incremental doses of aspirin orally, which may lead to an improvement in the severity of asthma and particularly of rhinitis. The mechanism of AIA may depend upon inhibition of cyclooxygenase, resulting in an increased generation of spasmogenic leukotrienes. In subjects with AIA, ingestion of aspirin was accompanied by the release of immunoreactive LTC_4 into nasal secretion (Ferreri *et al.*, 1988). In addition, an asthma attack caused by aspirin challenge leads to enhanced release of the sulphidopeptide leukotrienes as indicated by the increased levels of LTE_4 secreted in the urine.

Apart from AIA, sulphidopeptide leukotrienes are also released in allergen- and exercise-induced asthma, as well as nocturnal asthma and acute asthmatic attacks. The critical role of these mediators in asthma is now supported by the finding that sulphidopeptide leukotriene receptor antagonists, and 5-lipoxygenase inhibitors improve airflow obstruction in asthmatic patients (*see* Chapter 12).

The finding that SRS-A could enhance the contractile response of guinea-pig ileum to histamine prompted a number of investigators to evaluate the capacity of the sulphidopeptide leukotrienes to enhance airways smooth muscle responsiveness both *in vitro* and *in vivo*. Pretreatment of guinea-pig tracheal spirals with LTE_4, but not LTC_4 or LTD_4, enhanced the subsequent contractile response to histamine via an augmentation of acetylcholine release from cholinergic neurones (Lee *et al.*, 1984). Several studies have evaluated the capacities of LTC_4 and LTD_4 to enhance airway smooth muscle responsiveness *in vivo*. In those with asthma the inhalation of bronchoconstricting doses of LTC_4 did not enhance airway response to inhalation of distilled water. In normals, the inhalation of a dose of LTD_4 that did not elicit bronchoconstriction did not significantly enhance airway responsiveness to histamine or to isocapnic hyperventilation, although it increased the sensitivity of the airways to inhaled $PGF_{2\alpha}$. Inhalation of a bronchoconstricting dose of LTD_4 in normal people produced an approximate twofold increase in airway methacholine responsiveness but did not increase the airway response to exercise. Because LTC_4 and LTD_4 are converted to LTE_4 and as LTE_4 may persist at the site of contraction for the longest period of time, the capacity of LTE_4 to enhance airways histamine responsiveness was studied in both asthmatic and normal people (Arm *et al.*, 1988b). Inhalation of LTE_4 led to a mean 3.5-fold decrease in the dose of histamine required to elicit a 35% fall in specific airways conductance (sG_{AW}) in asthmatic but not normal individuals. Inhalation of methacholine to elicit a comparable fall in sG_{AW} was not followed by any significant change in airways histamine responsiveness. Changes in airways histamine responsiveness were maximal at 4–7 hours after inhalation of LTE_4 and had returned to baseline values by 1 week. Recent work suggests that airways responsiveness to histamine is also enhanced to a comparable degree in asthmatics following the prior inhalation of LTC_4 and LTD_4.

The pathological features of asthma include mucus plugging, epithelial sloughing, airways oedema and infiltration of the airways by a mixed population of leucocytes, most prominent amongst which is the eosinophil. The association between airways inflammation and the development of airways hyperresponsiveness is well described in both animal models and in human airways. The mechanism by which leucocytes are recruited to the airways in asthma is an area of considerable interest. Recent studies demonstrate that CHO (Chinese hamster ovary) cells expressing exogenous leukotriene B4 receptor showed marked chemoattractant responses to low concentrations of LTB_4 and recent studies in mice support these data (Yokomizo *et al.*, 1997; Huang *et al.*, 1998). Other mechanisms of likely importance are discussed below. While the possible contribution of LTB_4 to the pathophysiology of bronchial asthma is suggested by its potent pro-inflammatory properties, specific LTB_4 receptor antagonists have not been effective in attenuating the allergen-induced asthmatic response.

Other lipoxygenases, in addition to 5-lipoxygenase, have been identified and their products may also play a role in asthma. The 12- and 15-lipoxygenase form 12- and 15-hydroxyeicosatetraenoic acids (HETEs) respectively; 15-HETE increases airways mucus secretion in animals. Considering 15-HETE is a major product of arachidonic acid metabolism in human lung, it could play a significant role in asthma, either alone or after transformation to lipoxins (Lee *et al.*, 1990).

Prostaglandins

Almost all cells are able to generate cyclooxygenase products, although the specificity varies from cell to cell. Human mast cells preferentially generate PGD_2, macrophages generate $PGF_{2\alpha}$, PGE_2 and thromboxane, whereas vascular endothelial cells produce PGI_2 (prostacyclin). $PGF_{2\alpha}$ and PGD_2 are potent bronchoconstrictors. Recent studies comparing wild type and mice deficient in expression of the PGD_2 receptor, show that following sensitization and aerosol challenge the latter show reduced concentrations of Th2 cytokines, lymphocyte accumulation, eosinophil infiltration and airway hyperreactivity (Matsuoka *et al.*, 2000). Studies in humans implicate a role for PGE_2 in regulating Th2 cytokine production (reviewed by Kalinski *et al.*, 1999). PGE_2, which produces bronchodilatation in normal subjects *in vivo*, provokes bronchoconstriction in asthmatic individuals because it stimulates afferent nerves in airways. PGI_2 has little effect on bronchial smooth muscle but is a potent systemic and pulmonary vasodilator. Prostaglandins may have an important regulatory role in the lung. Thus, PGE_2 may modulate cholinergic neural effects. Thromboxane A_2 has been implicated in the BHR resulting from ozone exposure in dogs, and a thromboxane analogue has been shown to enhance acetylcholine release in dog airways. Thromboxane may, therefore, potentiate cholinergic bronchoconstriction.

Despite the evidence that has implicated cyclooxygenase products in asthma, there is little evidence that cyclooxygenase inhibitors, such as aspirin and indomethacin, are beneficial to the majority of patients with this disease. Perhaps the relative ineffectiveness of cyclooxygenase blockers may be due to the fact that concentrations of the drug in the airways are inadequate to inhibit local production of prostaglandins. In a proportion of asthmatics (approximately 3%), cyclooxygenase inhibitors actually cause a worsening of asthma ('aspirin-sensitive asthma'), either by blocking the production of bronchodilator prostaglandins, or by diverting arachidonic acid metabolism down lipoxygenase pathways with the formation of leukotrienes and other bronchoconstrictor products, as discussed earlier in this chapter.

Platelet activating factor

In several animal species, platelet activating factor (PAF) may cause a prolonged increase in bronchial responsiveness. Inhaled PAF in humans causes an increased bronchial response to methacholine in normals but not asthmatics, whereas its inactive precursor, lyso-PAF, is without effect (Cuss *et al.*, 1986). The maximal effect is observed 3 days after inhalation and may persist for up to 4 weeks.

PAF-induced BHR is platelet-dependent in guinea-pigs, since it may be prevented by prior depletion of platelets. Inhaled PAF has no effect on circulating platelets in man, but causes a profound fall in circulating neutrophils and eosinophils. PAF, like antigen, stimulates accumulation of eosinophils in lung and it selectively releases basic proteins from eosinophils. This selective recruitment and activation of eosinophils provides a mechanism for PAF-induced increases in airways responsiveness, as eosinophil basic proteins may lead to damage and shedding of airway epithelium. PAF has other properties that may be relevant in asthma. In animals, PAF is a potent inducer of airway microvascular leak, which may result in airway oedema and plasma extravasation contributing to BHR.

Specific antagonists of PAF have now been tested in asthma and they are not efficacious, suggesting that endogenous PAF may have little or no role in the mechanism of asthma and BHR.

Chemotactic factors

The release of chemotactic mediators contributes to the recruitment of a cellular reaction at allergic and asthmatic lesions, which is characterized by cellular infiltration and may include release of lysosomal enzymes and cationic proteins, superoxide anion generation and subsequent amplification of the humoral phase of inflammation.

In the skin, Atkins and colleagues have demonstrated that the first infiltrating cell is the neutrophil, which appears approximately 2 hours after mast cell activation (Atkins *et al.*, 1973). Subsequently, eosinophils and mononuclear cells infiltrate the area over a 2–8 hour interval. The cellular infiltration of the lesions may be prevented by the prior administration of corticosteroids, which do not prevent the initial wheal-and-flare reaction. In contrast, the administration of most antihistamines prevents the wheal-and-flare reaction but not the cellular response. The exact events that occur in the lung during a dual phase asthmatic response are less certain, although the late phase reaction is substantially inflammatory in nature. Recent studies using lavage or bronchial biopsy material have studied cellular infiltration in the lung: following bronchial challenge with allergen; monitoring atopic asthmatic individuals before and during natural seasonal allergen challenge; and analysis of post-mortem material from mild, moderate and severe asthmatics. These studies underline the infiltration of CD4[+] T lymphocytes, mast cells and eosinophils (Gerblich *et al.*, 1984; Gonzalez *et al.*, 1987; Djukanovic *et al.*, 1996; Synek *et al.*, 1996). Less marked infiltration of monocytes/macrophages and neutrophils are also observed (Poston *et al.*, 1992). In the last decade, clues to the relationships between mediator release and cellular recruitment to the target organ have emerged from numerous studies demonstrating the existence and release of several potent chemotactic factors with varying leucocyte specificities.

The chemoattractant properties of molecules such as formulated peptides (e.g. f-Met-Leu-Phe), complement fragments (e.g. C5a) and arachidonic acid metabolites (e.g. LTB_4; Ford-Hutchinson *et al.*, 1980) has long been recognized, although their mode of action does not explain the selective recruitment of distinct cell lineages. Studies of the role of a large family of small protein mediators (typically 8–10 kD) termed chemokines that recruit white blood cells to inflammatory sites have, however, progressed rapidly in less than 10 years. This has been fuelled by the recognition of their role in determining susceptibility to HIV-1 infection but has resulted in a search for specific inhibitors of the chemokines or their receptors that block destructive cellular infiltrates to the lung in asthma and other conditions (Fig. 6.2). Chemokines are produced by almost any nucleated cell although, in asthma, epithelial cells, fibroblasts and mononuclear phagocytes may represent important sources which are synthesized in response to bacterial products and pro-inflammatory cytokines. In general they act on several different cell types, albeit with differing selectivity. Dissecting the importance of individual chemokines must reflect both their demonstrated *in vitro* potencies and the pattern of ligand and receptor expression *in vivo*. Nevertheless, animal studies are encouraging and suggest that despite the redundancy in action blocking a single chemokine *in vivo*, chemokines can greatly reduce inflammatory responses (Sekido *et al.*, 1993). In particular, in allergic asthma there is great interest in eotaxin and its receptor which appear to be selective to eosinophils and basophils and therefore a highly attractive target for immunotherapy.

Estimates based on the use of bioinformatics technology suggest that 50 or more chemokines may exist. Classification to distinct families is based on the position of N-terminal cysteine residues, with the two major families expressing four conserved cysteine residues and clustering on chromosomes 4 and 17, respectively. The first family has two N-terminal cysteine residues separated by a single non-conserved residue – the CXC or α chemokine family. The second has two adjacent N-terminal cysteines and is called the CC or β family. Two additional families have a single conserved N-terminal cysteine residue (the C or γ family) or two cysteines separated by three non-conserved residues (CX_3C). The CXC chemokines act predominantly on polymorphonuclear phagocytes although some also act on lymphocytes. The CC family preferentially acts on mononuclear phagocytes, lymphocytes, eosinophils and basophils and have therefore been most extensively studied in asthma.

The chemokine receptors show similar complexity. All so far described represent 7 transmembrane-spanning, G-protein coupled glycoprotein receptors. In humans to date, 4 CXC chemokine-specific (CXCR1–4) and 8 CC chemokine-specific (CCR1–8) receptors have been described. Receptor expression is complex with examples of narrow and broad patterns of cellular expression and of constitutive versus regulated expression. Most receptors bind several chemokines (reviewed in Luster, 1998).

The enormous array of chemokines and their receptors already described, the likelihood of more yet to be described and the rate at which new data on their physical and functional properties are emerging suggest that we are only beginning to understand the importance of this family and their potential for manipulation in asthmatic disease.

Cell type	Receptors	Chemokines

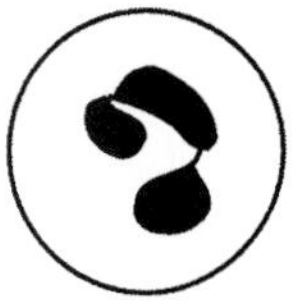

Eosinophil

CCR1 — MCP-3 and 4, MIP-1α, RANTES
CCR3 — MCP-3 and 4, eotaxin 1 and 2, RANTES

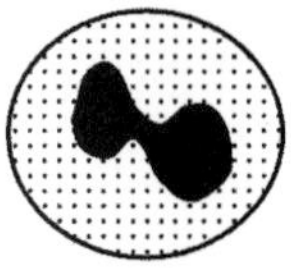

Basophil

CCR2 — MCP-1 to 5
CCR3 — MCP-3 and 4, eotaxin 1 and 2, RANTES

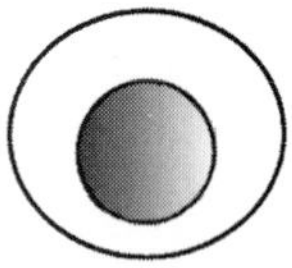

Memory/ activated T lymphocyte

CCR1 — MCP-3 and 4, MIP-1α, RANTES
CCR2 — MCP-1 to 5
CCR4 — TARC
CCR5 — MIP-1α and β, RANTES
CCR7 — MIP-3β

CX$_3$CR1 — Fractaline

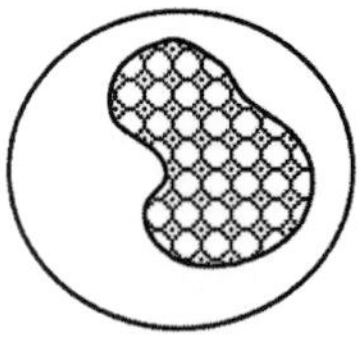

Monocyte

CCR1 — MCP-3 and 4, MIP-1α, RANTES
CCR2 — MCP-1 to 5
CCR5 — MIP-1α and β, RANTES
CCR8 — I-309

CX$_3$CR1 — Fractaline

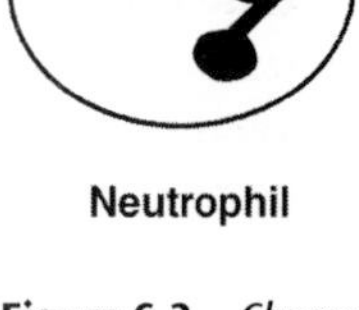

Neutrophil

CXCR1 — IL-8
CXCR2 — IL-8, GROα, β and γ, ENA-78, NAP-2

Figure 6.2 *Chemokines likely to regulate cellular recruitment at sites of allergic inflammation. Key cell types that regulate allergy and the chemokine receptors they express are shown together with chemokines known to bind those receptors. MCP, monocyte chemoattractant protein; MIP, macrophage inflammatory protein; RANTES, regulated upon activation, normal T-cell expressed and secreted; TARC, thymus and activation-regulated chemokine. For further explanation, see text.*

NEUTROPHIL-DIRECTED CHEMOTACTIC FACTORS

Early studies identified activities displaying chemotactic specificity for neutrophils *in vitro* as being released from human leukaemic basophils, rat mast cells, mononuclear cells and extracts of human lung tissue. These mediators not only attracted but could also activate neutrophils: enhancing C3b receptors; stimulating the release of lysozyme and to a lesser extent myeloperoxidase; and also enhancing neutrophil-mediated, complement-dependent killing of helminth larvae. They could be detected *in vivo* in the serum of patients undergoing experimentally induced physical urticarias and allergic and non-allergic bronchoconstriction. Atkins and colleagues described a heat-stable neutrophil chemotactic factor (NCF) that was released into the circulation of patients with bronchial asthma after inhalation of specific antigen (Atkins *et al.*, 1977) and was associated with a peripheral blood neutrophilia. NCF release was suppressed by disodium cromoglycate and β-agonists. A number of subsequent studies (Metzger *et al.*, 1986) demonstrated release of such activities by specific antigen (Schenkel *et al.*, 1982), anti-IgE (O'Driscoll *et al.*, 1983), after cold immersion of patients with cold urticaria (Wasserman *et al.*, 1977, 1982) and during exercise-induced asthma (Lee *et al.*, 1982a,b).

It seems likely that much of these activities can now be explained by the CXC chemokines. The majority of CXC chemokines possess an ELR (glutamate-leucine-arginine) motif between the N-terminus and the first cysteine residue which appears necessary for neutrophil chemoattractant function. The best defined CXC chemokine is IL-8, which is subject to N-terminal processing for optimal functional activity. Originally described as monocyte-derived, it is also made by T-cells, neutrophils, endothelial cells, fibroblasts and epithelial cells. Intradermal challenge with IL-8 induces neutrophil accumulation in humans (Douglass *et al.*, 1996). Expression of IL-8 genes and proteins is increased in bronchial epithelium of symptomatic asthmatic individuals (Marini *et al.*, 1992). Additionally, immunostaining of BAL cell cytospins showed the macrophage to be the major cell expressing immunoreactive IL-8, whilst BAL fluid from intrinsic asthmatics compared to non-atopic controls showed significantly elevated IL-8 (Folkard *et al.*, 1997). However, a study by Teran *et al.* (1996) suggested that IL-8 expression and neutrophil recruitment, unlike eosinophil influx, was a non-specific response to bronchoscopy and lavage.

A number of other neutrophil-specific chemokines have been described including GROα which was also defined as monocyte-derived and has similar potency to IL-8. In addition the related products GROβ and GROγ also act on neutrophils. A number of additional chemokines have been reported, although the relative importance of all of these in their capacity to attract and activate neutrophils and their role in asthma await definition (reviewed in Rollins, 1997).

EOSINOPHIL-DIRECTED CHEMOTACTIC FACTORS

The association of eosinophilia with IgE mast cell-dependent allergic reactions was noted early this century. Eosinophil chemotactic factors (ECFs) have been identified in supernatants from anaphylactic patients, and tissue extracts of human and animal lung tissues (Kay and Austen, 1971; Goetzl and Austen, 1975), human leukaemic basophils, rat and human mast cells as well as the serum of patients with antigen-induced bronchoconstriction and physical urticarias after the appropriate challenge. Much of the data from these earlier studies is most likely explained by the action of chemokines.

A number of chemokines have been to shown to act on eosinophils, with considerable interest in eotaxin and its newly described homologue eotaxin-2 (White *et al.*, 1997). These appear the most potent of the chemokines acting primarily on eosinophils and basophils. Animal studies suggest eotaxin is important in the early phase of the late response. Unlike other CC family members, the eotaxins only signal via the CCR3 receptor, which is expressed on eosinophils and basophils. Expression of eotaxin and CCR3 mRNA and protein in bronchial mucosal biopsy samples has been shown to be significantly elevated in atopic asthmatic patients versus non-atopic, non-asthmatic controls. Epithelial cells and endothelial cells appeared to be the major source of eotaxin mRNA, whilst CCR3 expression was mainly detected on the eosinophil population (Ying *et al.*, 1997). Furthermore, animal studies highlight co-operativity between eotaxin and IL-5, a cytokine which also shows selectivity to eosinophils, in promoting tissue eosinophilia (Collins *et al.*, 1995)

In addition to the eotaxins, a number of other chemokines act upon eosinophils and basophils although they are frequently not as potent and some act through a second major receptor expressed by eosinophils, CCR1. For eosinophils, MCP-2 and MCP-3 appear to both attract and activate (Dahinden *et al.*, 1994; Weber *et al.*, 1995); MCP-4 shares a common receptor with, and is equally potent to, eotaxin (Uguccioni *et al.*, 1996); MCP-5 which has only been described in mice so far (Jia *et al.*, 1996); MIP-1α (Dahinden *et al.*, 1994); RANTES stimulates secretion of eosinophil cationic protein and superoxide and makes eosinophils hypodense (Rot *et al.*, 1992). MCP-1, RANTES, MCP-2 and MCP-3 are all active upon basophils and several of these also induce histamine release (Dahinden *et al.*, 1994) as does eotaxin (Elsner *et al.*, 1996). The contribution of chemokines versus allergen-IgE complexes in stimulating mediator release is unknown, but may well prove significant. The expression of many of these mediators is increased in lavage and mucosal biopsy samples from non-atopic and atopic asthma patients (Sousa *et al.*, 1994; Alam *et al.*, 1996; Humbert *et al.*, 1997).

Animal studies using either antibodies that neutralize specific chemokines (Jia *et al.*, 1996) or gene targeted mice (Rothenberg *et al.*, 1997) suggest that all these mediators participate in eosinophil recruitment to the lung. However CCR3 not only contributes to eosinophil activation by eotaxin, but is also used by other CC chemokines acting upon eosinophils including MCP-4, RANTES and MCP-3, albeit generally with decreased affinity. Although the action of these chemokines is not restricted to eosinophils, and they also signal through other receptors, these studies highlight the considerable potential for targeting CCR3 to inhibit eosinophilic accumulation and mediator release to ameliorate the symptoms associated with allergic and asthmatic disease.

MONONUCLEAR CELL-DIRECTED CHEMOTACTIC FACTORS

In studies of the histology of the late phase response in immediate hypersensitivity reactions in which participation of IgG immune complexes was carefully excluded, a preponderance of mononuclear cell infiltration was noted. The greatest percentage of the cells was made up of CD4+ T lymphocytes. A number of early studies demonstrated the release, generally following activation, by lymphocytes, macrophages, peritoneal and pleural mast cells of uncharacterized chemoattractant factors which acted variously on monocytes/macrophages, granulocytes, basophils, eosinophils and T and B lymphocytes (e.g. Cohen and Ward, 1971; David and David, 1972; Altman *et al.*, 1975; Center and Cruikshank, 1982; van Epps *et al.*, 1983).

Recent developments in the chemokine field define several mediators active upon T lymphocytes and monocytes and it is likely that these explain many of the early observations described above. For monocytes, important chemotactic mediators include MCP-1, 2, 3 and 4 of which MCP-1 is the most potent. RANTES also acts upon monocytes and shows similar potency to MCP-1. MIP-1α and to a lesser extent MIP-1β are also active. All attract monocytes, whilst many also induce activation such as inducing exocytosis (Uguccioni *et al.*, 1995).

A broad range of chemokines act upon T lymphocytes including both CXC and CC chemokines. Recently T-cells with distinct effector functions based on patterns of cytokine secretion have been demonstrated to exhibit flexible programmes of chemokine receptor expression (Sallusto *et al.*, 1998). T-cells in the lung predominantly express a memory phenotype and it is therefore chemokines with known activity upon this subset that are likely to be important. The CXC chemokine IL-8 (Larsen *et al.*, 1989) is a potent activator of T-cell movement and other non-ELR CXC chemokines are clearly also active (reviewed in Rollins, 1997). CC chemokines with well defined T-cell activity include MCP-1 to 5, MIP-1α, β and γ and RANTES. Mediators active upon memory T-cells are MCP-1, 2 and 3 and RANTES and many are reportedly upregulated in asthma as discussed above. Studies of pulmonary inflammation following challenge with aerosolized ovalbumin in sensitized mice demonstrate the early appearance of MCP-1 and influx of monocytes/macrophages. This is followed by detection of eotaxin and RANTES and T-cell and eosinophil accumulation. Influx of the latter is partially reduced by treatment with anti-eotaxin antibodies (Gonzalo *et al.*, 1996).

Adenosine

Several different cell types have now been shown to have the capacity to release adenosine, which appears to act as a local regulatory factor. Adenosine given by inhalation causes bronchoconstriction in asthmatics, yet has little effect on isolated human airways *in vitro*, suggesting that its bronchoconstrictor action is indirect and may involve the release of histamine from airway mast cells (Church *et al.*, 1988)

Bradykinin

Bradykinin is a nine amino-acid peptide formed from high molecular weight kininogen via the enzymatic action of kallikrein and kininogenase. It is formed in inflammatory reactions and has been detected in nasal secretions after allergen challenge. Isolated human mast cells release a kininogenase on immunological stimulation. Bradykinin is a potent bronchoconstrictor when given by inhalation but has little effect on human airways *in vitro* (Fuller *et al.*, 1987). In animals, bradykinin selectively activates C-fibre afferent nerve endings in the airways and causes marked dyspnoea in humans, so it is possible that some of the constrictor effect of bradykinin is caused by the release of sensory neuropeptides, via an axon reflex. Bradykinin is also a potent inducer of bronchial oedema and airway secretion.

Neuropeptides

Neuropeptides such as substance P, neurokinin A and calcitonin gene-related peptide (CGRP) are localized to sensory nerves in airways and are released by a local axon reflex (summarized in Chapter 5). Neurokinin A may lead to bronchoconstriction, substance P to microvascular leakage and mucus secretion and CGRP to the chronic hyperaemia of asthmatic airways.

Cytokines

In both extrinsic (allergic) and more recently demonstrated in intrinsic (non-allergen-associated; Humbert *et al.*, 1996, 1997) asthma there is an increase in pro-inflammatory cytokine expression (e.g. GM-CSF, IL-1, IL-6, TNF) and Th2-derived cytokines (IL-4, IL-5). IL-13, IL-4, IL-5, IL-3 and GM-CSF together with other genes are located in close proximity on the long arm of human chromosome 5 (Fig. 6.3). This suggests a common origin and/or some common regulatory elements for the expression of these genes since several are

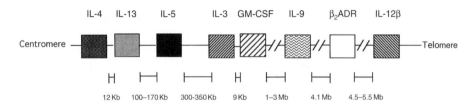

Figure 6.3 *The IL-4 gene cluster on the long arm of human chromosome 5. ADR, adrenoceptor; GM-CSF, granulocyte-macrophage colony stimulating factor; IL, interleukin.*

co-expressed in atopic disease. In contrast expression of the anti-inflammatory cytokine IL-10 is downregulated whilst levels of the IL-1 receptor antagonist (IL-1ra) are unchanged. The role of the Th2 cytokines in disease has been extensively reviewed (Kay, 1998) and is discussed above. Recent interest has focussed on what controls Th2 development and the role of locally derived signals including those derived from antigen-presenting cells (Kapsenberg *et al.*, 1998]. Recently, IL-12, a regulatory cytokine that derives from antigen-presenting cells, namely dendritic cells and monocytes/macrophages, promotes Th1 development and inhibits Th2 cells and has been shown to be decreased in blood monocytes from atopic asthmatic individuals (van der Pouw Kraan *et al.*, 1997).

There is increasing interest in the possibility that selected cytokines may amplify eosinophil recruitment and function in asthma. IL-3, IL-5 and GM-CSF have all been reported to change the phenotype of a normodense eosinophil to that of a hypodense cell. This is associated with an enhanced capacity of the cell to produce eicosanoid and granule-derived mediators, a phenomenon known as priming. In addition, the cytokines increase the survival of eosinophils, thereby providing a mechanism for the perpetuation of eosinophilic inflammation. IL-4 selectively promotes the adhesion of eosinophils to vascular endothelium. IL-3, IL-5 and GM-CSF stimulate the differentiation and maturation of eosinophils from bone marrow precursors. These cytokines are produced by a variety of cell types, including macrophages, lymphocytes, mast cells and the eosinophil itself. In mast cells and macrophages cytokine release can occur as a result of IgE-dependent stimulation.

SUMMARY

The pathology of bronchial asthma is characterized by significant inflammation of the airway mucosa and demonstrates a multicellular process. The biological properties of inflammatory mediators secreted by these cells support a role for mediators in the pathophysiology of the disease. There is increasing information about the biochemistry and the biosynthetic cascades for mediator generation and there is substantial information available about their pharmacology. However, this vast array of information has only yielded a limited number of potent and selective receptor antagonists for testing in man. This problem has hampered attempts to define the role of mediators in the disease.

There is now increasing interest in the interactions between different mediators and between humoral mediators and neurogenic reflexes. The mechanisms by which one agonist augments responsiveness of the airways to another agent are still poorly defined. This phenomenon adds to the complexity of elucidating the role of mediators in disease and to the possibility of using receptor antagonists to treat the asthmatic patient. The possibility of receptor heterogeneity for different mediators, as suggested for both the sulphidopeptide leukotrienes and PAF, implies that development of agents to inhibit the synthesis of mediators may be more appropriate than those which antagonize specific receptors. The recent discovery that rodent mast cells secrete cytokines as a result of an IgE-dependent stimulus is a major advance. It clearly links immediate hypersensitivity events with chronic immunological responses and provides a mechanism for the perpetuation of allergic inflammation.

REFERENCES

Adelroth E, Morris MM, Hargreave FE, *et al.* (1986) Airway responsiveness to leukotrienes C_4 and D_4 and to methacholine in patients with asthma and normal controls. *N Engl J Med*, **315**, 480–4.

Alam R, York J, Boyars M, Stafford S, *et al.* (1996) Increased MCP-1, RANTES and MIP-1α in bronchoalveolar lavage fluid of allergic asthmatic patients. *Am J Resp Crit Care Med*, **153** (4 Pt 1), 1398–404.

Altman LC, Chassy B, Mackler BF. (1975) Physicochemical characterization of chemotactic lymphokines produced by human T and B lymphocytes. *J Immunol*, **115**, 18–21.

Arm JP, Horton CE, House F, *et al.* (1988a) Enhanced generation of leukotriene B_4 by neutrophils stimulated by unopsonised zymosan and by calcium ionophore after exercise-induced asthma. *Am Rev Respir Dis*, **138**, 47–53.

Arm JP, Spur BW, Lee TH. (1988b) The effects of inhaled leukotriene E_4 on the airways responsiveness to histamine in asthmatic and normal subjects. *J Allergy Clin Immunol*, **82**, 654–60.

Arm JP, O'Hickey SP, Spur BW, *et al.* (1989) Airways responsiveness to histamine and leukotriene E_4 in subjects with aspirin-induced asthma. *Am Rev Respir Dis*, **140**, 148–53.

Arm JP, O'Hickey SP, Hawksworth RJ, *et al.* (1990) Asthmatic airways have a disproportionate hyperresponsiveness to LTE_4 as compared to normal airways, but not to LTC_4, LTD_4, methacholine and histamine. *Am Rev Respir Dis*, **142**, 1112–18.

Atkins PA, Green GR, Zweiman B. (1973) Histologic studies of human skin test response to ragweed compound 48/80 and histamine. *J Allergy Clin Immunol*, **51**, 263–73.

Atkins PC, Norman M, Weiner M, Zweiman B. (1977) Release of neutrophil chemotactic activity during immediate hypersensitivity reactions in humans. *Ann Intern Med*, **86**, 415–18.

Barnes PJ. (1990) Molecular biology and respiratory disease. Molecular biology of receptors: implications for lung disease. *Thorax*, **45**(6), S482–8.

Borish L, Aarons A, Rumbyrt J, Cvietusa P, *et al.* (1996) Interleukin-10 regulation in normal subjects and patients with asthma. *J Allergy Clin Immunol*, **97**,1288–96.

Busse WW, Coffman RL, Gelfand EW, Kay AB, Rosenwasser LJ. (1995) Mechanisms of persistent airway inflammation in asthma. A role for T cells and T cell products. *Am J Respir Crit Care Med*, **152**(1), 388–93.

Campbell AM, Vachier I, Chanez P, *et al.* (1998) Expression of the high-affinity receptor for IgE on bronchial epithelial cells of asthmatics. *Am J Respir Cell Mol Biol*, **19**(1), 92–7.

Center DM, Cruikshank W. (1982) Modulation of lymphocyte migration by human lymphokines. Identification and characterization of chemoattractant activity for lymphocytes from mitogen-stimulated mononuclear cells. *J Immunol*, **128**, 2563–8.

Church MK, Cushley MJ, Holgate ST. (1988) Adenosine, a positive modulator of the asthmatic response. In: Barnes PJ, Rodger IW, Thomson NC, eds. *Asthma: Basic Mechanisms and Clinical Management*. London: Academic Press, 273–84.

Cohen S, Ward PA. (1971) In-vitro and *in-vivo* activity of a lymphocyte and immunocomplex dependent chemotactic factor for eosinophils. *J Exp Med*, **133**, 133–46.

Collins PD, Marleau S, Griffiths-Johnson DA, Joce PJ, Williams TJ. (1995) Cooperation between interleukin-5 and the chemokine eotaxin to induce eosinophil accumulation *in vivo*. *J Exp Med*, **182**, 1163–72.

Cuss FM, Dixon CMS, Barnes PJ. (1986) Effects of inhaled platelet activating factor on pulmonary function and bronchial responsiveness in man. *Lancet*, **ii**, 189.

Dahinden CA, Geiser T, Brunner T, von Tscharner V, *et al.* (1994) Monocyte chemotactic protein 3 is a most effective basophil- and eosinophil-activating chemokine. *J Exp Med*, **179**, 751–6.

David JR, David RR. (1972) Cellular hypersensitivity and immunity. Inhibition of macrophage migration and the lymphocyte mediators. *Prog Allergy*, **16**, 300–449.

Djukanovic R, Feather I, Gratziou C, Walls A, *et al.* (1996) Effect of natural allergen exposure during the grass pollen season on airways inflammatory cells and asthma symptoms. *Thorax*, **51**(6), 575–81.

Douglass DJ, Dhami D, Bulpitt M, Lindley JJ, *et al.* (1996) Intradermal challenge with interleukin-8 causes tissue oedema and neutrophil accumulation in atopic and non-atopic human subjects. *Clin Exp Allergy*, **26**(12), 1371–9.

Drazen JM, Austen KF. (1987) Leukotrienes and airway responses. *Am Rev Respir Dis*, **136**, 985–98.

Elsner J, Hochstetter R, Kimmig D, Kapp A. (1996) Human eotaxin represents a potent activator of the respiratory burst of human eosinophils. *Eur J Immunol*, **26**(8),1919–25.

Ferreri NR, Howland WC, Stevenson DD, *et al.* (1988) Release of leukotrienes, prostaglandins and histamine into nasal secretions of aspirin-sensitive asthmatics during reaction to aspirin. *Am Rev Respir Dis*, **137**, 847–54.

Folkard SG, Westwick J, Millar AB. (1997) Production of interleukin-8, RANTES and MCP-1 in intrinsic and extrinsic asthmatics. *Eur Respir J*, **10**(9), 2097–104.

Ford-Hutchinson AW, Bray MA, Doig MV, *et al.* (1980) Leukotriene B, a potent chemokinetic and aggregating substance from polymorphonuclear leukocytes. *Nature*, **286**, 264–5.

Frigas E, Gleich GJ. (1986) The eosinophil and the pathology of asthma. *J Allergy Clin Immunol*, **77**, 527–37.

Fuller RW, Dixon CMS, Dollery CT, Barnes PJ. (1986) Prostaglandin D_2 potentiates airway responses to histamine and methacholine. *Am Rev Respir Dis*, **133**, 252–4.

Fuller RW, Dixon CMS, Cuss FMC, Barnes PJ. (1987) Bradykinin-induced bronchoconstriction in man: mode of action. *Am Rev Respir Dis*, **135**, 176–80.

Gerblich AA, Campbell AE, Schuyler MR. (1984) Changes in T lymphocyte subpopulations after antigenic bronchial provocation in asthmatics. *N Engl J Med*, **310**, 1349–52.

Goetzl EJ, Austen KF. (1975) Purification and synthesis of eosinophilotactic tetrapeptide of human lung and tissue: identification of eosinophil chemotactic factor of anaphylaxis. *Proc Natl Acad Sci USA*, **72**, 4123–7.

Gonzalez C, Diaz P, Galleguillos F, Ancic P, Kay AB. (1987) Allergen-induced recruitment of bronchoalveolar lavage T helper (OKT4) and T suppressor (OKT8) cells in asthma: relative increases in OKT8 cells in single early- as compared to late-phase responders. *Am Rev Respir Dis*, **136**, 600–4.

Gonzalo JA, Lloyd CM, Kremer L, Finger E, *et al.* (1996) Eosinophil recruitment to the lung in a murine model of allergic inflammation. The role of T cells, chemokines and adhesion receptors. *J Clin Invest*, **98**, 2332–45.

Huang SK, Xiao HQ, Kleine-Tebbe J, Paciotti G, *et al.* (1995) IL-13 expression at sites of allergen challenge in patients with asthma. *J Immunol*, **155**(5), 2688–94.

Huang W-W, Garcia-Zepeda EA, Sauty A, Oettgen HC, Rothenberg ME, Luster AD. (1998) Molecular and biological characterization of the murine leukotriene B₄ receptor expressed on eosinophils. *J Exp Med*, **188**(6), 1063–74.

Humbert M, Durham SR, Ying S, *et al.* (1996) IL-4 and IL-5 mRNA and protein in bronchial biopsies from patients with atopic and nonatopic asthma: evidence against 'intrinsic' asthma being a distinct immunopathologic entity. *Am J Respir Crit Care Med*, **154**(5), 1497–504.

Humbert M, Ying S, Corrigan C, Menz G, *et al.* (1997) Bronchial mucosal expression of the genes encoding chemokines RANTES and MCP-3 in symptomatic atopic and nonatopic asthmatics: relationship to the eosinophil active cytokines interleukin (IL-)5, granulocyte-macrophage colony stimulating factor and IL-3. *Am J Respir Cell Mol Biol*, **16**(1), 1–8.

Ichinose M, Stretton D, Barnes PJ. (1989) Histamine H$_3$-receptors inhibit cholinergic neurotransmission in guinea pig and human airways. *Am Rev Respir Dis*, **139**, 259 (Abstract).

Jia GQ, Gonzalo JA, Lloyd C, Kremer L, *et al.* (1996) Distinct expression and function of the novel mouse monocyte chemotactic protein 5 in lung allergic inflammation. *J Exp Med*, **184**, 1939–51.

John M, Lim S, Seybold J, Jose P, Robichaud A, *et al.* (1998) Inhaled corticosteroids increase interleukin-10 but reduce macrophage inflammatory protein 1α, granulocyte-macrophage colony-stimulating factor, and interferon-γ release from alveolar macrophages in asthma. *Am J Respir Crit Care Med*, **157**, 256–62.

Joseph M, Tonnel AB, Tarpier G, Capron A. (1983) Involvement of immunoglobulin E in the secretory process of alveolar macrophages from asthmatic patients. *J Clin Invest*, **71**, 221–30.

Kalinski P, Hilkins CMU, Wierenga EA, Kapsenberg ML. (1999) T-cell priming by type-1 and type-2 polarized dendritic cells: the concept of a third signal. *Immunol Today*, **20**(12), 561–7.

Kapsenberg ML, Hilkens CM, Wierenga EA, Kalinski P. (1998) The role of antigen-presenting cells in the regulation of allergen-specific T cell responses. *Curr Opin Immunol*, **10**(6), 607–13.

Kay AB, Austen KF. (1971) The IgE-mediated release of an eosinophil leukocyte chemotactic factor from human lung. *J Immunol*, **107**, 899–903.

Kay AB, Barata L, Meng Q, Durham SR, Ying S. (1997) Eosinophils and eosinophil-associated cytokines in allergic inflammation. *Int Arch Allergy Immunol*, **113**(1–3), 196–9.

Kay AB. (1998) Role of T cells in asthma. *Chem Immunol*, **71**, 178–91.

Laberge S, Ernst P, Ghaffar O, Cruickshank WW, *et al.* (1997) Increased expression of interleukin-16 in bronchial mucosa of subjects with atopic asthma. *Am J Respir Cell Mol Biol*, **17**(2), 193–202.

Lamkhioued B, Renzi PM, Abi-Younes S, Garcia-Zepada EA, *et al.* (1997) Increased expression of eotaxin in bronchoalveolar lavage and airways of asthmatics contributes to the chemotaxis of eosinophils to the site of inflammation. *J Immunol*, **159**(9), 4593–601.

Larsen CG, Anderson AO, Appella E, Oppenheim JJ, Matsushima K. (1989) Neutrophil activating protein (NAP-1) is also chemotactic for T lymphocytes. *Science*, **243**, 1464–6.

Lee TH, Brown MJ, Nagy L, Causon R, Walport MJ, Kay AB. (1982a) Exercise-induced release of histamine and neutrophil chemotactic factor in atopic asthmatics. *J Allergy Clin Immunol*, **70**, 73–81.

Lee TH, Nagy L, Nagajura T, Walport MJ, Kay AB. (1982b) Identification and partial characterization of an exercise-induced neutrophil chemotactic factor in bronchial asthma. *J Clin Invest*, **69**, 889–99.

Lee TH, Austen KF, Corey EJ, *et al.* (1984) Leukotriene E$_4$-induced airway hyperresponsiveness of guinea pig tracheal smooth muscle to histamine and evidence for three separate sulfidopeptide leukotriene receptors. *Proc Natl Acad Sci USA*, **81**, 4922–4.

Lee TH, Crea AEG, Gant V, *et al.* (1990) Identification of lipoxin A4 and its relationship to the sulfidopeptide leukotrienes C4, D4 and E4 in the bronchoalveolar lavage fluids obtained from patients with selected pulmonary diseases. *Am Rev Respir Dis*, **141**, 1453–8.

Luster AD. (1998) Chemokines – chemotactic cytokines that mediate inflammation. *N Engl J Med*, **338**(7), 436–45.

Marini M, Vittori E, Hollemberg J, Mattoli S. (1992) Expression of the potent inflammatory cytokines, granulocyte-macrophage colony stimulating factor and interleukin 6 and interleukin 8 in bronchial epithelial cells of patients with asthma. *J Allergy Clin Immunol*, **89**(5), 1001–9.

Matsuoka T, Hirata M, Tanaka H, *et al.* (2000) Prostaglandin D2 as a mediator of allergic asthma. *Science*, **287**(5460), 2013–7.

Maurer D, Fiebiger E, Reininger B, Wolff-Winiski B, *et al.* (1994) The high affinity IgE receptor (FcεRI) on monocytes of atopic individuals. *J Exp Med*, **179**, 745–50.

Metzger WJ, Richerson HB, Wasserman SI. (1986) Generation and partial characterization of eosinophil chemotactic activity and neutrophil chemotactic activity during early and late phase asthmatic response. *J Allergy Clin Immunol*, **78**, 282–90.

Nishizuka Y. (1992) Intracellular signalling by hydrolysis of phospholipids and activation of protein kinase C. *Science*, **258**(5082), 607–14.

O'Driscoll BR, Lee TH, Kay AB. (1983) Immunological release of neutrophil chemotactic activity from isolated lung fragments. *J Allergy Clin Immunol*, **72**, 695–701.

Ordonez CL, Shaughnessy TE, Matthay MA, Fahy JV. (2000) Increased neutrophil numbers and IL-8 levels in airway secretions in acute severe asthma: clinical and biologic significance. *Am J Respir Crit Care Med*, **161** (4 Pt 1), 1185–90.

Poston RN, Chanez P, Lacoste JY, Litchfield T, *et al.* (1992) Immunohistochemical characterization of the cellular infiltration in asthmatic bronchi. *Am Rev Respir Dis*, **145**, 918–21.

Rollins BJ. (1997) Chemokines. *Blood*, **90**(3), 909–28.

Rot A, Krieger M, Brunner T, Bischoff SC, *et al.* (1992) RANTES and macrophage inflammatory protein 1α induce the migration and activation of normal human eosinophil granulocytes. *J Exp Med*, **176**, 1489–95.

Rothenberg ME, MacLean JA, Pearlman E, Luster AD, Leder P. (1997) Targeted disruption of the chemokine eotaxin partially reduces antigen-induced tissue eosinophilia. *J Exp Med*, **185**(4), 785–90.

Sallusto F, Lenig D, Mackay CR, Lanzavecchia A. (1998) Flexible programmes of chemokine receptor expression on human polarized T helper 1 and 2 lymphocytes. *J Exp Med*, **187**(6), 875–83.

Samuelsson B. (1983) Leukotrienes: mediators of hypersensitivity reactions and inflammation. *Science*, **220**, 568–75.

Schenkel E, Atkins PC, Yost R, Zweiman B. (1982) Antigen-induced neutrophil chemotactic activity from sensitised lung. *J Allergy Clin Immunol*, **70**, 321–5.

Sekido N, Mukaida N, Harada A, Nakanishi I, *et al.* (1993) Prevention of lung reperfusion injury in rabbits by a monoclonal antibody against interleukin-8. *Nature*, **365**, 654–7.

Sousa AR, Poston RN, Lane SJ, Nakhosteen JA, Lee TH. (1993) Detection of GM-CSF in asthmatic bronchial epithelium and decrease by inhaled corticosteroids. *Am Rev Respir Dis*, **147**(6 Pt 1), 1557–61.

Sousa AR, Lane SJ, Nakhosteen JA, Yoshimura T, *et al.* (1994) Increased expression of the monocyte chemoattractant protein-1 on bronchial tissue from asthmatic subjects. *Am J Respir Cell Mol Biol*, **10**(2), 142–7.

Sousa AR, Trigg CJ, Lane SJ, Hawksworth R, *et al.* (1997) Effect of inhaled glucocorticoids on IL-1 beta and IL-1 receptor antagonist (IL-1ra) expression in asthmatic bronchial epithelium. *Thorax*, **52**(5), 407–10.

Synek M, Beasley R, Frew AJ, Goulding D, *et al.* (1996) Cellular infiltration of the airways in asthma of varying severity. *Am J Respir Crit Care Med*, **154**(1), 224–30.

Teran LM, Carroll MP, Frew AJ, Redington AE, *et al.* (1996) Leukocyte recruitment after local endobronchial allergen challenge in asthma. Relationship to procedure and to airway interleukin-8 release. *Am J Respir Crit Care Med*, **154**(2 Pt 1), 469–76.

Uguccioni M, D'Apuzzo M, Loetscher M, Dewald B, Baggiolini M. (1995) Actions of the chemotactic cytokines MCP-1, MCP-2, MCP-3, RANTES, MIP-1α and MIP-1β on human monocytes. *Eur J Immunol*, **25**, 64–8.

Uguccioni M, Loetscher P, Forssman U, Dewald B, *et al.* (1996) Monocyte chemotactic protein 4 (MCP-4), a novel structural and functional analogue of MCP-3 and eotaxin. *J Exp Med*, **183**, 2379–84.

van der Pouw Kraan TC, Boeije LC, de Groot ER, *et al.* (1997) Reduced production of IL-12 and IL-12-dependent IFN-gamma release in patients with allergic asthma. *J Immunol*, **158**(11), 5560–5.

van Epps DR, Potter JW, Durant DA. (1983) Production of a human lymphocyte chemotactic factor by T-cell subpopulations. *J Immunol*, **130**, 2727–31.

Wasserman SI, Soter NA, Center DM, Austen KF. (1977) Cold urticaria. Recognition and characterization of a neutrophil chemotactic factor which appears in serum during experimental cold challenge. *J Clin Invest*, **60**, 189–96.

Wasserman SI, Austen KF, Soter AN. (1982). The functional and physicochemical characterization of three eosinophilotactic activities released into the circulation of patients with cold urticaria. *Clin Exp Immunol*, **479**, 570–8.

Weber M, Uguccioni M, Ochensberger B, Baggiolini M, *et al.* (1995) Monocyte chemotactic protein 2 activates human basophil and eosinophil leukocytes similar to MCP-3. *J Immunol*, **154**, 4166–72.

Weller P. (1997) Updates on cells and cytokines: human eosinophils. *J Allergy Clin Immunol*, **100**, 283–7.

White JR, Imburgia C, Dul E, Appelbaum E, *et al.* (1997) Cloning and functional characterization of a novel human CC chemokine that binds to the CCR3 receptor and activates human eosinophils. *J Leuk Biol*, **62**, 667–75.

Yamaguchi Y, Hayashi Y, Sugara Y, Yasusada M, *et al.* (1988) Highly purified murine interleukin 5 (IL-5) stimulates eosinophil function and prolongs *in vitro* survival. *J Exp Med*, **167**, 1737–42.

Ying S, Robinson DS, Meng Q, Rottman J, *et al.* (1997) Enhanced expression of eotaxin and CCR3 mRNA and protein in atopic asthma. Association with airway hyperresponsiveness and predominant co-localization of eotaxin mRNA to bronchial epithelial and endothelial cells. *Eur J Immunol*, **27**(12), 3507–16.

Yokomizo T, Izumi T, Chang K, Takuwa Y, Shimizu T. (1997) A G-protein-coupled receptor for leukotriene B4 that mediates chemotaxis. *Nature*, **387**(6633), 620–4.

7

Genetics of asthma

GERARD H. KOPPELMAN, GERDA G. MEIJER, EUGENE R. BLEECKER AND
DIRKJE S. POSTMA

INTRODUCTION

Asthma and allergies have long been recognized to have a familial basis. In a paper published in 1916, Cooke and Vanderveer studied family histories of 504 patients with allergy and concluded 'that inheritance is a definite factor in human sensitisation' (Cooke and Vanderveer, 1916). However, the exact mechanisms that underlie this familial basis remained unknown. This situation has changed in the last two decades since new tools in molecular biology and genetic epidemiology have become available to facilitate genetic studies. The cystic fibrosis gene, discovered in 1989, follows Mendel's laws for single gene transmission. Mendelian genes show recessive or dominant patterns of inheritance in families. A current challenge is the genetic dissection of traits and diseases that do not show these Mendelian patterns. Such traits and diseases are called genetic complex diseases, which are influenced both by genes and environmental factors (Lander and Schork, 1994). Examples of genetic complex diseases are multiple sclerosis, diabetes and asthma.

In general, genetic complex diseases show no simple relation of genotype and phenotype. This may be due to different genes causing the same phenotype (genetic heterogeneity) or the same genotype resulting in different phenotypes (pleiotropy). Some individuals with the mutated gene may not express the phenotype (incomplete penetrance), whereas others without the gene do show the specific phenotype (phenocopy). Furthermore, it is likely that in asthma some traits may require the presence of mutations in different genes at the same time (polygenic inheritance). These genes in turn can have different gene–gene and gene–environment interactions. Thus, mutated genes in genetic complex diseases can be regarded as risk factors for a disease comparable with other generally recognized risk factors for the development of diseases. This can be illustrated by the example of airway responsiveness. Hypothetically, genetic regulation of airway responsiveness may be influenced by two major genes. Different variants of these genes may lead to susceptibility for airway hyperresponsiveness. Environmental factors, such as smoking and allergen exposure, may act as exogenous factors, resulting in airway hyperresponsiveness in susceptible individuals by different gene–environmental interactions. The purpose of this chapter is to review the definition of asthma in genetic studies, the genetic basis of asthma and the current evidence on the localization of asthma susceptibility genes. A glossary of some genetic terms is listed in Table 7.1.

Table 7.1 *Explanations of genetic terms*

Affected relative pair:	A set of individuals related by blood, each of whom is affected with the trait in question. The most common types of affected relative pairs include affected sibling pairs, affected cousins and affected avuncular pairs
Affected sibling pair:	*See* affected relative pair
Allele:	Alternative variant of a gene or marker due to changes at the DNA level
Ascertainment:	The selection of individuals for inclusion in a genetic study
Autosome:	In humans any chromosome other than the sex chromosomes
Candidate gene:	A gene that has been implicated in causing or contributing to the development of a particular disease
CentiMorgan:	A measure of genetic distance, equivalent to 1% recombination
Chromosome:	Macromolecular complex of DNA and protein. Humans have 46 chromosomes (23 pairs)
Codon:	A triplet of three bases in a DNA and RNA molecule, specifying a single amino acid
Concordant:	A pair of relatives, mostly twins, in which both members exhibit the same phenotype or trait
Complex trait	A trait which has a genetic component, that is not inherited in a strictly Mendelian fashion (dominant, recessive or sex-linked)
Crossing-over:	Reciprocal breaking and rejoining of homologous chromosomes in meiosis that results in exchange of chromosomal segments
Discordant:	A pair of relatives, mostly twins, in which both members exhibit different phenotypes or traits
DNA:	Deoxyribonucleic acid, the molecule that encodes the genetic information in virtually all organisms
DNA marker:	A cloned chromosomal locus with allelic variation that can be followed directly by a DNA-based assay such as polymerase chain reaction
Epistasis:	Two or more genes interacting with each other in a multiplicative fashion
Exon:	The portion of the genome that is expressed as processed mRNA
Gamete:	Any mature germ cell
Gene:	An individual unit of heredity. It is a specific instruction that directs the synthesis of a mRNA product
Genome:	The sum of all genetic information of an organism
Genotype:	The observed alleles at a genetic locus for an individual
Haploid:	The chromosome number of a normal gamete. In a gamete, only one of the two chromosomes of a chromosome pair is present
Haplotype:	The linear, ordered arrangement of alleles on a chromosome

Table 7.1 *Explanations of genetic terms – contd*

Heterozygote:	A diploid organism with two distinguishable alleles at a particular locus
Homozygote:	A diploid organism with two identical alleles at a particular locus
Identity-by-descent:	Two alleles are identical by descent when it can be determined that they have been inherited from a common ancestor
Imprinting:	A phenomenon in which the phenotype depends on which parent passed the disease gene
Intron:	The non-coding regions of genes. The introns are spliced out of the mRNA following transcription
Linkage:	Co-inheritance of two or more loci because of close proximity on the same chromosome, so that after meiosis they remain associated more often than the 50% expected for unlinked loci
Linkage disequilibrium:	The preferential association of a particular allele, for example, a mutant allele for a disease with a specific allele at a nearby locus
LOD score:	A statistical method that tests whether a set of linkage data indicates two loci are unlinked or linked. The LOD score is the logarithm to the base 10 of the odds favouring linkage
Mapping:	The process of determining the position of a locus on the chromosome relative to other loci
Marker:	*See* DNA marker
Meiosis:	The specialized form of a cell division that creates germ cells
Microsatellite:	A class of DNA polymorphisms arising from a short base-pair sequence that is tandemly repeated a variable number of times; microsatellites are used as genetic markers in linkage analysis
mRNA:	Messenger RNA, a type of RNA molecule that carries the information copied from a gene and serves as a template for the production of proteins
Multifactorial:	A trait is considered to be multifactorial in origin when two or more genes, together with an environmental effect, work together to lead to a phenotype
Mutation:	A change, deletion, or rearrangement of the DNA sequence
Nucleotide:	The building block of RNA and DNA
Oligogenic:	A few genes work together to produce the phenotype. Contrasted to polygenic, which implies that many genes are involved
PCR:	Polymerase chain reaction, a technique for amplifying short stretches of DNA
Penetrance:	The probability of expressing a phenotype given a genotype
Phenocopy:	A trait which appears to be identical to a genetic trait, but which is caused by non-genetic factors
Phenotype:	The observed manifestation of a genotype
Polymorphism:	Loci at which there are two or more alleles that are each present at a frequency of at least 1% in the population
Power:	The probability of correctly rejecting the null hypothesis
Proband:	An individual, through which a family is ascertained for a genetic study, mostly an affected individual
Recombination:	The formation of a new combination of genes during meiosis

Table 7.1   *Explanations of genetic terms – contd*

Restriction enzymes:	A group of enzymes isolated from bacteria that cut DNA molecules at specific sites characterized by specific nucleotide sequences
RNA:	Ribonucleic acid, a ribonucleotide polymer into which DNA is transcribed
Segregation analysis:	A method of genetic analysis that tests whether an observed pattern of phenotypes in families is comparable with an explicit model of inheritance
Sequencing:	The process of determining the order of nucleotides in a nucleic acid or amino acids in a protein

DEFINITION OF ASTHMA IN GENETIC STUDIES

Asthma is a respiratory disease characterized by variable airway obstruction, airway inflammation and airway hyperresponsiveness. A major issue in genetic studies is how to define the asthma phenotype (Kauffmann *et al.*, 1997). Ideally, this definition would separate 'true' asthma from other lung diseases such as chronic obstructive pulmonary disease (COPD) or healthy status. An accurate definition of asthma in genetic studies is important, as misclassification of individuals reduces the power of genetic studies to a great extent.

In defining the asthma phenotype for genetic studies, one has to recognize the marked clinical heterogeneity of the disease, with regard to its age of onset and variations in symptoms over time, its severity and the association of asthma and atopy. Furthermore, an overlap may exist between asthma and COPD. There are some clear differences between asthma and COPD, such as age of onset (asthma mainly in childhood and adolescence, COPD in older age). An example of a similarity is airway hyperresponsiveness, a central feature of asthma, which can be detected in the majority of patients with COPD. Furthermore, both diseases are characterized by airway obstruction. Airway obstruction is reversible spontaneously or after the use of β_2-agonists in most patients with asthma, but not all. In contrast, airway obstruction is not reversible in most patients with COPD. However, in a 25 years follow-up study of adult asthmatic patients about 30% of these patients developed irreversible airway obstruction (Panhuysen *et al.*, 1997). These patients do have asthma with irreversible airways obstruction, but without any clinical history one could easily diagnose them as patients with COPD. This example illustrates that the classification of patients with obstructive airways disease is not always easily made.

Possible approaches in defining the asthma phenotype

In genetic studies the asthma phenotype can be studied by a questionnaire that assesses self-reported wheeze or asthma, or a doctor's diagnosis of asthma. A clear advantage is that this is an easy and feasible approach which can be used in large scale studies. However, a disadvantage is that self-reported wheeze has a high population frequency and may overestimate the asthma prevalence, as some children wheeze during the course of a viral upper airway infection, but do not develop asthma (Martinez *et al.*, 1995). Furthermore, wheeze is also present in a considerable proportion of patients with COPD. The use of a doctor's diagnosis of asthma or the use of asthma medication for classifying asthmatics has been criticized, because some evidence suggests that doctors are more likely to diagnose asthma in females, non-smokers and children who have a positive family history of allergy (Sibbald *et al.*, 1994). Furthermore, one may misclassify individuals with mild, intermittent disease because they do not attend a doctor. Thus, questionnaire-based approaches appear to have their limitations. Therefore, current studies are now directed at measuring clinical and objective characteristics, which constitute a marker of, or are associated with asthma. Examples of these traits are airway hyper-responsiveness, reversibility of airway obstruction after inhaling a β-agonist, and markers of atopy such as total serum IgE or allergen-specific IgE levels, the number of eosinophils in peripheral blood and skin-prick tests for common aeroallergens.

Airway hyperresponsiveness (AH) to inhaled bronchoconstrictor agents is a central feature in asthma, which can be detected in virtually all symptomatic patients. Longitudinal studies have indicated that AH is a risk factor for the development of asthma and respiratory symptoms. It can be studied by inhalation provocation either using a direct stimulus (histamine or methacholine) or indirect stimulus (adenosine-5-monophosphate, cold air, exercise or hypertonic saline).

Reversibility of airway obstruction after inhalation of a β$_2$-agonist is often taken as a surrogate marker for AH in patients who cannot perform this test due to low lung function. However, a recent study showed that these two phenotypes are not interchangeable in the general population (Douma et al., 1997). Variability of airway obstruction can also be assessed with serial peak expiratory flow (PEF) measurements. International guidelines have advised the use of increased variability of PEF during the day as a diagnostic tool for asthma, and to use it in clinical management for adjusting therapy. Although AH and variability of PEF are correlated, their different associations to allergy markers in the general population may indicate that they cannot be used interchangeably (Boezen et al., 1996). Furthermore, the genetic component of peak flow variability and reversibility has not been formally studied, and the value of this phenotype remains to be established.

Asthma has a close relation with atopy, especially in children and adolescents. Atopy can be defined as a prolonged increased production of IgE as a reaction on exposure to common antigens. Its clinical expression includes asthma, allergic rhinitis (hay fever) and atopic dermatitis (eczema). Atopy is reflected in elevated levels of total serum IgE, allergen-specific IgE levels and positive skin tests to common allergens. Atopy is often accompanied by raised numbers of eosinophils in peripheral blood. The phenotypes of asthma and atopy are often interrelated (Fig. 7.1) (Burrows et al., 1989; Xu et al., 1997). Therefore, in this chapter

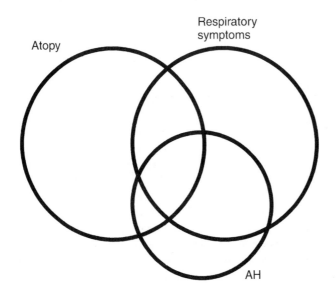

Figure 7.1 *Venn diagram showing the interrelation of airway hyperresponsiveness (AH), atopy and respiratory symptoms in asthma, such as wheeze, dyspnoea, cough and nocturnal asthma. This figure shows the interrelationship of these three phenotypes, which are often found together in individuals with asthma. However, these phenotypes can occur separately in individuals who do not have asthma.*

attention will be given to the complex asthma phenotype, as well as the distinct intermediate phenotypes of asthma, such as AH, reversibility, total serum IgE, allergen-specific IgE, positive skin-prick tests and the total number of eosinophils in peripheral blood.

ASTHMA AS A GENETIC DISEASE

Asthma clusters in families. The risk that a first-degree family member of a patient with asthma will develop asthma has been calculated to be less than two to almost six times higher than the risk for individuals in the general population (Sandford *et al.*, 1996; Schonberger and van Schayck, 1998; Wjst *et al.*, 1999). Both shared genes and shared environment could account for such an excess risk. Two approaches, twin studies and segregation analyses, can separate the relative contribution of genes and environment to a certain trait and are discussed below.

Twin studies

The main goal in the study of twins is to estimate the genetic and environmental contributions to a specific trait or disease. Similarities or differences are compared in monozygotic (MZ) and dizygotic (DZ) twins. Since MZ twins share 100% of their genetic information and DZ twins 50%, higher similarity in MZ co-twins is explained by their greater genetic similarity. The main assumptions of twin studies are: that the environment for both MZ and DZ twins is similar; that they are representative of the general population; and, in questionnaire-based studies, that self-reported zygosity is correct.

The first large twin study published on asthma was a Swedish population-based study of 6996 twin pairs (Edfors-Lubs, 1971). In this study MZ concordance for self-reported asthma was 19.0% and DZ concordance was 4.8%. This indicated that both genetic and environmental factors are important in asthma. The genetic influence is illustrated by the higher concordance in MZ twins compared with DZ twins. In contrast, environmental influences are evidenced by the finding that in genetically similar MZ twins sometimes one of a twin pair has asthma and the other not. Since then, several other twin studies in different populations have confirmed this finding (Table 7.2) (Hopp *et al.*, 1984; Duffy *et al.*, 1990; Nieminen *et al.*, 1991; Sarafino and Goldfedder, 1995; Lichtenstein and Svartengren, 1997; Harris *et al.*, 1997; Laitinen *et al.*, 1998). These twin studies provide strong evidence for the hereditary basis of asthma. Furthermore, from these twin studies one can conclude that both airway hyperresponsiveness and total serum IgE are under significant genetic control. Data of twin studies on the genetic regulation of allergen-specific IgE and skin test sensitivity are, at the moment, scanty. The currently available evidence suggests that whereas the ability to produce IgE is regulated genetically, the specificity of the IgE response is governed mainly by environment (Table 7.2) (Wutrich *et al.*, 1981; Hopp *et al.*, 1984; Hanson *et al.*, 1991).

Segregation analysis

Segregation analysis tests the hypothesis that the aggregation of a trait in families is the result of the action of a major gene. It does not include molecular biological techniques or DNA analyses. This analysis compares the number of individuals with a certain trait under study in a family with the expected numbers using different genetic models of inheritance. Examples of these models are models with a Mendelian component (a dominant gene model, a recessive

Table 7.2 *Twin studies of asthma and asthma-associated phenotypes*

Phenotype	First author, year of publication	Population	Number of twin pairs	MZ correlation[+]	MZ concordance[#]	DZ correlation[+]	DZ concordance[#]	Definition of phenotype/comments
Asthma	Edfors-Lubs, 1971	Swedish	6996		0.19~		0.05~*	Questionnaire/population-based study.
	Hopp, 1984	US	107		0.50~		0.33~	'History of asthma' by questionnaire.
	Duffy, 1990	Australian	3808	0.65		0.24*		Questionnaire.
	Nieminen, 1991	Finnish	13 888	0.43		0.25*		Hospitalization, medication or cause of death/population-based study.
	Sarafino, 1995	US	94		0.59		0.24*	Questionnaire.
	Lichtenstein, 1997	Swedish	434♂		0.62♂		0.26♂ *	Questionnaire (ever wheezing with shortness of breath, wheezing without a cold, or parental-reported asthma)/twins aged 7–9 years.
			456♀		0.41♀		0.18♀ *	
	Harris, 1997	Norwegian	2559		0.45		0.12*	Questionnaire/population-based study of twins aged 18–25 years.
	Laitinen, 1998	Finnish	1713		0.42		0.17*	Questionnaire/population-based study of twins aged 16 years.
AH	Hopp, 1984	US	107	0.67		0.34*		AH to methacholine.
Total IgE	Hopp, 1984	US	107	0.82		0.52*		
	Hanson, 1991	US apart	70	0.64		0.49*		Twins reared apart.
		US together	61	0.42		0.26		Twins reared together.
		Finnish	158	0.56		0.37*		
Specific IgE	Wütrich, 1981	German	50		0.60		0.23	At least one allergen RAST positive.
	Hanson, 1991	US apart	26		0.50		0	Specific IgE antibodies for *Ambrosia artemisiifolia*, *P. pratense* and *Alternaria teni* were measured by RAST/apart: reared apart; together: reared together.
		US together	14		0.50		0.33	
Skin test	Hopp, 1984	US	107	0.82	0.55	0.46*	0.50	Sum of positive intracutaneous (skin) tests.
	Hanson, 1991	US apart	39		0.55		0.50	≥One intracutaneous (skin) test with wheal size > 5 mm
		US together	41		0.70		0.28	

*, Statistically significant differences between monozygous (MZ) and dizygous (DZ) pairs; +, correlation, intrapair correlation; #, concordance, probandwise concordance; ~, pairwise concordance; AH, airway hyperresponsiveness; RAST, radioallergosorbent test to measure specific IgE.

gene model), or non-Mendelian models such as a polygenic model (multiple genes with small effect), a mixed model (a single major gene on a polygenic background) or a non-genetic, environmental model (no evidence for genetic factors). The result of segregation analysis is the genetic model with the highest likelihood, i.e. the model that gives the best description of the segregation of the trait under study in the family data. From this model, one can estimate the mode of inheritance and parameters such as the penetrance, the heritability and allele frequencies (Khoury et al., 1993).

Segregation of the asthma phenotype has been studied in several large, questionnaire-based studies (Table 7.3). The self-reported family history of 13 963 asthma patients participating in the European Community Respiratory Health Survey was analyzed with a complex segregation analysis. This study reveals further support for genetic regulation of asthma and provides evidence for a two-allele gene with codominant inheritance (European Community Respiratory Health Survey Group, 1997). Four other studies, each with less participants, have also shown the familial aggregation of asthma and wheeze. However, the segregation of asthma in these families was consistent with the action of multiple genes with a small effect (Lawrence et al., 1994; Holberg et al., 1996; Jenkins et al., 1997; Chen et al., 1998).

Few family studies on airway hyperresponsiveness (AH) have been published. Longo et al., studied AH to carbachol in non-asthmatic parents of patients with asthma and a sample of healthy controls. Ten per cent of the normal population showed AH, whereas 50% of the non-asthmatic parents of asthmatic children had AH. These different distributions indicate a familial clustering of AH (Longo et al., 1987). Complex segregation analysis of AH was performed by Townley et al., in 83 families from the USA and by Lawrence et al., in 131 randomly selected families from the United Kingdom (Table 7.3). These analyses illustrate the genetic contribution to AH, but no evidence for a single major gene for AH was found (Townley et al., 1986; Lawrence et al., 1994).

Segregation of total serum IgE has been studied most extensively (Table 7.3). First, segregation analyses of total serum IgE confirmed the results of twin studies indicating major genetic regulation of total serum IgE levels. Second, the mode of inheritance was assessed in several studies. These studies provide evidence for different genetic models. Using a single locus approach, best fitting models were for a major Mendelian gene, either codominant (Meyers et al., 1982; Martinez et al., 1994), recessive (Dizier et al., 1995), mixed model of recessive inheritance (Meyers et al., 1987), dominant (Gerrard et al., 1978) or, in two other studies, for polygenic inheritance (Lawrence et al., 1994; Hasstedt et al., 1983). Dizier et al. (1995), studied total serum IgE levels in 234 Australian nuclear families. Evidence for recessive inheritance of total serum IgE levels and significant residual familial correlations were found. However, these correlations were no longer significant when the presence of the specific immune response was accounted for in the analysis. This study suggested that regulation of total serum IgE is independent from the regulation of allergen-specific IgE.

Xu et al., were the first to perform a two-locus approach to the fit the total serum IgE data in 92 Dutch families ascertained through a proband with asthma. This resulted in a significantly better fit of the data than a one-locus model, thereby providing evidence for two unlinked loci regulating total serum IgE in these families. The first locus alone explained 50.6% of the variance of the level of total serum IgE, the second 19.0%. Considered jointly, the two loci account for 78.4% of the variability of total serum IgE levels (Xu et al., 1995). To date, there are no data on the segregation of other asthma-associated phenotypes in families.

In summary, segregation analyses of asthma and AH confirm their genetic background, but are not conclusive on the mode of inheritance and the number of genes involved. Evidence for a major gene regulating total serum IgE was provided by studies in different countries, and evidence for different genetic models was obtained. Several explanations may be given for

Table 7.3   *Segregation analyses of asthma and asthma-associated phenotypes*

Phenotype	First author, year	Number of families	Genetic model	Definition of phenotype/comments
Asthma	Lawrence, 1994	131	Common genes of small effect	Questionnaire/population-based sample
	Holberg, 1996	906	Polygenic or oligogenic model, not a single two-allele gene	Questionnaire, physician-diagnosed asthma
	ECRHSG, 1997	13 963	Two-allele gene with codominant inheritance could not be rejected	Questionnaire, family history of asthma was reported by proband
	Jenkins, 1997	7394	Oligogenic model	Questionnaire/population of school children
	Chen, 1998	309	Single locus explains a portion of wheeze that is related to respiratory allergy. Also contribution of environmental factors and/or polygenes	Questionnaire defined self-reported wheeze
AH	Townley, 1986	83	Environmental hypothesis rejected, no single autosomal locus	AH to methacholine, families with and without asthma
	Longo, 1987	40	Autosomal dominant pattern of inheritance	AH to carbachol, no formal segregation analysis performed
	Lawrence, 1994	131	Common dominant genes of small effect	AH to histamine, random population sample
Total IgE	Gerrard, 1978	173	Dominant model, dominant allele suppresses high levels of IgE	In Caucasian Americans
	Meyers, 1982	23	Mendelian codominant model	In US-Amish population not selected for allergy
	Hasstedt, 1983	5	No major gene, polygenic inheritance	Families selected through breast cancer probands
	Meyers, 1987	42	Mixed model with recessive inheritance of high IgE levels	In families not selected for allergic disease
	Martinez, 1994	291	Codominant inheritance of a major gene for high IgE levels	In hispanic and non-hispanic families
	Lawrence, 1994	131	Polygenic model	Random population sample
	Xu, 1995	92	Two-locus recessive model with epistasis	Families ascertained through a proband with asthma
	Dizier, 1995	234	Recessive major gene controlling high IgE levels	Independent from specific response to allergens

ECRHSG, European Community Respiratory Health Survey Group. AH, airway hyperresponsiveness.

these contradictory results. A first explanation may be the definition of the phenotype. The definition of asthma and BHR varies between studies (Table 7.3). A second explanation may be the ascertainment of families for segregation studies. In families ascertained for asthma, estimates on allele frequencies of alleles regulating total serum IgE may be higher than in families sampled randomly from the general population. A final explanation may be genetic heterogeneity. This means that in different populations, different genes act in the regulation of these phenotypes. To date, this cannot be investigated since the exact localizations of these genes are still unknown.

FINDING GENES FOR ASTHMA

The human genome

The haploid human genome consists of approximately 3×10^9 base pairs. Generally, genetic distances are expressed in centiMorgans (cM), one cM corresponding to 1% recombination and approximately 1 000 000 base pairs on a physical map. One per cent recombination means that a crossing-over between two loci occurs every one in a hundred meioses. Roughly, every one cM contains 50 genes. DNA is organized into 22 pairs of autosomes and two sex-specific chromosomes. Each chromosome comprises two arms, the short arm denoted as 'p' and the long arm as 'q'. Every region of a chromosome has been assigned a number, for example for chromosome 1, the regions are called 1q21, 1q22, 1q23, etc.

The total number of genes is estimated to be between 65 000 and 80 000 (Antequera and Bird, 1994). At a given place in the genome, called a locus, different variants are called alleles. Many genes have a number of alleles in the population and are therefore said to be polymorphic. The majority of the DNA is not coding for any biological product. In these non-coding regions, polymorphisms can also be detected. These polymorphisms are typically used as markers for genetic studies. Thus, in this respect the words 'markers' and 'polymorphisms' are used interchangeably.

In general, two different strategies have been used to identify susceptibility genes for asthma and atopy. The first strategy is positional cloning, the second is the candidate gene approach.

POSITIONAL CLONING

The first step is to identify chromosomal regions of interest that may harbour disease genes by linkage analysis. The second step in positional cloning is to narrow down the region of interest as far as possible. Finally, in the last step the genes in this specified region are checked for mutations associated with the disease.

The principles of linkage analysis are shown in Fig. 7.2. Finding linkage is to determine a chromosomal region (sometimes millions of base pairs in length) which cosegregates with a certain trait within families. The likelihood that a trait cosegregates with a marker is expressed as a LOD score. The LOD score is the logarithm of the likelihood ratio of linkage versus no linkage. To study linkage using a LOD score approach, a model has to be specified for different genetic parameters such as mode of inheritance, penetrance, and allele frequencies. These parameters can sometimes be estimated from segregation analyses. However, given that in most studies these parameters are unknown, most investigators prefer non-parametric approaches. A non-parametric approach is a method that does not need specification of a genetic model. Examples are affected sibling pair analysis and affected relative pair analysis. These non-parametric approaches test whether the inheritance of a chromosomal region is not consistent with random segregation. If this is the case, affected relatives inherit identical

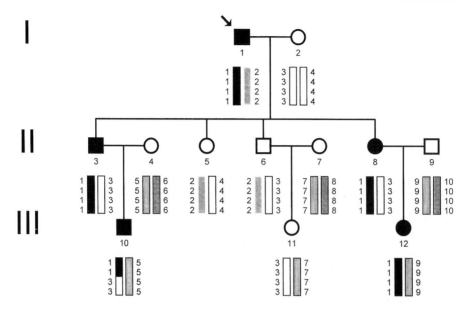

Figure 7.2 *Pedigree of a family with asthma. A fictive family with asthma: affected family members are shown as black boxes (males) or black circles (females); unaffected individuals are represented by the open boxes (males) and open circles (females). The proband is indicated by an arrow (individual 1). This family consists of three generations, as indicated by the roman capitals I, II, and III. The grandfather (individual 1), the oldest son (individual 3) and the youngest daughter (individual 8) and two grandchildren (individuals 10 and 12) are affected. On a chromosome, four subsequent markers are typed. The different alleles are coded by different numbers. In this example, the trait asthma cosegrates with the haplotype of four markers with allele 1 (black chromosome). It is said that this trait is linked to the marker. Furthermore, a crossing-over is observed in individual 10. From the fact, that this person is still affected, one can deduce that the gene causing this trait is located upstream of the third marker.*

copies of alleles in this region more often than would be expected by chance (Lander and Schork, 1994). The observed and expected distributions of alleles can be tested with a χ^2-test.

CANDIDATE GENE APPROACH

Candidate genes can be detected in the process of positional cloning. In addition, investigators may choose a certain, known, gene as a plausible candidate gene for asthma. In general, candidate genes are tested with the use of association analysis in which alleles of candidate genes are tested using a case-control design. The frequency of an allele in a gene or a marker is compared between affected individuals and unaffected individuals. The finding of a positive association of an allele and a trait can be interpreted in three ways (Lander and Schork, 1994):

- the allele of interest is the relevant mutation in the disease gene;
- the allele is in linkage disequilibrium, that means it is physically very close to the disease gene;
- the association is a result of population admixture. This occurs if a certain trait has a higher prevalence in an ethnic subgroup within a mixed population. Any allele with a higher frequency within this subgroup will show association with the trait.

A method of testing for linkage and association is the transmission disequilibrium test (TDT) (Spielman *et al.*, 1993). Alleles of heterozygote parents are divided in transmitted and non-transmitted alleles, and the preferential transmission of a certain allele to an affected child is tested.

Results of linkage studies in asthma and atopy

The most frequently studied chromosomal regions that may harbour asthma and/or atopy susceptibility genes are on chromosomes 11q, 5q and 12q (Table 7.4).

CHROMOSOME 11q

Cookson et al. (1989) were the first to report linkage of atopy on chromosome 11q. In this study, atopy was defined as one of either elevated total serum IgE, raised allergen-specific IgE or the presence of one or more positive skin-prick tests. Seven families were studied, whereas most of the LOD score was contributed by a single family using an autosomal dominant mode of inheritance. These authors replicated this finding in other samples, one of which was an Australian sample (Young et al., 1992; Moffatt et al., 1992; Daniels et al., 1996). In addition, in other studies from the Netherlands, Germany, Japan and Australia, evidence for linkage was found between different asthmatic and/or atopic phenotypes and markers on chromosome 11q. In a Dutch sample of 26 sib-pairs linkage was found between 11q and asthma and atopy, defined as the presence of two respiratory symptoms and elevated specific or total serum IgE levels (Collee et al., 1993). In a German study linkage was found between 11q and a clinical history of atopy and an elevated total serum IgE level (Folster Holst et al., 1998), and in a Japanese study linkage was found between 11q and severe atopy (total serum IgE > 400 IU/mL; three or more positive intradermal skin tests > 9 mm or three or more positive *RAST* (radioallergosorbent test) scores) in four selected families (Shirakawa et al., 1994a). In an Australian study no linkage between chromosome 11q and atopy was found. However, airway hyperresponsiveness to methacholine appeared to be linked to 11q (van Herwerden et al., 1995).

Linkage of chromosome 11q to atopy and asthma is still controversial due to multiple failures to replicate this finding in several other populations (Table 7.4) (Lympany et al., 1992; Rich et al., 1992; Hizawa et al., 1992; Coleman et al., 1993; Brereton et al., 1994; Martinati et al., 1996; Noguchi et al., 1997; Amelung et al., 1998). Cookson et al. (1992) suggested that maternal inheritance of atopy may have obscured linkage in other studies; excess sharing of maternal, not paternal, alleles on chromosome 11q was shown in atopic children. Possible explanations for maternal inheritance of atopy are paternal imprinting or maternal modification of the developing immune response. A candidate gene for atopy in this chromosomal region, the β-chain of the high-affinity IgE receptor, will be discussed in the next section (Sandford et al., 1993).

CHROMOSOME 5q

Chromosome 5q31–q33 contains numerous candidate genes for asthma and atopy, such as a cluster of cytokine genes (interleukin-3 (IL-3), IL-4, IL-5, IL-9, IL-13, the β-chain of IL-12) and the genes coding for the β_2-adrenergic receptor, CD-14, the corticosteroid receptor and the granulocyte-macrophage colony stimulating factor.

In 1994, linkage between total serum IgE levels and chromosome 5q was first reported in a US Amish population (Marsh et al., 1994). This finding was replicated by Meyers et al. (1994) in a study of Dutch families who were ascertained with asthma through a proband. In 1995, Postma et al., showed in the latter population that AH to histamine was linked between the same region of chromosome 5q as total serum IgE (Fig. 7.3). These findings indicated that a gene governing AH is located near a gene regulating total serum IgE (Postma et al., 1995).

Table 7.4 Linkage analyses of asthma and airway hyperresponsiveness

Phenotype	Chromosome, + or – result	First author, year	Number	Genetic analysis	Definition of phenotype/comments
Asthma	5q +	Noguchi, 1997	41 s	Sib-pair	Intermittent episodes of wheeze and dyspnoea.
		CSGA, 1997	79 f	Affected relative pair	Two of three symptoms (cough, wheeze, dyspnoea) and AH to methacholine or reversibility/modest evidence of linkage.
		Ober, 1998	361 n	TDT, LR test	Bronchial hyperresponsiveness to methacholine and/or symptoms of asthma.
	5q –	Kamitani, 1997	45 s	Sib-pair	Wheeze or use of asthma medication in past year/random population sample.
		Laitinen, 1997	157 f	Affected relative pair, association	History of asthma, wheezing by auscultation, reversibility and/or AH.
	11q +	van Herwerden, 1995	123 s	Sib-pair	Episode of asthma in the past 12 months, nocturnal shortness of breath or use of asthma medication.
	11q –	Noguchi, 1997	44 s	Sib-pair	Intermittent episodes of wheeze and dyspnoea.
	12q +	Barnes, 1996	29 f	Sib-, relative pair, TDT	Reported history of asthma, confirmed by a doctor diagnosis.
		CSGA, 1997	79 f	Relative pair	Two of three symptoms (cough, wheeze, dyspnoea) and AH to methacholine or reversibility after bronchodilator use.
		Ober, 1998	361 n	TDT, LR test	Bronchial hyperresponsiveness to methacholine and/or symptoms of asthma.
		Wilkinson, 1998	240 f	Sib-pair	Wheeze and asthma, defined as a quantitative asthma score.
AH	5q +	Postma, 1995	35 s	Sib-pair	AH to methacholine/families ascertained through a proband with asthma.
	5q –	Doull, 1996	131 f	Association	AH to histamine/random population.
		Kamitani, 1997	51 s	Sib-pair	AH to methacholine/random population.
		Mansur, 1998	181 n	Association	AH to methacholine/random population, weak association.
	11q +	Doull, 1996	131 f	Association	AH to histamine/random population.
		van Herwerden, 1995	123 s	Sib-pair	AH to methacholine/linkage even in absence of atopy.
	11q –	Lympany, 1992	9 f	LOD	AH to methacholine/in children aged 2–8 years exercise challenge test.
		Amelung, 1998	83 f	Sib-pair	AH to histamine/one marker at 11q had a modest significance level.

–, negative or not confirmative results; +, positive results.

f, number of families; s, number of sib-pairs; n, number of individuals.

Sib-pair, affected sibling pair analysis; Association, association analysis; TDT, transmission disequilibrium test; LOD, LOD score analysis;

LR test, likelihood ratio test, a semiparametric test for linkage; AH, airway hyperresponsiveness; CSGA, Collaborative Study on the Genetics of Asthma.

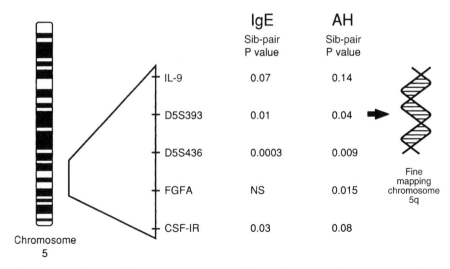

Figure 7.3 *Linkage analysis for total serum IgE and airway hyperresponsiveness (AH). Results of affected sib-pair analysis of chromosome 5q in a Dutch sample.*

Studies of asthma in Japan (Noguchi *et al.*, 1997), the UK (Doull *et al.*, 1996) and the USA (CSGA, 1997; Ober *et al.*, 1998) also implicated chromosome 5q as a region containing one or more susceptibility genes for asthma. However, in Australian (Kamitani *et al.*, 1997), Finnish (Laitinen *et al.*, 1997), British (Mansur *et al.*, 1998) and German (Ulbrecht *et al.*, 1997) populations and in four US families (Blumenthal *et al.*, 1996) chromosome 5q did not appear to be linked to asthma or atopy.

CHROMOSOME 12q

Chromosome 12q is an interesting region for both asthma and atopy, because of several candidate genes, including interferon-γ (an inhibitor of IL-4 production by Th2 lymphocytes), a mast cell growth factor, and the β subunit of nuclear factor-Y which possibly upregulates transcription of both IL-4 and the human leucocyte antigen class D-genes.

Barnes *et al.* studied individuals with doctor-diagnosed asthma and individuals with elevated total serum IgE levels in two different populations: an Afro-Caribbean population from Barbados, and Caucasian Amish kindreds from Pennsylvania, USA. Evidence for linkage and association to this chromosomal region was found for both elevated total serum IgE (Barbados and Amish) and for doctor-diagnosed asthma (Barbados) (Barnes *et al.*, 1996). Linkage of high serum IgE levels to 12q15–q24.1 was replicated in a German population sample of 52 children selected for high serum IgE levels (Nickel *et al.*, 1997). Finally, evidence for linkage of asthma and 12q was shown in 240 families from the UK (Wilkinson *et al.*, 1998) and a study in the Hutterites from the USA (Ober *et al.*, 1998).

An interesting finding is that the chromosomal regions on 12q implicated in these studies are not exactly the same. Further studies are needed to fine-map this region. These studies will have to answer the question of whether one or more regions on 12q are implicated in asthma and atopy.

Other chromosomal regions detected by genome-wide searches

To date, four genome-wide searches on asthma and atopy have been published. In genome-wide searches, the whole genome is scanned with markers spaced every 10 to 20 cM. The goal

Table 7.5 *Results of linkage analyses of atopy and total IgE*

Phenotype	Chromosome, + or − result	First author, year	Number, type	Genetic analysis	Definition of phenotype/comments
Atopy	5q +	Noguchi, 1997	71 s	Sib-pair	Total IgE > 1 SD of the Japanese mean and/or elevated allergen-specific IgE.
	5q −	Kamitani, 1997	103 s	Sib-pair	Skin-prick test positivity to common aeroallergens.
		Laitinen, 1997	157 f	Affected relative pair, association	
	11q +	Cookson, 1989	7 f	LOD	Either of ≥ 1 positive skin-prick test, elevated specific or total serum IgE.
		Cookson, 1992	70 f	Sib-pair	*Idem*/increased sharing of maternal, not paternal alleles.
		Young, 1992	64 f	LOD	≥ 1 positive skin-prick test, elevated specific or tota seruml IgE.
		Collee, 1993	26 s	Sib-pair	≥ 2 respiratory symptoms and elevated total serum IgE or elevated specific IgE.
		Shirakawa, 1994	4 f	LOD	Serum IgE > 400 IU/mL, ≥ 3 positive intradermal skin tests or ≥ 3 positive RAST scores.
		Daniels, 1996	80 f	Sib-pair	Sum of the skin-prick tests to grasses and house dust mite/genome-wide search.
		Folster Holst, 1998	12 f	Affected relative pair, LOD	Clinical diagnosis of atopy and elevated total serum IgE levels/families with atopic dermatitis, two-locus analysis with recessive-dominant model showed linkage in 2 of 12 families.
	11q −	Lympany, 1992	9 f	LOD	Positive skin-prick test and/or positive allergen-specific IgE.
		Rich, 1992	3 f	Sib-pair, LOD	Either of ≥ 1 positive skin-prick test, elevated specific or total serum IgE.
		Hizawa, 1992	4 f	LOD	Either of ≥ 1 positive skin-prick test, elevated specific or total serum IgE, other definitions tested.
		Coleman, 1993	95 f	Sib-pair, LOD	*Idem*/family ascertainment through two first degree family members with atopic eczema.

	Reference	n	Analysis	Notes
	Brereton, 1994	12 f	Sib-pair, LOD	≥ 1 positive skin-prick test.
	Martinati, 1996	45 f	Sib-pair	Either of ≥ 1 positive skin-prick test, elevated specific or total serum IgE.
	Noguchi, 1997	70 s	Sib-pair	Total serum IgE > 1 SD of the mean of the Japanese population and/or elevated allergen-specific IgE.
	Amelung, 1998	83 f	Sib-pair, LOD	Elevated total serum IgE or number of positive skin tests.
Total IgE 5q +	Marsh, 1994	11 f	Sib-pair, LOD	Eleven Amish extended families.
	Xu, 1995	92 f	Two locus LOD	First locus at 5q, second locus not mapped. (Also Meyers, 1994.)
	Doull, 1996	131 f	Association	Random population sample.
	Noguchi, 1997	71 s	Sib-pair	Families ascertained through asthmatic children.
5q –	Blumenthal, 1996	4 f	Sib-pair, LOD	
	Ulbrecht, 1997	395 n	Association	Population sample.
	Mansur, 1998	181 n	Association	Population sample.
11q +	Daniels, 1996	80 f	Sib-pair	Genome-wide search.
11q –	Watson, 1995	131 f	LOD	Random selected families with a minimum of three children.
	Amelung, 1998	83 f	Two locus LOD	Families ascertained through a proband with asthma.
12q +	Barnes, 1996	29 f	Sib-pair, TDT	Afro-Caribbean families ascertained through a proband with asthma.
	Barnes, 1996	24 f	Sib-pair, TDT	Amish families ascertained through one child with detectable allergen-specific IgE.
	Nickel, 1997	52 n	TDT	German children ascertained from population study for high total serum IgE levels.

–, negative or not confirmative results; +, positive results.
f, number of families; s, number of sib-pairs; n, number of individuals.
Sib-pair, affected sibling pair analysis; Association, association analysis; TDT, transmission disequilibrium analysis; LOD, LOD score analysis;
SD, standard deviation.

of a genome-wide search is to detect regions of interest for asthma and atopy using modest criteria of significance. These criteria could lead to the detection of new regions that contain susceptibility genes, as well as some regions that could represent false-positive results. Therefore, these regions need to be followed-up by additional mapping studies before a definitive conclusion can be drawn. The results from the four genome-wide searches on asthma and atopy will be discussed in this section. In the first published genome-wide search in an Australian and British sample, evidence for linkage was found on chromosome 4 (AH), chromosome 6 (eosinophils), chromosome 7 (AH), chromosome 11 (skin tests, total serum IgE) and chromosome 16 (total serum IgE) (Daniels et al., 1996).

The second genome-wide search was a US multicenter study in 140 asthma families ascertained through two or more affected siblings with asthma. Three different racial groups, namely Hispanics, Caucasians and Afro-Americans were studied (CSGA, 1997). An interesting result is that different regions appeared to be linked in these different racial groups. Regions of interest for asthma were chromosome 5p and 17p in Afro-Americans; 11p and 19q in Caucasians and 2q and 21q in Hispanics.

A third genome-wide search was performed in the Hutterites. This is a religious sect that originated in Europe. In 1870, 900 members of this population moved to the USA. The current Hutterite population originates from less than 90 ancestors, and is therefore a homogeneous population. In this study, asthma was defined as 'strict' asthma if the subjects showed AH to methacholine and reported asthma symptoms. Asthma was defined as 'loose' asthma if subjects had either AH to methacholine or reported asthma symptoms. Regions of interest for 'strict' asthma were chromosome 19q and 21q. In addition, regions of interest for 'loose' asthma were 5q and 12q. Furthermore, a region of interest for 'loose' asthma, not reported in other studies, was chromosome 3p. In conclusion, even in a homogeneous population such as the Hutterites, multiple susceptibility genes may influence asthma phenotypes (Ober et al., 1998).

Finally, a fourth genome screen was performed in German families with asthma. Asthma was defined by clinical history and supported by questionnaire data of a history of at least 3 years of recurrent wheezing in children over age 3. For asthma, four possible linkages were reported at chromosomes 2p, 6p, 9q and 12q. These linkage results for asthma were repeated with the study of intermediate phenotypes of asthma and atopy. For chromosome 2p, evidence for linkage was found for airway responsiveness to methacholine, specific and total IgE; for chromosome 6p for total and specific IgE and eosinophils; for chromosome 9q for total and specific IgE; and lastly, for chromosome 12q for specific IgE (Wjst et al., 1999).

Having reviewed the linkage results for asthma and atopy, some conclusions can be drawn. First, chromosome 5q, 11q and 12q are the most cited regions of interest for asthma and atopy. These findings of linkage are an important step towards the actual identification of susceptibility genes for asthma and atopy in these regions. Second, replication of linkages in other populations has proven to be difficult. Several possible reasons may explain this difficulty. One explanation may be that the definition of the phenotypes and genotypes under study are often different between studies (Table 7.4). For example, atopy has been defined in one study as a positive history of atopic disease, in another study as a positive skin-prick test, and in some other studies as a combination of elevated total serum IgE, allergen-specific IgE or positive skin-prick tests in different studies. Another explanation may be a high degree of genetic heterogeneity. This means that different genes are important in different populations; and each of these genes is sufficient to express the phenotype. In addition, several major and minor genes may interact in order to express the phenotype (oligogenic inheritance). One gene may be more prevalent in one population, whereas the second or third gene is more prevalent in other populations. Nevertheless, they provide the same phenotype. Yet another explanation may be that some of the published linkage results represent false-positive results.

A final explanation could be that some studies did not have a sufficient sample size to detect linkage, which may have led to false-negative results.

Therefore, it is crucial that linkage results are replicated by different investigators in different populations of sufficient size. Thereafter, confirmed regions can be studied in detail and candidate genes can be detected.

CANDIDATE GENES FOR ASTHMA

After determining linkage between asthma and a chromosomal region, the next challenge is to screen this region for candidate genes. A candidate gene for asthma has to meet four criteria: (i) the gene product must be functionally relevant to asthma; (ii) mutations within the gene must alter the function of the gene; (iii) asthma needs to be linked to the chromosomal region harbouring the candidate gene; and (iv) asthma has to show association with different alleles of this candidate gene. To date, a number of candidate genes for asthma and atopy have been studied. These include the gene encoding the β_2-adrenergic receptor and genes from the cytokine cluster at chromosome 5q31–q33; the gene encoding the β chain of the high-affinity IgE receptor at chromosome 11q13, the gene encoding the IL-4 receptor α chain at chromosome 16p, and the major histocompatibility complex and the gene encoding tumour necrosis factor-α at chromosome 6. Some other candidate genes for asthma and atopy will also be discussed in this section.

The β_2-adrenergic receptor

The β_2-adrenergic receptor was hypothesized to play a role in the pathogenesis of asthma by Szentivanyi (1968). β_2-Adrenergic receptors are localized in several human tissues and cells, including lung tissue (for instance, in airway smooth muscle and epithelium) and inflammatory cells (mast cells, macrophages, eosinophils and T lymphocytes). β_2-Adrenergic receptor function is mainly regulated by circulating epinephrine and mediates most of the effects of β_2-agonists on airway function (Barnes, 1995).

The gene coding for the β_2-adrenergic receptor is situated on chromosome 5q31. This receptor is a protein of 413 amino acids. In this gene, nine polymorphisms were identified, of which four lead to altered amino-acid sequences at positions 16, 27, 34 and 164. (Fig. 7.4) In most studies on polymorphisms of the β_2-adrenergic receptor, none of these polymorphisms contributes to the risk of developing asthma (Reihsaus et al., 1993; Dewar et al., 1997; Martinez et al., 1997). Current evidence suggests that the polymorphisms at positions 16 and 27 may play an important role in modifying the clinical severity of asthma.

Amino-acid 16 of the β_2-adrenergic receptor can either be glycine (Gly) or arginine (Arg). The Gly-16 variant of the receptor might be associated with nocturnal asthma and with more severe asthma, as evidenced by the finding that patients with the Gly-16 variant were more likely to use corticosteroids and immunotherapy (Turki et al., 1995; Reihsaus et al., 1993). Furthermore, in a population study of children, individuals with the Gly-16 variant showed a decreased short-term bronchodilation after the use of a short-acting β-agonist compared to individuals with the Arg-16 allele. The investigators suggest that the low response of the Gly-16 variant following β-agonist stimulation could be a reason for an increased use of inhaled corticosteroids (Martinez et al., 1997). The Gly-16 and Arg-16 variants of the β_2-adrenergic receptor may also regulate receptor downregulation after long-term exposure. Studies in airway smooth muscle cell cultures showed that long-term β-agonist exposure downregulates the Gly-16 variant of the β_2-adrenergic receptor to a greater extent than the Arg-16 variant

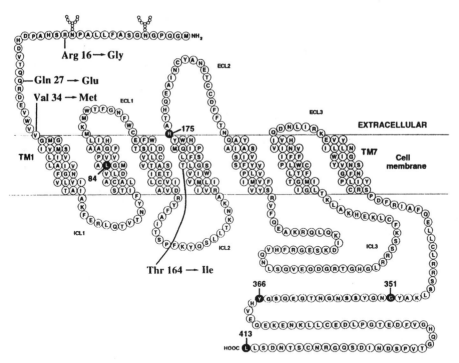

Figure 7.4 *Primary amino-acid sequence and proposed membrane topography of the human β₂-adrenergic receptor. The darkened circles indicate codons where degenerate polymorphisms of the receptor gene were found. The four polymorphisms which result in changes in the amino-acid sequence are indicated. Source: Liggett SB. (1995) Genetics of β₂ receptor variants in asthma.* Clin Exp Allergy, **25**(2), *89–94. (Reproduced with permission.)*

(Green *et al.*, 1995). Another study in patients with asthma showed that a greater degree of agonist-promoted receptor downregulation was associated with the Gly-16 variant, not with the Arg-16 variant (Tan *et al.*, 1997).

The amino-acid 27 of the β₂-adrenergic receptor can either be a glutamine (Gln) or a glutamate (Glu) residue. The Gln-27 variant was associated with elevated levels of total serum IgE in a study of 60 families having a proband with asthma. This variant was associated with more severe airway responsiveness compared to the Glu-27 variant as well (Hall *et al.*, 1995; Dewar *et al.*, 1997). The Glu-27 variant of the β₂-adrenergic receptor showed an attenuated downregulation after the use of a long-acting β-agonist in another study; however, this 'protective' effect seemed less important than the effects of downregulation of the Gly-16 allele (Tan *et al.*, 1997).

In general, it is difficult to study these variants in human populations separately, as in most populations these alleles are in linkage disequilibrium. This means that the alleles at the 16 and 27 positions of the β₂-adrenergic receptor are not distributed randomly in the population. Since new polymorphisms have been detected recently in a regulatory region of the β₂-adrenergic receptor, more studies may be expected on the role of polymorphisms of this gene in asthma (McGraw *et al.*, 1998).

The β chain of the high-affinity IgE receptor

The high-affinity IgE receptor (FcεRI) is composed of three subunits: one α, one β and two γ subunits. This αβγ₂ complex is found on the surface of mast cells, basophils, eosinophils and

Langerhans cells. The binding of allergen to receptor-bound IgE on mast cells leads to activation and excretion of cytokines such as IL-4, thus upregulating IgE production by B lymphocytes. The α subunit is responsible for ligand binding and the γ dimer mediates for both the assembly of the receptor as well as signal transduction. The β subunit amplifies the signal strength mediated by the γ subunit (Ravetch, 1994).

Whereas the α and γ chains did not appear to be associated to asthma or atopy (Doull *et al.*, 1996), the β chain has received considerable interest (Sandford *et al.*, 1993). The gene encoding the β chain is situated on chromosome 11q. As we have reported in the section on linkage (p. 157), this chromosomal region was linked to asthma and/or atopy in several studies. In 1994, Shirakawa *et al.*, reported that in a random British population sample an isoleucine (IIe) to leucine (Leu) change at position 181 in this protein was significantly associated with atopy if the Leu-181 variant had been inherited maternally. Of the 60 families of allergic asthmatic probands under study, this variant was detected in 10 families. In addition, at position 183 a valine (Val) to leucine (Leu) change was found (Shirakawa *et al.*, 1994b). The combination of Leu-181/Leu-183 was found in 4.5% of 1004 members of 230 two-generation families in Western Australia. When inherited maternally, the Leu-181/Leu-183 variant was associated with atopy (Hill *et al.*, 1995). However, the Leu-181/Leu-183 variants were not detected in other populations from Japan (Shirakawa *et al.*, 1996a), the UK (Hall *et al.*, 1996), Italy (Martinati *et al.*, 1996) or the Netherlands (Amelung *et al.*, 1998).

Other polymorphisms in this gene result in two restriction sites for the restriction enzyme *Rsa*I. One of these variants was associated with atopic disease in a Japanese population (Shirakawa *et al.*, 1996b) and atopic dermatitis in a British population (Cox *et al.*, 1998). However, in another Japanese study the association between these variants and atopy could not be confirmed (Fukao *et al.*, 1996). The most recent mutation reported is a substitution of Glu for Gly at amino-acid 237 (E237G). The population frequency of this mutation is about 5% in Australian and Japanese populations. In two studies this mutation was strongly associated with asthma, and in the Australian study with airway hyperresponsiveness as well (Hill and Cookson, 1996; Shirakawa *et al.*, 1996a). In summary, the question remains if the Ile-181 and Ile-183 variants in the gene that codes for the β chain of the high-affinity IgE receptor can account for the linkage reported by several groups, as it is detected in a subset of families or not detected at all in some populations. In addition, little is known on altered function of one of these variants in relation to atopy. It is therefore plausible, that other variants of this gene, such as the E237G variant, or other genes on chromosome 11q, are more important in atopy and atopic asthma.

The interleukin 4-receptor α chain

Both interleukins 4 and 13 and their receptors are candidate genes for asthma and atopy, given that IL-4 and IL-13 are central in the switch of B-cells to produce IgE and IL-4 stimulates the maturation of Th0- to Th2-type lymphocytes. The IL-4 receptor and the IL-13 receptor share the IL-4 receptor α chain. The interleukin 4 receptor α gene resides at chromosome 16p. In a study from Germany, this chromosomal region was linked to markers of atopy. Only alleles inherited from the mother appeared to increase the risk of atopy in children (Deichmann *et al.*, 1998). The IL-4 receptor α chain has 13 known polymorphisms. Most data are available of one extracellular variant (Ile50Val), and two intracellular variants (Pro478Ser and Arg551Gln) (Shirakawa *et al.*, 2000). The Ile50 allele was associated with atopic asthma in one Japanese population (Mitsuyasu *et al.*, 1998), but this could not be confirmed in another Japanese population (Noguchi *et al.*, 1999). The Arg551 allele was associated with high total serum IgE levels in a study of patients with hyper-IgE syndrome and eczema (Hershey *et al.*, 1997). In these studies other polymorphisms of the IL-4 receptor α chain were not investigated. In a German population, the combination of Pro478 and the Arg551 allele was associated with lowered total serum IgE levels. Arg551Gly and Pro478Ser are in linkage disequilibrium in most populations; therefore, the association of one allele with total IgE or asthma cannot be studied separately. Given the multiple polymorphisms in this gene, and the contradictory association results, several groups have attempted to study the functional role of these polymorphisms. First, from *in vitro* studies with transfected cell lines, Mitsuyasu and coworkers provided evidence that Ile50 allele, but not Arg551 allele, is involved in increased STAT-6 activation and proliferation and transcription of the IgE promoter by IL-4 (Mitsuyasu *et al.*, 1999). Second, from *in vivo* immunoassays using T-cells of individuals with different alleles of the Pro468Ser and the Arg551Gly, Kruse and coworkers suggested that the phosphorylation status of transcription factors IRS-1, IRS-2 and STAT6 was changed in the presence of these polymorphisms (Kruse *et al.*, 1999). In conclusion, although the genetic associations and the available functional data indicate the importance of the IL-4R gene, more research is needed to clarify the role and the interaction of these polymorphisms in the regulation of IgE levels.

The human leucocyte antigen region

At chromosome 6p resides the human leucocyte antigen (HLA) region and the gene for tumour necrosis factor-α (TNF-α) as well. The HLA molecules are membrane-bound glycoproteins which bind processed antigenic peptides and present them to T-cells. Two HLA classes can be distinguished: class I is expressed on virtually every somatic cell; class II is merely expressed on B-cells, activated T-cells and monocytes/macrophages.

Polymorphisms in genes encoding the HLA class II molecules are associated with the specific IgE responses to several small allergens, such as ragweed pollen (Howell and Holgate, 1995). Other studies have failed to extend this finding to common major allergens, such as house dust mite (Young *et al.*, 1994; Holloway *et al.*, 1996). Certain HLA class II alleles may be important in susceptibility to isocyanate-induced asthma, the most common cause of industrial asthma (Bignon *et al.*, 1994). In a collaborative US study, in Caucasian pairs of siblings with asthma, an increased sharing of alleles was found at chromosome 6p (CSGA, 1997). However, it is questionable whether the HLA region is implicated in asthma, considering that several other studies could not identify significant associations between asthma and the HLA region (Li *et al.*, 1995; Aron *et al.*, 1995). Thus, as atopy was present in over 75% of the US sample, the finding of linkage of asthma on 6p may, in fact, reflect the known association of the specific IgE response and the HLA region on 6p.

Tumour necrosis factor-α

TNF-α is a potent modulator of the immune inflammatory response and elevated levels can be detected in sputum and bronchoalveolar lavage fluid of patients with asthma during asthmatic attacks. Therefore, polymorphisms in this gene that may upregulate TNF-α production have been studied by Albuquerque *et al.* (1998). In the promoter region of TNF-α on chromosome 6p, a polymorphism was detected at position 308 (G to A substitution), called the TNF1 allele. This polymorphism could be associated with a six- to sevenfold upregulation in transcription of TNF-α. In a sample of 124 Australian schoolchildren, aged 6–12 years, this polymorphism resulted in a fivefold increased risk to asthma, defined as *physician-diagnosed* asthma requiring the use of prophylactic medication. Moreover, all patients had positive skin-prick tests to one or more common aeroallergens and a family history of asthma and/or atopic disease in first degree relatives (Albuquerque *et al.*, 1998).

Within 7 cM of the TNF-α gene, a polymorphism in the first intron of the lymphotoxin-α gene (LTα*2 allele) showed a similar association. Furthermore, at chromosome 6p, the HLA region may also be involved in these atopic individuals.

On the contrary, Moffat and Cookson (1997) found positive associations between asthma (questionnaire-defined) and TNF2 and LTα*1 alleles. This illustrates, that a positive association needs to be supported by linkage studies and functional studies before definitive conclusions can be drawn regarding the role of these polymorphisms in the pathogenesis of asthma.

The cytokine gene cluster and other candidate genes

The cytokine gene cluster at chromosome 5q31−33 contains several pro-inflammatory cytokines (IL-3, IL-4, IL-9, IL-13), the glucocorticoid receptor, leukotriene C_4 synthase (LTC$_4$ synthase), CD14 and several other candidate genes. Much interest has been given to cytokines produced by Th2-like lymphocytes, and therefore promote IgE production and airway inflammation. In general, studies in patients with asthma showed elevated IL4, IL-5, IL-9 and IL-13 production, and reduced IFN-γ production. These elevations may be due to polymorphisms that upregulate regulation of cytokine production. It is also possible that changes in other cytokine genes or transcription factors that regulate these cytokines are responsible for these elevations. To date, there is some evidence for a possible role of a change in the promoter region of the IL-4 gene (Walley and Cookson, 1996; Rosenwasser and Borish, 1997), the IL-9 gene (Doull et al., 1996; Nicolaides et al., 1997), and the IL-13 gene (van der Pouw Kraan et al., 1999), but not the IL-5 gene (Pereira et al., 1998).

The CD14 gene resides in the vicinity of the cytokine gene cluster on chromosome 5q and encodes for a high-affinity lipopolysaccharide receptor. This receptor is present as membrane-bound CD14 on monocytes, macrophages and neutrophils, and in a soluble form (sCD14) in serum. Baldini and coworkers studied this CD14 gene based on the hypothesis that bacterial wall components could influence the Th1-Th2 balance, and thus the development of atopy, through a CD14-dependent pathway. In a population study of children in the USA, a promoter polymorphism in the CD14 gene was associated with levels of sCD14 in serum, total IgE levels and number of positive skin tests (Baldini et al., 1999). This interesting finding merits further study.

Other candidate genes for asthma and atopy include the IFN-γ gene at chromosome 12, and the T-cell receptor genes at chromosome 7 and 14. A screening of the IFN-γ gene on chromosome 12 revealed no sequence variants in patients with asthma and controls (Hayden et al., 1997). Other groups have studied the genetics of the T-cell receptor. In most individuals, this receptor is made up of α chains (gene at chromosome 14) and β chains (gene at chromosome 7). Around the α chain, increased sharing of alleles was found for the specific immune response in a UK and Australian population (Moffatt et al., 1994). Around the β chain gene, increased sharing of alleles was found for childhood asthma and total serum IgE in a Japanese study (Noguchi et al., 1998). This study could not confirm the linkage to the region of the α chain of the T-cell receptor gene. Further studies are needed to confirm these findings.

In summary, association studies of candidate genes have led to interesting new insights into the genetics of asthma. Two polymorphisms of the β$_2$-adrenergic receptor most likely do not cause asthma, but modify the severity of asthma. An interesting feature is that these polymorphisms might be involved in the response to medication. The high-affinity IgE receptor could play a role in atopy and asthma in some populations. The E237G polymorphism of the high-affinity IgE receptor especially needs to be studied in other populations. The IL-4 receptor α chain is a strong candidate for atopy, based on different association and functional studies. Finally, numerous other candidate genes have been studied. None of these candidate genes meets all four criteria as stated in the first paragraph of this section (p. 167). It is clear that in the near future more genetic and functional studies are needed to clarify the role of these candidate genes in asthma and atopy.

SUMMARY AND FUTURE DEVELOPMENTS

The genetics of asthma has become a promising new field of research. In the pathogenesis of asthma multiple genes interact with each other and the environment. In different populations, different genes may have a major effect in the clinical manifestation of asthma. To date, several candidate genes have been identified. Polymorphisms in the β_2-adrenergic receptor do not cause asthma, but modify asthma into a more severe phenotype. Furthermore, polymorphisms in the β chain of the high-affinity IgE receptor could play a role in a subset of patients with atopy. However, most of the susceptibility genes for asthma and atopy remain to be determined. The recent identification of multiple linkages between asthma and different chromosomal regions represents a first step towards the identification of these asthma genes. However, in recent years, the procession from linkage to the actual identification of the gene has proved to be difficult.

In the coming years, developments in molecular biology and genetic epidemiology may accelerate the process of the identification of genes for asthma and atopy. In the field of molecular biology, the Human Genome Project has the ultimate goal to sequence the human genome by 2003, and to identify single nucleotide polymorphisms throughout the genome. This project will aid genetic studies to a great extent (Collins *et al.*, 1998). Furthermore, one may anticipate new observations from animal studies, leading to further understanding of the genetics of human asthma. A genome-wide search for airway hyperresponsiveness in mice has been completed, and has resulted in two possible linked regions on the mouse genome (De Sanctis *et al.*, 1995). This approach could identify genes important in the regulation of airway hyperresponsiveness in mice, and possibly in humans, by searching for their homologous genes in human DNA.

In the field of genetic epidemiology, an interesting new method is the mapping of genes through the systematic analysis of shared haplotypes of affected individuals in founder populations. This approach is based on the idea that current asthmatics have identical copies of parts of chromosomes from a common ancestor. If one is able to identify such a chromosomal region which is identical by descent, it is likely that this chromosomal region contains an asthma susceptibility gene (Te Meerman and van der Meulen, 1997).

The potential benefits of the identification of susceptibility or modifier genes for asthma are numerous. First of all, identification of persons at risk for asthma provides the opportunity for early prevention, such as allergen avoidance or early introduction of medication. Second, protein products of these genes are potential drug targets, opening the way to causative rather than symptomatic treatment. Another clinical application may be that certain polymorphisms could result in a more severe asthmatic phenotype or predict resistance to therapy (pharmacogenetics). The latter is illustrated by the recent finding in a clinical trial of an experimental 5-lipoxygenase inhibitor in 325 patients with asthma. In this study, variants in the promoter region of the 5-lipoxygenase gene were associated with response to this anti-asthma treatment (Drazen *et al.*, 1999).

In conclusion, although considerable progress regarding the genetics of asthma has been made, important questions remain to be answered. Which genes are the susceptibility genes for asthma? Are the genes for airway hyperresponsiveness and atopy the same or different? What is the biological function of asthma susceptibility genes? How do these genes interact with each other and with the environment? It will be a major challenge to unravel this complex genetic disease in the coming years.

ACKNOWLEDGEMENT

This work is supported by the Netherlands Asthma Foundation, AF 95.09.

REFERENCES

Albuquerque RV, Hayden CM, Palmer LJ *et al.* (1998) Association of polymorphisms within the tumour necrosis factor (TNF) genes and childhood asthma. *Clin Exp Allergy*, **28**, 578–84.

Amelung PJ, Postma DS, Xu J, Meyers DA, Bleecker ER. (1998) Exclusion of chromosome 11q and the FCERIB gene as aetiological factors in allergy and asthma in a population of Dutch asthmatic families. *Clin Exp Allergy*, **28**, 397–403.

Antequera F, Bird A. (1994) Predicting the total number of human genes. *Nat Genet*, **8**, 114.

Aron Y, Swierczewski E, Lockhart A. (1995) HLA class II haplotype in atopic asthmatic and non-atopic control subjects. *Clin Exp Allergy*, **25** (Suppl 2), 65–7.

Baldini MC, Lohman CI, Halonen M, Erickson RP, Holt PG, Martinez FG. (1999) A polymorphism in the 5′ flanking region of the CD14 gene is associated with circulating soluble CD14 levels and with total serum immunoglobulin E. *Am J Resp Mol Cell Biol*, **20**, 976–83.

Barnes KC, Neely JD, Duffy DL, *et al.* (1996) Linkage of asthma and total serum IgE concentration to markers on chromosome 12q: evidence from Afro-Caribbean and Caucasian populations. *Genomics*, **37**, 41–50.

Barnes PJ. (1995) Beta-adrenergic receptors and their regulation. *Am J Respir Crit Care Med*, **152**, 838–60.

Bignon JS, Aron Y, Ju LY, *et al.* (1994) HLA class II alleles in isocyanate-induced asthma. *Am J Respir Crit Care Med*, **149**, 71–5.

Blumenthal MN, Wang Z, Weber JL, Rich SS. (1996) Absence of linkage between 5q markers and serum IgE levels in four large atopic families. *Clin Exp Allergy*, **26**, 892–6.

Boezen HM, Postma DS, Schouten JP, Kerstjens HAM, Rijcken B. (1996) PEF variability, bronchial responsiveness and their relation to allergy markers in a random population (20–70 yr). *Am J Respir Crit Care Med*, **154**, 30–5.

Brereton HM, Ruffin RE, Thompson PJ, Turner DR. (1994) Familial atopy in Australian pedigrees: adventitious linkage to chromosome 8 is not confirmed nor is there evidence of linkage to the high affinity IgE receptor. *Clin Exp Allergy*, **24**, 868–77.

Burrows B, Martinez FD, Halonen M, Barbee R, Cline MG. (1989) Association of asthma with serum IgE levels and skin-test reactivity to allergens. *N Engl J Med*, **320**, 271–7.

Chen Y, Rennie DC, Lockinger LA, Dosman JA. (1998) Evidence for major genetic control of wheeze in relation to history of respiratory allergy: Humboldt Family Study. *Am J Med Genet*, **75**, 485–91.

Coleman R, Trembath RC, Harper JI. (1993) Chromosome 11q13 and atopy underlying atopic eczema. *Lancet*, **341**, 1121–2.

Collee JM, ten Kate LP, de Vries HG, *et al.* (1993) Allele sharing on chromosome 11q13 in sibs with asthma and atopy. *Lancet*, **342**, 936.

Collins FS, Patrinos A, Jordan E, Chakravarti A, Gesteland R, Walters L, members of the DOE and NIH planning groups. (1998) New goals for the US Human Genome Project: 1998–2003. *Science*, **282**, 682–9.

Cooke RA, Vanderveer AJ. (1916) Human sensitization. *J Immunol*, **1**, 201–39.

Cookson WO, Sharp PA, Faux JA, Hopkin JM. (1989) Linkage between immunoglobulin E responses underlying asthma and rhinitis and chromosome 11q. *Lancet*, **1**, 1292–5.

Cookson WOCM, Young RP, Sandford AJ, Nakumuura Y, *et al.* (1992) Maternal inheritance of atopic IgE responsiveness on chromosome 11q. *Lancet*, **340**, 381–4.

Cox HE, Moffatt MF, Faux JA, *et al.* (1998) Association of atopic dermatitis to the β subunit of the high affinity immunoglobulin E receptor. *Br J Dermatol*, **138**, 182–7.

CSGA. (1997) A genome-wide search for asthma susceptibility loci in ethnically diverse populations. The Collaborative Study on the Genetics of Asthma (CSGA). *Nat Genet*, **15**, 389–92.

Daniels SE, Bhattacharrya S, James A, *et al.* (1996) A genome-wide search for quantitative trait loci underlying asthma. *Nature*, **383**, 247–50.

De Sanctis GT, Merchant M, Beier DR, *et al.* (1995) Quantitative locus analysis of airway hyperresponsiveness in A/J and C57BL/6J mice. *Nat Genet*, **11**, 150–4.

Deichmann A, Heinzmann A, Forster J, *et al.* (1998) Linkage and allelic association of atopy and markers flanking the IL4-receptor gene. *Clin Exp Allergy*, **28**, 151–5.

Dewar JC, Wilkinson J, Wheatley A, *et al.* (1997) The glutamine 27 β_2-adrenoceptor polymorphism is associated with elevated IgE levels in asthmatic families. *J Allergy Clin Immunol*, **100**, 261–5.

Dizier MH, Hill M, James A, *et al.* (1995) Detection of a recessive major gene for high IgE levels acting independently of specific response to allergens. *Genet Epidemiol*, **12**, 93–105.

Doull IJ, Lawrence S, Watson M, *et al.* (1996) Allelic association of gene markers on chromosomes 5q and 11q with atopy and bronchial hyperresponsiveness. *Am J Respir Crit Care Med*, **153**, 1280–4.

Douma WR, de Gooijer A, Rijcken B. (1997) Lack of correlation between bronchoconstrictor response and bronchodilator response in a population-based study. *Eur Respir J*, **10**, 2772–7.

Drazen JM, Yandava CN, Dubé L, *et al.* (1999) Pharmacogenetic association between ALOX5 promoter genotype and the response to anti-asthma treatment. *Nat Genet*, **22**, 168–70.

Duffy DL, Martin NG, Battistutta D, Hopper JL, Mathews JD. (1990) Genetics of asthma and hay fever in Australian twins. *Am Rev Respir Dis*, **142**, 1351–8.

Edfors-Lubs, ML. (1971) Allergy in 7000 twin pairs. *Acta Allergol*, **26**, 249–85.

European Community Respiratory Health Survey Group. (1997) Genes for asthma? An analysis of the European Community Respiratory Health Survey. *Am J Respir Crit Care Med*, **146**, 1773–80.

Fölster Holst R, Moises HW, Yang L, Fritsch W, Weissenbach J, Christophers E. (1998) Linkage between atopy and the IgE high-affinity receptor gene at 11q13 in atopic dermatitis families. *Hum Genet*, **102**, 236–9.

Fukao T, Kaneko N, Teramoto T, Tashita H, Kondo N. (1996) Association between FcεRIβ and atopic disorder in Japanese population? *Lancet*, **348**, 407.

Gerrard JW, Rao DC, Morton NE. (1978) A genetic study of immunoglobulin E. *Am J Hum Genet*, **30**, 46–58.

Green SA, Turki J, Bejarano P, Hall IP, Liggett SB. (1995) Influence of β_2-adrenergic receptor genotypes on signal transduction in human airway smooth muscle cells. *Am J Respir Cell Mol Biol*, **13**, 25–33.

Hall IP, Wheatley A, Wilding P, Liggett SB. (1995) Association of Glu 27 β_2-adrenoceptor polymorphism with lower airway reactivity in asthmatic subjects. *Lancet*, **345**, 1213–14.

Hall IP, Wheatley A, Dewar J, Wilkinson J, Morrison J. (1996) FcεRI-β polymorphisms unlikely to contribute substantially to genetic risk of allergic disease. *BMJ*, **312**, 311.

Hanson B, McGue M, Roitman Johnson B, Segal NL, Bouchard TJ Jr, Blumenthal MN. (1991) Atopic disease and immunoglobulin E in twins reared apart and together. *Am J Hum Genet*, **48**, 873–9.

Harris JR, Magnus P, Samuelsen SO, Tambs K. (1997) No evidence for effects of family environment on asthma. A retrospective study of Norwegian twins. *Am J Respir Crit Care Med*, **156**, 43–9.

Hasstedt SJ, Meyers DA, Marsh DG. (1983) Inheritance of immunoglobulin E: genetic model fitting. *Am J Med Genet*, **14**, 61–6.

Hayden C, Pereira E, Rye P. (1997) Mutation screening of interferon-γ (IFN-γ) as a candidate gene for asthma. *Clin Exp Allergy*, **27**, 1412–16.

Hershey GKK, Friedrich MF, Esswein LA, Thomas ML, Chatila TA. (1997) The association of atopy with a gain-of-function mutation in the α subunit of the interleukin-4 receptor. *N Engl J Med*, **337**, 1720–5.

Hill MR, James AL, Faux JA, *et al.* (1995) FcεRI-β polymorphism and risk of atopy in a general population sample. *BMJ*, **311**, 776–9.

Hill MR, Cookson WO. (1996) A new variant of the β subunit of the high-affinity receptor for immunoglobulin E (FcεRI-β E237G): associations with measures of atopy and bronchial hyper-responsiveness. *Hum Mol Genet*, **5**, 959–62.

Hizawa N, Yamaguchi E, Ohe M, *et al.* (1992) Lack of linkage between atopy and locus 11q13. *Clin Exp Allergy*, **22**, 1065–9.

Holberg CJ, Elston RC, Halonen M, *et al.* (1996) Segregation analysis of physician-diagnosed asthma in Hispanic and non-Hispanic white families. A recessive component? *Am J Respir Crit Care Med*, **154**, 144–50.

Holloway JW, Doull I, Begishvili B, Beasley R, Holgate ST, Howell WM. (1996) Lack of evidence of a significant association between HLA-DR, DQ and DP genotypes and atopy in families with house dust mite allergy. *Clin Exp Allergy*, **26**, 1142–9.

Hopp RJ, Bewtra AK, Watt GD, Nair NM, Townley RG. (1984) Genetic analysis of allergic disease in twins. *J Allergy Clin Immunol*, **73**, 265–70.

Howell WM, Holgate ST. (1995) HLA genetics and allergic disease. *Thorax*, **50**, 815–18.

Jenkins MA, Hopper JL, Giles GG. (1997) Regressive logistic modeling of familial aggregation for asthma in 7394 population-based nuclear families. *Genet Epidemiol*, **14**, 317–32.

Kamitani Z, Wong ZYH, Dickson P, *et al.* (1997) Absence of genetic linkage of chromosome 5q31 with asthma and atopy in the general population. *Thorax*, **52**, 816–17.

Kauffmann F, Dizier MH, Pin I, *et al.* (1997) Epidemiological study of the genetics and environment of asthma, bronchial hyperresponsiveness, and atopy: phenotype issues. *Am J Respir Crit Care Med*, **156**, S123–9.

Khoury MJ, Beaty TH, Cohen BH. (1993) Genetic approaches to familial aggregation. II. Segregation analysis. In: Khoury MJ, Beaty TH, Cohen BH, eds. *Fundamentals of genetic epidemiology*. New York and Oxford: Oxford University Press, 233–83.

Kruse S, Japha T, Tedner M, Sparholt S, Forster J, Kuehr J, Diechmann KA. (1999) The polymorphisms S503P and Q576R in the interleukin-4 receptor alpha gene are associated with atopy and influence signal transduction. *Immunology*, **96**, 365–71.

Laitinen T, Kauppi P, Ignatius J. (1997) Genetic control of serum IgE levels and asthma: linkage and linkage disequilibrium studies in an isolated population. *Hum Mol Genet*, **6**, 2069–76.

Laitinen T, Rasanen M, Kaprio J, Koskenvuo M, Laitinen LA. (1998) Importance of genetic factors in adolescent asthma. *Am J Respir Crit Care Med*, **157**, 1073–8.

Lander ES, Schork NJ. (1994) Genetic dissection of complex traits. *Science*, **265**, 2037–48.

Lawrence S, Beasley R, Doull I, *et al.* (1994) Genetic analysis of atopy and asthma as quantitative traits and ordered polychotomies. *Ann Hum Genet*, **58**, 359–68.

Li PK, Lai CK, Poon AS, Ho AS, Chan CH, Lai KN. (1995) Lack of association between HLA-DQ and -DR genotypes and asthma in southern Chinese patients. *Clin Exp Allergy*, **25**, 323–31.

Lichtenstein P, Svartengren M. (1997) Genes, environments, and sex: factors of importance in atopic diseases in 7–9-year-old Swedish twins. *Allergy*, **52**, 1079–86.

Longo G, Strinati R, Poli F, Fumi F. (1987) Genetic factors in nonspecific bronchial hyperreactivity: an epidemiologic study. *Am J Dis Child*, **141**, 331–4.

Lympany P, Welsh K, MacCochrane G, Kemeny DM, Lee TH. (1992) Genetic analysis using DNA polymorphism of the linkage between chromosome 11q13 and atopy and bronchial hyperresponsiveness to methacholine. *J Allergy Clin Immunol*, **89**, 619–28.

Mansur AH, Bishop DT, Markham AF, Britton J, Morrison JFJ. (1998) Association study of asthma and atopy traits and chromosome 5q cytokine cluster markers. *Clin Exp Allergy*, **28**, 141–50.

Marsh DG, Neely JD, Breazeale DR, *et al.* (1994) Linkage analysis of IL4 and other chromosome 5q31.1 markers and total serum immunoglobulin E concentrations. *Science*, **264**, 1152–6.

Martinati LC, Trabetti E, Casartelli, A, Boner AL, Pignatti PF. (1996) Affected sib-pair and mutation analyses of the high affinity IgE receptor β chain locus in Italian families with atopic asthmatic children. *Am J Respir Crit Care Med*, **153**, 1682–5.

Martinez FD, Holberg CJ, Halonen M, Morgan WJ, Wright AL, Taussig LM. (1994) Evidence for Mendelian inheritance of serum IgE levels in Hispanic and non-Hispanic white families. *Am J Hum Genet*, **55**, 555–65.

Martinez FD, Wright AL, Taussig LM, Holberg CJ, Halonen M, Morgan WJ, the Group Health Medical Associates. (1995) Asthma and wheezing in the first six years of life. *N Engl J Med*, **332**, 133–8.

Martinez FD, Graves PE, Baldini M, Solomon S, Erickson R. (1997) Association between genetic polymorphisms of the β_2-adrenoreceptor and response to albuterol in children with and without a history of wheezing. *J Clin Invest*, **100**, 3184–8.

McGraw DW, Forbes SL, Kramer LA, Liggett SB. (1998) Polymorphisms of the 5′ leader cistron of the human β_2-adrenergic receptor regulate receptor expression. *J Clin Invest*, **102**, 1927–32.

Meyers DA, Bias WB, Marsh DG. (1982) A genetic study of total IgE levels in the Amish. *Hum Hered*, **32**, 15–23.

Meyers DA, Beaty TH, Freidhoff LR, Marsh DG. (1987) Inheritance of total serum IgE (basal levels) in man. *Am J Hum Genet*, **41**, 51–62.

Meyers DA, Postma DS, Panhuysen CI, *et al.* (1994) Evidence for a locus regulating total serum IgE levels mapping to chromosome 5. *Genomics*, **23**, 464–70.

Mitsuyasu H, Izuhara K, Mao X-Q, *et al.* (1998) Ile50Val variant of IL4Rα upregulates IgE synthesis and associates with atopic asthma. *Nat Genet*, **19**, 119–20.

Mitsuyasu H, Yanagihara Y, Mao X-Q, *et al.* (1999) Dominant effect of Ile50Val variant of the human IL-4 receptor α-chain in IgE synthesis. *J Immunol*, **163**, 1227–31.

Moffatt MF, Sharp PA, Faux JA, Young RP, Cookson WO, Hopkin JM. (1992) Factors confounding genetic linkage between atopy and chromosome 11q. *Clin Exp Allergy*, **22**, 1046–51.

Moffatt MF, Hill MR, Cornelis F, *et al.* (1994) Genetic linkage of T-cell receptor α/δ complex to specific IgE responses. *Lancet*, **343**, 1597–600.

Moffatt MF, Cookson WO. (1997) Tumour necrosis factor haplotypes and asthma. *Hum Mol Genet*, **6**, 551–4.

Nickel R, Wahn U, Hizawa N, *et al.* (1997) Evidence for linkage of chromosome 12q15–q24.1 markers to high total serum IgE concentrations in children of the German Multicenter Allergy Study. *Genomics*, **46**, 159–62.

Nicolaides NC, Holroyd KJ, Ewart SL, *et al.* (1997) Interleukin 9: a candidate gene for asthma. *Proc Natl Acad Sci USA*, **94**, 13175–80.

Nieminen MM, Kaprio J, Koskenvuo M. (1991) A population-based study of bronchial asthma in adult twin pairs. *Chest*, **100**, 70–5.

Noguchi E, Shibasaki M, Arinami T, *et al.* (1997) Evidence for linkage between asthma/atopy in childhood and chromosome 5q31–q33 in a Japanese population. *Am J Respir Crit Care Med*, **156**, 1390–3.

Noguchi E, Shibasaki M, Arinami T, Takeda K, Kobayashi K, Matsui A, Hamaguchi H. (1998) Evidence for linkage between the development of asthma in childhood and the T-cell receptor β chain gene in Japanese. *Genomics*, **47**, 121–4.

Noguchi E, Shibasaki M, Arinami T, *et al.* (1999) No association between atopy/asthma and the Ile50Val polymorphism of IL-4 receptor. *Am J Respir Crit Care Med*, **160**, 342–5.

Ober C, Cox NJ, Abney M, *et al.* and Collaborative Study on the Genetics of Asthma. (1998) Genome-wide search for asthma susceptibility loci in a founder population. *Hum Mol Genet*, **7**, 1393–8.

Panhuysen CIM, Vonk JM, Koeter GH, *et al.* (1997) Adult patients may outgrow their asthma. A 25-year follow-up study. *Am J Respir Crit Care Med*, **155**, 1267–72.

Pereira E, Goldblatt J, Rye P, Sanderson C, LeSouef P. (1998) Mutation analysis of Interleukin-5 in an asthmatic cohort. *Hum Mutat*, **11**, 51–4.

Postma DS, Bleecker ER, Amelung PJ, *et al.* (1995) Genetic susceptibility to asthma-bronchial hyperresponsiveness coinherited with a major gene for atopy. *N Engl J Med*, **333**, 894–900.

Ravetch JV. (1994) Atopy and Fc receptors: mutation is the message? *Nat Genet*, **7**, 117–18.

Reihsaus E, Innis M, MacIntyre N, Liggett SB. (1993) Mutations in the gene encoding for the β_2-adrenergic receptor in normal and asthmatic subjects. *Am J Respir Cell Mol Biol*, **8**, 334–9.

Rich SS, Roitman-Johnson B, Greenberg B, Roberts S, Blumenthal MN. (1992) Genetic analysis of atopy in three large kindreds: no evidence of linkage to D11S97. *Clin Exp Allergy*, **22**, 1070–6.

Rosenwasser LJ, Borish L. (1997) Genetics of atopy and asthma: the rationale behind promoter-based candidate gene studies (IL-4 and IL-10). *Am J Respir Crit Care Med*, **156**, S152–5.

Sandford A, Weir T, Pare P. (1996) The genetics of asthma. *Am J Respir Crit Care Med*, **153**, 1749–65.

Sandford AJ, Shirakawa T, Moffatt MF, *et al.* (1993) Localisation of atopy and β subunit of high-affinity IgE receptor (FcεRI) on chromosome 11q. *Lancet*, **341**, 332–4.

Sarafino EP, Goldfedder J. (1995) Genetic factors in the presence, severity, and triggers of asthma. *Arch Dis Child*, **73**, 112–16.

Schonberger HJAM, van Schayck CP. (1998) Prevention of asthma in genetically predisposed children in primary care – from clinical efficacy to a feasible intervention programme. *Clin Exp Allergy*, **28**, 1325–31.

Shirakawa T, Deichmann KA, Mao XQ, Adra CI, Hopkin JM. (2000) Atopy and asthma: genetic variants of IL-4 and IL-13 signalling. *Immunology Today*, **21**(2), 60–4.

Shirakawa T, Hashimoto T, Furuyama J, Takeshita T, Morimoto K. (1994a) Linkage between severe atopy and chromosome 11q13 in Japanese families. *Clin Genet*, **46**, 228–32.

Shirakawa T, Li A, Dubowitz M, (1994b) Association between atopy and variants of the β subunit of the high-affinity immunoglobulin E receptor. *Nat Genet*, **7**, 125–9.

Shirakawa T, Mao XQ, Sasaki S, *et al.* (1996a) Association between atopic asthma and a coding variant of FcεRIβ in a Japanese population. *Hum Mol Genet*, **5**, 1129–30.

Shirakawa T, Mao XQ, Sasaki S, Kawai M, Morimoto K, Hopkin JM. (1996b) Association between FcεRI-β and atopic disorder in a Japanese population. *Lancet*, **347**, 394–5.

Sibbald B, Kerry S, Strachan DP, Anderson HR. (1994) Patient characteristics associated with the labelling of asthma. *Fam Pract*, **11**, 127–32.

Spielman RS, McGinnis RE, Ewens WJ. (1993) Transmission test for linkage disequilibrium: the insulin gene region and insulin dependent diabetes. *Am J Hum Genet*, **52**, 506–16.

Szentivanyi A. (1968) The β-adrenergic theory of the atopic abnormality in bronchial asthma. *J Allergy*, **42**, 203–32.

Tan S, Hall IP, Dewar J, Dow E, Lipworth B. (1997) Association between β_1-adrenoceptor polymorphism and susceptibility to bronchodilator desensitisation in moderately severe stable asthmatics. *Lancet*, **350**, 995–9.

Te Meerman GJ, van der Meulen MA. (1997) Genomic sharing surrounding alleles identical by descent: effects of genetic drift and population growth. *Genet Epidemiol*, **14**, 1125–30.

Townley RG, Bewtra A, Wilson AF, *et al.* (1986) Segregation analysis of bronchial response to methacholine inhalation challenge in families with and without asthma. *J Allergy Clin Immunol*, **77**, 101–7.

Turki J, Pak J, Green SA, Martin RJ, Liggett SB. (1995) Genetic polymorphisms of the β_2-adrenergic receptor in nocturnal and non-nocturnal asthma. Evidence that Gly 16 correlates with the nocturnal phenotype. *J Clin Invest*, **95**, 1635–41.

Ulbrecht M, Eisenhut T, Bonisch J, *et al.* (1997) High serum IgE concentrations: association with HLA-DR and markers on chromosome 5q31 and 11q13. *J Allergy Clin Immunol*, **99**, 828–36.

van der Pouw Kraan TCTM, van Veen A, Boeije LCM, *et al.* (1999) An IL-13 promoter polymorphism associated with an increased risk of allergic asthma. *Genes Immunity*, **1**, 61–5.

van Herwerden L, Harrap SB, Wong ZY, *et al.* (1995) Linkage of high-affinity IgE receptor gene with bronchial hyperreactivity, even in absence of atopy. *Lancet*, **346**, 1262–5.

Walley AJ, Cookson WO. (1996) Investigation of an interleukin-4 promoter polymorphism for associations with asthma and atopy. *J Med Genet*, **33**, 689–92.

Watson M, Lawrence S, Collins A, Beasley R, Douii I, Begishvili B, Lampe F, Holgate ST, Morton NE. (1995) Exclusion from proximal 11q of a common gene with megaphenic effect on atopy. *Ann Hum Genet*, **59**, 403–11.

Wilkinson J, Grimley S, Collins A, Thomas NS, Holgate ST, Morton N. (1998) Linkage of asthma to markers on chromosome 12 in a sample of 240 families using quantitative phenotype scores. *Genomics*, **53**, 251–9.

Wjst M, Fischer G, Immervoll T, *et al.* (1999) A genome-wide search for linkage to asthma. *Genomics*, **58**, 1–8.

Wütrich B, Baumann E, Fries RA, Schnyder UW. (1981) Total and specific IgE (RAST) in atopic twins. *Clin Allergy*, **11**, 147–54.

Xu J, Levitt RC, Panhuysen CI, *et al.* (1995) Evidence for two unlinked loci regulating total serum IgE levels. *Am J Hum Genet*, **57**, 425–30.

Xu X, Rijcken B, Schouten JP, Weiss ST. (1997) Airway responsiveness and development and remission of chronic respiratory symptoms in adults. *Lancet*, **350**, 1431–4.

Young RP, Sharp PA, Lynch JR, *et al.* (1992) Confirmation of genetic linkage between atopic IgE responses and chromosome 11q13. *J Med Genet*, **29**, 236–38.

Young RP, Dekker JW, Wordsworth BP, *et al.* (1994) HLA-DR and HLA-DP genotypes and immunoglobulin E responses to common major allergens. *Clin Exp Allergy*, **24**, 431–9.

8

Pathology of asthma

PETER K. JEFFERY

INTRODUCTION

This chapter focuses on the pathology of asthma and makes comparisons with chronic obstructive pulmonary disease (COPD) in order to assist in an understanding of what is characteristic of asthma *per se*. Asthma and COPD are not disease entities but rather each is a complex of conditions that have in common airflow limitation (syn. obstruction). The distinction between asthma and COPD is a difficult but important one to the clinician and a challenge to the pathologist and research scientist (Jeffery, 1991, 2000). An understanding of whether or not there are fundamental differences between these two conditions is relevant to clinical decisions regarding treatment and patient management. In the longer term it is of value to both the design of specific therapy and to the prevention of disease. The definitions of asthma and COPD highlight the differences of variability and reversibility of airflow (Siafakas *et al.*, 1995; American Thoracic Society, 1995, 1987). However, with age, there is often overlap and a progression from the reversible airflow obstruction of the young asthmatic to the more irreversible or 'fixed' obstruction of the older patient with COPD. Indeed the Dutch hypothesis encompasses the idea that both conditions are extreme ends of a single condition (Orie *et al.*, 1961). The present author subscribes to the hypothesis that the two syndromes are distinct in regard to their pathogenesis and in this chapter they are largely contrasted, based on the observations of: (i) bronchial fluids and sputum, (ii) studies of tissues obtained post-mortem and of (iii) mucosal biopsies of relatively large airways obtained at rigid or flexible fibreoptic bronchoscopy (FOB), which has provided the means by which the early inflammatory and structural alterations of asthma have been ascertained (Jeffery, 1996). As we shall see, the distinction based on histo-, immuno-, and molecular pathology is not always clear and in this respect there is some overlap at both the structural and functional levels.

SPUTUM AND BRONCHOALVEOLAR LAVAGE FLUID

The examination of spontaneously produced or saline-induced sputum has become a much used and relatively non-invasive method for determining the extent of inflammation in the asthmatic airway (Hargreave et al., 1993a, 1993b, 1995; Pizzichini et al., 1996; Peleman et al., 1999). Corkscrew-shaped twists of condensed mucus (Curschmann's spirals) (Curschmann, 1883), clusters of surface airway epithelial cells (referred to as Creola bodies and named after the first patient in whom they were described; Naylot, 1962), and the presence of Charcot–Leyden crystals, composed of eosinophil cell and granule membrane lysophospholipase (Plates 1 and 2) (Weller et al., 1984), together with eosinophils and metachromatic cells, are characteristic features of sputa obtained from asthmatic, but not bronchitic patients (Gibson et al., 1989a). Sputum eosinophilia has, however, also been reported in non-asthmatics in the absence of the airways hyperresponsiveness (AH) characteristic of asthma (Gibson et al., 1989). In contrast, sputa from bronchitic patients may be mucoid or, during infective exacerbations, purulent when neutrophils may be present in large numbers (Peleman et al., 1999). Bronchoalveolar lavage fluid in mild (allergic) asthma demonstrates the presence of sloughed epithelial cells, the numbers of which show an association with AH (Beasley et al., 1989), and of eosinophils and their highly charged secreted products, such as eosinophil cationic protein and major basic protein (Wardlaw et al., 1988). By contrast, in smokers' bronchitis, macrophages predominate (Glynn and Michaels, 1960) and neutrophils are numerous (Thompson et al., 1989) as is their secreted product, myeloperoxidase (Riise et al., 1995).

AIRWAY PLUGGING

Post-mortem examination of cases of fatal asthma has shown that the lungs are hyperinflated and remain so on opening the pleural cavities, owing to the widespread presence of markedly tenacious airway 'plugs' in both large (segmental) and small bronchi (Plate 3). Even intrabronchial inflation with fixative to a 1.5 metre head of pressure hardly moves these sticky lumenal plugs (Dunnill, 1960; Dunnill et al., 1969). Histologically the airway plugs in asthma are composed predominantly of inflammatory exudate together with mucus in which lie desquamated surface epithelial cells, lymphocytes and eosinophils (Fig. 8.1). The arrangement of the cellular elements of the plug is often as concentric, multiple lamellae suggesting that several episodes have led to their formation rather than a single terminal event (Plate 4). The non-mucinous, proteinaceous contribution is the result of increased vascular permeability and includes fibrin. Electrostatic interaction of serum constituents and mucin probably contributes to the particular stickiness of the airway plug (List et al., 1978). There are, however, reports of sudden death in asthmatics in which intra-lumenal plugs are absent (Reid, 1987) but these are rare (Cardell and Pearson, 1959; Messer et al., 1960). In chronic bronchitis, there is also an excess of intralumenal mucus but this lacks the marked eosinophilia and obvious epithelial content seen in asthma and, if mucoid, is usually less tenacious than that characteristic of asthma. In the absence of a history of smoking, there is little evidence of destructive emphysema in fatal asthma and right ventricular hypertrophy is uncommon. However, areas of atelectasis and petechial haemorrhages may be present in asthma caused by

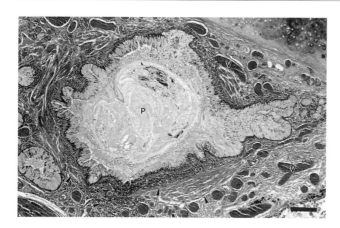

Figure 8.1 *Light micrograph of an haematoxolin and eosin stained section through a bronchial plug (P) that consists of exudate and mucus and cellular elements in a case of fatal asthma. There is marked inflammatory cell infiltrate (arrows), enlargement of the mass of bronchial smooth muscle (arrowheads), and vasodilation of the bronchial vessels (V) (scale, 180 μm).*

bronchial obstruction, reabsorption collapse and repeated forced inspiratory efforts. Clearly the asthmatic who has smoked will likely have features which overlap between asthma and COPD and in these cases, there may be focal evidence of centri-acinar (bronchocentric) alveolar destruction (i.e. emphysema) (*see* Plate 3).

MUCUS-SECRETING ELEMENTS

Submucosal gland enlargement and bronchial goblet cell hyperplasia have been reported as the histological hallmarks and the correlate of mucus hypersecretion in chronic bronchitis (Reid, 1954). There is also submucosal gland enlargement in fatal asthma (Dunnill *et al.*, 1969) and excessive production of mucus which, together with the inflammatory exudate, forms the sticky tenacious plugs which block the airways (Wanner, 1988). There is dilatation of gland ducts, referred to as bronchial gland ectasia (Cluroe *et al.*, 1989). Whilst the condensed twists of mucus referred to as Curschmann's spirals are often said to represent the casts of small airways, their size is more in keeping with that of gland ducts which are, therefore, their more likely origin. In chronic bronchitis there is thought to be replacement of submucosal gland serous by mucous acini (Glynn and Michaels, 1960). Serous acini normally contain antibacterial substances such as lysozyme, lactoferrin and a small molecular weight antiprotease: the reduction in these factors in COPD favours bacterial colonization and proteolytic damage to airways: such a change in the proportion of serous and mucous acini is, however, reported not to occur in asthma (Glynn and Michaels, 1960).

Goblet cell hyperplasia is a feature of both asthma (Aikawa *et al.*, 1992) and bronchitis (Reid, 1954). The appearance and increase in number of newly differentiated epithelial goblet cells (referred to as mucous metaplasia) in small bronchi and bronchioli of less than 2 mm diameter, where they are normally absent or sparse, is a characteristic of small airways disease in COPD (Ebert and Terracio, 1975; Cosio *et al.*, 1980; Jeffery, 1990). Whether mucous metaplasia also occurs in asthma is debated. It is considered by some that the mucus present at this distal site in asthma is aspirated from larger airways. The mucus secreted from surface epithelial goblet cells appears to adhere and to maintain a continuity between the cells' secretions and the plug, suggesting the secretory process or the mucin itself is altered in fatal asthma (Aikawa *et al.*, 1992; Shimura 1996).

SURFACE EPITHELIUM

Histologically, damage and shedding of the airway surface epithelium are reported in asthma post-mortem (Plates 5 and 6) but this change is highly variable with loss of epithelium in some airways whilst others have completely intact surface epithelium in the presence of marked inflammation and other structural changes (*see* Fig. 8.1). Subepithelial oedema has been suggested to be one mechanism responsible for lifting of the overlying surface epithelium where this occurs (Dunnill, 1960). Repeated loss of the epithelium induces a healing process as evidenced by squamous cell metaplasia and/or goblet cell hyperplasia. Histologically, damage and shedding of airway surface epithelium appears to be an early feature of asthma as it is prominent in biopsy specimens of patients with stable mild disease and is not a feature of smokers with bronchitis or COPD (Plates 7 and 8) (Laitinen *et al.*, 1985; Beasley *et al.*, 1989; Jeffery *et al.*, 1989). Loss of superficial epithelium is accompanied by mitotic activity in the remaining cells (*see* Ayers and Jeffery, 1988). There is repeated epithelial regeneration in the form of simple and then stratified cells prior to restoration of the normal ciliated and goblet cell phenotypes, the entire process taking approximately two weeks (Wilhelm, 1953). Aggregations of platelets together with fibrillary material, thought to be fibrin, have been observed in association with the damaged surface (Jeffery *et al.*, 1989). Such fibrin deposits are also seen during the late phase response following allergen challenge (P.K. Jeffery, unpublished results). The greater the loss of surface epithelium in biopsy specimens, the greater appears to be the degree of airways hyperresponsiveness (Jeffery *et al.*, 1989). It is recognized that there is inevitably artefactual loss of surface epithelium during the taking and preparation of such small biopsy pieces, even normally, which makes interpretation of the epithelial loss seen in bronchial biopsies controversial (Soderberg *et al.*, 1990). In the author's opinion, the observed loss reflects the fragility of the epithelium *in vivo* which facilitates sloughing during the bronchoscopy procedure. The fragility of the epithelium *in vivo* in asthma is supported by the frequent appearance of clusters of sloughed epithelial cells in sputa (*see* Plate 1) (Naylor, 1962) and the increased presence of bronchial epithelial cells in bronchoalveolar lavage fluid of asthmatics with mild disease (Beasley *et al.*, 1989). Other researchers have found no significant increase in the loss of epithelium in biopsies of mild asthmatics (Lozewicz *et al.*, 1990) and this may be related to differing methods of measurement of such loss or to differences in the severity of the patients sampled. The fragility of the surface may involve disruption of epithelial cell tight junctions (Elia *et al.*, 1988; Godfrey *et al.*, 1995) which normally act as a selective barrier to the passage of ions, molecules and water between cells: their disruption may lower the threshold for stimulation of intra-epithelial nerves leading to axonal reflexes, stimulation of mucus-secreting submucosal glands, vasodilatation and oedema through the release of sensory neuropeptides (i.e. referred to as neurogenic inflammation) (Jeffery 1994; Barnes, 1986). Experimentally there is also evidence that the sensitivity of bronchial smooth muscle to substances placed in the airway lumen correlates strongly with the integrity of the surface epithelium (Sparrow and Mitchell, 1991). Loss or damage of surface epithelium would thus lead to a reduction in the concentration of factors normally relaxant to bronchial smooth muscle with resultant increased sensitivity and 'reactivity' of bronchial smooth muscle (Hogg and Eggleston, 1984; van Houtte, 1989; Sparrow and Mitchell, 1991).

Apart from their role as stem cells, the basal cells of normal pseudostratified surface epithelium have been suggested to act as a bridge, enhancing the adhesion of 'superficial' cells to epithelial basement membrane (Evans and Plopper, 1988). When superficial cells are lost in asthma the preferential plane of cleavage appears to be between superficial and basal cells (Montefort *et al.*, 1992), leaving basal cells still attached to their basement membrane (*see*

Plates 6 and 7). Epithelial cells also act as effector cells by their synthesis and release of cytokines such as IL-6, IL-8 and GM-CSF and chemokines such as RANTES (Bellini *et al.*, 1993) and eotaxin (Li *et al.*, 1997; Sun *et al.*, 1997) (*see* Chapter 6). Disruption of the epithelium and attempts at repair may increase production of these pro-inflammatory cytokines by those cells which remain.

RETICULAR BASEMENT MEMBRANE

Thickening of the reticular basement membrane (i.e. the lamina reticularis) which lies external to (or below) the epithelium has long been recognized as a consistent change in allergic, non-allergic and occupational forms of asthma (Crepea and Harman, 1955; Dunnill, 1960; Callerame *et al.*, 1971; Nowak, 1969; Sabonya, 1984; Jeffery *et al.*, 1989; Roche *et al.*, 1989; Mullen *et al.*, 1985). This may occur in response to repeated loss and healing of the surface epithelium (*see* Plates 6 and 7). Whilst there may be focal and variable thickening of the reticular layer in COPD and other inflammatory chronic diseases of the lung such as bronchiectasis and tuberculosis (Crepea and Harman, 1955), the lesion, when homogeneous and hyaline in appearance, is highly characteristic of asthma and is not usually found in COPD (*see* Plate 8). The reticular layer appears to be absent in the foetus (at least up to 18 weeks of gestation) (Jeffery, 1998) but develops in normal, healthy individuals, presumably during childhood: its thickening in asthma occurs very early on in the condition, even before asthma is diagnosed. The thickening remains even when asthma is mild and well controlled by anti-asthma treatment (O'Shaughnessy *et al.*, 1996) and is present in patients with a long history of asthma but who have not died of their asthma (Sobonya, 1984) (Fig. 8.2). The extent of thickening is maximal early on in the development of asthma and does not appear to increase significantly with time or severity, albeit the latter is debated. Using a model system it has been predicted that the thickening and hence increased rigidity of the reticular basement membrane may reduce its capacity to fold during bronchial smooth muscle contraction: it is suggested that reduced folding would result in increased airway responsiveness (Lambert, 1991).

It should be emphasized that the 'true' epithelial basement membrane (i.e. the basal lamina) which consists mainly of type IV collagen, glycosaminoglycans and laminin, is not thickened in either asthma or COPD (Fig. 8.3). The thickening of the reticular basement membrane,

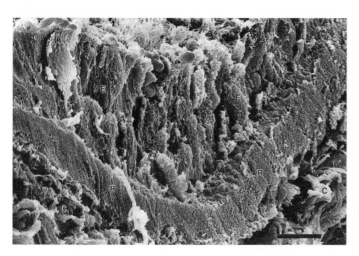

Figure 8.2 *Scanning electron micrograph of surface epithelium (E) and a thickened reticular basement membrane (R) that appears as a homogeneous band, distinct from the underlying collagen (C) in a patient with 25 years' history of asthma who died of another cause (scale, 10 μm).*

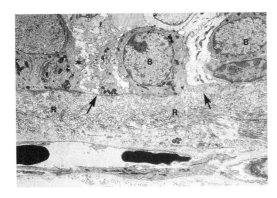

Figure 8.3 *Transmission electron micrograph of a bronchial biopsy showing a thickened reticular basement membrane (R) and a basal lamina (arrows), also referred to as the 'true' basement membrane, to which the epithelial basal cells (B) attach (scale, 2 μm).*

which is immunopositive for collagen types III and V together with fibronectin but not laminin, has been referred to as 'subepithelial fibrosis' (Roche *et al.*, 1989). In the author's opinion this is an unfortunate use of the term, as the thickened layer of reticulin is ultrastructurally different to the banded collagen which lies deeper in the airway wall or that which is characteristic of scarring. Much research effort, therefore, has been put into examining mechanisms of fibrosis in asthma which the author believes is inappropriate to the condition. The reticular layer is comprised of thinner fibres of reticulin linked to a tenascin-rich matrix (Laitinen *et al.*, 1997) in which there are sugars together with entrapped molecules such as heparin sulphate and serum-derived components such as fibronectin: these molecules may modulate the state of differentiation and function of overlying epithelium. Swelling of this subepithelial reticular layer may also contribute to its thickening in asthma. Interestingly, the thickened layer does not behave as a barrier to the transmigration of inflammatory cells which, by the release of enzymes (e.g. metalloproteases), can pass through it with apparent ease (Fig. 8.4). An association between the numbers of myofibroblasts underlying the reticular layer and thickening of the reticular layer has been demonstrated in asthma (Brewster *et al.*, 1990).

In contrast to asthma, a study of bronchial biopsies in patients with COPD, has reported that the reticular layer is not thickened (Ollerenshaw and Woolcock, 1992). A recent report confirms this and demonstrates that the reticular layer in smokers' COPD is similar to that in normals and is even significantly thinner than that of asthmatics who had been treated with

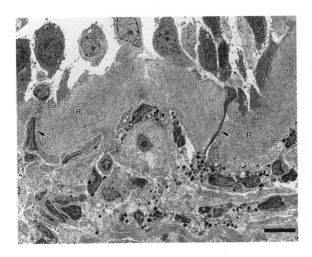

Figure 8.4 *Transmission electron micrograph showing the thickened reticular basement membrane (R) in a bronchial biopsy from an allergic asthmatic subject after allergen challenge. Inflammatory cells appear to be in the process of migrating across the thickened layer (arrows) (scale, 10 μm).*

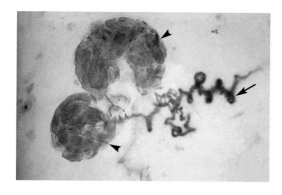

Plate 1 *A Light micrograph of sputum showing a Curschmann's spiral (arrow) and Creola bodies (arrowheads) in a case of asthma (approximate scale, 20 μm).*

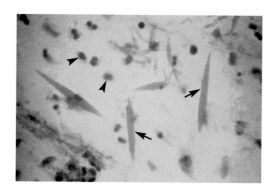

Plate 2 *Charcot–Leyden crystals (arrows) and eosinophils (arrowheads) in sputum in a case of asthma (stained with eosin) (approximate scale, 20 μm).*

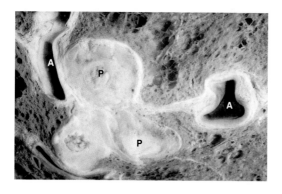

Plate 3 *Gross appearance of an airway plug (P) in a bronchus with adjacent arteries (A) in a case of fatal asthma (approximate scale, 400 μm; courtesy of Prof. B. Heard).*

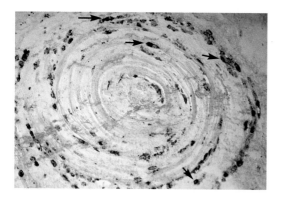

Plate 4 *Immunohistologic staining of bronchial plug showing concentric lamellae in which there are EG2+ (i.e. activated) eosinophils (scale, 50 μm).*

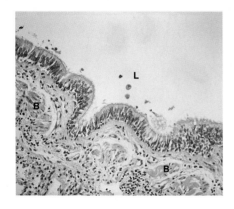

Plate 5 *Light micrograph of haematoxolin and eosin stained section of normal bronchial mucosa taken from a road traffic accidental death showing a lumen (L) free of exudate, intact surface epithelium and normal amounts of bronchial smooth muscle (B) (scale, 80 μm).*

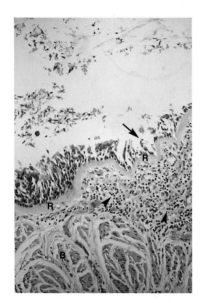

Plate 6 *In contrast, a light micrograph of haematoxolin and eosin stained mucosa from an asthma death showing loss of surface epithelium (arrow), hyaline and homogeneous thickening of the reticular basement membrane (R), and increases in subepithelial inflammatory cells (arrowheads) and bronchial smooth muscle mass (B) (scale, 80 μm).*

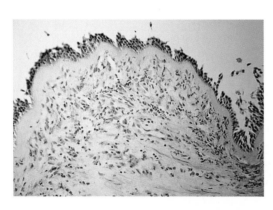

Plate 7 *Bronchial biopsy of the airway mucosa in a patient with mild allergic asthma showing the loss of surface epithelium and the homogeneous thickening of the reticular basement membrane (scale, 50 μm).*

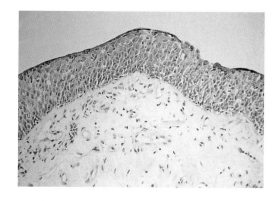

Plate 8   *Bronchial biopsy of the airway mucosa of a heavy smoker (FEV$_1$ of 40% of predicted) demonstrating an intact epithelium (uppermost) which has undergone squamous metaplasia. In contrast to the asthmatic (Plate 7), the underlying reticular basement membrane is relatively thin (scale, 50 μm).*

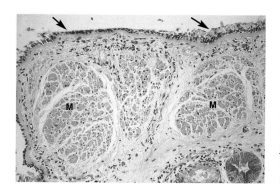

Plate 9   *Light micrograph of an haematoxylin and eosin stained section of bronchial mucosa from an asthma death demonstrating increased muscle mass (M) and sloughed epithelial cells (arrows) (scale, 80 μm).*

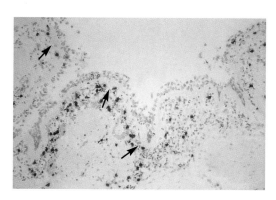

Plate 10   *EG2+ immunopositive (i.e. activated) subepithelial eosinophils in an area of bronchus from an asthma death. The eosinophils are stained blue and lie immediately beneath the reticular basement membrane (arrows) (scale, 80 μm).*

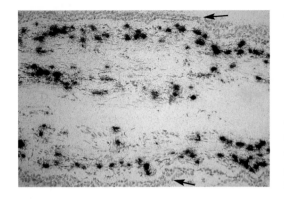

Plate 11   In situ *hybridization of a bronchial biopsy to demonstrate IL-5 gene expression in a case of acute severe asthma. Each cell expressing the gene is densely labelled. The position of the epithelium is shown (arrows) (scale, 50 μm).*

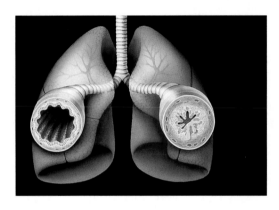

Plate 12   *Diagrammatic representation of the differences exhibited in the lumen and underlying mucosa of the normal bronchial airway (to the left) and the asthmatic airway (to the right). The asthmatic airway has mucus in the lumen and a wall thickened by increases of reticular basement membrane, vessels, mucus-secreting glands and bronchial smooth muscle.*

inhaled corticosteroids (O'Shaughnessy *et al.*, 1996). There are, however, data showing that there is a subpopulation of patients with COPD defined by their smoking history, and irreversibility to inhaled β_2-agonist: but who show significant airways reversibility (into the asthma range) to a 14-day course of oral prednisolone. This subpopulation demonstrates thicker reticular basement membranes than normal and shows evidence of BAL eosinophilia (Chanez *et al.*, 1997) demonstrating the potential overlap between asthma and COPD, even at the tissue level.

BRONCHIAL SMOOTH MUSCLE

The percentage of bronchial wall occupied by bronchial smooth muscle is usually increased in fatal asthma (Dunnill *et al.*, 1969) (Plate 9 and Fig. 8.5). The absolute increase in muscle mass is reported to be particularly striking in large intrapulmonary bronchi of lungs obtained following a fatal attack as compared with that in asthmatic subjects dying of other causes (Carroll *et al.*, 1993). It is an important contributor to the thickening of the airway wall and hence to the marked increase in resistance to airflow which may be life-threatening (Moreno *et al.*, 1986; James *et al.*, 1989; Wiggs *et al.*, 1990, 1992). Using a morphometric technique Dunnill showed that approximately 12% of the wall in segmental bronchi obtained from cases of fatal asthma is comprised of muscle compared with about 5% in normals. Hogg and colleagues (Pare *et al.*, 1991; Hogg, 1993) have confirmed this trend in airways larger than 2 mm diameter and demonstrated a 3–4-fold increase over normal in the area of the wall occupied by bronchial smooth muscle. In asthma the increase in muscle mass does not appear to extend to airways of less than 2 mm in diameter (Carroll *et al.*, 1993). In contrast, there may be increases in bronchiolar smooth muscle in smokers and in some patients with emphysema (Cosio *et al.*, 1980; Saetta, 1998). In the absence of wheeze, values for muscle mass in segmental bronchi in chronic bronchitis and emphysema fall largely within the normal range but intermediate levels are present in so-called wheezy bronchitis (Takizawa and Thurlbeck, 1971; Thurlbeck, 1985). Whether the increase in muscle mass in asthma is due to muscle fibre hyperplasia (Heard and Hossain, 1983) or hypertrophy is at present unclear. Two patterns of distribution of increased muscle mass have been described in asthma: one in which the increase occurs throughout the airways and another in which the increase is restricted to the largest airways; it is suggested that in the former there is muscle fibre hyperplasia and hypertrophy, and in the latter hypertrophy alone (Ebina *et al.*, 1990, 1993).

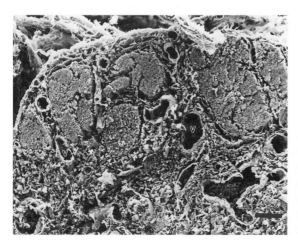

Figure 8.5 *Scanning electron micrograph of part of the bronchial wall showing enlarged blocks of bronchial smooth muscle (B) in a case of fatal asthma. Dilated bronchial vessels (V) also contribute to the increased thickness of the airway wall (scale, 50 μm).*

We have observed recently that solitary contractile cells appear in substantial numbers during the late phase response to allergen challenge (Figs 8.6 and 8.7) and we have suggested that, with repeated exposure to allergen, they may contribute not only to increased production of reticulin but also to the increased mass of bronchial smooth muscle seen in the airway wall in severe asthma (Gizycki *et al.*, 1997). It is now likely that de-differentiation of existing smooth muscle and its migration to a subepithelial site occurs in asthma (Gizycki *et al.*, 1997). This process may parallel the changes to vascular smooth muscle described in atherosclerosis (Jeffery, 1994).

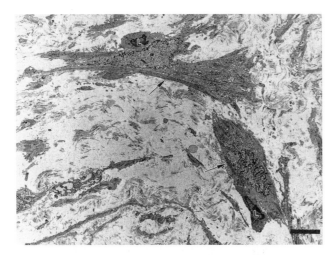

Figure 8.6 *Transmission electron micrograph of myofibroblasts, with adjacent lymphocyte (L), in the subepithelial matrix of the airway wall. Contractile filaments (arrows) can be observed at the periphery of the myofibroblast: there is also much dilated rough endoplasmic reticulum indicating both the contractile and secretory nature of this phenotype (scale, 5 μm).*

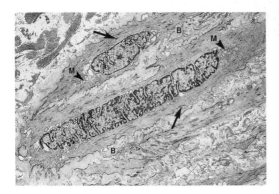

Figure 8.7 *Transmission electron micrograph of a bronchial smooth muscle cell showing the characteristic envelopment by basement membrane (B). Most of the cytoplasm has contractile filaments (arrows) and there are also many mitochondria (M) (scale bar, 5 μm).*

AIRWAY VESSELS

The increase in thickness of the bronchial wall in severe asthma is not accounted for by the increase in bronchial smooth muscle and mucous gland mass alone. Dilatation of bronchial mucosal blood vessels, congestion and wall oedema are also consistently reported features of fatal asthma and these can account for considerable swelling of the airway wall (see Figs 8.1 and 8.5) (Lambert *et al.*, 1991; Kuwano *et al.*, 1993; Jeffery, 1994; Carrol *et al.*, 1997). The onset of vasodilation, congestion and mucosal oedema in response to a variety of mediators of inflammation (Widdicombe, 1993) can be rapid and, probably can also be relatively rapidly reversed. There are indications that there may also be new growth of bronchial vessels which contribute to the increased vascularity of the airway wall and that this change may occur even in mild asthma (Charan *et al.*, 1997; Orsida *et al.*, 1999).

INFLAMMATION

It is now recognized that both asthma (Azzawi *et al.*, 1990; Saetta *et al.*, 1991; Azzawi *et al.*, 1992) and COPD (Saetta *et al.*, 1993; Mullen *et al.*, 1997; O'Shaughnessy *et al.*, 1997) are inflammatory conditions, albeit the relative magnitude and site of the inflammatory infiltrate and the predominant inflammatory cell phenotype may differ. In fatal asthma there is a marked infiltrate throughout the airway wall and also in the occluding plug (*see* Figs 8.1 and 8.4; Plate 6): lymphocytes are abundant (Dunnill, 1960; Azzawi *et al.*, 1992; Saetta *et al.*, 1991) and eosinophils are characteristic (Azzawi *et al.*, 1992; Carroll *et al.*, 1996; Synek *et al.*, 1996) (Plate 10). Neutrophils are often absent albeit they are reported to be present in relatively large numbers in cases of status asthmaticus where death is sudden (i.e. within 24 hours of the attack) (Sur *et al.*, 1993). The inflammation of the airway wall may spread to surrounding alveolar septae (Kraft *et al.*, 1996) and affect the adjacent pulmonary artery (Saetta *et al.*, 1991). Alveolar walls may thus show evidence of eosinophilic infiltration and alveolar spaces may contain a fibrillary-rich component, most likely, fibrin. The association of tissue eosinophilia and asthma is a strong one, but the extent of tissue eosinophilia varies greatly with each case and the duration of the terminal episode (Gleich *et al.*, 1980; Saetta *et al.*, 1991; Sur *et al.*, 1993). The variation may be due, in part, to eosinophil degranulation which makes cell identification difficult. In comparison with mild asthma, fatal asthma is reported to be associated with a higher concentration of eosinophils in the large airways and a reduction of lymphocytes in the peripheral (smaller) airways (Synek *et al.*, 1996). Post-mortem studies by Heard and colleagues have shown that the apparent reduction of mast cell number in asthmatic bronchi is also seen in the lung parenchyma (Heard *et al.*, 1989).

The inflammation and airway wall remodelling process of asthma appears therefore to occur in much larger airways than was thought previously whereas small bronchi and bronchioles are considered the major site of increased airflow resistance in COPD (Hogg *et al.*, 1968; van Brabandt *et al.*, 1983). Niewoehner and colleagues (Niewoehner *et al.*, 1974) have described lesions in young smokers dying suddenly: inflammation in bronchioles and a respiratory bronchiolitis consisting of pigmented macrophages were described. In more severe patients these changes were associated with mucous metaplasia, smooth muscle hypertrophy, mural oedema, peribronchiolar fibrosis and an excess of airways <400 μm diameter (Cosio *et al.*, 1980). In contrast macrophages are not usually present in increased numbers in asthma.

In COPD, elastolytic destruction of alveolar wall attachments, probably following microvascular sequestration of neutrophils and release of elastase (MacNee and Selby, 1992) leads to loss of radial traction, a tendency to early small airway closure and increased tortuosity of unsupported bronchioli (Saetta *et al.*, 1985; Lamb *et al.*, 1993). There is controversy as to whether there is loss of elastic tissue in asthma, one group demonstrating there is not (Jeffery *et al.*, 1992) and another group indicating that there is elastolysis (Bousquet *et al.*, 1996).

Studies of biopsies obtained by fibre-optic bronchoscopy (FOB) or at open lung biopsy in asthma demonstrate the presence of an inflammatory cell infiltrate even in patients with newly diagnosed asthma (Laitinen *et al.*, 1993). The infiltrate comprises CD3 immunopositive (T) lymphocytes of the CD4 (helper) subset and eosinophils (Fig. 8.8) (Laitinen *et al.*, 1985; Beasley *et al.*, 1989; Jeffery *et al.*, 1989, 1992). Our own studies of bronchial biopsies in asthma have shown that the increase in leucocytes, including lymphocytes and eosinophils, occurs in

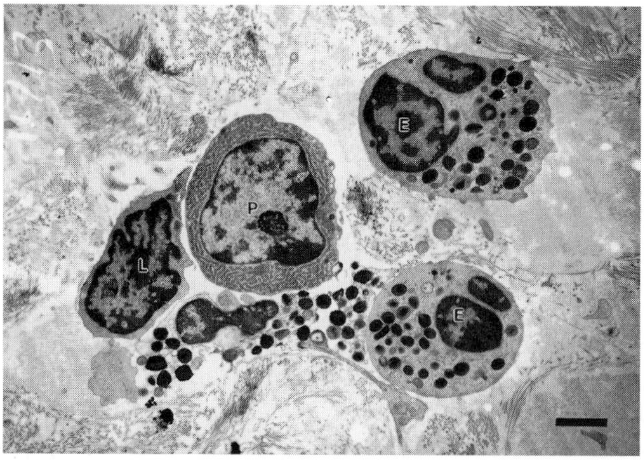

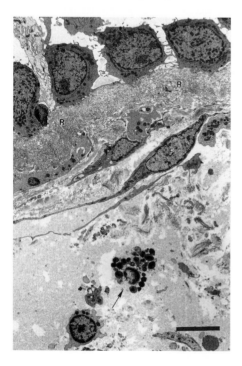

Figure 8.8 *Transmission electron micrograph of bronchial biopsy of a mild asthmatic showing the close association of a lymphocyte (L), plasma cell (P) and eosinophils (E) (scale, 2 μm).*

relatively mild atopic, occupational and intrinsic asthma and that it is associated with an increase of 'activation' markers for both lymphocytes (CD25+ cells) and eosinophils (EG2+ cells) (Jeffery *et al.*, 1989; Azzawi *et al.*, 1990; Bentley *et al.*, 1992a, 1992b; Jeffery *et al.*, 1992). In symptomatic atopic asthmatics, irregularly shaped lymphomononuclear cells appear and these may represent ultrastructural forms of the CD25+ (activated) lymphocyte. EG2 is a marker for the cleaved ('secreted') form of eosinophil cationic protein which can be found both within eosinophils and diffusely in the wall, often in association with the reticular layer beneath the epithelium. Eosinophil-derived products such as major basic protein (Filley *et al.*, 1982) together with toxic oxygen radicals and proteases probably all contribute to the epithelial fragility discussed above. Eosinophil cytolysis or disintegration and release of granules (Persson and Erjefalt, 1997; Erjefalt *et al.*, 1998) and of cytokines may also stimulate nearby fibroblasts to produce additional reticulin and so induce thickening of the reticular basement membrane (Fig. 8.9).

Figure 8.9 *Transmission electron micrograph of biopsy of a mild asthmatic showing lysis of an eosinophil (arrow) close to a fibroblast (F) beneath the reticular basement membrane (R) (scale, 5 μm).*

The role of the activated T-helper lymphocyte in controlling and perpetuating the chronic inflammatory reaction in asthma has received much attention (Jeffery *et al.*, 1989; Kay, 1991). The T lymphocyte is thought to effect its control of allergic inflammation via the selective release of the pro-inflammatory cytokines (interleukins) IL-4 and IL-5 which characterize the T-helper (type 2) phenotype (Robinson *et al.*, 1993). IL-5 gene expression has been shown to be increased in bronchial biopsies from symptomatic mildly atopic asthmatics (Hamid *et al.*, 1991) (Plate 11), and this is supported by studies of cells obtained at bronchoalveolar lavage (Robinson *et al.*, 1992; Ohnishi *et al.*, 1993) and peripheral blood (Corrigan *et al.*, 1993). IL-5 appears to be a key cytokine required to induce terminal differentiation of eosinophils and enhances their vascular retention and longevity in tissues. It is also a key cytokine in the late-phase reaction to allergen challenge (Ohnishi *et al.*, 1993). IL-4 is also increased in atopic asthma (Walker *et al.*, 1992; Ackerman *et al.*, 1994) and may be important in both the initiation and persistence of allergic inflammation. IL-4 encourages the selective recruitment of eosinophils by upregulating adhesion molecules (V-CAM) on bronchial endothelium whose ligand on the eosinophil cell surface is VLA-4. The latter is absent from the surface of neutrophils and helps to explain the eosinophil predominance in asthma. There is currently debate as to the involvement of IL-4 in asthma of the intrinsic (i.e. non-atopic) form (Humbert *et al.*, 1996). IL-4 and IL-5 are not, however, unique to asthma and may occur in other inflammatory conditions such as fibrosing alveolitis (Jeffery *et al.*, 1993). Interestingly, IL-5 gene expression has recently been reported in smokers' chronic bronchitis and COPD (Zhu *et al.*, 1999). Whilst IL-5 may be important in promoting eosinophil terminal differentiation, and the release of eosinophils into the blood from bone marrow, it is likely that other molecules such as eotaxin and RANTES are involved as selective chemokines inducing eosinophil diapedesis (Jose *et al.*, 1994; Collins *et al.*, 1995; Li *et al.*, 1997). The same or distinct molecules may be involved in eosinophil activation, a process about which little is as yet known. Symptomatic asthma is associated with the production of additional cytokines including tumour necrosis factor-α, GM-CSF, IL-1, IL-2 and IL-6 (Broide *et al.*, 1992; Robinson *et al.*, 1993). GM-CSF has also been reported to increase during the late-phase reaction to allergen (Wooley *et al.*, 1995). In addition to their production of toxins and lipid-derived mediators, eosinophils themselves may also produce pro-inflammatory cytokines and growth factors as evidenced by their gene expression for TGFβ IL-6 and GM-CSF (Hamid *et al.*, 1992; Holgate *et al.*, 1993; Robinson *et al.*, 1993). Macrophages have been reported to increase in number in more severe asthma of the intrinsic form (Bentley *et al.*, 1992).

Mast cells have long been thought to play a key role in the immediate (type 1 sensitivity) reaction in asthma through their release of a variety of mediators including those which bronchoconstrict, i.e. histamine and prostaglandin D$_2$. Mast cells are now thought to act as an important source of IL-4 and other pro-inflammatory cytokines whose secretion may act as a trigger to the induction of subsequent persistent production of IL-4 and IL-5 by lymphocytes (Bradding *et al.*, 1992, 1993). Early biopsy studies have demonstrated an apparent reduction in bronchial mast cell numbers in asthma due to their degranulation (Salvato, 1968). Studies of bronchoalveolar lavage show increased numbers of T-helper cells and eosinophils and there is evidence of increased intralumenal mast cell and eosinophil degranulation and histamine release (Gerblich *et al.*, 1984; Wardlaw *et al.*, 1988; Adelroth *et al.*, 1990). However, recent morphometric studies of mast cells in bronchial biopsies taken from symptomatic mildly extrinsic asthmatics show no evidence for their degranulation when compared with those in normal healthy mucosa (Jeffery *et al.*, 1993). In a recent morphometric analysis of bronchial biopsies taken during the late-phase reaction (i.e. a 24 h post-allergen challenge), there was also no change in mast cell size or in the number of secretory granules or their area, expressed as a percentage of cell cytoplasm (P. K. Jeffery, unpublished observations). Little is known of the role of basophils in these conditions, albeit there is evidence for increased recruitment of basophils and their precursors to sites of allergic reaction in atopic patients (Denburg *et al.*, 1985).

In smoking-related conditions, bronchial mast cell numbers are reported to be increased (Lamb and Lumsden, 1982). Immunohistochemical and electron microscopic techniques are beginning to be applied to examine the airway inflammation of smokers' bronchitis (CB) and COPD. In an early study by Mullen and colleagues of lungs resected for cancer in patients with a history of chronic bronchitis (Mullen *et al.*, 1985, 1987), airway wall inflammation bore a stronger relationship to mucus hypersecretion (i.e., sputum volume) than did gland enlargement. In bronchial biopsies of subjects with COPD there is also evidence of an increase of inflammatory cells (Ollerenshaw and Woolcock, 1992; Saetta *et al.*, 1993; O'Shaugnessy *et al.*, 1997; Jeffery, 1997). In COPD, mononuclear cells are frequent and neutrophils are scarce (in the absence of an exacerbation of infection) and there are few eosinophils: the mononuclear component comprises lymphocytes, plasma cells and macrophages. Saetta and colleagues have examined bronchial biopsies obtained from patients with chronic sputum production and a history of cigarette smoking. Compared with non-smoking healthy people, there are significant increases in the numbers of CD45 (total leucocytes), CD3 (T lymphocytes), CD25 (interleukin-2-receptor) and VLA-1 (late activation) positive cells and of macrophages (Saetta *et al.*, 1993). The increase in COPD of the numbers of T lymphocytes and macrophages is confirmed in a report by O'Shaughnessy and colleagues (O'Shaughnessy *et al.*, 1997). Interestingly, these workers found that, unlike asthma, which is a CD4 (helper) T lymphocyte-driven disorder, the predominant T lymphocyte subset in the airway wall of patients with COPD was the CD8 (i.e. cytotoxic/suppressor) subset (O'Shaugnessy *et al.*, 1997). The high CD8:CD4 ratio has also been found in the area of the wall occupied by submucosal glands (Saetta *et al.*, 1997) and this is also true of peripheral blood and of cells (Costabel *et al.*, 1986) recovered at bronchoalveolar lavage (BAL). Thus the CD8:CD4 ratio appears to be a fundamental distinction between the CD4, allergen-driven process of allergic asthma and the CD8, cigarette smoked-induced inflammation of COPD. Interestingly, the numbers of CD8+ cells in the airway mucosa bear a statistically significant negative relationship with the measurements of forced expiratory volume (FEV_1) in the group of bronchitic smokers whose bronchial biopsies were studied (O'Shaugnessy *et al.*, 1997). The biopsy findings in relatively large airways appear to reflect those described in small bronchi, bronchioli and alveolated portions of the lung (Finkelstein *et al.*, 1995; Majo *et al.*, 1996; Lams *et al.*, 1998; Saetta, 1998) in COPD which again contrasts with the allergic pattern of inflammation described thus far in the small airways and alveolar attachments in asthma (Kraft *et al.*, 1996; Hamid *et al.*, 1997). A relatively small but significant number of eosinophils may also be identified in bronchial biopsies obtained from patients diagnosed as having COPD: however, in contrast to asthma the eosinophil cationic protein concentrations in BAL fluid are not increased, suggesting that the eosinophils which are present have not degranulated (Lacoste *et al.*, 1993). However, eosinophils may increase substantially in cases of COPD where there are exacerbations of chronic bronchitis, defined on the basis of a worsening of their condition, requiring patients to seek medical attention (Saetta *et al.*, 1994). In these cases of bronchitis, gene expression for IL-4, IL-5 and eosinophil chemoattractants such as eotaxin and MCP-4 can be found (Zhu *et al.*, 1999) and IL-4 and IL-5 gene expression has been described in the airway submucosa of non-asthmatic smokers whose lungs have been resected for cancer (Zhu *et al.*, 1999).

These results of IL-4 and IL-5 expression in smokers' bronchitis make the distinction between allergic asthma and smokers' COPD less clear. Further studies of the distinctive patterns of inflammation, cytokine gene expression and protein secretion in the airways of asthma and COPD should prove to be of scientific and clinical interest. However, the relationships between the inflammatory/structural changes and symptoms/airways hyperresponsiveness and asthma severity are still unclear (van Krieken *et al.*, 1996) and require further investigation.

AIRWAY WALL NERVES

The topic of airway wall innervation and its relation to asthma is a large one (Barnes, 1986; Jeffery, 1994). There are data showing that in *fatal* asthma there is an absence of (relaxant) vasoactive intestinal polypeptide (VIP)-containing nerve fibres and an increase in the numbers of substance P-containing fibres (stimulatory to bronchial smooth muscle), contrasting markedly with the innervation of the control lungs taken at resection from chronic smokers (Ollerenshaw and Woolcock, 1993; Ollerenshaw *et al.*, 1991). The reduction has not, however, been confirmed in examination of bronchial biopsies in mild asthma (Haworth *et al.*, 1995). Whilst Sharma and colleagues have described a reduction of airway VIP and β-adrenoreceptors in cystic fibrosis, the densities of both VIP receptors and β-adrenoreceptors are reported to be similar in asthma to those of grossly normal tissue of the lungs of smokers resected for carcinoma (Sharma and Jeffery, 1990; Sharma *et al.*, 1990).

AIRWAYS HYPERRESPONSIVENESS

Airways hyperresponsiveness (AH; also referred to as hyperreactivity) is a feature of asthma but is not unique to it. The factors that contribute to AH are probably multiple and vary from person to person: (i) increased bronchial smooth muscle sensitivity and contracture occur, as evidenced by the effectiveness of inhaled β_2-agonists which relax airway muscle and usually relieve an acute attack of asthma. Although there is increased bronchial smooth muscle mass in asthma there is no evidence that it behaves abnormally in isolation: accordingly there is no correlation between AHR *in vivo* and increased airway muscle sensitivity measured *in vitro* (Vincens *et al.*, 1983; Armour *et al.*, 1984; Cerrina *et al.*, 1986); (ii) increased maximal contraction of bronchial muscle may also occur *in vivo* as a consequence of reduction in, or uncoupling from, the forces which normally oppose contraction, such as the elastic recoil of the lung parenchyma which surrounds membraneous intrapulmonary airways. The effect of airway wall oedema in asthma may result in a 'functional' detachment of alveolar walls, whose elastic recoil maintains patent non-cartilagenous airways (bronchioli) (Ding *et al.*, 1987). Similarly functional loss of lung elastic recoil would allow bronchial smooth muscle to contract maximally and with greater net force. However, Godfrey and colleagues have found no reduction in the staining for elastic fibre, either in the alveolar walls of patients who died following an asthmatic attack or in the airway wall of specimens obtained in mild asthma (Godfrey *et al.*, 1992). In contrast loss of alveolar wall attachments due to elastolytic destruction occurs in COPD and likely contributes to early closure of small airways, particularly during expiration (Saetta *et al.*, 1985; Lamb *et al.*, 1987, 1993) and to the development of AHR which may be detected also in some patients with COPD. Loss of elastic recoil in COPD also likely occurs as 'microscopic' emphysema develops prior to the development of macroscopic lesions: this microscopic alteration is probably an important contributor to reduced FEV_1 (Gillooly, 1993; Hogg *et al.*, 1994); (iii) thickening of the airway wall, due to chronic inflammation, and inappropriate remodelling of the airway wall (James *et al.*, 1989) results in an increased resistance to airflow due to encroachment of the airway lumen, particularly when bronchial smooth muscle contracts (Plate 12). James and colleagues have shown that airway wall thickening need only be relatively minor to have dramatic consequences on airflow limitation (James *et al.*, 1989). The increased wall thickness in airways greater than 2 mm diameter has long been described in fatal asthma since 1922 when interesting comparisons with bronchitis were also made (Huber and Koessler, 1922). The relevance of the airway wall thickening to reduced airflow and AH in asthma has been much discussed (Freedman, 1972; Benson, 1975). It has been suggested that for a given degree of smooth muscle shortening the effect on reduction of airway radius and increased resistance to airflow (to the power 4) would be considerably greater if the airway wall were thickened.

This concept and link of airway geometry to AH has been confirmed by computer modelling: the model predicts that when the airway wall is thickened in the absence of muscle contraction there will be only moderate effects to baseline airflow resistance but, by contrast, there will be profound effects when bronchial smooth muscle shortens even normally (Moreno *et al.*, 1986; Wiggs *et al.*, 1990; 1992). Indeed, James and colleagues have shown that smooth muscle need only shorten by about 40% to completely occlude the airway lumen. A further consideration is that the smooth muscle which surrounds intrapulmonary airways is not truly circular: it encircles the airway arranged as two opposing spirals (a so-called geodesic pattern). Normally muscle contraction thus has the effect of both shortening and constricting the airway. Prevention of airway shortening by thickening of the reticular basement membrane or wall oedema may result in a greater proportion of the force generated by bronchial smooth muscle shortening being redirected to airway constriction.

Finally, alterations of the physical properties of airway fluid may be important in the airways of asthmatics. Macklem and colleagues have shown that the stability of the peripheral airways is partially determined by their lining of surfactant (Macklem *et al.*, 1970). When such a surface tension-reducing lining layer is replaced by a plasma exudate (as in asthma) or by mucus (as in COPD), the surface tension may increase from nearly 0 to about 90 dynes/cm. Such an increase of surface tension could narrow the peripheral airways even without shortening of airway smooth muscle. The plugs of exudate seen in the lumen in asthma might represent collections behind sites where the airways have become unstable or closed and the tendency for asthmatic patients to breath at high lung volumes may be an attempt to prevent such airways closure.

SUMMARY AND CONCLUSION

We have considered the structural and inflammatory basis of asthma and examined tissue-based distinctions between asthma and COPD: none is, as yet, diagnostic. There is evidence of airway inflammation in both asthma and COPD but there are marked differences in terms of the site and consequence of such inflammation between these two airway conditions. Between subject variation is high in both asthma and COPD and, in part, indicates the heterogeneity of both these inflammatory conditions (Richmond *et al.*, 1996). The distinctions are of interest to the researcher who seeks to understand the basic mechanistic differences between asthma and COPD and these may prove to be of importance in diagnosis and in the design of rationale for effective treatment and prevention of these inflammatory conditions in the future.

Further studies of bronchial biopsies obtained from patients with asthma but who have well-defined clinical and smoking histories are required to determine the effects of smoking on the inflammation of asthmatics. Further studies are also required in smokers with exacerbations of COPD and eosinophilia in order to determine which inflammatory cell phenotypes express the genes for IL-5 and for the chemoattractants needed for eosinophilic recruitment. Cases of non-asthmatic eosinophilic bronchitis without evidence of airways hyperresponsiveness form a valuable group whose airway mucosa has not yet been studied. These studies may help us to understand the complex relationships between the clinical signs and symptoms of asthma, bronchitis, airways hyperresponsiveness and eosinophilic inflammation.

ACKNOWLEDGEMENTS

I thank Leone Oscar for invaluable secretarial assistance and Andy Rogers for his expert assistance with the illustrations. I am grateful to the National Asthma Research Campaign and Cystic Fibrosis Trust (UK) for their support and I thank the numerous clinical and research colleagues with whom I have worked.

REFERENCES

Ackerman V, Marini M, Vittori E, Bellini A, Vassali G, Mattoli S. (1994) Detection of cytokines and their cell sources in bronchial biopsy specimens from asthmatic patients: relationship to atopic status, symptoms and level of airway hyperresponsiveness. *Chest*, **105**, 687–96.

Adelroth E, Rosenhall L, Johansson S-A, Linden M, Venge P. (1990) Inflammatory cells and eosinophilic activity in asthmatics investigated by bronchoalveolar lavage: the effects of anti-asthmatic treatment with budesonide or terbutaline. *Am Rev Respir Dis*, **142**, 91–9.

Aikawa T, Shimura S, Sasaki H, Ebina M, Takishima T. (1992) Marked goblet cell hyperplasia with mucus accumulation in the airways of patients who died of severe acute asthma attack. *Chest*, **101**, 916–21.

American Thoracic Society Medical Section of the American Lung Association. (1995) Standards for the diagnosis and care of patients with chronic obstructive pulmonary disease. *Am J Respir Crit Care Med*, **152**, S77–S120.

American Thoracic Society. (1987) Standards for the diagnosis and care of patients with chronic obstructive pulmonary disease (COPD) and asthma. *Am Rev Respir Dis*, **136**, 225–44.

Armour CL, Lazar NM, Schellenberg RR, *et al.* (1984) A comparison of an in vivo and in vitro human airway reactivity to histamine. *Am Rev Respir Dis*, **129**, 907–10.

Ayers M, Jeffery PK. (1988) Proliferation and differentiation in adult mammalian airway epithelium: a review. *Eur Respir J*, **1**, 58–80.

Azzawi M, Bradley B, Jeffery PK, *et al.* (1990) Identification of activated T lymphocytes and eosinophils in bronchial biopsies in stable atopic asthma. *Am Rev Respir Dis*, **142**, 1407–13.

Azzawi M, Johnston PW, Majumdar S, Kay AB, Jeffery PK. (1992) T lymphocytes and activated eosinophils in asthma and cystic fibrosis. *Am Rev Respir Dis*, **145**, 1477–82.

Barnes PJ. (1986) State of art: neural control of human airways in health and disease. *Am Rev Respir Dis*, **134**, 1289–314.

Beasley R, Roche W, Roberts JA, Holgate ST. (1989) Cellular events in the bronchi in mild asthma and after bronchial provocation. *Am Rev Respir Dis*, **139**, 806–17.

Bellini A, Yoshimura H, Vittori E, Marini M, Mattoli S. (1993) Bronchial epithelial cells of patients with asthma release chemoattractant factors for T-lymphocytes. *J Allergy Clin Immunol*, **92**, 412–24.

Benson MK. (1975) Bronchial hyperreactivity. *Br J Dis Chest*, **69**, 227–39.

Bentley AM, Maestrelli P, Saetta M, *et al.* (1992a) Activated T lymphocytes and eosinophils in the bronchial mucosa in isocyanate-induced asthma. *J Allergy Clin Immunol*, **89**, 821–9.

Bentley AM, Menz G, Storz C, *et al.* (1992b) Identification of T-lymphocytes, macrophages and activated eosinophils in the bronchial mucosa in intrinsic asthma: relationship to symptoms and bronchial responsiveness. *Am Rev Respir Dis*, **146**, 500–6.

Bousquet J, Lacoste J-Y, Chanez P, Vic P, Godard P, Michel F-B. (1996) Bronchial elastic fibers in normal subjects and asthmatic patients. *Am J Resp Crit Care Med*, **153**, 1648–54.

Bradding P, Feather IH, Howarth PH, *et al.* (1992) Interleukin 4 is localized to and released by human mast cells. *J Exp Med*, **176**, 1381–6.

Bradding P, Feather IH, Wilson S, *et al.* (1993) Immunolocalization of cytokines in the nasal mucosa of normal and perennial rhinitic subjects. *J Immunol*, **151**, 3853–65.

Brewster CEP, Howarth PH, Djukanovic R, Wilson J, Holgate ST, Roche WR. (1990) Myofibroblasts and subepithelial fibrosis in bronchial asthma. *Am J Respir Cell Mol Biol*, **3**, 507–11.

Broide DH, Lotz M, Cuomo AJ, Coburn DA, Federman EC, Wasserman SI. (1992) Cytokines in symptomatic asthma airways. *J Allergy Clin Immunol*, **89**, 958–67.

Callerame MD, Condemi MD, Bohrod MD, Vaughan JH. (1971) Immunologic reactions of bronchial tissues in asthma. *N Engl J Med*, **284**, 459–64.

Cardell BS, Pearson RSB. (1959) Deaths in asthmatics. *Thorax*, **14**, 341–52.

Carroll N, Carello S, Cooke C, James A. (1996) Airway structure and inflammatory cells in fatal attacks of asthma. *Eur Respir J*, **9**, 709–15.

Carroll N, Elliot A, Morton A, James A. (1993) The structure of large and small airways in nonfatal and fatal asthma. *Am Rev Respir Dis*, **147**, 405–10.

Carroll NG, Cooke C, James AL. (1997) Bronchial blood vessel dimensions in asthma. *Am J Respir Crit Care Med*, **155**, 689–95.

Cerrina J, Ladurie ML, Labat C, Raffestin B, Bayol A, Brink C. (1986) Comparison of human bronchial muscle responses to histamine *in vivo* with histamine and isoproterenol *in vitro*. *Am Rev Respir Dis*, **134**, 51–61.

Chanez P, Vignola AM, O'Shaughnessy T, *et al.* (1997) Corticosteroid reversibility in COPD is related to features of asthma. *Am J Resp Crit Care Med*, **155**, 1529–34.

Charan NB, Baile EM, Pare PD. (1997) Bronchial vascular congestion and angiogenesis. *Eur Respir J*, **10**, 1173–80.

Cluroe A, Holloway L, Thomson K, Purdie G, Beasley R. (1989) Bronchial gland duct ectasia in fatal bronchial asthma: association with interstitial emphysema. *J Clin Pathol*, **42**, 1026–31.

Collins PD, Marleau S, Griffiths-Johnson DA, Jose PJ, Williams TJ. (1995) Cooperation between interleukin-5 and the chemokine eotaxin to induce eosinophil accumulation *in vivo*. *J Exp Med*, **182**, 1169–74.

Corrigan CJ, Haczku A, Gemou-Engesaeth V, *et al.* (1993) CD4 T-lymphocyte activation in asthma is accompanied by increased serum concentrations of interleukin-5. *Am Rev Respir Dis*, **147**, 540–7.

Cosio MG, Hale KA, Niewoehner DE. (1980) Morphologic and morphometric effects of prolonged cigarette smoking on the small airways. *Am Rev Respir Dis*, **122**, 265–71.

Costabel U, Bross KJ, Reuter C, Ruhle K-H, Matthys H. (1986) Alterations in immunoregulatory T-cell subsets in cigarette smokers. A phenotypic analysis of bronchoalveolar and blood lymphocytes. *Chest*, **89**, 39–44.

Crepea SB, Harman JW. (1955) The pathology of bronchial asthma. I. The significance of membrane changes in asthmatic and non-allergic pulmonary disease. *J Allergy*, **26**, 453–60.

Curschmann H. (1883) Uber bronchiolitis exsudatira und ihr verhaltuis zum asthma nervosum. *Dtsch Arch Klin Med*, **32**, 1–34.

Denburg JA, Telizyn S, Belda A, Dolovich J, Bienenstock J. (1985) Increased numbers of circulating basophil progenitors in atopic patients. *J Allergy Clin Immunol*, **76**, 466–72.

Ding DJ, Martin JG, Macklem PT. (1987) Effects of lung volume on maximal methacholine-induced broncho-constriction in normal humans. *J App Physiol*, **62**, 1324.

Dunnill MS, Massarella GR, Anderson JA. (1969) A comparison of the quantitative anatomy of the bronchi in normal subjects, in status asthmaticus, in chronic bronchitis, and in emphysema. *Thorax*, **24**, 176–9.

Dunnill MS. (1960) The pathology of asthma, with special reference to changes in the bronchial mucosa. *J Clin Pathol*, **13**, 27–33.

Ebert RV, Terracio MJ. (1975) The bronchiolar epithelium in cigarette smokers: observations with the scanning electron microscope. *Am Rev Respir Dis*, **111**, 4–11.

Ebina M, Takahashi T, Chiba T, Motomiya M. (1993) Cellular hypertrophy and hyperplasia of airway smooth muscles underlying bronchial asthma – a 3-D morphometric study. *Am Rev Respir Dis*, **148**, 720–6.

Ebina M, Yaegashi H, Chiba R, Takahashi T, Motomiya M, Tanemura M. (1990) Hyperreactive site in the airway tree of asthmatic patients revealed by thickening of bronchial muscles. *Am Rev Respir Dis*, **141**, 1327–32.

Elia C, Bucca C, Rolla G, Scappaticci E, Cantino D. (1988) A freeze-fracture study of tight junctions in human bronchial epithelium in normal, bronchitic and asthmatic subjects. *J Submic Cytol Pathol*, **20**, 509–17.

Erjefalt JS, Andersson M, Greiff L, *et al.* (1998) Cytolysis and piecemeal degranulation as distinct modes of activation of airway mucosal eosinophils. *J Allergy Clin Immunol*, **102**, 286–94.

Evans MJ, Plopper CG. (1988) The role of basal cells in adhesion of columnar epithelium to airway basement membrane. *Am Rev Respir Dis*, **138**, 481–3.

Filley WV, Holley KE, Kephart GM, Gleich GJ. (1982) Identification by immunofluorescence of eosinophil granule major basic protein in lung tissue of patients with bronchial asthma. *Lancet*, **1**, 11–16.

Finkelstein R, Fraser RS, Ghezzo H, Cosio MG. (1995) Alveolar inflammation and its relation to emphysema in smokers. *Am J Respir Crit Care Med*, **152**, 1666–72.

Freedman BJ. (1972) The functional geometry of the bronchi. *Bull Physiopathol Respir*, **8**, 545–51.

Gerblich AA, Campbell AE, Schuyler MR. (1984) Changes in T-lymphocyte subpopulations after antigenic bronchial provocation in asthmatics. *N Engl J Med*, **310**, 1349–52.

Gibson PG, Dolivich J, Denburg J, Ramsdale EH, Hargreave FE. (1989b) Chronic cough: eosinophilic bronchitis without asthma. *Lancet*, **1**, 1346–8.

Gibson PG, Girgis-Gabardo A, Morris MM, *et al.* (1989) Cellular characteristics of sputum from patients with asthma and chronic bronchitis. *Thorax*, **44**, 693–9.

Gibson PG, Hargreaves FE, Girgis-Gabardo A, Morris M, Denburg JA, Dolovich J. (1995) Chronic cough with eosinophilic bronchitis and examination for variable airflow obstruction and reponse to corticosteroid. *Allergy*, **25**, 127–32.

Gillooly M, Lamb D. (1993) Microscopic emphysema in relation to age and smoking habit. *Thorax*, **48**, 491–5.

Gizycki MJ, Adelroth E, Rogers AV, O'Byrne PM, Jeffery PK. (1997) Myofibroblast involvement in the allergen-induced late response in mild atopic asthma. *Am J Respir Cell Mol Biol*, **16**, 664–73.

Gleich GJ, Motojima S, Frigas E, Kephart GM, Fujisawa T, Kravis LP. (1980) The eosinophilic leucocyte and the pathology of fatal bronchial asthma: evidence for pathologic heterogeneity. *J Allergy Clin Immunol*, **80**, 412–15.

Glynn AA, Michaels L. (1960) Bronchial biopsy in chronic bronchitis and asthma. *Thorax*, **15**, 142–53.

Godfrey RW, Lorimer S, Majumdar S, Adelroth E, Johnston PW, Rogers AV, Johansson SA, Jeffery PK. (1995) Airway and lung elastic fibre is not reduced in asthma nor in asthmatics following corticosteroid treatment. *Eur Respir J*, **6**, 922–7.

Godfrey RWA, Severs NJ, Jeffery PK. (1992) Freeze-fracture morphology and quantification of human bronchial epithelial tight junctions. *Am J Respir Cell Mol Biol*, **6**, 453–8.

Hamid Q, Azzawi M, Ying S, *et al.* (1991) IL-5 mRNA in bronchial biopsies from asthmatic subjects. *J Clin Invest*, **87**, 1541–6.

Hamid Q, Barkans J, Meng Q, *et al.* (1992) Human eosinophils synthesize and secrete interleukin-6, in vitro. *Blood*, **80**, 1496–501.

Hamid Q, Song Y, Kotsimbos TC, *et al.* (1997) Inflammation of small airways in asthma. *J Allergy Clin Immunol*, **100**, 44–51.

Hargreave FE, Popov T, Kidney J, Dolovich J. (1993a) Sputum measurements to assess airway inflammation in asthma. *Allergy*, **48**, 81–3.

Hargreave FE, Wong BJO, Popov T, Dolovich J. (1993b) Noninvasive methods to examine the anti-inflammatory effects of drugs. In: Hansel T, Morley J, eds. *New drugs in allergy and asthma*. Basel: Birkhauser Verlag, 291–5.

Haworth PH, Djukanovic R, Wilson JW, Holgate ST, Springall DR, Polak JM. (1995) Neuropeptide-containing nerves in endobronchial biopsies from asthmatic and non-asthmatic subjects. *Am J Cell Molec Biol*, **13**, 288–96.

Heard BE, Hossain S. (1983) Hyperplasia of bronchial muscle in asthma. *J Pathol*, **110**, 319–31.

Heard BE, Nunn AJ, Kay AB. (1989) Mast cells in human lungs. *J Pathol*, **157**, 59–63.

Hogg JC. (1993) The pathology of asthma. In: Austen KF, Lichtenstein L, Kay AB, Holgate ST, eds. *Asthma*, Vol. IV, *Physiology, immunopharmacology and treatment*. Oxford: Blackwell Scientific Publications, 17–25.

Hogg JC, Eggleston PA. (1984) Is asthma an epithelial disease? *Am Rev Respir Dis*, **129**, 207–8.

Hogg JC, Macklem PT, Thurlbeck WM. (1968) Site and nature of airway obstruction in chronic obstructive lung disease. *N Engl J Med*, **278**, 1355–60.

Hogg JC, Wright JL, Wiggs BR, Coxson HO, Saez AO, Pare PD. (1994) Lung structure and function in cigarette smokers. *Thorax*, **49**, 473–8.

Holgate ST, Howarth PH, Church MK, Djukanovic R, Roche W, Montefort S. (1993) Mechanisms of acute and chronic mucosal inflammation in asthma. In: Austen KF, Lichtenstein L, Kay AB, Holgate ST, eds. *Asthma*, Vol. IV, *Physiology, immunopharmacology and treatment*. Oxford: Blackwell Scientific Publications, 287–98.

Huber H, Koessler KK. (1922) The pathology of bronchial asthma. *Arch Intern Med*, **30**, 689–760.

Humbert M, Durham SR, Ying S, *et al.* (1996) IL-4 and IL-5 mRNA and protein in bronchial biopsies from atopic and non-atopic asthma. Evidence against 'intrinsic' asthma being a distinct immunopathological entity. *Am J Resp Crit Care Med*, **154**, 1497–504.

James AL, Pare PD, Hogg JC. (1989) The mechanics of airway narrowing in asthma. *Am Rev Respir Dis*, **139**, 242–6.

Jeffery PK, Godfrey RWA, Adelroth E, Nelson F, Rogers A, Johansson S-A. (1992) Effects of treatment on airway inflammation and thickening of reticular collagen in asthma: a quantitative light and electron microscopic study. *Am Rev Respir Dis*, **145**, 890–9.

Jeffery PK, Heard BE, Kay AB. (1993) Do mast cells degranulate in the bronchial mucosa of mildly symptomatic atopic asthmatic subjects? *Am Rev Respir Dis*, **145**, A23.

Jeffery PK, Wardlaw A, Nelson FC, Collins JV, Kay AB. (1989) Bronchial biopsies in asthma: an ultrastructural quantification study and correlation with hyperreactivity. *Am Rev Respir Dis*, **140**, 1745–53.

Jeffery PK. (1990) Tobacco smoke-induced lung disease. In: Cohen RD, Lewis B, Alberti KGMM, Denman AM, eds. *The metabolic and molecular basis of acquired disease*. London: Ballière Tindall, 466–95.

Jeffery PK. (1991) Morphology of the airway wall in asthma and chronic obstructive pulmonary disease. *Am Rev Respir Dis*, **143**, 1152–8.

Jeffery PK. (1994) Innervation of the airway mucosa: Structure, function and changes in airway disease. In: Goldie R, ed. *Immunopharmacology of epithelial barriers*, Vol 8 of the *Handbook of Immunopharmacology* (series ed. C Page). London: Academic Press, 85–118.

Jeffery PK. (1994) Structural changes in asthma. In: Page C, Black J, eds. *Airways and vascular remodelling in asthma and cardiovascular disease*. London: Academic Press, 3–19.

Jeffery PK. (1996) Bronchial biopsies and airway inflammation. *Eur Respir J*, **9**, 1583–7.

Jeffery PK. (1998) The development of large and small airways. *Am J Respir Crit Care Med*, **157**, S174–S180.

Jose PJ, Griffiths-Johnson DA, Collins PD, *et al.* (1994) Eotaxin: a potent eosinophil chemoattractant cytokine detected in a guinea pig model of allergic airways inflammation. *J Exp Med*, **179**, 881–7.

Kay AB. (1991) Asthma and inflammation. *J Allergy Clin Immunol*, **87**, 893–910.

Kraft M, Djukanovic R, Wilson S, Holgate ST, Martin RJ. (1996) Alveolar tissue inflammation in asthma. *Am J Respir Crit Care Med*, **154**, 1505–10.

Kuwano K, Bosken CH, Pare PD, Bai TR, Wiggs BR, Hogg JC. (1993) Small airways dimensions in asthma and in chronic obstructive pulmonary disease. *Am J Resp Crit Care Med*, **148**, 1220–23.

Lacoste JY, Bousquet J, Chanez P, *et al.* (1993) Eosinophilic and neutrophilic inflammation in asthma, chronic bronchitis, and chronic obstructive pulmonary disease. *J Allergy Clin Immunol*, **92**, 537–48.

Laitinen A, Altraja A, Kampe M, Linden M, Virtanen I, Laitinen L. (1997) Tenascin is increased in airway basement membrane of asthmatics and decreased by an inhaled steroid. *Am J Respir Crit Care Med*, **156**(3 Pt 1), 951–8.

Laitinen LA, Heino M, Laitinen A, Kava T, Haahtela T. (1985) Damage of the airway epithelium and bronchial reactivity in patients with asthma. *Am Rev Respir Dis*, **131**, 599–606.

Laitinen LA, Laitinen A, Haahtela T. (1993) Airway mucosal inflammation even in patients with newly diagnosed asthma. *Am Rev Respir Dis*, **147**, 697–704.

Lamb D, Lumsden A. (1982) Intra-epithelial mast cells in human airway epithelium: evidence for smoking-induced changes in their frequency. *Thorax*, **37**, 334–42.

Lamb D, Mclean A, Gould G, MacNee W, Warren P, Flenley DC. (1987) Airflow limitation *in vivo* relates to alveolar attachment to membranous airways but not to small airway calibres. *Am Rev Respir Dis*, **135**, A510.

Lamb D, McLean A, Gillooly M, Warren PM, Gould GA, MacNee W. (1993) The relationship between distal airspace size, bronchiolar attachments and lung function. *Thorax*, **48**, 1012–17.

Lambert RK. (1991) Role of bronchial basement membrane in airway collapse. *J App Physiol*, **71**(2), 666–73.

Lambert RK, Wiggs BR, Kuwano K, Hogg JC, Pare PD. (1991) Functional significance of increased airway smooth muscle in asthma and COPD. *J Appl Physiol*, **74**, 2771–81.

Lams BEA, Sousa AR, Rees PJ, Lee TH. (1998) Immunopathology of the small-airway submucosa in smokers with and without chronic obstructive pulmonary disease. *Am J Respir Crit Care Med*, **158**, 1518–23.

Li D, Wang D, Griffiths-Johnson DA, Wells TNC, *et al.* (1997) Eotaxin protein gene expression in guinea-pigs: constitutive expression and upregulation after allergen challenge. *Eur Respir J*, **10**, 1946–54.

List SJ, Findlay BP, Forstner GG, Forstner JF. (1978) Enhancement of the viscosity of mucin by serum albumin. *Biochem J*, **175**, 565–71.

Lozewicz S, Wells C, Gomez E, *et al.* (1990) Morphological integrity of the bronchial epithelium in mild asthma. *Thorax*, **45**, 12–15.

Macklem PT, Proctor DF, Hogg JC. (1970) The stability of peripheral airways. *Resp Physiol*, **8**, 191–203.

MacNee W, Selby C. (1992) New perspectives on basic mechanisms in lung disease. Neutrophil traffic in the lungs: role of haemodynamics, cell adhesion and deformability. *Thorax*, **48**, 79–88.

Majo J, Ghezzo H, Hogg J, Cosio MG. (1996) Alveolar wall inflammation in lungs of smokers. *Am J Respir Crit Care Med*, **153**(4), A821.

Majumdar S, Li D, Ansari T, Pantelidis P, Black CM, Gizycki M, du Bois RM, Jeffery PK. (1999) Different cytokine profiles in cryptogenic fibrosing alveolitis and fibrosing alveolitis associated with systemic sclerosis: a quantitative study of open lung biopsies. *Eur Respir J*, **2**, 251–7.

Messer JW, Peters GA, Bennett WA. (1960) Causes of death and pathologic findings in 304 cases of bronchial asthma. *Dis Chest*, **38**, 616–24.

Montefort S, Roberts JA, Beasley R, Holgate ST, Roche WR. (1992) The site of disruption of the bronchial epithelium in asthmatic and non-asthmatic subjects. *Thorax*, **47**, 499–503.

Moreno RH, Hogg JC, Pare PD. (1986) Mechanisms of airway narrowing. *Am Rev Respir Dis*, **133**, 1171–80.

Mullen JBM, Wright JL, Wiggs BR, Pare PD, Hogg JC. (1985) Reassessment of inflammation of airways in chronic bronchitis. *BMJ*, **291**, 1235–9.

Mullen JBM, Wright JL, Wiggs BR, Pare PD, Hogg JC. (1987) Structure of central airways in current smokers and ex-smokers with and without mucus hypersecretion. *Thorax*, **42**, 843–6.

Naylor B. (1962) The shedding of the mucosa of the bronchial tree in asthma. *Thorax*, **17**, 69–72.

Niewoehner DE, Klienerman J, Rice D. (1974) Pathologic changes in the peripheral airways of young cigarette smokers. *N Engl J Med*, **291**, 755–8.(1974)

Nowak J. (1969) Anatomopathologic changes in the bronchial walls in chronic inflammation, with special reference to the basement membrane, in the course of bronchial asthma. *Acta Med Polona*, **2**, 151–72.

O'Shaughnessy TC, Ansari TW, Barnes NC, Jeffery PK. (1996) Reticular basement membrane thickness in moderately severe asthma and smokers' chronic bronchitis with and without airflow obstruction. *Am J Resp Crit Care Med*, **153**, A879 (Abstract).

O'Shaughnessy TC, Ansari TW, Barnes NC, Jeffery PK. (1997) Inflammation in bronchial biopsies of subjects with chronic bronchitis: inverse relationship of CD8+ T lymphocytes with FEV_1. *Am J Respir Crit Care Med*, **155**, 852–7.

Ohnishi T, Kita H, Weiler D, *et al.* (1993) IL-5 is the predominant eosinophil-active cytokine in the antigen-induced pulmonary late-phase reaction. *Am Rev Respir Dis*, **147**, 901–7.

Ollerenshaw SL, Jarvis D, Sullivan CE, Woolcock AJ. (1991) Substance P immunoreactive nerves in airways from asthmatics and non-asthmatics. *Eur Respir J*, **4**, 673–82.

Ollerenshaw SL, Woolcock AJ. (1992) Characteristics of the inflammation in biopsies from large airways of subjects with asthma and subjects with chronic airflow limitation. *Am Rev Respir Dis*, **145**, 922–7.

Ollerenshaw, SL, Woolcock AJ. (1993) Quantification and location of vasoactive intestinal peptide immunoreactive nerves in bronchial biopsies from subjects with mild asthma. *Am Rev Respir Dis*, **147**, A285.

Orie NGM, Sluiter HJ, De Vries K, Tammeling GJ, Witkop J. (1961) The host factor in bronchitis. In: Orie NGM, Sluiter HJ, eds. *Bronchitis, an international symposium*. Assen, The Netherlands: Royal Van Gorcum, 43–59.

Orsida BE, Li X, Ickey B, Thien F, Wilson JW, Walters EH. (1999) Vascularity in the asthmatic airways: relation to inhaled steroids. *Thorax*, **54**, 289–95.

Pare PD, Wiggs BR, James A, Hogg JC, Bosken C. (1991) The comparative mechanics and morphology of airways in asthma and chronic obstructive pulmonary disease. *Am J Resp Crit Care Med*, **143**, 1189–93.

Peleman RA, Rytila PH, Kips JC, Joos GF, Pauwels RA. (1999) The cellular composition of induced sputum in chronic obstructive pulmonary disease. *Eur Resp J*, **13**, 839–43.

Persson CGA, Erjefalt JS. (1997) Eosinophil lysis and free granules: an in-vivo paradigm for cell activation and drug development. *Trends Pharmacol Sci*, **18**, 117–23.

Pizzichini MNN, Pizzichini E, Morris M, *et al.* (1996) Indices of airway inflammation in sputum of smokers with non-obstructive and obstructive bronchitis. *Eur Respir J*, **9**, 126S.

Reid L. (1954) Pathology of chronic bronchitis. *Lancet*, **i**, 275–9.

Reid LM. (1987) The presence or absence of bronchial mucus in fatal asthma. *J Allergy Clin Immunol*, **80**, 415–16.

Richmond I, Booth H, Ward C, Walters EH. (1996) Intrasubject variability in the airway inflammation in biopsies in mild to moderate stable asthma. *Am J Respir Crit Care Med*, **153**, 899–903.

Riise GC, Ahlstedt S, Larsson S, Enander I, Jones I, Andersson B. (1995) Bronchial inflammation in chronic bronchitis assessed by measurement of cell products in bronchial lavage fluid. *Thorax*, **50**, 360–5.

Robinson DS, Durham SR, Kay AB. (1993) Cytokines: 3-cytokines in asthma. *Thorax*, **48**, 845–53.

Robinson DS, Hamid Q, Ying S, *et al.* (1992) Predominant Th2-like bronchoalveolar T-lymphocyte population in atopic asthma. *N Engl J Med*, **326**, 298–304.

Roche WR, Beasley R, Williams JH, Holgate ST. (1989) Subepithelial fibrosis in the bronchi of asthmatics. *Lancet*, **i**, 520–3.

Sabonya RE. (1984) Quantitative structural alterations in long-standing allergic asthma. *Am Rev Respir Dis*, **130**, 289–92.

Saetta M. (1998) CD8+ T-lymphocytes in peripheral airways of smokers with chronic obstructive pulmonary disease. *Am J Respir Crit Care Med*, **157**, 822–6.

Saetta M, Di Stefano A, Maestrelli P, *et al.* (1993) Activated T-lymphocytes and macrophages in bronchial mucosa of subjects with chronic bronchitis. *Am Rev Respir Dis*, **147**, 301–6.

Saetta M, Di Stefano A, Maestrelli P, *et al.* (1994) Airway eosinophilia in chronic bronchitis during exacerbations. *Am J Respir Crit Care Med*, **150**, 1646–52.

Saetta M, Di Stefano A, Rosina C, Thiene G, Fabbri LM. (1991) Quantitative structural analysis of peripheral airways and arteries in sudden fatal asthma. *Am Rev Respir Dis*, **143**, 138–43.

Saetta M, Ghezzo H, Wong Dong Kim, *et al.* (1985) Loss of alveolar attachments in smokers. A morphometric correlate of lung function impairment. *Am Rev Respir Dis*, **132**, 894–900.

Saetta M, Turato G, Facchini FM, *et al.* (1997) Inflammatory cells in the bronchial glands of smokers with chronic bronchitis. *Am J Respir Crit Care Med*, **156**, 1633–9.

Salvato G. (1968) Some histological changes in chronic bronchitis and asthma. *Thorax*, **23**, 168–72.

Sharma R, Jeffery PK. (1990) Airway B-adrenoceptor number in cystic fibrosis and asthma. *Clin Sci*, **78**, 409–17.

Sharma RK, Jeffery PK. (1990) Airway VIP receptor number is reduced in cystic fibrosis but not asthma. *Am Rev Respir Dis*, **141**, A726.

Shimura S, Andoh Y, Haraguchi M, Shirato K. (1996) Continuity of airway goblet cells and intralumenal mucus in the airways of patients with bronchial asthma. *Eur Respir J*, **9**, 1395–401.

Siafakas NM, Vermeire P, Pride NB, *et al.* (1995) Optimal assessment and management of chronic obstructive pulmonary disease (COPD). *Eur Respir J*, **8**, 1398–420.

Soderberg M, Hellstrom S, Sandstrom T, Lungren R, Bergh A. (1990) Structural characterization of bronchial mucosal biopsies from healthy volunteers: a light and electron microscopical study. *Eur Respir J*, **3**, 261–6.

Sparrow MP, Mitchell HW. (1991) The epithelium acts as a barrier modulating the extent of bronchial narrowing produced by substances perfused through the lumen. *Br J Pharmacol*, **103**, 1160–4.

Sun Y, Robinson DS, Qiu M, *et al.* (1997) Enhanced expression of eotaxin and CCR3 mRNA and protein in atopic asthma. Association with airway hyperresponsiveness and predominant colocalization of eotaxin mRNA to bronchial epithelial and endothelial cells. *Eur J Immunol*, **27**, 3507–16.

Sur S, Crotty TB, Kephart GM, *et al.* (1993) Sudden onset fatal asthma: a distinct entity with few eosinophils and relatively more neutrophils in the airway submucosa? *Am Rev Respir Dis*, **148**, 713–19.

Synek M, Beasley R, Frew AJ, *et al.* (1996) Cellular infiltration of the airways in asthma of varying severity. *Am J Resp Crit Care Med*, **154**, 224–30.

Takizawa T, Thurlbeck WM. (1971) Muscle and mucous gland size in the major bronchi of patients with chronic bronchitis, asthma and asthmatic bronchitis. *Am Rev Respir Dis*, **104**, 331–6.

Thompson AB, Daughton D, Robbins RA, Ghafouri MA, Oehlerking M, Rennard SI. (1989) Intraluminal airway inflammation in chronic bronchitis. Characterization and correlation with clinical parameters. *Am Rev Respir Dis*, **140**, 1527–37.

Thurlbeck WM. (1985) Chronic airflow obstruction. Correlation of structure and function. In: Petty TL, ed. *Chronic obstructive pulmonary disease*, 2nd edn. New York: Dekker, 129–203.

van Brabandt H, Cauberghs M, Verbeken E, Moerman PH, Lauweryns JM, van de Woestijne KP. (1983) Partitioning of pulmonary impedance in excised human and canine lungs. *J Appl Physiol: Respir Environ Exercise Physiol*, **55**, 1733–42.

van Krieken JHJM, Evertse CE, Hooijer R, Willems LNA, Sterk PJ. (1996) Relationship between the inflammatory infiltrate in bronchial biopsy specimens and clinical severity of asthma in patients treated with inhaled steroids. *Thorax*, **51**, 496–502.

van Houtte PM. (1989) Epithelium-derived relaxing factor(s) and bronchial reactivity. *J Allergy Clin Immunol*, **83**, 855–61.

Vincens KS, Black JL, Yan K, Armour CL, Donnelly PD, Woolcock AJ. (1983) A comparison of *in vivo* and *in vitro* responses to histamine in human airway. *Am Rev Respir Des*, **128**, 875–9.

Walker C, Bode E, Boer L, Hansel TT, Blaser K, Virchow J-C Jr. (1992) Allergic and nonallergic asthmatics have distinct patterns of T-cell activation and cytokine production in peripheral blood and bronchoalveolar lavage. *Am Rev Respir Dis*, **146**, 109–15.

Wanner A. (1988) Airway mucus and the mucociliary system. In: Middleton E, Reed CE, Ellis EF, Adkinson

NF, Uunginer JW, eds. *Allergy: principles and practice*. St Louis, Washington DC, Toronto: CV Mosby, 541–8.

Wardlaw AJ, Dunnett S, Gleich GJ, Collins JV, Kay AB. (1988) Eosinophils and mast cells in bronchoalveolar lavage in mild asthma: relationship to bronchial hyperreactivity. *Am Rev Respir Dis*, **137**, 62–9.

Weller PF, Bach DS, Austen KF. (1984) Biochemical characterization of human eosinophil Charcot–Leyden crystal protein (lysophospholipase). *J Biol Chem*, **259**, 15100–5.

Widdicombe J. (1993) New perspectives on basic mechanisms in lung disease. 4. Why are the airways so vascular? *Thorax*, **48**, 290–5.

Wiggs BR, Bosken C, Pare PD, James A, Hogg JC. (1992) A model of airway narrowing in asthma and in chronic obstructive pulmonary disease. *Am Rev Respir Dis*, **145**, 1215–18.

Wiggs BR, Moreno R, Hogg JC, Hilliam C, Pare PD. (1990) A model of the mechanics of airway narrowing. *J Appl Physiol*, **69**, 849–60.

Wilhelm DL. (1953) Regeneration of tracheal epithelium. *J Pathol*, **65**, 543–50.

Woolley KL, Adelroth E, Woolley MJ, Ellis R, Jordana M, O'Byrne PM. (1995) Granulocyte-macrophage colony-stimulating factor, eosinophils and eosinophil cationic protein in subjects with and without mild, stable atopic asthma. *Eur Resp J*, In press.

Zhu J, Majumdar S, Ansari T, *et al.* (1999) IL-4 and IL-5 mRNA in the bronchial wall of smokers. *Am J Resp Crit Care Med*, **159**, A450.

Zhu J, Majumdar S, Turato G, Fabbi L, Saetta M, Jeffery PK. (1999) Airway eosniophilia in bronchitis and gene expression for IL-4, IL-5, and eotaxin in bronchial biopsies. *Eur Resp J*, **14**, 360S.

9

Epidemiology

P.G.J. BURNEY

INTRODUCTION

There is accumulating evidence that asthma has been growing in prevalence and has imposed an increasingly large burden on the health services since at least the middle of the twentieth century. Although mortality rates attributed to asthma among older people have fallen steadily during the twentieth century, mortality from asthma in young people has remained unchanged or increased with some 'epidemics' of asthma death (Marks and Burney, 1998). In spite of this we still have only a sketchy idea of what causes asthma. Much work has been done recently, however, to standardize instruments and to harmonize protocols for studying the condition (Burney *et al.*, 1994; Asher *et al.*, 1995).

The earliest reports of an increasing prevalence of asthma came from surveys of schoolchildren in Birmingham, UK in the late 1960s (Morrison Smith, 1976), and Lower Hutt in New Zealand in the early 1980s (Mitchell, 1983). Apart from concerns about the comparability of methods in the Birmingham surveys, the principal concerns with these early studies were that changes might reflect local changes in the population, and/or that changes in the prevalence of 'diagnosed asthma' might simply reflect a change in the way that doctors were labelling children with symptoms related to the airway. Since this time, however, increases have also been reported from national samples in Sweden, England and Finland, and increases have been recorded not only in the prevalence of diagnosed asthma but also in the prevalence of airway responsiveness and in symptoms. Evidence for an increasing incidence of asthma from the USA suggests that this increase in prevalence is not due to fewer remissions.

This increase in prevalence has been accompanied by an increased, use of services. Hospitalizations for asthma have increased, particularly among children, against the trend for most other diseases. This trend has been reported in England and Wales, New Zealand, and the USA, as well as other countries. Changing admission rates are not simply explained by changes in prevalence or changes in the threshold of severity for admission. In Finland, for instance, admission rates remained unchanged while prevalence rates increased, while in Croydon, south London, admission rates rose much faster than the prevalence of wheeze. The increase was not due to a lower threshold of severity for admission (Anderson *et al.*, 1980). More recently, admission rates have steadied or declined and this has happened in spite of a continuing increase in episodes of asthma.

The proportion of people who are seeing their doctor for asthma has also been increasing (Gerstman *et al.*, 1989) as have sales of drugs for asthma (Department of Health, 1995a). Gerstman *et al.* have also shown that the average number of anti-asthma treatments per case of asthma increased in the Michigan Medicaid programme over the period 1980–86.

DEFINITION AND DIAGNOSIS IN EPIDEMIOLOGICAL STUDIES

One problem that has greatly hindered progress in the epidemiology of asthma is the lack of clear definition with a well-standardized instrument for detecting the condition. The first international attempt to agree a definition of asthma was made in 1958 at the CIBA guest symposium, which defined asthma as 'widespread narrowing of the bronchial airways, which changes its severity over short periods of time either spontaneously or under treatment, and is not due to cardiovascular disease' (Anon, 1959). Three years later the American Thoracic Society introduced the characteristic of hyperresponsiveness into the definition: 'Asthma is a disease characterized by an increased responsiveness of the trachaea and bronchi to various stimuli and manifested by a widespread narrowing of the airways that changes in severity either spontaneously or as a result of therapy'. This definition also excluded explicitly 'bronchial narrowing which results solely from widespread bronchial infection. . . . from destructive disease of the lung . . . or from cardiovascular disorders'.

Such definitions are inadequate because they leave room for various interpretations. A true definition must give clear criteria for deciding whether any particular individual has asthma. In 1971 a further CIBA study group (Porter and Birch, 1971) attempted to provide such a definition but concluded that, on the information then available, asthma could not be defined. This conclusion remains essentially unchanged as greater specificity in the definition leads either to disagreement or to counterintuitive conclusions. Nevertheless, 'asthma' can be studied indirectly be defining proxy conditions and studying those instead. The appropriateness of these proxy conditions depends on the nature and purpose of the study. Variation in the definition is likely to lead to inconsistent results between different studies.

Three principal methods have been used to define asthma in epidemiological studies. These are: a positive answer to a question asking whether the subject has asthma, sometimes qualified by a further question on whether this has been confirmed by a doctor; a physiological measurement of increased bronchial responsiveness; and a positive answer to a question on symptoms, almost always a question on wheeze in the English language studies of asthma.

Definitions based on a diagnosis of asthma

Questions about asthma rarely elicit a positive answer from someone who does not, in the opinion of a doctor, have asthma. However, many people who do have asthma, in the opinion of a doctor, will deny that they have asthma. For instance, in a study undertaken in four different countries only half of the people studied who were thought by the clinicians to have asthma, said that they had asthma (Burney *et al.*, 1989). This under-reporting may lead to important biases, and it has been shown that children at any rate are less likely to be labelled by their parents as asthmatics if they are not being treated for asthma. Any other variable used to explain the distribution of 'asthma' that is itself determined by or correlated with the use of health services, such as age, sex, social class or place of residence, may therefore also be spuriously associated with asthma if it is defined in this way. Dodge and Burrows (1980) have also shown in their longitudinal study in Tucson, AZ, that women are more likely than men to be labelled as having asthma, even when differences in symptoms, cigarette smoking and lung function have been taken into account. Finally, there is evidence from studies of death certification that there are consistent differences between countries in the way that the term is used as a diagnostic label at the time of death. These studies are discussed in more detail below.

Definitions based on symptoms

Asthma may also be defined in terms of symptoms. These do not depend on a doctor's diagnosis and so are not subject to the same bias as questionnaires asking about 'asthma'. However, asthma not only presents a heterogeneous clinical picture but also shares many symptoms with other conditions. It has been recognized since the 1930s, for instance, that asthma may present as chronic cough and several groups have shown that bronchial hyperresponsiveness may be associated independently with several different symptoms including cough, shortness of breath, morning tightness and nocturnal dyspnoea. Asthma is not distinguished from smokers' bronchitis by the production of sputum. Part of this diversity may be due to a diverse pathophysiology, differences in severity of disease or to differences in perception.

Definitions based on airway responsiveness

The American Thoracic Society included airway hyperresponsiveness in its definition of asthma, and the relation of hyperresponsiveness to other clinical features of asthma, such as the presence of symptoms, the variation in peak flow, and the amount of treatment required to control symptoms, has been used to justify its use in this way.

Several tests of airway responsiveness have been proposed including response to various bronchoconstrictors or exercise, variation in peak flow rates and response to bronchodilators. Unfortunately, these different methods give different results. There is a relatively good association between the responses to histamine and methacholine, though even here differences have been suggested comparing the tests among children. There is less agreement between other tests. Substantial disagreement has been shown between the results of tests using methacholine or histamine and exercise (Sierstedt *et al.*, 1996), ultrasonically nebulized distilled water and exercise, cold air and methacholine, and diurnal variation in peak flow and response to histamine. Some measures of airway hyperresponsiveness have also been criticized because they are not specific for asthma. In infancy it has been suggested that hyperresponsiveness to histamine is normal. Smokers who have impaired lung function also show hyperresponsiveness to inhaled agonists, as well as having an increased diurnal variation in peak flow and a response to inhaled bronchodilators. Yet the mechanism of this hyper-responsiveness would appear to be different from that seen in asthma. Though this lack of specificity has raised problems of interpretation, these are not generally insuperable. Many physiological characteristics including, for instance, blood pressure are useful markers of disease even though they are not the specific result of a single mechanism. There are strong arguments to suggest that tests based on challenge with exercise, cold air or adenosine are more specific for asthma (*see* Chapter 3: Exercise and environmentally-induced asthma).

CLASSIFICATION OF ASTHMA

Asthma is most commonly classified as 'extrinsic' or 'intrinsic' depending largely on whether an extrinsic allergen can be shown to be involved. Many studies from around the world have now shown an association between airway hyperresponsiveness and atopy, whether this is defined as a raised serum IgE or as a positive skin response to common inhalant allergens (Burney *et al.*, 1987). The association is strong and the more marked the atopy, the greater is the hyperresponsiveness.

Rare exceptions to this association have been reported. The association between airway responsiveness and skin sensitivity to three common inhalant allergens has been reported to weaken with age (Burney *et al.*, 1987), and a few studies that have included only, or predominantly, older subjects have shown no association. Other studies showing no association between airway response and skin sensitivity have selected samples in a way that is likely to have obscured the relationship. Recent assessments of the role of atopy in asthma have suggested that the proportion of 'asthma' attributable to atopy is in the order of 30% (Pearce *et al.*, 1999). Such estimates need to be interpreted with due regard to the ambiguities of the definition of 'asthma' and the complex aetiology of the condition. It is clear that atopy is not a sufficient cause of asthma and that many atopic people do not get asthma. It is also clear that many people get symptoms similar to those with asthma who have a non-atopic cause for their symptoms. The extent to which these people would be regarded as 'asthmatic' is contentious.

Intrinsic asthma is defined by the lack of evidence for an external allergic cause. It is generally of late onset and more severe and is often associated with eosinophilia and nasal polyps. The principal negative criterion for its definition has led some to doubt whether 'intrinsic asthma' really exists as a separate condition, and this view has been supported by two observations. The first is the close association at all ages of diagnosed 'asthma' with a high age-standardized serum IgE (Burrows *et al.*, 1989). The second is the observation that some patients with many of the characteristics of 'intrinsic' asthma have atopic responses to unusual 'intrinsic' allergens such as Trichophyton. In this case 'intrinsic' should not be used to imply 'non-allergic'. Too sharp a divide between the two types of asthma may not be justified on the current evidence.

Because of the importance of atopy in the aetiology of asthma, but also because there are clearly risk factors for asthma other than atopy, the discussion of the distribution and determinants of asthma will deal with the two conditions separately.

DISTRIBUTION OF ATOPY AND ASTHMA

Atopy

The term 'atopy' is used to mean different things. The underlying concept is of an abnormal reaction to environmental allergens. This has been defined clinically as a history of asthma, eczema or hay fever, or by skin testing as an abnormal response to at least one common inhaled allergen, or as an abnormally high total serum IgE level not explained by parasitic infestation, or by the presence of serum IgE to specific inhalant allergens. Standardized definitions are not yet agreed but the methods for skin testing are becoming more standardized with the use of purified allergens and standard lancets. Data are now being collected on large samples using standardized methods.

A large survey of skin sensitivity was undertaken in the second National Health and Nutrition Examination Survey (NHANES II) in the USA between 1976 and 1980 (Gergen and Turkeltaub, 1986). This survey examined skin sensitivity in over 15 000 individuals in a national representative sample of non-institutionalized civilians aged 6–74 years living in the USA. This confirmed for the most part the distribution of skin sensitivity that had been established in other earlier but smaller studies. Skin sensitivity, defined as an erythematous reaction of at least 10.5 mm diameter to at least one of eight common allergens, reaches a peak in early adulthood (18–24 years) with approximately 30% of white men being positive by this definition. The age-adjusted prevalence rates were about 20% higher in men than in women, though this difference between the sexes has not always been observed.

Among blacks the prevalence of positive skin tests tended to be slightly higher and the excess prevalence in males was less obvious and appeared to vary with age. Higher levels of skin sensitivity were also found among the rich than among the poor and in the well-educated compared with the less well-educated. Both these associations appeared to hold through a broad range of values. Positive skin tests were more common in urban than in rural areas, though the prevalence tended to be slightly higher in the suburbs than in the city centres. There were considerable variations in prevalence between different regions, though these did not seem to be explained by differences in the prevalence of exposure to specific allergens, with the exception of ragweed sensitivity. Sensitivity to oak and Bermuda grass were more evenly distributed, possibly because of greater cross-reactivity between these and other allergens. The sensitivity to allergens appeared to be slightly greater in the months following the season of greatest exposure compared to the months of exposure and the months prior to exposure.

Measurements of IgE vary markedly worldwide, as does the prevalence of sensitivity to common inhalant allergens (Burney *et al.*, 1997). The community prevalence of specific IgE to common inhalant allergens does not, however, correlate with the geometric mean total serum IgE levels in the population.

Asthma

Ambiguity in the definition of asthma makes it difficult to obtain a clear picture of the distribution of the disease or to give an authoritative estimate of its absolute prevalence. However, we do have a clear idea of the relative prevalence of the condition now from standardized international surveys. The prevalence of symptoms associated with asthma vary markedly around the world in both adults (Burney *et al.*, 1996) and children (The International Study of Asthma and Allergies in Childhood (ISAAC) Steering Committee, 1998). These findings are supported by information on bronchial responsiveness in adults and children.

In children, both asthma and wheeze are commoner in boys than girls, with convergence between rates in the two sexes during adolescence (Gergen *et al.*, 1988). In adults there is greater equality between the sexes. There appear to be considerable regional variations in western countries (Gergen *et al.*, 1988), but even more so in developing countries where underdeveloped rural areas have a low prevalence of the condition (Keeley and Galivan, 1991). Prevalence is higher in urban than in rural areas (Gergen *et al.*, 1988). Racial differences have been noted in a number of studies. In the USA, rates of wheeze and diagnosed asthma are higher in blacks (Gergen *et al.*, 1988). In New Zealand, Maori children have been reported to have more symptoms but less hyperresponsiveness than Europeans, whereas Pacific Islanders have a lower prevalence of hyperresponsiveness than Europeans, but no fewer symptoms (Pattemore *et al.*, 1989). Melia *et al.* (1988) found slightly lower prevalence of 'asthma' and wheezing in Afro-Caribbean children than in white children in a sample of 5–11-year-olds living in 20 inner city areas of England. Among Asian children, however, they found a lower prevalence of wheeze but, if anything, a slightly higher prevalence of reported asthma. Other studies of South Asian children living in England have tended to confirm the lower prevalence of symptoms but have given mixed results on airway reactivity (Jones *et al.*, 1996).

Social class has a very inconstant relation to asthma prevalence with most studies showing no effect. Although earlier studies suggested that asthma was more common in higher social classes, severe disease was also reported to be more common in poorer children. Mitchell *et al.* (1989) found little difference in hyperresponsiveness or diagnosis of asthma in 8–10-year-old children by social class, but significantly more common history of wheeze or exercise-induced wheeze among those of lower social class. More recently, studies have identified severe asthma with areas of social deprivation, and this seems to be a better marker than social class (Duran-Tauleria and Rona, 1999; Salmond *et al.*, 1999).

GENETIC INFLUENCES

The familial nature of atopic disease was recognized early, as was the heterogeneity within families of both the clinical presentation, and the allergens triggering attacks. Community-based twin studies estimate the heritability of asthma to lie between 36% and over 60%, though heritability does not have a straightforward interpretation. Family studies suggest that the risk of all the atopic diseases is increased by the presence of any of them in the family, but that the individual diseases themselves also run in families. This and the finding that atopy is not more common in the families of those with asthma (Sibbald *et al.*, 1980) suggest that there may be separate genetic factors influencing atopy and asthma.

An important stimulus was given to the study of the genetics of atopy by the discovery of IgE in the 1960s. Early studies of rodents suggested the presence of two important genes: one regulating the overall response to antigen and linked to the major histocompatability complex (MHC) genes, a so-called immune response gene (Ir); the other a gene regulating the basal level of IgE. Much of the epidemiological research on the genetics of asthma since the early 1970s has been linked to these two findings.

Control of immunoglobulin E

There is consistent evidence from twin studies, family studies and animal experiments that the level of serum IgE is under genetic control. It has been much more difficult to establish the mode of inheritance of this control mechanism. Studies have suggested dominant, codominant, recessive and polygenic transmission. There are a number of significant obstacles to progress in this field, including the poor definition of the abnormal phenotype, the wide overlap in serum IgE between normal and diseased, the high environmental contribution to serum IgE levels and the impossibility of establishing basal levels in human studies.

Studies using a broader definition of allergy, that is, a high total serum IgE, or a positive specific IgE to a common inhalant allergen or a positive skin test to a common inhalant allergen, initially established linkage to a marker on the long arm of chromosome 11 (Cookson and Hopkin, 1988). The gene near this point is dominant for the allergic response.

Response to specific allergens

Research on the skin response to highly purified low molecular weight allergens suggests that response to these, especially in those who have low total serum IgE levels, is associated with specific human leucocyte antigen (HLA) phenotypes. The most extensively studied allergen is the ragweed allergen Ra5. Sensitivity to this allergen is closely associated to the HLA-Dw2 phenotype. Responses to rye grass allergens have also been studied, though less extensively. These have been associated with HLA-DR2. The proliferative response of leucocytes to artificial low molecular weight polypeptides is also linked within pedigrees to the inheritance of extended HLA haplotypes, suggesting linkage of these specific responses to a gene near to the HLA genes on chromosome 6. The practical impact of these findings is unclear as most of the associations are to small polypeptides. As most responses to allergens involve several of these, restriction of the ability to raise antibody to any one of them may not be critical. Nevertheless, Tovey et al. (1998) have found evidence for limited inheritance of allergen-specific sensitivity measured by skin tests.

In addition to those associations already cited above, a weak association has been noted between HLA-A1 and -B8 and asthma associated with nasal polyps. Caraballo and Hernandez (1990) found no association between intrinsic asthma and HLA phenotype.

Other genetically controlled mechanisms

Relatively small family studies originally suggested that wheeziness might be inherited independently of atopy (Sibbald et al., 1980), and this has also been shown for the airway response to cholinergic agents. The increased airway response in relatives of asthmatics is independent of atopy and a history of smoking. Although this is evidence for an independent genetic transmission of hyperresponsiveness to these agents, it has not so far been possible to show a specific Mendelian pattern of inheritance.

More recently changes in genetic technology have led to an increased use of whole genome scans to establish possible linkage with different asthma phenotypes (The Collaborative Study on the Genetics of Asthma (CSGA), 1997; Daniels et al., 1996). These have found associations with an area on chromosome 5q previously linked to bronchial hyperreactivity in two earlier linkage studies (Marsh et al., 1994; Postma et al., 1995) which contains candidate genes including those for interleukins 3, 4, 5, 9, 13, granulocyte-macrophage colony-stimulating factor, the β_2-adrenoceptor and the lymphocyte glucocorticoid receptor. Several authors have linked specific mutations of the β_2-adrenoceptor gene with particular asthma phenotypes. Other linkages that have been noted in some populations have been with chromosome 6p, 11q, 12q, 13 and 14q. All of these areas have potential candidate genes but the consistency among studies is disappointing.

ENVIRONMENTAL INFLUENCES

Atopy

EXPOSURE TO ALLERGENS

An atopic response to an allergen depends not only on exposure to the allergen but also on the dose. For instance, abnormal levels of specific IgE against mite antigens are rare when the environmental exposure is less than 2 pg antigen per gram of dust but increasingly common thereafter (Lau et al., 1989). Skin sensitivity to mite allergen is also less common in areas such as the French Alps where mite populations are low and levels of specific IgE against mite antigens fall when children are taken to areas with low mite populations. On the other hand, there are groups such as farmers who have evidently high exposure to allergens who do not have a high prevalence of sensitization (Braun-Fahrlander et al., 1999) and there is evidence that though exposure to allergen is necessary, it is not the rate limiting factor in the development of sensitization. First, where increases in sensitization have been noted, these are to all allergens tested, not to individual allergens to which exposure might have increased (Gassner, 1992; Nakagomi et al., 1994). Second, though sensitization to allergens varies greatly between different areas, this does not seem to be much influenced by allergens that are locally important (Burney *et al.*, 1997). Finally, though exposure to allergen is quantitatively linked to the likelihood of sensitization to dust mite allergens, this is only the case for those who are already sensitized to other allergens (Kuehr *et al.*, 1994).

EARLY EXPOSURE TO ALLERGEN

It has been suggested that the timing of allergen exposure is important as well as the dose. In particular, it has been suggested that exposure around the time of birth may be important in stimulating a life-long sensitivity to an allergen. The major part of the evidence for this comes from studies of month of birth in people with known atopy to seasonal allergens.

These studies have had variable results, some finding associations and others not, and the associations that have been found have not always favoured the same months. In general, mite-allergic subjects have been found to be more likely to be born in the latter part of the year (Warner and Price, 1978; Businco *et al.*, 1988), though mite allergen is not generally a seasonal exposure in temperate climates.

Studies of pollen-allergic people have been less consistent. Businco *et al.* (1988) found an excess of grass-sensitive people born in March–May in central Italy, and Rugtveit (1990) found an excess of grass-sensitive people born between March and August in Norway, but no increase in birch-sensitive people in those born between January and June. Finnish studies have shown that people allergic to birch pollen are more likely to be born between February and April and grass- and mugwort-sensitive individuals are more likely to be born in April–May, and have also suggested that sensitization was more likely to occur in years with high pollen counts. However, Reed and Corvallis (1958), and many other authors since, have shown no seasonal preference for month of birth in pollen-allergic people.

An earlier Finnish study showed an excess of grass-allergic people born in March–June, but only among boys, and no seasonal differences in the births of birch-, mugwort-, or other pollen-allergic groups. Pearson *et al.* (1977) found an excess of pollen-sensitive people born in December–January but only after excluding either females or those with perennial as well as seasonal symptoms. Suoniemi *et al.* (1981) also found an excess of pollen-sensitive patients born in December-May but again the effect was confined to boys. Carosso *et al.* (1986) found an excess of grass-sensitive persons born in March–June in northern Italy, but not in the south, the difference between regions being statistically significant. Aberg *et al.* (1989) found no association between atopic history and month of birth in 18-year-old Swedish conscripts born in 1953. For those born in 1963 he found an excess of rhinitic patients born in May–June but this excess was at least as great in the non-atopic as in the atopic rhinitics. There are important differences between all these studies including the age of the individuals and their country of residence.

A seasonal pattern in the month of birth has also been shown for children admitted to hospital with asthma in England. The month of birth of children most likely to be admitted to hospital with asthma coincides with the month of birth of children admitted with bronchiolitis (Strachan *et al.*, 1994). The significance of this is unclear.

Other investigators have tested the association between early exposure to perennial allergens and current sensitivity to them, though some of these workers have not paid adequate attention to the later exposure to the same allergens, clearly an important potential confounder. Even during the first year of life, Burr *et al.* (1989) noted an association between a history of prolonged colds and the concentration of the mite allergen *Der p 1* in the homes of these infants, though this association was no longer significant after adjusting for the number of siblings and the number of weeks for which the children were breast-fed. Sporik *et al.* (1990) showed that the age of onset of symptoms of asthma was directly related to the level of mite allergen in the homes of the children, those with high exposure having an earlier onset of symptoms. They also reported an almost fivefold higher prevalence of asthma at age 11 years in those children who had been exposed to more than 10 pg of *Der p 1* per gram of dust at age 1 year. These results are not, however, adjusted for current levels of exposure, which may be closely related to levels at the time of birth if the children have not moved house.

Suoniemi *et al.* (1981) found a strong association between sensitivity to cats and having had a cat in the home during the first 6 months of life, but no similar association for dogs. Rugtveit (1990) failed to show an association between skin sensitivity and cat or dog ownership during the first 6 months of life in 8-year-old asthmatic children. Since then most of the evidence has suggested that ownership of pets in early childhood, particularly dogs, reduces the risk of sensitization to cats and other allergens (Svanes *et al.*, 1999). The explanation for this may be related less to exposure to the allergen than to other exposures related to pet keeping.

Migrant studies suggest that sensitization to local allergens occurs fairly rapidly in migrants coming from areas with relatively low prevalence of sensitization (Leung *et al.*, 1994). This suggests that early exposure may not be a rate limiting factor in the development of allergy.

INFANT FEEDING

There is little consensus on the effects of infant feeding on the incidence of atopy, but some studies have suggested a protective effect from breast-feeding and allergen avoidance. A randomized trial of breast milk in premature neonates (Lucas *et al.*, 1990) has shown a reduction in atopic disease in early life but only among those with a family history of atopic disease. Zeiger *et al.* (1989) found that a rigid regime of allergen avoidance by both mother and baby did reduce food-associated allergy during infancy and up to 24 months of age. Savilahti *et al.* (1987), by way of contrast, studying older children, showed a trend towards more atopic disease in those breast-fed for longest, particularly among those with no family history of atopy.

SMOKING

Since 1980 many reports have shown an increased serum level of IgE in smokers (Gerrard *et al.*, 1980). This increase is most marked in moderate smokers and in some studies does not persist in ex-smokers. Although Taylor *et al.* (1985) found both higher levels of IgE and a more prevalent response to skin-prick tests in ex-smokers, this could be because atopic subjects are more likely to give up smoking. They also found higher basophil counts and a trend towards higher eosinophil counts in smokers. There is considerable evidence that workers who smoke are more likely to be sensitized to occupational allergens, though not to common inhalant allergens (Zetterstrom and Johansson, 1981).

On the other hand, there are now data suggesting that smoking may reduce the probability of sensitization to common allergens, though this is not entirely consistent across all allergens (Omebans *et al.*, 1994). Most of these data are from cross-sectional studies and could be interpreted as a reluctance for atopic subjects to take up smoking, but there is some evidence from prospective studies indicating that smokers are also less likely to develop new sensitizations (Barbee *et al.*, 1987).

AIR POLLUTION

Although there are some animal experiments suggesting that specific pollutants can increase the probability of sensitization to allergen, there is relatively little epidemiological evidence that this is an important mechanism. Particulates and diesel exhaust particularly have been shown to enhance IgE production in mice.

A few small ecological studies suggest that higher levels of air pollution are associated with increased levels of sensitization. However, studies comparing Eastern Europe with Western Europe which had lower levels of particulates showed that there was a lower prevalence of atopy in the East (von Mutius *et al.*, 1994), and areas with relatively low levels of pollution such as New Zealand have high levels of sensitization.

INFECTIONS AND INFESTATIONS

Interest in a possible association between infection and allergy extends back to the beginning of the century but attention has recently been focused on the possibility that viruses and bacteria may promote or suppress an IgE response. Experimental studies in animals show that pertussis vaccine can potentiate IgE responses in animals, though there is no evidence that infection with *Bordetella pertussis* leads to persistent respiratory disease (Johnston *et al.*, 1983). Almost 70% of infants respond to infection by respiratory syncytial virus (RSV) with cell-bound IgE on days 1–2 of the infection. However, those with clinical bronchiolitis have a more persistent IgE response than those who develop upper respiratory symptoms only or pneumonia (Welliver *et al.*, 1980), and a persistent IgE response over 5 weeks is three times as likely in those with a personal or family history of wheeze. This suggests that an IgE response to RSV is normal and that some other factors, possibly genetic, are needed to explain persistent IgE and severe airway disease.

More recently, attention has been focused on the potentially protective effect of infections, particularly infections in early life. The hypothesis that infections might be protective was a potential explanation for the association between atopy, particularly hay fever, and small families (Strachan, 1989). It has been difficult to find evidence to support this hypothesis based on common infections of childhood and infections of infancy. However, there is some evidence for the hypothesis from a study in West Africa which showed lower levels of sensitization to house dust mite in those who had been infected in one of the last serious outbreaks of measles in West Africa (Shaheen *et al.*, 1996), and a study of Italian recruits which found an inverse association between sensitization to allergens and evidence of Hepatitis A infection (Matricardi *et al.*, 1998). A recent study from Germany has shown that early placement in nursery education is protective for children from small families, but not for children from larger families, a finding that is also compatible with the original hypothesis (Kramer *et al.*, 1999).

The relation of parasites to asthma has variously been claimed to be causative and protective. The hypothesis that parasitic infection might produce a 'blocking' antibody and so prevent a response to common inhalant allergens was given some support by *in vitro* studies. Stanworth *et al.* inhibited the Prausnitz–Kustner reaction by 'blocking' mast cells with myeloma protein and Godfrey and Gradidge (1976) were similarly able to block the passive sensitization of human lung fragments to IgE against grass pollen by first exposing them to serum from West African patients with high levels of IgE. The epidemiological evidence that parasitic infestation prevents atopic sensitization is weak, being for the most part from ecological studies relying on small and selected populations. However, one experimental study has shown that treatment of patients with antihelminthics may worsen asthma (Lynch *et al.*, 1993).

Asthma and airway hyperresponsiveness

EXPOSURE TO ALLERGEN

Exposure of sensitized people to allergen increases bronchial hyperresponsiveness, as shown by experimental studies with allergen challenge. This increase is related to the occurrence of a late asthmatic response.

An increase in airway reactivity has been reported during the grass pollen season, though contradictory results have been reported with respect to the ragweed season, some reporting an increase in reactivity and others not. Britton *et al.* (1988) noted an increase in reactivity in the south of England between March and June and a further increase in reactivity in September, but failed to show any relation between skin sensitivity to grass pollen and the increased responsiveness in June. The increased responsiveness in September was associated with greater skin sensitivity to three common inhalant allergens but no individual allergen appeared to be particularly important. In contrast, Pollart *et al.* (1988) studying patients attending a medical centre in the USA with asthma during the spring 'epidemic', found a higher prevalence of specific IgE to ryegrass antigen than in serum taken from controls. There was no significant increase in specific IgE to three indoor allergens.

There is also evidence for an association between hyperresponsiveness or severe asthma and exposure to indoor allergens (Rosenstreich *et al.*, 1997). Pollart *et al.* (1989) have also shown high specific IgE levels (> 200 RAST units) to be strongly associated with emergency room visits with asthma, and that this association is stronger for IgE against the indoor allergens dust mite, cat and cockroach, than for grass and ragweed. The hypothesis that dust mites might be particularly important in determining the prevalence of airway disease was tested in Australia (Britton *et al.*, 1986). Although sensitivity to mites was much greater in coastal New South Wales than in the dry inland areas where mite counts are low, clinical asthma was more common inland, possibly because of a greater prevalence of sensitivity to pollens and moulds. When those sensitive to mite allergens were studied, hyperreactivity was greater in those with the greatest exposure to mite allergens.

SMOKING

Smoking has been associated with airway hyperresponsiveness in a number of population surveys (Burney *et al.*, 1987) as well as in many clinical studies. The association is stronger in older people or in those with a greater lifetime exposure to cigarettes which is strongly correlated with age in smokers. There is also a strong relation between baseline lung function and airway responsiveness in smokers, and one prospective study (Lim *et al.*, 1988) has shown that continued decline in lung function over time in smokers is associated with increasing responsiveness, while the reduced rate of decline in forced expiratory volume in 1 second (FEV_1) in those who stop smoking is associated with a constant response to histamine over time. This hyperresponsiveness does not reverse on quitting smoking, suggesting that the origin of the hyperresponsiveness in smokers is in the geometrical changes in the airway rather than in some more transitory mechanism such as inflammation. However, this may not be the whole explanation. There may be an element of hyperresponsiveness associated with smoking that is independent of these structural changes and baseline lung function

Smoking causes temporary increase in airway responsiveness in normal people. Passive smoking increases airway responsiveness in adults with asthma and people with asthma who give up smoking have been shown to experience a fall in airway responsiveness. However, there is evidence that smoking among adults does not lead to any increased risk of developing asthma (Vesterinen *et al.*, 1988).

Murray and Morrison (1986) reported more airway responsiveness in the children of smoking parents, but other studies have been more equivocal. Some have found no association and others have found no overall association but some association in selected subgroups. Strachan *et al.* (1990) found no association between airway response to exercise in 7-year-old children and salivary cotinine.

Several studies have reported a higher prevalence of asthma or wheeze in the children of smoking parents, though some of these have reported inconsistent results for the two sexes and Strachan *et al.* (1990) found no association between either wheeze or night-time cough and salivary cotinine levels in 7-year-olds. Asthmatic children from families who smoke are reported to require an increased use of emergency rooms for the management of asthma (Evans *et al.*, 1987), though this could be related to unresolved confounding by other social factors.

Smoking is certainly the single most important preventable cause of respiratory ill health, but its role in the aetiology of asthma is still unclear. It is very likely that it causes considerable annoyance to the majority of asthmatics, it may well cause a temporary increase in airway responsiveness, it is unlikely that it causes asthma. The effects on the airway are likely to be confounded by the effects of smoking on sensitization (*see* p. 205 above).

AIR POLLUTION

Although there is a strong reason *a priori* to believe that air pollution could play an important role in asthma, it has been difficult to assemble convincing evidence that this role is of primary significance. Hyde Salter, who was aware of the importance of 'respirable irritants' in bringing on attacks of asthma, wrote nevertheless that, 'it is, one may almost say, a *law* of asthma for it to be better in the air of great cities' (Salter, 1870). In this he distinguished clearly between asthma and bronchitis, which he recognized was strongly affected by air pollution.

Air pollution is a loose term that refers to many different exposures. These exposures are themselves associated with other climatic and social factors that may in turn affect asthma. Air pollution has changed in character from a mixture of particles and sulphur dioxide predominantly derived from coal burning, to a mixture of particles and nitrogen dioxide derived from road traffic. Ozone is a secondary pollutant formed from nitrogen dioxide in sunlight.

Studies that have compared the prevalence of asthma in areas with different levels of pollution, taken together, provide no strong evidence that pollutant levels are a strong determinant of asthma (Department of Health, 1995b). The exception to this is a series of studies that have suggested an association between living close to main roads with a heavy density of traffic and asthma prevalence, though even here the evidence has been mixed. Asthma prevalence has been increasing at a time that pollution associated with coal burning has been declining and at a time that traffic density has been increasing. Even so, some of the highest prevalences of asthma are in areas such as New Zealand that do not have high levels of any pollutants. Air pollution is unlikely to be the main driving force behind the recent increase in prevalence.

A few exceptional episodes of air pollution where levels of pollutants reached very high levels provide some evidence on the acute effects of air pollution on asthma. These have generally been associated with increased overall mortality rates, but in the London smog of 1952, Fry (1953) noted that the younger asthmatics in his practice were not affected. This is consistent with observations on hospitalization rates during a more recent smog episode in the Ruhr in 1985 (Wichmann *et al.*, 1989). Hospitalizations with asthma did not increase at the time of this episode and in fact declined by an estimated 14% in the polluted area compared to a 4% decline in the control area. Two episodes occurring in the Meuse valley in 1930 and Donora, Pennsylvania, in 1948 were noted specifically to affect people with asthma, but post-mortem findings showed a high prevalence of acute cardiac failure and this may have confused the clinical picture.

Other investigations of acute effects have either considered individuals (panel studies) or have examined routine data on deaths, admissions to hospital or consultation rates at times of changing pollution levels. Although both of these types of study have shown evidence for deteriorations in asthma control when pollution levels are high the effects have been small and inconsistent. There is an additional difficulty in assessing the results of such studies in that there is considerable latitude given in most of them in the number of pollutants examined and the number of time 'lags' allowed between the change in pollution levels and the effects on asthma. The largest of the panel studies so far has been unable to show any effect of changing particle levels on children with asthma (Roemer *et al.*, 1998).

One potential confounder in all these studies of acute effects in patients with asthma is the presence of allergen in air. Allergen is a potent trigger of asthma and when there are weather conditions that trap air pollutants, these will trap any allergen present also. The major outbreaks of asthma that occurred in Barcelona caused by unloading of soya bean in the harbour during such conditions (Anto *et al.*, 1989) were initially attributed to increases in nitrogen dioxide in the air (Ussetti *et al.*, 1983).

There is plenty of positive evidence that allergens do cause such epidemics (Ordman, 1955), and that natural changes in the prevalence of fungal spores, one source of allergen, alter control of asthma and increase asthma mortality rates (Targonski *et al.*, 1995). In smaller quantities more unusual allergens can increase admission rates without causing epidemics (Soriano *et al.*, 1995). A recent Dutch study has suggested that only those who are both atopic and hyperresponsive react to air pollution changes (Boezen *et al.*, 1999), a finding that would be compatible with the hypothesis that much of this effect is due to allergen.

INFECTION

Viral infections have been shown to cause temporary increases in the bronchial response to citric acid and histamine. Such changes have been shown in normal adults following 'colds' (Empey *et al.*, 1976), and infections with respiratory syncytial virus, and influenza A. Selected adults with allergic rhinitis and low neutralizing antibody against rhinovirus show similar changes following experimental rhinovirus infections (Lemanske *et al.*, 1989). Airway responsiveness increases following immunization with live vaccine but not generally after the use of killed vaccines, though there are notable exceptions.

Clinical exacerbations of respiratory disease are commonly associated with viral infections in children and have been particularly linked with rhinovirus and parainfluenza virus infections. Storr and Lenney (1989) have shown that asthma admissions in schoolchildren occur in clusters which coincide with school terms and they have suggested that this is likely to be due to a high proportion of the attacks being due to viral infections. Improved virological techniques have demonstrated the importance of viral infections as a cause of asthma exacerbations in both children and adults. Duff (1993) has suggested that atopic children are more susceptible to the respiratory effects of viral infections.

Several authors have suggested that viral infections may cause more permanent wheeze. The principal model for this is respiratory syncytial virus infection in children (Pullan and Hey, 1982). Most of the studies investigating this do not have information on lung function or hyperresponsiveness prior to the infection. The causal nature of any relation between infection and subsequent hyperresponsiveness is therefore open to question. Moreover, children who have greater airway obstruction in the neonatal period are more likely to have clinical episodes of wheeze in the first year of life (Martinez *et al.*, 1988). This suggests that reactivity and clinical illness may both be caused by a prior abnormality in the airway.

Diet

FOOD INTOLERANCE AND SENSITIVITY

Diet was recognized early on to be a possible contributory factor in asthma. In the nineteenth century, Salter (1870) classified the provoking causes of asthma under three headings: respired irritants, alimentary irritants, and irritants immediately affecting the nervous system. By the early twentieth century, theories that asthma might be triggered by an anaphylactic reaction to food or the ingestion of pharmacologically-active substances, had already been advanced and dietary restriction was part of the standard advice to patients. However, in the late 1940s it was increasingly recognized that restrictive diets might do harm and a more critical appraisal of reported adverse reactions to food was introduced with the double-blind challenge (Loveless, 1950). This in turn may lead to over-conservative estimates of the prevalence of food sensitivity if response is measured as change in lung function rather than as the change in airway response to histamine.

Many different forms of food and drink have been implicated by patients as triggers for asthmatic attacks, though convincing scientific evidence that the foods are indeed the cause of attacks is more difficult to establish. Reliable estimates of the prevalence of food intolerance are difficult to find, and there are even fewer estimates of food-induced asthma. Young et al. (1987) found that 13% of adults complained of food-associated symptoms if those intolerant to aspirin were excluded. However, only 1.7% of them reported asthmatic symptoms following food and only between 1 and 23 per 10 000 were estimated to respond to double-blind challenge with food additives. Wilson (1985) has, however, suggested that the prevalence may well be underestimated and that higher levels of food-induced asthma may be found particularly in Asian children in Britain.

INFANT FEEDING

Burr et al. (1989) re-analysed data from a trial in which soy milk formula had been substituted for cow's milk, a substitution that had no effect on either eczema or wheeze. They noted that breast-feeding on any occasion, regardless of duration, was associated with half the incidence of wheeze during infancy, an association that persisted after adjustment for a wide selection of variables.

Most studies have, however, suggested that infant feeding may be less critical in asthma. Zeiger et al. (1989), for instance, were able to reduce food-associated atopic dermatitis, urticaria and gastrointestinal disease by strict food allergen avoidance in mothers and infants, but these measures had no influence on rhinitis or asthma, or on sensitization to inhalant allergens. Neither of the two large British cohorts showed any association between breast-feeding and wheeze or asthma (Taylor et al., 1983; Anderson et al., 1986). In the Melbourne cohort it has even been suggested that those with the worst asthma had been breast-fed for the longest (Martin et al., 1981).

OVERALL NUTRITION

There are few studies of the effects of overall nutrition on asthma but children with protein calorie malnutrition have a reduced skin sensitivity and, at an ecological level, children in Africa from rural areas with low levels of bronchial response to exercise are smaller and lighter than those from urban areas where a bronchial response to exercise is more common (Keeley and Gallivan, 1991). Such ecological data are hard to interpret but individual studies have also shown an association between fatness and respiratory symptoms or asthma (Somerville et al., 1984), particularly in women (Shaheen et al., 1999). Associations have also been shown between fatness and skin sensitivity (Huang et al., 1999), though not convincingly with hay fever and eczema (Shaheen et al., 1999).

DIETARY LIPID AND ASTHMA

Cod liver oil was widely recommended early on for the treatment of asthma. Martin (1898) attributed its effect on the general improvement of the patients' health, and held a strongly favourable view: 'The improvement if the oil can be taken is sometimes very marked, rendering possible the diminution, or even cessation of the inhalations which the patient considered his sheet-anchor'. Much later, the more specific hypothesis that fish oil might block the formation of lipid mediators led to a number of studies on this as a form of treatment. The studies did show a reduction in lipid mediators and a blunting of the late allergic response but little effect on clinical asthma. Aspirin-sensitive asthmatics appeared to deteriorate on this diet. Recent epidemiological studies have renewed interest in this area (Hodge *et al.*, 1996), though they have provided mixed results (Troisi *et al.*, 1995; Fluge *et al.*, 1998).

VITAMINS AND TRACE ELEMENTS

Many of the vitamins have been examined for a possible role in either the aetiology or management of asthma.

Vitamin B$_6$

Theophylline reduces pyridoxal-5-phosphate (PLP) levels but not pyridoxal levels or pyridoxic acid excretion in normal volunteers. It has been suggested that the drug may therefore inhibit the enzyme pyridoxal kinase. This may explain why studies in the USA, where theophyllines are a common mode of treatment, have shown evidence of vitamin B$_6$ deficiency in asthma whereas a study from Britain did not (Hall *et al.*, 1981).

Ascorbic acid

Ascorbic acid was first tried for asthma in Europe in the 1930s but was found to have little effect. There are several studies, however, showing reduced plasma levels (Akinkugbe and Ette, 1987) or reduced intake (Soutar *et al.*, 1997) of vitamin C in asthmatics as compared with controls. More recent trials of vitamin C in asthma have shown variable results. Neither Kreisman *et al.* (1977) nor Malo *et al.* (1986) were able to show an effect on either lung function or the response to histamine in asthmatics, but others have reported reductions in the number and severity of attacks (Anah *et al.*, 1980), the response to exercise (Schachter and Schlesinger, 1982), and the response to methacholine (Mohsenin *et al.*, 1983) following ascorbic acid.

Nicotinic acid

Early uncontrolled studies suggested that nicitonic acid might improve asthma (Melton, 1943). Although animal studies suggest this may be the case (Bekier and Czerwinska, 1973), there are no epidemiological assessments of whether this finding is relevant to the distribution and severity of the disease.

Selenium

Although an earlier study showed no difference in blood selenium levels and rather higher levels of whole blood glutathione peroxidase in asthmatic compared to healthy children (Ward *et al.*, 1984), several subsequent studies have suggested that selenium and/or glutathione peroxidase levels may be reduced in patients with asthma (Flatt *et al.*, 1990).

Electrolytes and asthma

Early interest in the role of electrolytes in asthma was based on Ringer's studies of the effects of different electrolyte solutions on spontaneous contractions, and a residual interest in hydrotherapy in Europe.

Magnesium

Cross-sectional studies suggest that asthma is associated with a low intake of magnesium (Britton *et al.*, 1994; Soutar *et al.*, 1997) and asthmatic patients have low levels of intracellular magnesium (Emelyanov *et al.*, 1999). However, although magnesium has been used since early in the century as a bronchodilator in patients with asthma, experimental studies using magnesium have been disappointing (Hill *et al.*, 1997).

Sodium

Dietary sodium, as estimated from 24-hour urinary excretion, has been shown to relate to the bronchial response to histamine in adult men; the higher the dietary sodium, the greater the response to histamine (Burney *et al.*, 1986). Subsequent cross-sectional studies have had mixed results and have not given overall support to this finding, though intervention studies (Carey *et al.*, 1989) have shown a change in hyperresponsiveness in response to experimental changes in dietary sodium in men though not in women (Burney *et al.*, 1986). An ecological study of asthma mortality in England and Wales (Burney, 1987) showed that purchases of table salt in the different regions related well to asthma mortality for men and children, but not for women. In this respect the analysis was consistent with experimental evidence and provided a possible explanation for the very different regional distribution of asthma deaths among women compared with those among men and children. The mechanism is unknown, though bronchial hyperresponsiveness has been associated with a serum factor that increases sodium movement into cells (Tribe *et al.*, 1994).

NATURAL HISTORY

Atopy

Cross-sectional surveys of atopic markers such as serum IgE and skin tests show an increase in the prevalence of atopy that continues into early adult life but which is followed by a lower prevalence in older age groups. Prospective studies (Gerritsen *et al.*, 1990) confirm the general increase in sensitization to allergens that occurs between childhood and early adult life, but the interpretation of the lower prevalence in older people is more controversial. The lower prevalence in older age groups seen in cross-sectional data could be due to an ageing effect, or to lower rates of sensitization in people born in the more distant past. Disentangling these two possibilities requires longitudinal data and such data are uncommon in adults. Barbee *et al.* (1987) surveyed the population of Tucson twice, eight years apart, using the same allergens in the same concentrations from the same supplier and showed that the prevalence of positive responses was higher in the second survey in all age groups and in people who had moved to Tucson in the previous 10 years. Though it is difficult to be sure precisely how closely the testing procedures compared during the two surveys these results do not support the view of a rapid decline in the prevalence of skin sensitivity with age and caution against a simple interpretation of results from cross-sectional surveys.

Prognosis of asthma in children

About one-quarter of all children wheeze at some time in their lives with a peak incidence in the second year of life. However, relatively few persist with severe respiratory problems. In the National Child Development Study, a complete cohort of children born in Great Britain in one week of March 1958 have been followed to the age of 16 years (Anderson *et al.*, 1986). At the age of 7, 8.3% of these children were said to have had an episode of asthma or wheeze in the previous 12 months. By the age of 11 this had fallen to 4.7% and by 16 it had fallen to 3.5%. In Australia, Peat *et al.* (1989) have followed a group of schoolchildren from age 8–10 to age

12–14. At age 8–10, 16.1% had an 'abnormal' response to inhaled histamine defined as a greater than 20% fall in FEV_1 in response to a dose of 7.8 μmol or less. Two years later only 8.8% were 'abnormal' and by age 12–14 years 6.3% were abnormal. Severe disease and signs of atopy, which are themselves associated with each other, are both associated with persistence of wheeze and bronchial hyperresponsiveness into later childhood. Poor lung function at an early age also carries a relatively poor prognosis, and low lung function and bronchial hyperresponsiveness in childhood are predictive of low lung function and bronchial hyperresponsiveness in early adult life (Gerritsen et al., 1989). However, although symptomatic children have low lung function, their lung growth may be normal (Borsboom et al., 1993).

There is disagreement as to whether an early onset of wheeze predicts a poor prognosis, a good prognosis or has no influence on prognosis by itself, although the number of attacks in infancy may still be important. Some have found that pneumonia before the age of 7 years is associated with a more persistent wheeze, though others (van Weel et al., 1987) have been unable to demonstrate any association between respiratory infections and asthma or chronic bronchitis at age 7 years.

Children who cough in early childhood have three times the risk of developing persistent wheeze than those who are asymptomatic, but they are also twice as likely to have a complete remission of their symptoms compared with children who wheeze (Giles et al., 1984). Children whose wheeze is associated with croup have a good prognosis with only 10% having a persistent problem at age 10, approximately half the prevalence in those with a non-specific diagnosis or a diagnosis of bronchitis. The worst prognosis is in those with a diagnosis of asthma, of whom about 50% are still wheezing at age 10 (Park et al., 1986).

Of those who have persistent symptoms in childhood only about 20% are symptom-free in early adult life (Martin et al., 1980). By the age of 14 years current symptoms have become a fairly accurate guide to the future; 68% of those with frequent wheezing at that age in the Melbourne cohort were still suffering asthma at 28 years (Kelly et al., 1987).

Prognosis of asthma in adults

There is controversy over whether uncomplicated asthma leads to a long-term decline in lung function with age. Burrows et al. (1987) studied a selected group aged 40–74 years old who were found to have poor lung function in a population survey. Those who had a diagnosis of asthma and who had either positive skin tests to allergens or a history of never smoking had an average loss of FEV_1 of 5 mL/year over the next 10 years. By contrast, those who had never been diagnosed as having asthma who had negative skin tests for allergies and who had a history of smoking had an average loss of lung function of 70 mL/year. An intermediate group had a loss of lung function of 20 mL/year. Some other studies support this finding (Annesi et al., 1987; Suppli Ulrik and Lange, 1994), though Annesi et al. did report an increased decline in lung function among smokers with either allergic- or cold air-induced rhinitis and both Peat (1987), and Schachter and colleagues (1984) found representative samples of asthmatic patients had an accelerated decline in lung function. Though many authors have reported an association between bronchial hyperresponsiveness and a rapid decline in lung function, this finding is difficult to interpret as hyperresponsiveness may itself simply reflect increased airflow obstruction (Lim et al., 1988).

Population-based studies demonstrate that asthma does carry an increased risk of death (Markowe et al., 1987). Under the age of 45 the excess risk in English patients with asthma is small but in those aged 55–59 years those with asthma have twice the risk of death compared to controls matched for age, sex and general practice (Markowe et al., 1987). There is some debate as to whether allergic diseases may confer protection against malignant disease. Markowe *et al.* (1987) found this to be the case only in the younger age groups, and only clearly so below the age of 45 years.

Mortality

COLLECTION OF MORTALITY DATA

Studies that have compared the cause of death as recorded on the death certificate with the opinion of experts asked to review the evidence have concluded that asthma is accurately recorded at least in the younger age groups (British Thoracic Association, 1984). However, these studies were undertaken in England and New Zealand, both of which have relatively high recorded asthma mortality rates. A study that had asked representative samples of doctors in eight European countries to fill in death certificates for 10 case histories, including two with asthma-like symptoms, showed that there were significant differences in certification practice between countries and that these differences related to the recorded mortality rates for asthma for the different countries (Burney, 1989). The conclusion that some countries under-report deaths from asthma even in young people is supported by the observations of Riou and Barriot (1990) in France. Mortality rates estimated from their study of asthmatics who died following calls to the emergency services in Paris were twice as high as the recorded national asthma mortality rates under the age of 55 years.

GEOGRAPHICAL VARIATIONS IN MORTALITY

Recorded asthma mortality varies considerably between countries (Holland, 1988), but it is difficult to interpret these figures in the light of the differences noted in the practice of certification. On the other hand, there remain substantial within-country differences in mortality rates that are significantly greater than would be expected by chance in England and Wales, France, Belgium and Germany (Holland, 1988). These within-country differences are unlikely to be due to the same biases. In studies of geographical variation in asthma mortality, these within-country differences may be more informative. In the USA, Weiss and Wagener (1990) have shown particularly high mortality from asthma in two poor inner-city areas. This coincides with findings from other countries of asthma being concentrated in deprived areas (Duran-Tauleria and Rona, 1999; Salmond *et al.*, 1999).

TRENDS IN MORTALITY

Time trends in mortality can also be affected by changes in the clinical definition of diseases, by changes in health care that alter the information that doctors have about their patients and by the methods used to code the deaths. The most fully investigated part of this process is the change that occurs when the method of coding is changed. Whenever the International Classification of Disease (ICD) has been revised in recent years, national coding centres have undertaken 'bridge-code' exercises in which a sample of deaths have been coded both by the old and the new codes and the differences analysed. Neither these exercises nor analysis of trends (Burney, 1986) have suggested that the change from ICD-8 to ICD-9 had much effect on the recorded asthma mortality rates for younger patients, though it did have a more profound effect on recorded rates in older subjects.

Transference from one diagnostic group to another at times other than the change in the ICD is much more difficult to assess. A declining recorded mortality rate in related diagnostic groups such as bronchitis and pneumonia, at a time when asthma mortality rates are increasing, may suggest diagnostic transfer but it is hardly convincing by itself. To conclude that this is evidence for transference is to suppose that mortality from other conditions should not be declining, and given the general fall in mortality rates this seems to be a weak premise. It is difficult to decide whether these are the same deaths by a different name, or different deaths and any tentative conclusion is bound to rely on indirect evidence.

In England and Wales, asthma mortality has fallen in the last century, but in 5–34 year olds rates have been relatively stable or have risen slightly (Marks and Burney, 1998). Further analysis of the trends in the UK suggests that some of the increase may be due to mortality increasing from one generation to another rather than to an increase in mortality among all age groups at the same time (Burney, 1988). In the younger age groups there was a major increase in deaths from asthma in several countries in the 1960s. From the mid-1970s to the mid 1980s there was a further more limited increase, which was more marked among males and which has since resolved in England and Wales, though not in the USA. Increases were also noted in other countries including, most notably, New Zealand where the increase reached a peak in the late 1970s, and the USA. In the presence of an increasing prevalence of asthma it is difficult to estimate whether case fatality from asthma is falling, rising or remaining constant, though it could be argued on the indirect evidence that case fatality has been falling (Burney, 1988).

CAUSES OF DEATH

Environment

It is likely that the death of asthmatics may be associated with the same factors that exacerbate the disease, but there is little direct evidence for this. Targonski et al., (1995) demonstrated that mortality was higher on days of high mould spore counts and deaths have been associated with some other instances of allergen pollution such as the episodes of asthma in Barcelona associated with soy bean allergen (Anto et al., 1989). Whether indoor allergens are also important in this context is unknown. Rosenstreich et al. (1997) were able to demonstrate an association between exacerbations of asthma and high exposure to cockroach allergen in inner city America where mortality rates are also high.

Treatment

The earliest drugs to be consistently reported as dangerous in asthma were central nervous system depressants and antiinflammatory agents. Case reports of deaths from asthma mentioning these drugs date from as early as the 1930s, though the implication that these may be dangerous was not always recognized. Benson and Perlman (1948) were the first to report an increased mortality in those using an inhaled adrenergic agent. Of 2236 cases of asthma treated by them in a decade, 648 had used adrenaline sprays and of these 48 (7.4%) had died. Among the other 1588 patients there had been only 22 deaths (1.4%). This amounts to more than a fivefold risk of death in those using the spray. The difficult question is whether there was selective use of sprays by those at greatest risk of death.

The increase in mortality from asthma that was noted in several countries in the 1960s was attributed early on to a change in management. Early enquiries into the circumstances of death seemed to implicate the use of bronchodilator aerosols. The increase in deaths began soon after the introduction of aerosols, and a high proportion (84%) of those who died of asthma had been taking aerosols. Furthermore, there were several case histories suggesting a particularly heavy use in the period before death. Inman and Adelstein (1969) were able to show that both the increase and the decrease in sales after June 1967, when the Committee on Safety of Medicines issued a warning to all doctors, coincided with changes in mortality rates in the UK and that sales of pressurized aerosols to each age group correlated well with the number of excess deaths in that age group. These observations were later extended to show a general trend of the same kind in six countries (Stolley and Schinnar, 1978), though the association was found only for the high dose isoprenaline aerosol, and this was not quite significant at the conventional 5% level of probability. However, the association did not seem to hold for Australia and the fall in mortality after 1967 was not as great as would have been expected if the increase in mortality was entirely due to the prescription of aerosols. Some of the weaknesses in the hypothesis have been reviewed by Lanes and Walker (1987) but alternative hypotheses seem to have even more difficulties and fewer data to support them.

In the 1980s, the hypothesis attracted renewed interest with the observation that asthma deaths in New Zealand were associated with the prescription of fenoterol, another β-agonist sold at a relatively high dose (Crane et al., 1989). The interpretation of this association depends on whether adequate account has been taken of differences in severity between the two patient groups, those who were on the drug and those who were not. As fenoterol was a new drug and was sold in higher doses it may have been prescribed more often to more severely ill patients. There is evidence that this did happen, though it is questioned whether it occurred within the group of hospitalized asthmatics studied, and therefore whether the selective prescribing affected the results of the case–control comparisons. A related problem has been the method of adjustment used in the studies to take account of any difference in severity between the cases who died and their controls. This relied on the treatment prescribed as a marker of the severity of the disease. This is at best an indirect measure and is itself confounded by the quality of the medical service provided to the patients. β-Agonists reduce serum potassium and it is hypothesized that this and other specific effects on the myocardium may lead to serious arrhythmias and so explain the deaths (Newhouse et al., 1996). Others have suggested that bronchodilators may themselves increase bronchial hyperresponsiveness (Sears et al., 1990). However, subsequent trials have cast doubt on the clinical importance of these effects (Drazen et al., 1996).

Poor treatment and undertreatment

From the early 1970s there have been several enquiries into the circumstances surrounding deaths from asthma. These were handicapped by the lack of any comparative information on those who had survived asthma attacks but they did document deviations from the currently recommended management of the condition. For the most part they reported a poor ability to recognize serious symptoms on the part of both patient and doctor and a general undertreatment, especially with steroids. Whether these noted defects in treatment were in fact responsible for the deaths is difficult to determine. Rea et al. (1986) compared patients dying of asthma with controls selected both from hospital records and from GP records and found that the severity of the asthma, poor medical care and psychosocial problems were all important in determining the outcome.

CURRENT QUESTIONS

Developments in genetics may add considerably to our ability to understand the mechanisms of asthma and these in turn may give further clues as to where to look in the environment for the large influences that this certainly has on the expression of the condition. Knowledge of gene products may also lead to further advances in treatment. However, it is unlikely that such knowledge can be used directly for the prevention of disease when the genes are as common as those involved in atopy and asthma.

Environmental allergen clearly has a major role in exacerbating asthma, but variation in the concentration of environmental allergen is not yet established as the critical factor in determining sensitization. Most environments are allergenic and man has lived at relative peace with potential allergens for thousands of years, and in some places evidently still does. There are important questions still to be asked about the possible role of other environmental factors in sensitization and the development of atopy.

There are also important questions relating to the development of asthma in atopic individuals. This area has been relatively neglected and has probably been influenced too greatly by rather naïve mechanistic models, particularly the notion that generic inflammation might cause asthma. The role of diet has been largely neglected, partly because diet therapy appeared redundant with the advent of specific therapy, and partly no doubt because of a reaction to the use of extreme and harmful diets in the 1930s.

Questions relating to mortality have been particularly difficult to resolve. Reliance on uncontrolled audits to provide answers to the question as to why people die of asthma is clearly unacceptable, though these still account for much of the quoted literature on this subject. Case–control studies have been a major advance on uncontrolled studies but still lack conviction in the absence of any credible independent markers for the severity of the disease. The development of such markers would provide a major advance in this area. Prospective studies would need to be large and would inevitably be expensive; they would only be justified by clear hypotheses.

REFERENCES

Aberg N. (1989) Asthma and allergic rhinitis in Swedish conscripts. *Clin Exp Allergy*, **19**(1), 59–63.

Akinkugbe FM, Ette SI. (1987) Role of zinc, copper, and ascorbic acid in some common clinical paediatric problems. *J Trop Pediatr*, **33**, 337–42.

American Thoracic Society. (1962) Chronic bronchitis, asthma and pulmonary emphysema: a statement by the committee on diagnostic standards and non-tuberculous respiratory disease. *Am Rev Respir Dis*, **85**, 762–8.

Anah CC, Jarike LN, Baig HA. (1980) High dose ascorbic acid in Nigerian asthmatics. *Trop Geogr Med*, **32**, 132–7.

Anderson HR, Bailey P, West S. (1980) Trends in the hospital care of acute childhood asthma. *BMJ*, **281**, 1191–4.

Anderson HR, Bland JM, Patel S, Peckham C. (1986) The national history of asthma in childhood. *J Epidemiol Community Health*, **40**, 121–9.

Annesi I, Neudirch F, Orvoen-Frija E, Oryszczyn MP, Korobaeff M, Kauffmann F. (1987) The relevance of hyperresponseiveness but not of atopy to FEV_1 decline. Preliminary results in a working population. *Bull Eur Physiopathol Respir*, **23**, 397–400.

Anon. (1959) Terminology, definitions, and classification of chronic pulmonary emphysema and related conditions: a report of the conclusions of a CIBA guest symposium. *Thorax*, **14**, 286–99.

Anto J, Sunyer J, Roderigo-Roisin R, Suarez-Cervera M, Vazquez L. (1989) Community outbreaks of asthma associated with inhalation of soybean dust. *N Engl J Med*, **320**, 1097–102.

Asher I, Keil U, Anderson HA, *et al*. (1995) International Study of Asthma and Allergies in Childhood (ISAAC): rationale and methods. *Eur Respir J*, **8**, 483–91.

Barbee RA, Kaltenborn W, Lebowitz MD, Burrows B. (1987) Longitudinal changes in allergen skin test reactivity in a community population sample. *J Allergy Clin Immunol*, **79**, 16–24.

Bekier E, Czerwinska U. (1973) The effect of nicotinamide on the experimental asthma in guinea pigs. *Acta Physiol Pol*, **24**, 887–9.

Benson RL, Perlman F. (1948) Clinical effects of epinephrine by inhalation. *J Allergy Clin Immunol*, **19**, 129–40.

Boezen HM, van der Zee SC, Postma DS, *et al*. (1999) Effects of ambient air pollution on upper and lower respiratory symptoms and peak expiratory flow in children. *Lancet*, **353**, 874–8.

Borsboom GJJM, van Pelt W, Quanjer PH. (1993) Pubertal growth curves of ventilatory function: relationship with childhood respiratory symptoms. *Am Rev Respir Dis*, **147**, 372–8.

Braun-Fahrlander C, Gassner M, Grize L, *et al*. (1999) Prevalence of hay fever and allergic sensitization in farmers' children and their peers living in the same rural community. *Clin Exp Allergy*, **29**, 28–34.

British Thoracic Association. (1984) Accuracy of death certificates in bronchial asthma. *Thorax*, **39**, 505–9.

Britton J, Chinn S, Burney P, Papacosta AO, Tattersfield A. (1988) Seasonal variation in bronchial reactivity in a community population. *J Allergy Clin Immunol*, **82**, 134–9.

Britton J, Pavord I, Richards K, *et al*. (1994) Dietary magnesium, lung function, wheezing, and airway hyperreactivity in a random adult population sample. *Lancet*, **344**, 357–62.

Britton WJ, Woolcock AJ, Peat JK, Sedgewick CJ, Lloyd DM, Leeder SR. (1986) Prevalence of bronchial hyperresponsiveness in children: the relationship between asthma and skin reactivity to allergens in two communities. *Int J Epidemiol*, **15**, 202–9.

Burney P. (1988) Asthma deaths in England and Wales 1931–85: evidence for a true increase in asthma mortality. *J Epidemiol Community Health*, **42**(4), 316–20.

Burney P, Chinn S, Jarvis D, Luczynska C, Lai E. (1996) Variations in the prevalence of respiratory symptoms, self-reported asthma attacks, and use of asthma medication in the European Community Respiratory Health Survey (ECRHS). *Eur Respir J*, **9**, 687–95.

Burney PGJ. (1986) Asthma mortality in England and Wales: evidence for a further increase, 1974–84. *Lancet*, **Aug 9**, 323–6.

Burney PGJ. (1987) A diet rich in sodium may potentiate asthma. *Chest*, **91**, 143S–148S.

Burney PGJ. (1989) The effect of death certification practice on recorded national asthma mortality rates. *Rev Epidemiol Sante Publique*, **37**, 385–9.

Burney PGJ, Britton JR, Chinn S, *et al*. (1986) Response to inhaled histamine and 24 hour sodium excretion. *BMJ*, **292**, 1483–6.

Burney PGJ, Britton JR, Chinn S, *et al*. (1987) Descriptive epidemiology of bronchial reactivity in an adult population: results from a community study. *Thorax*, **42**, 38–44.

Burney PGJ, Laitinen LA, Perdrizet S, *et al*. (1989) Validity and repeatability of the IUATLD (1984) Bronchial Symptoms Questionnaire: an international comparison. *Eur Respir J*, **2**, 940–5.

Burney PGJ, Luczynska C, Chinn S, Jarvis D. (1994) The European Community Respiratory Health Survey. *Eur Respir J*, **7**, 954–60.

Burney PGJ, Malmberg E, Chinn S, Jarvis D, Luczynska C, Lai E. (1997) The distribution of total and specific IgE in the European Community Respiratory Health Survey. *J Allergy Clin Immunol*, **99**, 314–22.

Burr M, Miskelly FG, Butland BK, Merrett TG, Vaughan-Williams E. (1989) Environmental factors and symptoms in infants at high risk of allergy. *J Epidemiol Community Health*, **43**, 125–32.

Burrows B, Martinez FD, Halonen M, Barbee RA, Cline MG. (1989) Association of asthma with serum IgE levels and skin-test reactivity to allergens. *N Engl J Med*, **320**(50), 271–7.

Burrows B, Bloom JW, Traver GA, Cline MG. (1987) The course and prognosis of different forms of chronic airways obstruction in a sample from the general population. *N Engl J Med*, **317**, 1309–47.

Businco L, Cantani A, Farinella F, Businco E. (1988) Month of birth and grass pollen or mite sensitization in children with respiratory allergy: a significant relationship. *Clin Allergy*, **18**, 269–72.

Caraballo LR, Hernandez M. (1990) HLA haplotype segregation in families with allergic asthma. *Tissue Antigens*, **35**, 182–6.

Carey OJ, Lock CR, Cookson JB. (1993) Effect of alterations of dietary sodium on the severity of asthma in men. *Thorax*, **48**, 714–18.

Carosso A, Ruffino C, Bugiani M. (1986) The effect of birth season on pollenosis. *Ann Allergy*, **56**, 300–3.

Collaborative Study on the Genetics of Asthma (CSGA). (1997) Collaborative study on the genetics of athma: a genome-wide search for asthma susceptibility loci in ethnically diverse populations. *Nat Genet*, **15**, 389–92.

Cookson WOC, Hopkin JM. (1988) Dominant inheritance of atopic immunoglobulin-E responsiveness. *Lancet*, **Jan 16**, 86–7.

Crane J, Flatt A, Jackson R, *et al*. (1989) Prescribed fenoterol and death from asthma in New Zealand, 1981–83: case-control study. *Lancet*, **i**, 917–23.

Daniels SE, Battacharrya S, James A, *et al*. (1996) A genome-wide search for quantitative trait loci underlying asthma. *Nature*, **383**, 247–50.

Department of Health. (1995a) Asthma: an epidemiological overview. *Central Health Monitoring Unit Epidemiological Overview Series*. London: HMSO.

Department of Health. (1995b) Committee on the Medical Effects of Air Pollutants. Asthma and outdoor air pollution. London: HMSO.

Dodge RR, Burrows B. (1980) The prevalence and incidence of asthma and asthma-like symptoms in a general population sample. *Am Rev Respir Dis*, **122**, 567–75.

Drazen JM, Israel E, Boushey HA, *et al*. (1996) Comparison of regularly scheduled with as-needed use of albuterol in mild asthma. *N Engl J Med*, **335**(12), 841–7.

Duff AL, Pomeranz ES, Gelber LE, *et al*. (1993) Risk factors for acute wheezing in infants and children: viruses, passive smoke, and IgE antibodies to inhalant allergens. *Pediatrics*, **92**, 535–40.

Duran-Tauleria E and Rona RJ. (1999) Geographical and socioeconomic variation in the prevalence of asthma symptoms in English and Scottish children. *Thorax*, **54**, 476–81.

Emelyanov A, Fedoseev G, Barnes PJ. (1999) Reduced intracellular magnesium concentrations in asthmatic patients. *Eur Respir J*, **13**, 38–40.

Empey DW, Laitinen LA, Jacobs L, Gold WM, Nadel JA. (1976) Mechanisms of bronchial hyperreactivity in normal subjects after upper respiratory tract infection. *Am Rev Respir Dis*, **113**, 131–9.

Evans D, Levison MJ, Feldman CH, *et al*. (1987) The impact of passive smoking on emergency room visits of urban children with asthma. *Am Rev Respir Dis*, **135**, 567–72.

Flatt A, Pearce N, Thomson CD, *et al*. (1990) Reduced selenium in asthmatic subjects in New Zealand. *Thorax*, **45**, 95–9.

Fluge O, Omenaas E, Eide GE, Gulsvik A. (1998) Fish consumption and respiratory symptoms among young adults in a Norwegian community. *Eur Respir J*, **12**, 336–40.

Fry J. (1953) Effects of a severe fog on a general practice. *Lancet*, **I**, 235–6.

Gassner M. (1992) Immunologische-allergologische reactionen unter veranderten umweltbedudngingen. *Schweiz Rundsch Med Prax*, **81**, 426–30.

Gergen PJ, Mullally DI, Evans R. (1988) National survey of prevalence of asthma among children in the United States, 1976 to 1980. *Pediatrics*, **81**, 1–7.

Gergen PJ, Turkeltaub PC. (1986) Percutaneous immediate hypersensitivity to eight allergens. Washington DC: US Department of Health, Education and Welfare: *Vital Health Stat (Series 11)*, **235**, 669–79.

Gerrard JW, Heiner DC, Mink J, Meyers A, Dosman JA. (1980) Immunoglobulin levels in smokers and non-smokers. *Ann Allergy*, **44**, 261–2.

Gerritsen J, Koeter GH, Monchy J, Knol K. (1990) Allergy in subjects with asthma from childhood to adulthood. *J Allergy Clin Immunol*, **85**, 116–25.

Gerritsen J, Koeter GH, Postma DS, Schouten FP, Knol K. (1989) Prognosis of asthma from childhood to adulthood. *Am Rev Respir Dis*, **140**, 1325–30.

Gerstman BB, Bosco LA, Tomita DK, Gross TP, Shaw MM. (1989) Prevalence and treatment of asthma in the Michigan Medicaid patient population younger than 45 years, 1980–1986. *J Allergy Clin Immunol*, **83**, 1032–9.

Giles GG, Gibson HB, Lickiss N, Shaw K. (1984) Respiratory symptoms in Tasmanian adolescents: a follow up of the 1961 birth cohort. *Aust NZ J Med*, **14**, 631–7.

Godfrey RC, Gradidge CF. (1976) Allergic sensitization of human lung fragments prevented by saturation of IgE binding sites. *Nature*, **259**, 484–6.

Hall MA, Thom H, Russell G. (1981) Erythrocyte aspartate amino transferase activity in asthmatic and non-asthmatic children and its enhancement by vitamin B6. *Ann Allergy*, **47**, 464–7.

Hill J, Micklewright A, Lewis S, Britton J. (1997) Investigation of the effect of short-term change in dietary magnesium intake in asthma. *Eur Respir J*, **10**, 2225–9.

Hodge L, Salome CM, Peat JK, Haby MM, Xuan W, Woolcock AJ. (1996) Consumption of oily fish and childhood asthma risk. *Med J Aust*, **164**, 137–40.

Holland WW, ed. (1988) *European community atlas of avoidable death*. Oxford: Oxford University Press.

Huang S-L, Shiao G-M, Chou P. (1999) Association between body mass index and allergy in teenage girls in Taiwan. *Clin Exp Allergy*, **29**, 323–9.

Inman WH, Adelstein AM. (1969) Rise and fall of asthma mortality in England and Wales in relation to use of pressurised aerosols. *Lancet*, **2**, 279–84.

International Study of Asthma and Allergies in Childhood (ISAAC) Steering Committee. (1998) Worldwide variations in the prevalence of asthma symptoms: the International Study of Asthma and Allergies in Childhood (ISAAC). *Eur Respir J*, **12**, 315–35.

Johnston EDA, Anderson HR, Lambert HP, Patel S. (1983) Respiratory morbidity and lung function after whooping-cough. *Lancet*, **2**, 1104–9.

Jones CO, Qureshi S, Rona RJ, Chinn S. (1996) Exercise-induced bronchoconstriction by ethnicity and presence of asthma in British nine year olds. *Thorax*, **51**, 1134–6.

Keeley DJ, Gallivan S. (1991) Comparison of the prevalence of reversible airways obstruction in rural and urban Zimbabwean children. *Thorax*, **46**, 549–53.

Kelly WJW, Hudson I, Phelan PD, Pain MCF, Olinsky A. (1987) Childhood asthma in adult life: a further study at 28 years of age. *BMJ*, **294**, 1059–61.

Kramer U, Heinrich J, Wjst M, Wichmann H-E. (1999) Age of entry to day nursery and allergy in later childhood. *Lancet*, **353**, 450–4.

Kreisman H, Mitchell C, Bouhuys A. (1977) Inhibition of histamine-induced airway constriction negative results with oxtriphylline and ascorbic acid. *Lung*, **154**, 223–9.

Kuehr J, Frischer T, Meinert R, *et al.* (1994) Mite allergen exposure is a risk for the incidence of specific sensitization. *J Allergy Clin Immunol*, **94**, 44–52.

Lanes S, Walker AM. (1987) Do pressurized bronchodilator aerosols cause death among asthmatics? *Am J Epidemiol*, **125**, 755–61.

Lau S, Falkenhorst G, Weber A, *et al.* (1989) High mite-allergen exposure increases the risk of sensitization in atopic children and young adults. *J Allergy Clin Immunol*, **84**, 718–25.

Lemanske RF, Dick EC, Swanson CA, Vrtis RF, Busse WW. (1989) Rhinovirus upper respiratory infection increases airway hyperreactivity and late asthmatic reactions. *J Clin Invest*, **83**, 1–10.

Leung RC, Carlin JB, Burdon JGW, Czarny D. (1994) Asthma, allergy and atopy in Asian immigrants in Melbourne. *Med J Aust*, **161**, 418–25.

Lim TK, Taylor RG, Watson A, Joyce H, Pride NB. (1988) Changes in bronchial responsiveness to inhaled histamine over four years in middle aged male smokers and ex-smokers. *Thorax*, **43**, 599–604.

Loveless MH. (1950) Milk allergy: a survey of its incidence: experiments with a masked ingestion diet. *J Allergy*, **21**, 489–99.

Lucas A, Brooke OG, Morley R, Cole TJ, Bamford MF. (1990) Early diet of preterm infants and development of allergic or atopic disease: randomised prospective study. *BMJ*, **300**, 837–40.

Lynch N, Hagel I, Perez M. (1993) Effect of antihelminthic treatment on the allergic reactivity of children in a tropical slum. *J Allergy Clin Immunol*, **92**, 404–11.

Malo J, Cartier A, Pineau L, L'Archeveque J, Ghezzo H, Martin RR. (1986) Lack of acute effects of ascorbic acid on spirometry and airway responsiveness to histamine in subjects with asthma. *J Allergy Clin Immunol*, **78**, 1153–8.

Markowe HLJ, Bulpitt CJ, Shipley MJ, Crombie DL, Fleming DM. (1987) Prognosis in adult asthma: a national study. *BMJ*, **295**, 949–52.

Marks G, Burney P. (1998) Diseases of the respiratory system. In: Charlton J, Murphy M, eds. *The Health of Adult Britain 1841–1991*. London: HMSO, 93–113.

Marsh DG, Neely JD, Breazeale DR, *et al*. (1994) Linkage analysis of IL4 and other chromosome 5q31.1 markers and total serum immunoglobulin E concentrations. *Science*, **264**, 1152–6.

Martin AJ, Landau LI, Phelan PD. (1980) Lung function in young adults who had asthma in childhood. *Am Rev Respir Dis*, **122**, 609–16.

Martin AJ, Landau LI, Phelan PD. (1981) Natural history of allergy in asthmatic children followed to adult life. *Med J Aust*, **2**, 470–4.

Martin S. (1898) Asthma and its treatment. *BMJ*, **2**, 1861–3.

Martinez FD, Morgan WJ, Wright AL, Holberg CJ, Taussig LM. (1988) Diminished lung function as a predisposing factor for wheezing respiratory illness in infants. *N Engl J Med*, **319**, 1112–17.

Matricardi PM, Franzinelli F, Franco A, *et al*. (1998) Sibship size, birth order, and atopy in 11,371 Italian young men. *J Allergy Clin Immunol*, **101**, 439–44.

Melia RJ, Chinn S, Rona RJ. (1988) Respiratory illness and home environment of ethnic groups. *BMJ*, **296**, 1438–41.

Melton G. (1943) Treatment of asthma by nicotinic acid. *BMJ*, **Vol. 1**, 600–1.

Mitchell EA. (1983) Increasing prevalence of asthma in children. *NZ Med J*, **96**, 463–4.

Mitchell EA, Stewart AW, Pattemore PK, Asher MI, Harrison AC, Rea H. (1989) Socioeconomic status in childhood asthma. *Int J Epidemiol*, **18**, 888–90.

Mohsenin V, Dubois AB, Douglas JS. (1983) Effect of ascorbic acid on response to methacholine challenge in asthmatic subjects. *Am Rev Respir Dis*, **127**, 143–7.

Morrison Smith J. (1976) The prevalence of asthma and wheezing in children. *Br J Dis Chest*, **70**, 73–7.

Murray AB, Morrison BJ. (1986) The effect of cigarette smoke from the mother on bronchial responsiveness and severity of symptoms in children with asthma. *J Allergy Clin Immunol*, **77**, 575–81.

Nakagomi T, Itaya H, Tominaga T, Yamaki M, Hisamatsu S-I, Nakagomi O. (1994) Is atopy increasing? *Lancet*, **343**, 121–2.

Newhouse MT, Chapman KR, McCallum AL, *et al*. (1996) Cardiovascular safety of high doses of inhaled fenoterol and albuterol in acute severe asthma. *Chest*, **110**, 595–603.

Omenaas E, Bakke P, Elsayed S, Hanoa R, Gulsvik A. (1994) Total and specific serum IgE levels in adults: relationship to sex, age and environmental factors. *Clin Exp Allergy*, **24**, 530–9.

Ordman D. (1955) An outbreak of bronchial asthma in South Africa affecting more than 200 persons caused by castor bean dust from an oil processing factory. *Int Arch Allergy Appl Immunol*, **7**, 10–24.

Park ES, Golding J, Carswell F, Stewart-Brown S. (1986) Preschool wheezing and prognosis at 10. *Arch Dis Child*, **61**, 642–6.

Pattemore PK, Asher MI, Harrison AC, Mitchell EA, Rea HH, Stewart AW. (1989) Ethnic differences in prevalence of asthma symptoms and bronchial hyperresponsiveness in New Zealand schoolchildren. *Thorax*, **44**(3), 168–76.

Pearce N, Pekkanen J, Beasley R. (1999) How much asthma is really attributable to atopy? *Thorax*, **54**, 268–72.

Pearson DJ, Freed DJ, Taylor G. (1977) Respiratory allergy and month of birth. *Clin Allergy*, **7**, 29–34.

Peat JK, Salome CM, Sedgwick CS, Kerrebijn J, Woolcock AJ. (1989) A prospective study of bronchial hyperresponsiveness and respiratory symptoms in a population of Australian schoolchildren. *Clin Exp Allergy*, **9**(3), 299–306.

Peat JK, Woolcock AJ, Cullen K. (1987) Rate of decline of lung function in subjects with asthma. *Eur J Resp Dis*, **70**, 171–9.

Pollart SM, Chapman MD, Fiocco GP, Rose G, Platts MT. (1989) Epidemiology of acute asthma: IgE antibodies to common inhalant allergens as a risk factor for emergency room visits. *J Allergy Clin Immunol*, **83**(5), 875–82.

Pollart SM, Reid MJ, Fling JA, Chapman MD, Platss-Mills TAE. (1988) Epidemiology of emergency room asthma in northern California: association with IgE antibody to ryegrass pollen. *J Allergy Clin Immunol*, **82**, 224–30.

Porter R, Birch JE. (1971) *Identification of asthma*. Edinburgh and London: Churchill Livingstone.

Postma DS, Bleecker ER, Amelung PJ, *et al.* (1995) Genetic susceptibility to asthma: bronchial hyperresponsiveness coinherited with a major gene for atopy. *N Engl J Med*, **333**, 894–900.

Pullan CR, Hey EN. (1982) Wheezing, asthma, and pulmonary dysfunction 10 years after infection with respiratory syncytial virus in infancy. *BMJ*, **284**, 1665–9.

Rea HH, Scragg R, Jackson R, Beaglehole R, Fenwick J, Sutherland D. (1986) A case-control study of deaths from asthma. *Thorax*, **41**, 833–9.

Reed C, Covallis MD. (1958) The failure of antepartum or neonatal exposure to grass pollen to influence the later development of grass sensitivity. *J Allergy Clin Immunol*, **29**, 300–1.

Riou B, Barriot P. (1990) Accuracy of asthma mortality in France. *Chest*, **97**, 507–9.

Roemer W, Hoek G, Brunekreef B, *et al.* (1998) Daily variations in air pollution and respiratory health in a multicentre study: the PEACE project. *Eur Respir J*, **12**, 1354–61.

Rosenstreich DL, Eggleston P, Kattan M, *et al.* (1997) The role of cockroach allergy and exposure to cockroach allergen in causing morbidity among inner-city children with asthma. *N Engl J Med*, **336**, 1356–63.

Rugtveit J. (1990) Environmental factors in the first months of life and the possible relationship to later development of hypersensitivity. *Allergy*, **45**, 154–6.

Salmond C, Crampton P, Hales S, Lewis S, Pearce N. (1999) Asthma prevalence and deprivation: a small area analysis. *J Epidemiol Community Health*, **53**, 476–80.

Salter HH. (1870) Diseases of the chest. *Lancet*, **1**, 183–7.

Savilahti E, Taino V-M, Salmenpera L, Simes MA, Perheentupa J. (1987) Prolonged exclusive breast feeding and heredity as determinants in infantile atopy. *Arch Dis Child*, **62**, 269–73.

Schachter EN, Doyle CA, Beck GJ. (1984) A prospective study of asthma in a rural community. *Chest*, **85**, 623–30.

Schachter EN, Schlesinger A. (1982) The attenuation of exercise-induced bronchospasm by ascorbic acid. *Ann Allergy*, **49**, 146–51.

Sears MR, Taylor DR, Print CG, *et al.* (1990) Regular inhaled beta-agonist treatment in bronchial asthma. *Lancet*, **336**, 1391–6.

Shaheen SO, Aaby P, Hall AJ, *et al.* (1996) Measles and atopy in Guinea-Bissau. *Lancet*, **347**, 1792–6.

Shaheen SO, Sterne JAC, Montgomery SM, Azima H. (1999) Birth weight, body mass index and asthma in young adults. *Thorax*, **54**, 396–402.

Sibbald B, Horn ME, Brain EA, Gregg I. (1980) Genetic factors in childhood asthma. *Thorax*, **35**, 671–4.

Sierstedt HC, Mostgaard G, Hyldebrandt N, Hansen HS, Boldsen J, Oxhoj H. (1996) Inter-relationships between diagnosed asthma, asthma like symptoms and abnormal airway behaviour in adolescence: the Odense schoolchild study. *Thorax*, **51**, 503–9.

Somerville SM, Rona RJ, Chinn S. (1984) Obesity and respiratory symptoms in primary school. *Arch Dis Child*, **59**, 940–4.

Soriano JB, Anto JM, Plasencia A, the Barcelona Soybean-asthma Group. (1995) Repeaters count: a sentinel method for asthma outbreaks. *Thorax*, **50**, 1101–3.

Soutar A, Seaton A, Brown K. (1997) Bronchial reactivity and dietary antioxidants. *Thorax*, **52**, 166–70.

Sporik R, Holgate T, Platts-Mills TAE, Cogswell JJ. (1990) Exposure to house-dust mite allergen (Der p I) and the development of asthma in childhood. *N Engl J Med*, **323**, 502–7.

Stolley PD, Schinnar R. (1978) Association between asthma mortality and isoproterenol aerosols: a review. *Prev Med*, **7**, 519–38.

Storr J, Lenney W. (1989) School holidays and admissions with asthma. *Arch Dis Child*, **64**, 103–7.

Strachan DP. (1989) Hay fever, hygiene and household size. *BMJ*, **299**(6710), 1259–60.

Strachan DP, Jarvis MJ, Feyerabend C. (1990) The relationship of salivary cotinine to respiratory symptoms, spirometry, and exercise-induced bronchospasm in seven-year-old children. *Am Rev Respir Dis*, **142**, 147–51.

Strachan DP, Seagroatt V, Cook DG. (1994) Chest illness in infancy and chronic respiratory disease in later life: an analysis by month of birth. *Int J Epidemiol*, **23**, 1060–8.

Suoniemi I, Bjorksten F, Haahtela T. (1981) Dependence of immediate hypersensitivity in the adolescent period on factors encountered in infancy. *Allergy*, **36**, 263–8.

Suppli Ulrik C, Lange P. (1994) Decline of lung function in adults with bronchial asthma. *Am J Resp Crit Care Med*, **150**, 629–34.

Svanes C, Jarvis D, Chinn S, Burney P. (1999) Childhood environment and adult atopy: results from the European Community Respiratory Health Survey. *J Allergy Clin Immunol*, **103**, 415–20.

Targonski PV, Persky VW, Ramekrishnan V. (1995) Effect of environmental molds on risk of death from asthma during the pollen season. *J Allergy Clin Immunol*, **95**, 955–61.

Taylor B, Wadsworth J, Golding J, Butler N. (1983) Breast feeding, eczema, asthma, and hayfever. *J Epidemiol Community Health*, **37**, 95–9.

Taylor RG, Gross E, Joyce H, Holland F, Pride NB. (1985) Smoking, allergy, and the differential white blood cell count. *Thorax*, **40**, 17–22.

Tovey ER, Sluyter R, Duffy D, Britton WJ. (1998) Immunoblotting analysis of twin sera provides evidence for limited genetic controls of specific IgE to house dust mite allergens. *J Allergy Clin Immunol*, **101**, 491–7.

Tribe RM, Barton JR, Poston L, Burney PGJ. (1994) Dietary sodium intake, airway responsiveness and cellular sodium transport. *Am J Resp Crit Care Med*, **149**, 1426–33.

Troisi RJ, Willett WC, Weiss ST, Trichopoulos D, Rosner, B, Speizer FE. (1995) A prospective study of diet and adult-onset asthma. *Am J Resp Crit Care Med*, **151**, 1401–8.

Ussetti P, Roca J, Agusti AGN, Montserrat JM, Rodriguez-Roisin R, Agusti-Vidal A. (1983) Asthma outbreak in Barcelona. *Lancet*, **2**, 280–1.

van Weel C, van den Bosch WJHM, van den Hoogen HJM, Smits AJA. (1987) Development of respiratory illness in childhood – a longitudinal study in general practice. *J R Coll Gen Pract*, **37**, 404–8.

Vesterinen E, Kaprio J, Koskenvuo M. (1988) Prospective study of asthma in relation to smoking habits among 14 729 adults. *Thorax*, **43**, 534–9.

von Mutius E, Martinez FD, Fritzsch C, Nicolai T, Roell G, Thiemann HH. (1994) Prevalence of asthma and atopy in two areas of West and East Germany. *Am J Respir Crit Care Med*, **149**(2pt1), 358–64.

Ward KP, Arthur JR, Russell G, Aggett PJ. (1984) Blood selenium content and glutathione peroxidase activity in children with cystic fibrosis, coeliac disease, asthma, and epilepsy. *Eur J Pediatr*, **142**, 21–4.

Warner JO, Price JF. (1978) House dust mite sensitivity in childhood asthma. *Arch Dis Child*, **53**, 710–13.

Weiss KB, Wagener DK. (1990) Changing patterns of asthma mortality: identifying target populations at high risk. *J Am Med Assoc*, **264**, 1683–7.

Welliver RC, Kaul T, Ogra PL. (1980) The appearance of cell-bound IgE in respiratory epithelium after respiratory-syncytial-virus infection. *N Engl J Med*, **303**, 1198–202.

Wichmann HE, Mueller W, Allhof P, *et al*. (1989) Health effects during a smog episode in West Germany in 1985. *Environ Health Perspect*, **79**, 89–99.

Wilson MN. (1985) Food related asthma: a difference between two ethnic groups. *Arch Dis Child*, **60**, 861–5.

Young E, Patel S, Stoneham M, Rona R, Wilkinson JD. (1987) The prevalence of reaction to food additives in a survey population. *J R Coll Physicians Lond*, **21**, 241–7.

Zeiger RS, Heller S, Mellon MH, *et al*. (1989) Effect of combined maternal and infant food-allergen avoidance on development of atopy in early infancy: a randomized study. *J Allergy Clin Immunol*, **84**(1), 72–89.

Zetterstrom O, Johansson SGO. (1981) IgE concentrations measured by PRIST in serum of healthy adults and in patients with respiratory allergy. *Allergy*, **36**, 537–47.

10

Occupational asthma

P. SHERWOOD BURGE

DEFINITION

Occupational asthma is due wholly or partly to agents met with at work. Once occupational asthma has developed, asthma is nearly always provoked in addition by non-specific factors such as exercise, cold air and respiratory infections, so that occupational exposure is rarely the only provoking factor in a worker with occupational asthma. Occupational asthma may also develop in workers with pre-existing asthma, where the consequences of a diagnosis may be equally as great as those with no pre-existing asthma. Those with pre-existing asthma are probably at increased risk of developing occupational sensitization to most occupational agents. In the UK, compensation by the government department for social security (under the Department of Health and Social Security Act of 1975) states that occupational asthma is asthma whose primary cause is a sensitizing agent inhaled at work. It is qualified by saying that there is usually a preliminary period ranging from days to years before the onset of symptoms, which occur during the working week and often remit during absence from work. Removal from exposure to the sensitizing agent may lead to remission of asthma, although sensitization can be permanent.

Some practitioners like to place qualifications on the diagnosis of occupational asthma and the following classification is suggested. The first three or four categories come within the traditional classification of occupational asthma.

1 **Occupational asthma** occurring for the first time after exposure to an occupational sensitizer, with specific IgE to the relevant occupational allergen. A latent period of exposure

without symptoms would be present, and symptoms with trivial exposure common after sensitization has occurred. Laboratory animal allergy would be a classical example.

2 **Occupational asthma** without specific IgE to a relevant occupational allergen, but with the other features of sensitization, such as a latent interval and subsequent symptoms with levels of exposure which do not affect non-sensitized asthmatics. Most isocyanate-induced asthma would come into this group, which is clinically and histologically indistinguishable from the first group.

3 **Occupational asthma** as above in an individual with previous non-occupational asthma. In this situation the occupational exposure would not be the cause of the underlying asthma, but the additional sensitization would necessitate a change of work practice or employment. A good example would be a doctor or nurse who has controlled asthma not interfering with work but develops latex sensitization. There is enough latex allergen in the air of many hospital wards to provoke asthma in a highly sensitized individual and preclude work in health care premises.

4 **Occupational asthma induced by a single large exposure.** Asthma induced by a single large exposure to an occupational agent with subsequent asthma induced by low level exposure. This is similar to occupational asthma with sensitization, but no latent interval is necessary. Several cases have followed isocyanate spills.

5 **Irritant-induced occupational asthma.** Asthma is work-related but occurs on first exposure to a recognized respiratory irritant, with persisting asthma and regular improvement away from exposure. Regular exposure to sulphur dioxide in a smelter would be an example. The consequences for the affected individual's work are the same as for a sensitizer, but exposure to very low levels should not cause problems.

6 **Irritant-induced asthma.** Asthma starting within 24 hours of a single large exposure, and persisting afterwards, usually accompanied by increased non-specific bronchial responsiveness. Subsequent usual level of exposure to the same agent does not provoke the asthma (and so continuing employment is not jeopardized). Large exposures to chlorine are the commonest cause. Some call this reactive airways dysfunction syndrome.

7 **Occupational bronchial hyperresponsiveness.** There are some workers with respiratory symptoms who do not have airflow obstruction or changes in peak expiratory flow, who have increased levels of non-specific responsiveness after work exposure, with improvement when away from exposure. These changes can also be reproduced with specific provocation testing. They do not fulfil even a broad definition of asthma, but nevertheless have work-related symptoms and abnormal physiology. It might represent the earliest evidence of disease in an individual who will later develop true occupational asthma, but this awaits confirmation.

EPIDEMIOLOGY

Estimates of the incidence of occupational asthma vary widely depending on the criteria for entry to the register. Data are available from statutory notification schemes, compensation registers and voluntary surveillance schemes.

STATUTORY NOTIFICATION FROM THE WORKPLACE

Cases always arise in a workplace, so it seems logical to make the employer responsible for notifying cases. Such a scheme is in operation in the UK, where the employer is required to notify cases under the Reporting of Injuries, Diseases and Dangerous Occurrences Regulations. The reports go to the Employment Medical Advisory Service, the group of government doctors who advise on health in the workplace. A notification usually results in a visit, and can result in prosecution. Not surprisingly there are few reports. In the some parts of the USA the SENSOR scheme works in a similar manner (Reilly *et al.*, 1994).

COMPENSATION REPORTS

The best register is in Finland where occupational diseases are notifiable by law, and a register has been in place since 1964. The register includes all cases notified by clinicians, all claims settled by insurance companies and all cases diagnosed by the Institute of Occupational Health. There was a large increase in notifications after 1982, when compensation was opened to self-employed farmers, the self-employed being otherwise excluded (Keskinen *et al.*, 1978; Kanerva and Vaheri, 1993; Reijula *et al.*, 1996). In other countries restrictions on the criteria for compensation have big effects on the agents identified as causes of occupational asthma and the numbers of cases identified. In the UK, occupational asthma has been a prescribed disease with no fault compensation from the government since 1981. The initial scheme included seven causes only, this was expanded by a further seven agents in 1986, the addition of wood dusts was the only cause that had an appreciable impact on the number of cases (the average number of annual cases increasing from 163 to 220). In 1991 an open category was introduced requiring greater proof of cause and effect. There were 532 cases per year in the first two years. Both these sources exclude the self-employed, who form about 12% of the workforce. At the same time the insurance industry was compensating around 800 cases a year, but does not publish any details.

Similar lists from other countries show different predominant causes. For instance, in Switzerland and Germany, flour in bakeries is by far the commonest cause recognized, while in Norway the commonest cause is related to aluminium smelting, which is not on the UK list of compensatable causes of occupational asthma, as many regard it as an example of irritant-induced occupational asthma. It appears that from the compensation data occupational asthma is not very common. When surveys are carried out in workplaces with identified index cases, further cases are commonly identified. For example, in the only epidemiological survey of workers exposed to the plastic blowing agent azodicarbonamide, a further 28 cases were identified among 141 exposed workers (Slovak, 1981); during the next 6 years only four of these were identified on compensation registers. There is substantial evidence that the great majority of patients with occupational asthma remain undiagnosed. This is partly because many physicians are content with the diagnosis of asthma without looking for specific aetiological agents.

VOLUNTARY SURVEILLANCE SCHEMES

An alternative approach is to set up a confidential reporting scheme, which cannot lead to prosecution or direct action. Such schemes are very dependent on the enthusiasm and appropriateness of those who report. A voluntary scheme called Shield is situated in the West Midlands region of the UK and run by the regional Midland Thoracic Society, to which all chest physicians and government compensation doctors report in that area, as well as some occupational physicians. When a report is received, information is then provided to the respondent as to whether other cases have been identified from the same employer (but not the patients' names), and the suspected cause; i.e. the process of reporting is of some benefit to the respondent. The area covered is around 10% of the UK, and averaged 90 reports per year from 1989 to 1992 (Gannon and Burge, 1993). Shield does not specify any particular agent or test necessary for reporting, merely that the diagnosis is the most likely one in the opinion of the respondent. Only 38% of the cases had a cause amongst the 14 available for government compensation at the time, and of these only 27% were reported from the government compensation board, implying that both groups were seeing largely distinct subsets of those with occupational asthma. Similar diagnostic criteria are required for SWORD, a UK national voluntary reporting scheme run jointly by the national societies of occupational and thoracic medicine, covering a total population of about 55 million (and recently extended to Eire). For the first 3 years (1989–92) there were 509 notifications per year (Meredith and McDonald, 1994), increasing to an estimated 977 per year for 1993–94 when a sampling system was used and the numbers multiplied by the sample proportion (Ross *et al.*, 1995, 1997). Occupational physicians report about 19% of the cases. The effects on the approximate number of reports per year for a population of 55 million are shown in Table 10.1.

These registers show a common group of agents responsible for most occupational asthma, particularly isocyanates which head all but the Finnish register; other commonly reported agents include flour and grain, colophony, laboratory animals and wood dusts (Table 10.2). There are also regional differences likely to be due to the particular local exposures, particularly cows in Finland, coolant oil aerosols in Shield, and western red cedar in British Colombia. The incidence by occupation can be calculated from the SWORD, Shield and

Table 10.1   *The effects of constraints on notification on the reported incidence of occupational asthma in the UK (population 55 million). Average number of reports per year (1989–92)*

RIDDOR Employer notification +/– regulatory visit	Government compensation; limited list (14)	Government compensation; open list	Shield: local voluntary scheme, mainly chest physicians	SWORD: national voluntary scheme, occupational and chest physicians
62	220	532	900	977

Table 10.2   *Common causes of occupational asthma. Percentages of total reports are given*

Agent	Shield: 1989–91	SWORD: 1989–91	Finland, 1992	Quebec, 1986–88	Michigan and New Jersey, 1988–92
Isocyanates	20	22	3	25	19
Animals	2	10	45	15	1
Flour/grain	10	7	25	14	2
Woods	6	4	2	13	1
Solder	8	6	–	2	1
Resins	5	5	2	–	7
Aldehydes	2	3	2	1	5
Welding	2	2	5	–	2
Drugs/pesticides	<1	2	–	5	2
Coolant oils	7	1	–	–	10
Co/Cr	5	1	1	–	4
Unknown	–	8	4	15	20

Finnish data (Meredith and Nordman, 1996). Spray painters usually head the list with an incidence per hundred thousand per year between 729 and 3111. Bakers, farmers and plastic makers all top the 1000/10⁶ in some registers. Some examples are shown in Table 10.3.

Table 10.3   *Incidence of occupational asthma from reporting schemes*

	Finland 1990		Shield: 1989–91		SWORD: 1989–91	
Occupation	Cases	Rate/10⁶/year	Cases	Rate/10⁶/year	Cases	Rate/10⁶/year
Baker	32	4000	20	445	64	285
Spray painter	14	3111	22	1833	108	729
Farmer	180	1401	8	44	43	34
Solderer/welder	30	1035	26	112	106	158
Plastic maker			38	1054	81	387
Chemical			3	143	77	346
Woodworker			18	130	65	45
Other	119	52	149	25	984	13
Total	375	152	284	42	1528	19

Table 10.4   *Incidence of inhalation injuries by occupation. Data from the UK SWORD surveillance scheme, 1990–1993*

Occupational group	Cases	Rate/million/year
Chemical processor	156	164
Engineering/electrical	343	32
Other manufacturing	163	15
Transportation/construction	100	10
Health and science professionals	59	9
Sales and services	163	6
Others	121	3

DIAGNOSIS OF OCCUPATIONAL ASTHMA

Occupational asthma should be considered in all patients with airways obstruction, as there is substantial confusion between the diagnosis of bronchitis and asthma, particularly when occurring in the older smoking population. The SWORD and Shield data show that the incidence of occupational asthma is highest in older workers, and several studies have shown that sensitization is more common in smokers than non-smokers (Juniper *et al.*, 1977; Burge *et al*, 1980; Zelterstrom *et al.*, 1981; Newman Taylor *et al.*, 1987; Venables *et al.*, 1989). All workers with airways obstruction should be asked two screening questions:

- Are you better on days away from work?
- Are you better on holiday?

It is important to ask about symptoms getting better away from work rather than symptoms deteriorating at work, as occupational asthma frequently comes on several hours after exposure and many workers have their maximum symptoms after work and during the night following work, rather than at work. Several workers therefore will state that they are not worse at work and yet have occupational asthma. Those with more severe occupational asthma do not improve significantly during a one-to-two day break at the weekend but require longer away from work. Recovery has nearly always started within a week of leaving work. Improvement on holidays is more complicated. Holidays away from home need to be differentiated from holidays at home as domestic allergens, such as animals, birds and moulds, may be avoided on holidays away from home.

About two-thirds of the workers with occupational asthma complain of cough, sputum and chest pain which frequently leads to the initial diagnosis of bronchitis (Burge, 1984). Some workers also have other organs affected and complain of rhinitis, eye irritation, dermatitis or, occasionally, bowel symptoms. A few workers have fever and joint aches and pains, which are more often the feature of alveolitis. Indeed some workers have symptoms of both diseases. However, systemic symptoms can be seen in workers without changes in gas transfer in whom the predominant part of the disease is in the airways (Paisley, 1969; Lemiere et al., 1996).

Other helpful items to identify in the history are the latent intervals between first exposure to the possible cause and the onset of disease. Many workers attribute their symptoms to materials that have recently been introduced and also to materials with strong smells, such as solvents, but even though these may be responsible, the offending agents may have been in the workplace for some time. If there is no latent interval the causative agent is likely to be acting as a direct irritant, such as sulphur dioxide (irritant-induced occupational asthma). Some occupational allergens, such as laboratory animals or complex salts of platinum, are associated with short latent intervals averaging a few months. Some, such as isocyanates, have a latent interval averaging 2 years, and longer in those exposed to colophony, which has a mean latent interval of 4 years. In bakers, sensitization may occur for the first time more than 20 years after first exposure. It is likely that the latent interval is longer when exposures are lower. Occupational asthma is not usually associated with catastrophic attacks of asthma on minimal exposure at work, although there are a few well publicized cases where this has happened (and indeed a few deaths due to unexpected exposures). Those with the most extreme sensitivity are frequently exposed to platinum salts, antibiotics and laboratory animals. In these circumstances workers may bring home sufficient allergen on their hair or clothing to induce attacks in an individual with whom they have contact only outside the workplace (Newman Taylor et al., 1989). The majority of workers, however, show much less sensitivity than this and can tolerate 8-hour exposures to materials to which they are sensitized day-by-day (much in the same way as individuals sensitized to house dust mites and grass pollens).

Although the diagnosis can often be made with a reasonable degree of certainty on history alone, further confirmation should be obtained before decisions are made about change of work practices, change of employment, or improvements at work are suggested. Few employers are prepared to spend money on their process solely after a diagnosis made from the account of an individual worker. Objective confirmation of a diagnosis is much easier at the early stage of the disease when treatment is minimal and the political situation unclouded. The best way of proceeding to make an objective diagnosis of occupational asthma is with serial measurements of peak flow, as described below (Burge, 1982; Bright and Burge, 1996; Gannon et al., 1996). These do not usually identify the precise cause of the occupational asthma for which immunological techniques, bronchial provocation testing or epidemiological studies are required. Nevertheless, there is often enough information from serial measurements of peak flow on which to base clinical decisions.

Serial measurements of peak flow

International guidelines are available (Moscato et al., 1995). Workers with extreme sensitivity, who can easily be identified from their history, are *not* suitable for unsupervised re-exposure at work, which is a necessary part of serial peak flow measurements. In these patients the diagnosis can often be confirmed by skin-prick tests or specific IgE measurements, or, occasionally, by bronchial provocation testing by skilled and experienced investigators, the levels and duration of exposure being carefully controlled.

The aims of serial measurements of peak flow are to investigate the effects of work on peak flow. They are substantially more difficult to interpret in those who are changing their treatment at the same time, and they are less sensitive in workers who are on inhaled steroids or cromoglycate when the records are made (Burge *et al.*, 1979a,b). It is therefore preferable to carry out these recordings before treatment is instituted. If prophylactic treatment is being taken it is important to keep the treatment the same on days at and away from work. It is also best to make pre-bronchodilator measurements and to keep bronchodilator treatment the same on work and rest days. The records are more suited to those who are exposed regularly at work rather than those who have intermittent and irregular exposures.

The best records are obtained by measuring peak expiratory flow two-hourly from waking to sleeping over several weeks, and to include similar records on days at and away from work (Gannon *et al.*, 1998). Individuals should be taught to make reproducible measurements of their peak flow, making at least three readings on each occasion, the best two to be within 20 L/min of each other or else further readings should be made. The best is recorded. It is also important to record the times of arriving at and leaving work, and any unusual exposures. Workers who change shifts will also need to record waking and sleeping times, as the diurnal variation in airway calibre is superimposed upon that related to occupational exposure. These records are by their nature unsupervised and are potentially liable to falsification. Logging meters have allowed assessment of incorrectly recorded and prefabricated measurements. Inaccuracies in time are more common than completely prefabricated readings, which have been measured between 7% (Gannon *et al.*, 1993) and 24% (Quirce *et al.*, 1995).

INTERPRETATION OF SERIAL MEASUREMENTS OF PEAK FLOW

When these records are plotted sequentially as a traditional treatment record they are more difficult to interpret than after replotting, as shown in Figs 10.1–10.3; plotting the daily maximum, minimum and mean peak flow. The 'day' should start with the first reading at work and continue until the last reading before work the next day (or equivalent). OASYS is a commercially available computer-assisted diagnostic aid for the plotting and interpretation of occupation peak expiratory flow records which includes the ability to plot 'days' as above, linearize non-linear meters and provided summary plots and an assessment of the likelihood of an occupational effect (Gannon *et al.*, 1996). The format of the plot is shown in Fig. 10.2. Visual inspection of these records has been shown to lead to more sensitive and specific diagnoses than statistical analysis, principally because of the varying interval between stopping work and the onset of improvement, and between starting work and the onset of deterioration (Burge, 1982). If it takes several days to improve away from work and several days to deteriorate at work it may be that the first day or two of work exposure are better than the first day or two away from work. This substantially complicates statistical analysis. The

---

Figure 10.1 (opposite) *Serial plot of peak expiratory flow (PEF) in an injection moulder with isocyanate (MDI) exposure. The periods of work have a shaded background, the vertical lines denote waking and sleeping. The workday is from 6 a.m. to 2 p.m. in the upper panel; the PEF improves over the working period, and declines during sleep. The workday is from 2 p.m. to 10 p.m. in the lower panel, when PEF declines, with little change while sleeping. The PEF improves during the days off work at the start of the lower panel.*

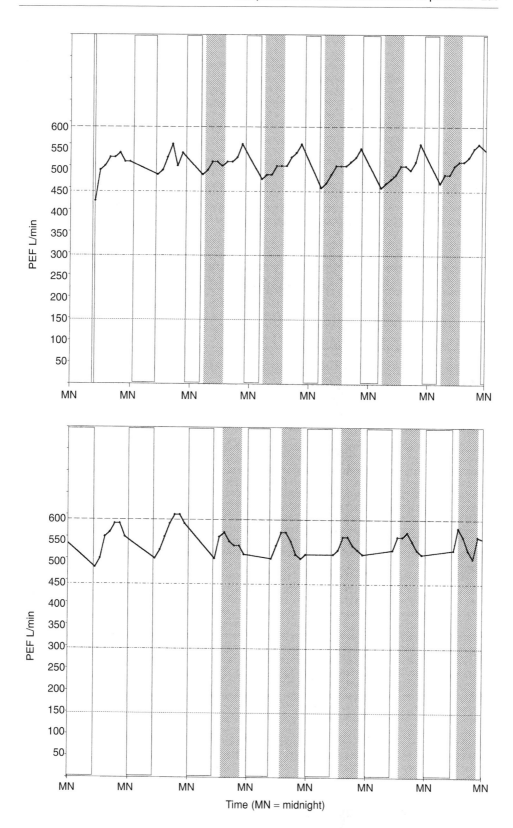

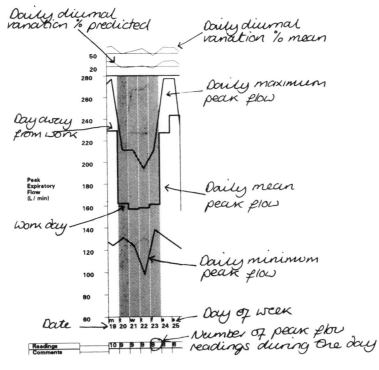

Figure 10.2 *Format of the* OASYS *plot, showing the daily maximum, mean and minimum peak expiratory flow.*

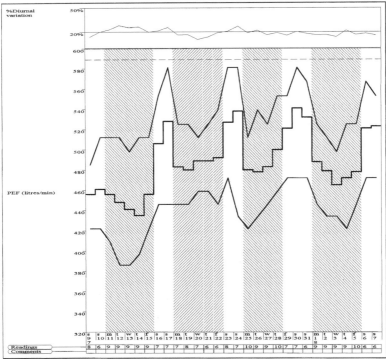

Figure 10.3 OASYS *plot of the same record as shown in Fig. 10.1 (with a further 2 weeks), showing equivalent daily deterioration in each work week, with rest day improvement, which is usually greater on the second day off work than on the first. The lower values on the first few days of the record may be due to a learning effect. The record shows definite occupational asthma.*

basis of the visual inspections is to identify patterns of deterioration and improvement related to work exposure.

PATTERNS OF REACTION

In workers regularly exposed to an occupational agent the pattern of reaction depends principally on the speed of recovery after each reaction. The patterns of reaction can be divided into those that occur from hour-to-hour in a particular work day, those that occur from day-to-day within a work week and those with longer periodicity.

Hourly patterns

Some workers have classical immediate reactions within a few minutes of coming to work. This usually progresses while work exposure continues and improves substantially in the evening at home (Fig. 10.4). However, late asthmatic reactions are more common. They usually start more than an hour after arrival at work, typically 4–8 hours after arrival. Some do not start until the following night, although this is unusual. The patterns of the daily reaction are superimposed on the normal diurnal variations such that immediate reactions are more common on afternoon shifts when the occupational exposure is superimposed on the declining part of the normal diurnal variation, and late reactions are more common on the morning shift (Fig. 10.5). After repeated exposures many workers develop a situation where they do not deteriorate acutely at work nor improve immediately on leaving work (the

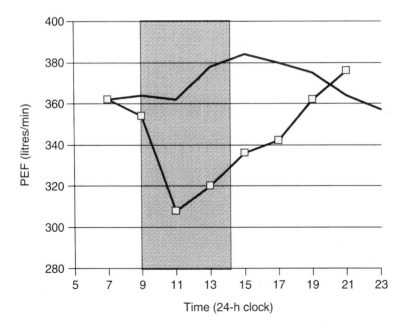

Figure 10.4   *Mean two-hourly peak expiratory flow (PEF) from the OASYS summary plot in a swimming teacher working between 9 a.m. and 2 p.m. (lower line), showing an immediate reaction with the start of recovery on leaving work. The upper line shows the mean PEF on days away from work, showing the usual diurnal variation.*

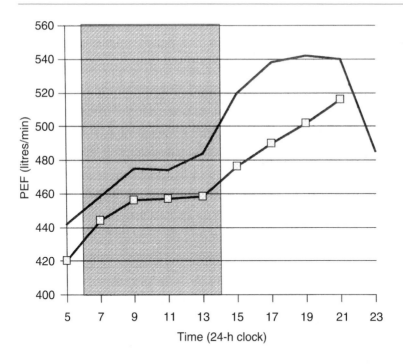

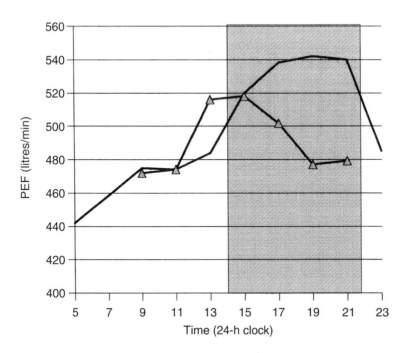

Figure 10.5   *Mean two-hourly peak expiratory flow (PEF) from the OASYS summary plot in the moulder shown in Figs 10.1 and 10.3. The upper panel shows the morning shift (■), where the PEF on workdays rises throughout the day and falls overnight. The days away from work (plain trace) have a maximum value between 5 p.m. and 9 p.m., which is later than usual. The lower panel shows the mean afternoon shift values (△) when the PEF falls within 3 hours of coming to work.*

so-called flat reaction, Fig. 10.6). Similar records are found in many patients with chronic airflow obstruction unrelated to work. The only way of differentiating these is to remove the worker from exposure for 2–3 weeks while records are maintained (Fig. 10.7).

Weekly patterns

Weekly patterns relate to the speed of recovery. If recovery is rapid and effectively complete by the following morning, each work day will result in equivalent deterioration and there will be rapid improvement on the first day away from work at a weekend (Fig. 10.3). If recovery is incomplete by the following morning but is substantial within the 2–3 day period away from work, then symptoms become progressively severe day-by-day at work (Fig. 10.8). Symptoms may be present only at the end of the working week, progression of symptoms with daily exposure being the most common pattern seen.

A few workers have symptoms and declines in peak flow that are maximal at the beginning of the working week, or in the middle of the working week, and improve despite continued exposures. These patterns are more common in a few specific situations such as workers exposed to cotton dust, contaminated humidifiers and coolant oil aerosols. In all of these situations there is a substantial bio-aerosol including endotoxin, where tolerance seems to develop with repeated exposures.

Long time interval patterns

When recovery is not complete within 2–3 days away from work, repeated weeks of exposure may lead to progressive deterioration of the person with asthma. Fortunately, this

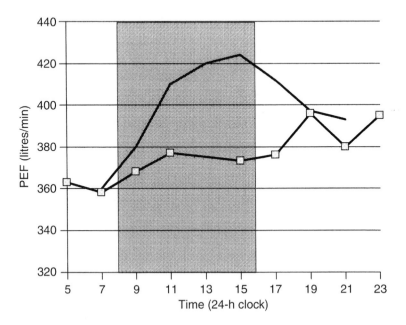

Figure 10.6   *Mean two-hourly peak expiratory flow (PEF) from the OASYS summary plot in a sodium manufacturer exposed to chlorine and intermittently to burning sodium. It shows a flat reaction on workdays (▢), where the normal midday increase in PEF shown on days away from work (plain trace) has been blunted.*

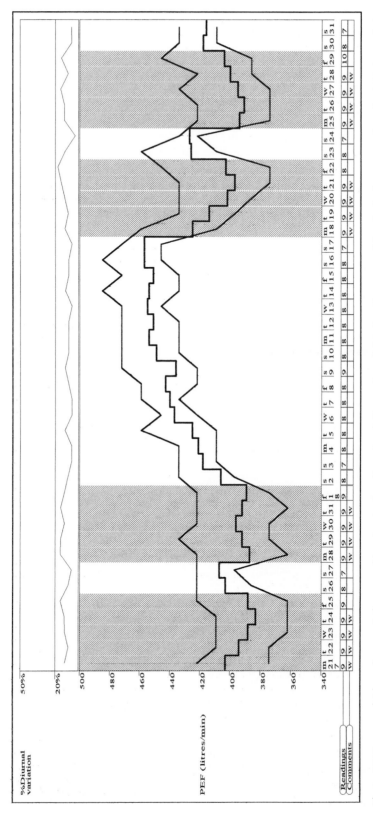

Figure 10.7 OASYS plot in an isocyanate foam moulder, showing low diurnal variation and small deteriorations on workdays in the first two work weeks. A 16-day period off work shows an improvement in PEF taking 10 days to plateau. On return to work the deterioration is more obvious.

deterioration does not continue and a plateau is reached. At this stage diurnal variation in peak flow may be reduced and improvements on days away from work may be minimal. On leaving work some workers continue to improve for up to 6 weeks after leaving work (Fig. 10.7).

INTERPRETATION OF SERIAL PEAK FLOW RECORDS

The simplest method is to inspect plotted records and to decide subjectively whether each consecutive block of work exposure shows a decline in peak flow, and whether each consecutive period away from work shows improvement. The original validation of this method was designed to be sensitive rather than specific (Burge *et al.*, 1979a,b). If deterioration at work and improvement away from work occurs in 75% or more of possible occasions, the records have been shown to be 100% specific. Sensitivity goes down to around 50% on those taking cromoglycate or inhaled steroids during these records. It is likely that the criteria for the subjective assessment of a positive record could be reduced substantially maintaining satisfactory specificity.

Recent work has shown again that visual inspection of the records is more helpful than statistical testing (Cote *et al.*, 1990; Perrin *et al.*, 1992). Perrin and co-workers showed that a subjective assessment of the records achieved 87% sensitivity (by undefined criteria) and 84% specificity. A 3.2-fold change in methacholine reactivity while off work was 48% sensitive and 64% specific, whereas the best statistical analysis achieved 76% sensitivity and 58% specificity. Agreement among readers is important but not always appreciated. In studies to date looking at relatively clear-cut cases Liss quoted agreement as measured by a kappa score of 0.62–0.83 for inter-reader agreement (Liss and Tarlo, 1991), while Malo *et al.* (1993) quoted intra-reader agreement as 83–100%.

Expert interpretation requires experts, who do not always agree and are not always consistent in their interpretation. The OASYS software overcomes some of these problems. The analyses split the record up into a series of overlapping elements containing either a period at work, a period away from work and a period at work (a work–rest–work complex), or its counterpart, a rest–work–rest complex. Discriminant analyses have been developed to mimic the effects of an expert, and tested against a wide range of workers' records. OASYS-2 has a sensitivity of 69% and a specificity of 94% when applied to records from workers with a final diagnosis made independently of the peak flow record (Gannon *et al.*, 1996). A neural net version with increased sensitivity is under development (Bright and Burge, 1995).

The interpretation of equivocal records can be enhanced by including measurements of non-specific bronchial responsiveness before and after a two-week period away from exposure (Cartier *et al.*, 1984; Kongerud *et al.*, 1992), or after removal from exposure (Malo *et al.*, 1988). A fourfold increase in the dose of histamine or methacholine required to drop the FEV_1 by 20% after a period without exposure increases the probability of occupational asthma. Failure to show an improvement in non-specific reactivity, or measurements within the normal range at work, are however both relatively frequent in workers with genuine occupational asthma (Burge, 1982).

It is unclear as yet whether these records can differentiate between irritant and allergic asthmatic reactions, largely because of the problems of differentiating between these types of mechanisms using other criteria. There are some workers who have quite large day-by-day changes at work, with very low diurnal variations throughout (Fig. 10.8). It seems unlikely that smooth muscle constriction in the bronchi is a prominent feature in this type of reaction. Large diurnal variations can certainly be due to non-allergic mechanisms, for instance, the classical asthmatic reaction to exercise. Identifications of patterns of reactions from serial peak

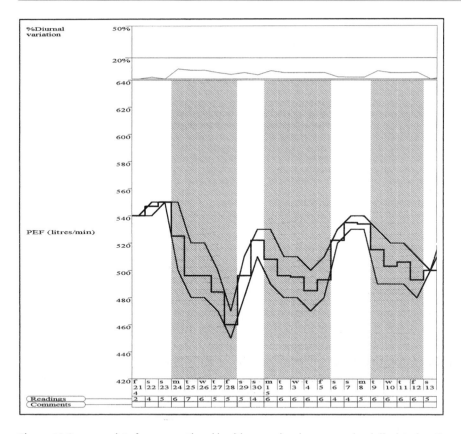

Figure 10.8 OASYS *plot of an occupational health nurse showing progressive daily deterioration with a two-day recovery pattern at weekends. The diurnal variation is low throughout. She was exposed intermittently to a very large number of agents, but had regular deterioration at work, which resolved when she was transferred to a different work site. The next occupant of her office also developed work-related symptoms, which were due to a floor cleaner used in the department.*

flow records allow the separation of reactions into different groups suitable for mechanistic evaluation.

MEASUREMENTS OF BRONCHIAL HYPERRESPONSIVENESS

Bronchial hyperresponsiveness may be induced for the first time by occupational sensitization. Alternatively, occupational asthma may develop in somebody with pre-existing bronchial hyperresponsiveness. At presentation about 80% of workers with occupational asthma have increased responsiveness (Burge, 1982). It is therefore not a useful method of screening workers for further investigation. Hyperresponsiveness is closely associated with the late asthmatic reaction seen on bronchial provocation testing. An immediate reaction alone rarely alters bronchial responsiveness. Workers who are going to develop a late asthmatic reaction develop their hyperresponsiveness following exposure before the fall in lung function (Durham *et al.*, 1987). Many are still hyperresponsive the following day and such hyperresponsiveness may occasionally last for a month or more following a single exposure.

In some individuals, however, the responsiveness returns to normal within 24 hours. Follow-up studies have shown that responsiveness returns to or towards normal in the majority of those who are completely removed from exposure but improves less in workers with a reduced exposure (Burge, 1982; Soyseth *et al.*, 1995). These tests are more useful when carried out serially, than on an individual occasion. There are workers who have symptoms and no change in peak flow who nevertheless have changes in responsiveness related to work exposure. These patients do not fulfil the usual definition of occupational asthma. Nevertheless, the work exposure may induce the hyperresponsiveness which may allow reactions to non-specific triggers such as exercise and cold air that would not have occurred otherwise.

IDENTIFICATION OF A SPECIFIC CAUSE

A specific cause can often be assumed when a worker with occupational asthma confirmed with serial peak expiratory flow measurements is exposed to a well recognized cause of occupational asthma in a high risk environment, e.g. in car spray painters exposed to isocyanates or platinum refiners exposed to complex salts of platinum. However, sometimes the individual with occupational asthma comes from a workforce without known problems and it is then important to make the specific diagnosis so that remedial action can take place. The simplest method (from the point of view of the patient) of making the diagnosis is by finding specific IgE antibodies to a relevant occupational allergen. However, before the results can be interpreted, the sensitivity and specificity of the IgE antibodies must be known. As there are very few standardized occupational allergens, some care is needed in interpreting the results. There are some situations where the sensitivity and specificity are poor (e.g. some locust antigens) (Burge *et al.*, 1980), and some where the specificity is good but the sensitivity is poor, such as with isocyanates (Tee *et al.*, 1998). There are other situations where IgE antibodies have never been found, e.g. with colophony. In some situations workers have IgE antibodies and some do not, e.g. with plicatic acid/human serum albumin antibodies in western red cedar workers (Chan-Yeung, 1982). There seems little difference in the disease in those with or without IgE antibodies. In some situations workers have IgE antibodies to more than one antigen, e.g. some bakers have antibodies both to the flour and to the enzyme amylase added to the flour (Baur *et al.*, 1986). Sometimes there are cross-reacting antibodies, particularly between different isocyanates (Cartier *et al.*, 1989) and different acid anhydrides (Bernstein *et al.*, 1984). Occasionally, immunological testing identifies antigens in unlikely situations, e.g. an outbreak of occupational asthma in makers of felt for flooring who were shown to have IgE antibodies to extracts of the felt; this was caused by contamination of sacking that was used in the felt by castor beans that had previously been contained in the sacks. The antigen in the felt was shown to be the castor bean antigen by RAST inhibition studies (Topping *et al.*, 1982).

In some situations skin-prick testing with characterized antigens is more appropriate than looking for IgE antibodies. This particularly applies to the complex salts of platinum, which produce positive skin-prick tests when the platinum salts are used in unconjugated forms (Murdoch *et al.*, 1986). The tests for serum antibodies using platinum conjugates are difficult to reproduce. The RAST assays sometimes have a problem with non-specific binding when the total IgE is high, which may lead to false-positive results.

IgE antibodies have been relatively disappointing when rhinitis is a principal symptom. For instance, they are negative in many laboratory animal workers with work-related rhinitis. IgE antibodies decrease once exposure ceases: those due to tetrachlorphthalic anhydride (an epoxy cross-linking agent) have been shown to have a half-life of approximately one year (Venables *et al.*, 1987). These tests are therefore less useful in those who have left work but are helpful if measured serially to see if a recurrence of symptoms is due to unknown exposure.

BRONCHIAL PROVOCATION TESTING

Bronchial provocation testing is regarded as the gold standard in the diagnosis of occupational asthma; international guidelines are available (Cartier *et al.*, 1989). However there are many problems with these tests and both false-positive and false-negative results are easy to obtain (Burge, 1987). Testing is laborious both from the point of view of the patient and the medical attendants and should only be done in centres with experience of occupational allergens. Before bronchial provocation starts, the exact materials to which a worker is exposed, the exposure levels and the form in which they are present in the workplace should be known. It often takes a long time to find out what workers are exposed to even in relatively simple situations such as bread baking, which is becoming a relatively chemical process. If materials are heated in the workplace their temperatures should be reproduced in the challenge chamber, as well as the particle size of any particulate material. False-positive tests are easy to produce if exposure levels are excessive. This particularly applies to fungal antigens, many of which are irritant at high concentrations. The tests may be falsely negative, either because the wrong materials have been tested or because the circumstances to exposure in the challenge chamber are wrong, e.g. the wrong particle size with a dust. The finding of a negative challenge test in the worker with a good history and positive peak flow record is more likely to be due to a problem with the challenge testing than with an incorrect diagnosis.

The aim of bronchial provocation testing is to expose the worker to one substance at a time at levels initially substantially less than those encountered at work, with durations of exposure that are far less than those encountered at work. It is rarely necessary to expose a worker for more than an hour in the challenge chamber, and most initial exposures should be of the order of a minute, unless the material has been heated when shorter exposures than this are needed to start with. The levels of antigen in the challenge chamber should be measured before the worker is exposed and care taken not to exceed occupational exposure levels or the levels encountered at work. If a new material is being tested (e.g. a new fungal extract), it is important to make sure that the reactions are specific, i.e. that unexposed individuals with a similar degree of asthma do not react to exposure.

Immediate reactions are usually relatively obvious (Fig. 10.9). Late asthmatic reactions frequently start 4–8 hours after exposure. If the testing has been done later in the morning this will be at a time when lung function is declining due to normal diurnal variation. It is therefore very important to have controlled exposures with measurements for 24 hours afterwards so that comparisons can be made with lung function measurements after an active challenge (Fig. 10.10). If there is doubt about a late asthmatic reaction, re-measurement of bronchial responsiveness when lung function has returned to normal the following day will often help confirm a significant late reaction. Despite all these problems well-performed bronchial provocation testing has been invaluable in the identification of new causes of occupational asthma and the unravelling of complex situations where multiple exposures are present at work. Occupational asthma is a problem in workers exposed to aerosols from cutting oils used in metal cutting, drilling and grinding. Challenge testing has shown that reactions may be due to constituents of the clean unused oil such as the reodorant (pine oil) but are sometimes due to the used oil which contains both the metal dissolved from the cutting tools and the piece being worked and also is usually heavily contaminated with bacteria (Robertson *et al.*, 1988). Control measures are clearly completely different in these two situations.

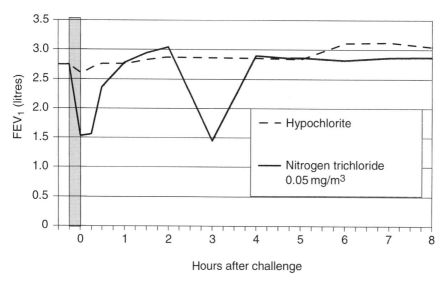

Figure 10.9 *Specific challenge test in the swimming teacher shown in Fig. 10.4. On the control day she painted a solution of calcium hypochlorite, the pool sterilizing agent used at work. There was no reaction. Exposure to chemically-generated nitrogen trichloride at levels below those at work resulted in an immediate reaction which resolved within 90 minutes, and a single low reading at 3 hours, at which time she was symptomatic and wheezy. Late asthmatic reactions usually develop and resolve more slowly than this, raising the possibility of another unidentified exposure causing a second immediate reaction (such as exercise or exposure to another hospital source of nitrogen trichloride).*

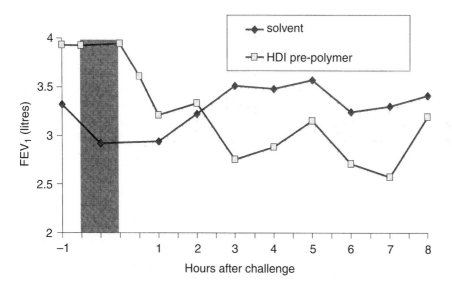

Figure 10.10 *Specific challenge to an isocyanate pre-polymer based on hexamethylene diisocyanate in a paint maker showing a late asthmatic reaction maximal 7 hours post-exposure (▢). The control day with exposure to the paint solvents two days previously starts with a lower FEV_1 making it difficult to interpret the isocyanate challenge (◆). If a worker has been recently exposed to the causative agent at work, they may still be reacting to this for several days in hospital confounding control exposures. If this occurs the control exposure should be repeated when the baseline has stabilized.*

CAUSES OF OCCUPATIONAL ASTHMA

There are over 400 recognized causes of occupational asthma. There are two broad groups: small molecular weight chemicals, which form the minority, and biologically-derived products, which form the great majority. It is likely that the biological products are mainly complete antigens, while small molecular weight chemicals act as haptens and require conjugation before they are active. All require to be inhaled before they cause occupational asthma. The agents can be divided into a number of broad categories.

Biologically-derived products

FUNGAL AND BACTERIAL ANTIGENS

Fungi appear to be commoner antigens than bacteria. The fungi may be a contaminant of vegetable matter, such as cereal crops being harvested where *Cladosporium*, *Alternaria* and *Didymella exitialis* are common causes of asthma during harvest time (Darke *et al.*, 1976; Harries *et al.*, 1985; Lander *et al.*, 1988). Fungi may contaminate wood bark and be a problem in sawmill workers, may contaminate growing fruit or tobacco (Lander *et al.*, 1988) or may sometimes be used to produce proteins in biotechnology plants (Cornillon *et al.*, 1976; Topping *et al.*, 1985).

ARTHROPODS

Arthropods produce a huge number of agents causing occupational asthma. Many of the sensitized workers are actually working with these in laboratories (particularly locusts; Burge *et al.*, 1980). Others are sensitized by storage mites, which contaminate grain and have caused occupational asthma in farmers (Cuthbert *et al.*, 1979; van Hage-Hamsten *et al.*, 1987; Blainey *et al.*, 1988; Iversen *et al.*, 1990).

CRUSTACEANS

Crustaceans are common causes of asthma in exposed workers. Many are exposed preparing these for food, such as workers extracting meat from crabs (Cartier *et al.*, 1984), prawns (Gaddie *et al.*, 1980), shrimps (Desjardins *et al.*, 1995) and lobsters (Lemiere *et al.*, 1996). Similar problems occur in some workers handling fish (Droxzcz *et al.*, 1981; Tomaszunas *et al.*, 1988).

ANIMALS

Many animals cause occupational asthma, particularly laboratory rats, mice, guinea pigs and rabbits (Newman Taylor, 1982). Cows are a common cause of occupational asthma in Finland (Virtanen *et al.*, 1996) and horses a potent antigen in veterinarians and ostlers (Dowaliby, 1992). Birds are usually non-occupational allergens but some workers develop occupational asthma from chickens and turkeys (Thelin *et al.*, 1984).

WOODS

There are a very large number of wood dusts that cause occupational asthma, the most important of which is western red cedar, the commonest identified cause of occupational asthma in western Canada (Chan-Yeung, 1982; Chan Yeung *et al.*, 1987). Apart from this, occupational asthma is more common with hardwoods than softwoods, the problem being seen usually in cabinet makers rather than building carpenters, who are exposed to larger particle dusts.

PLANTS AND PLANT PRODUCTS

Flour is the most common cause of occupational asthma in this group, being a major problem in bakers (Thiel, 1983; Musk *et al.*, 1989). Soya is a potent allergen responsible for environmental cases, but also for some cases in bakeries (Lavaud *et al.*, 1994). Many other agents have caused problems in horticulturists and market gardeners. Spices are a particular problem in those grinding and preparing them for consumption (Uragoda, 1984; Lankatilake and Uragoda, 1993).

ENZYMES

Enzymes are potent causes of asthma when they are in a form that can be inhaled. Amylase is the commonest recognized enzyme causing occupational asthma. It may be present in bakeries (Baur *et al.*, 1986; Houba *et al.*, 1996), used as a drug and in meat tenderising (Baur and Fruhmann, 1979). Enzymes derived from *Bacillus subtelis* were a problem in biological detergent manufacture but this has now largely been controlled (Juniper *et al.*, 1977; Flindt, 1996; Cathcart *et al.*, 1997).

LATEX

Health care workers are the group with the most rapidly increasing incidence of occupational asthma at present (Hunt *et al.*, 1995; Vandenplas *et al.*, 1995), and much of it is due to latex which gets into the air of ordinary hospital wards, mostly from powdered gloves. Contact urticaria and rhinitis are more common than asthma, but highly sensitized workers may have anaphylactic reactions. Latex cross-reacts with a number of foods, particularly bananas (Moller *et al.*, 1998).

COTTON

Byssinosis is an airway disease that occurs after prolonged contact with usually high levels of exposure, which has at least some of the features of asthma. Symptoms are worse at the beginning of the working week, with subsequent tolerance developing. Other workers with the same exposures develop traditional occupational asthma, without tolerance developing, and sometimes after much shorter exposures. There is also an increased risk of occupational COPD in the same group (Fishwick *et al.*, 1992, 1994).

Low molecular weight agents

ADHESIVES

Many low molecular weight allergens are reactive and adhesive in nature. The most important group are the isocyanates, which are cross-linking agents used in polyurethane manufacture (Davies, 1984). They are a particular problem in those who spray cars and aeroplanes but there are many other situations of exposure, such as in polyurethane foam manufacture and moulding, the soldering of polyurethane-coated wires, making cores for casting moulds and as surface lacquers. There is some cross-reactivity between the different isocyanates. IgE antibodies often recognize some part of the carrier protein as well as the isocyanate hapten. The acid anhydrides are less widely used but are also potent allergens, frequently sensitizing at least 5% of the workforce (Newman Taylor *et al.*, 1987). Their main use is as an epoxy resin cross-linking agent used in paints, surface coatings, encapsulating materials and adhesives. Acrylics are less common causes of occupational asthma in this group (Lozewicz *et al.*, 1985).

SOLDERING FLUXES

Soldering fluxes are common causes of occupational asthma; the principal cause being colophony present in non-corrosive electronic soldering fluxes (Burge, 1984). Acid fluxes containing ammonium chloride have also sensitized some workers (Weir *et al.*, 1989). Aminoethylethanolamine was a potent cause of occupational asthma in aluminium soldering but has now largely been replaced (Pepys and Pickering, 1972).

DRUGS

Many drugs cause occupational asthma, particularly in those who make them or sometimes in those who dispense them in bulk form (Machado *et al.*, 1979). Antibiotics are by far the commonest group (Davies *et al.*, 1974; Carlesi *et al.*, 1979; Malo and Cartier, 1988), and some workers develop extreme sensitivity to them. There is a lack of good epidemiological studies of pharmaceutical workers.

DYES

Both biological dyes such as carmine (Burge *et al.*, 1979) and small molecular weight reactive dyes cause occupational asthma (Alanko *et al.*, 1978). Reactive dyes can be used for skin-prick testing.

METALS

One of the few small molecular weight chemicals that produce positive skin-prick tests are the charged complex salts of platinum. They are some of the most potent antigens responsible for occupational asthma. In some situations at least 30% of a workforce has been affected (Venables *et al.*, 1989; Calverley *et al.*, 1995). Other metals include cobalt in hard metal (Gheysens *et al.*, 1985; Shirakawa *et al.*, 1989), chrome in electroplaters and welders of stainless steel (Keskinen *et al.*, 1980; Bright *et al.*, 1997), nickel (Malo *et al.*, 1982; Nieboer *et al.*, 1984) and zinc. Aluminium smelters have a substantial problem with occupational asthma (Kongerud and Samuelson, 1991, 1992; Soyseth and Kongerud, 1992). The exact cause of this is unclear but may be related to aluminium fluoride.

BIOCIDES AND STERILIZING AGENTS

Several of these cause occupational asthma, perhaps by altering proteins, although their exact mechanism is unknown. None sensitizes large numbers of workers in a single situation but a large number of chemically different materials have caused problems in this group including formaldehyde (Burge *et al.*, 1985), glutaraldehyde (Gannon *et al.*, 1995), chloramine (Bourne *et al.*, 1979), ethylene oxide (Deschamps *et al.*, 1992), benzalkonium chloride (Burge and Richardson, 1994), chlorhexidine (Waclawski *et al.*, 1989) and isothiazolinones (Nagorka *et al.*, 1990). They are present in many floor cleaning materials and can cause asthma in those occupying buildings where such cleaners are used.

AMINES

Many reactive amines are used as curing agents for cold-curing epoxy systems and are widely present in drugs, surface coatings and photographic chemicals. Ethylene diamine was an early recognized cause of occupational asthma (Lam and Chen-Yeung, 1980; Aldrich *et al.*, 1987). Triethylene tetramine is an important agent in this group (Fawcett *et al.*, 1977).

PROGNOSIS

It is often assumed that removing the single cause for asthma will result in complete recovery. This is rarely the case. Most studies have shown persisting asthma, particularly related to exercise and infection but sometimes also with persisting airflow obstruction in workers who have been removed from exposure (Burge, 1982; Lozewicz *et al.*, 1987; Gannon *et al.*, 1993; Cannon *et al.*, 1995; Ross and McDonald, 1998). This has been best studied in workers sensitized to western red cedar (Chan-Yeung *et al.*, 1987). Factors that predispose to a poor prognosis are a longer period between first exposure and first symptoms, a long period between first symptoms and removal from exposure, poor lung function at presentation and a dual asthmatic reaction on bronchial provocation testing. Few studies have shown any improvement in FEV$_1$ at follow-up compared with measurements made on days away from work at presentation. There is a greater improvement in non-specific responsiveness in those removed completely from exposure rather than those in whom reduced exposure continues (Burge, 1982; Chan-Yeung *et al.*, 1987). The reason for continuing symptoms is not completely clear. It may be that antigen inhaled at work persists for a long time, particularly if that antigen is combined with body proteins. The work with tetrachlorphthalic anhydride has shown that there is synthesis of specific IgE after removal from exposure, although this falls off with increasing time from last exposure (Venables *et al.*, 1987). Finally, it is possible that there is some domestic exposure to a number of common occupational allergens. Colophony is present in many domestic products such as pine oil, which is widely used as a deodorant. There may also be natural exposures in pine woods. Polyurethanes are widely used and it is possible that isocyanates are liberated either spontaneously or when they become hot, for instance in new cars. Flour is clearly in daily use in many households and the bacteria and fungi present in contaminated humidifiers are widely present in the environment. The physical reasons for the continuing symptoms in exposed workers are probably continuing bronchial inflammation (Saetta *et al.*, 1992, 1995; Maestrelli *et al.*, 1997). This has been shown in workers sensitized to western red cedar who had persisting symptoms after removal from exposure. Bronchial lavage demonstrated increased protein in the lavage, sloughing of epithelium and increase in eosinophils, all consistent with bronchial inflammation. Similar changes were present in patients with intrinsic asthma. Workers sensitized to complex salts of platinum and to laboratory animals seem to improve more than other groups; few remain symptomatic more than a year after exposure has ceased. This may be because of routine surveillance, which removed workers from exposure as soon as their skin tests to platinum salts became positive, or because exposure to these agents is rare outside the occupational situation.

ACTION ONCE THE DIAGNOSIS IS MADE

It is very easy to advise a worker to leave his or her job. However, this usually leaves the patient unemployed, a situation also associated with poor health. Once the specific cause has been found the medical advice should be to cease exposure. The most satisfactory method of doing this is to remove that particular material from the workplace so that other workers are protected from sensitization. It may be possible to remove the material completely or to substitute it for some other material that causes fewer problems. Alternatively, it may be possible to reduce exposures at work by better engineering and exhaust ventilation. Some workers need relocation within their workplace or retraining. These are all decisions that are best made by an occupational physician rather than a clinician caring for a patient. Some workers choose to remain exposed knowing the increased risks. Personal protection and drug treatment can sometimes allow this to happen in those who are not severely sensitized. However, it is likely the ultimate prognosis is less good in this situation.

PREDISPOSING FACTORS

Both personal factors and additional agents to which the worker is exposed may increase the incidence of occupational asthma. Early work concentrated on personal factors predisposing to occupational asthma, with the hope that the industrial process could remain unchanged and non-susceptible workers could be employed. This approach has not controlled occupational asthma and recent research has turned to cofactors to which the worker is also exposed. The principal determinants of sensitization still remain the levels of exposure and perhaps the duration of exposure.

Role of respiratory irritants

Some occupational sensitizers are also irritants in their own right, especially in high concentrations. This particularly applies to grain dust, which may activate the alternate pathway of complement, isocyanates, colophony, phthalic anhydride, and formaldehyde. All of these may induce sensitization at much lower concentrations in some circumstances. It may be that the irritant properties of these materials help enhance their sensitizing capability. Both colophony and plicatic acid (the main allergen in western red cedar) have been shown to cause epithelial damage in tracheal explants (Ayars et al., 1989).

The relationship between non-specific responsiveness and the threshold dose of an occupational allergen can be used to elucidate the mechanisms (irritant versus hypersensitivity). The relationship between the threshold doses of two irritants capable of inducing asthma is usually fairly close. If the threshold dose of an occupational agent required to induce asthma is closely related to non-specific responsiveness, it is likely that the mechanism is predominantly irritant. Studies of this sort show that isocyanates at levels below the occupational exposure standards do not cause irritant reactions, and that colophony may cause irritant reactions in those with the most marked non-specific reactivity (but is otherwise likely to be acting as a sensitizer) (Burge, 1982).

Cigarette smoke is likely to work as a non-specific irritant in two ways. It can both increase the incidence of sensitization (and production of specific IgE) or it can increase the incidence of asthma in sensitized workers. There are now several situations where increased sensitization has been found in cigarette smokers similarly exposed to an agent as compared to non-smokers. This particularly applies to green coffee beans (Zetterstrom et al., 1981) and tetrachlorphthalic anhydride (Newman Taylor et al., 1987). Smoking has been shown to increase occupational asthma in workers exposed to platinum salts (Venables et al., 1989) and colophony (Burge et al., 1979).

In several situations the exposure to an occupational sensitizing agent is accompanied by exposure to a known irritant. For example in the studies of platinum refiners where the allergen is a complex charged salt of platinum, the workers are also exposed to chlorine, a recognized irritant. Electronic soldering flux containing colophony as the main sensitizing agent also contains amine activators, which have been shown to be directly irritant and capable of inducing asthma (Burge, 1984). Aluminium smelters (where the precise cause of the asthma is as yet unclear) are also exposed to sulphur dioxide and hydrogen fluoride. Indeed, there is a fairly close association between fluoride exposure and asthma (Kongerud and Samuelson, 1991; Soyseth and Kongerud, 1992). However, there is good evidence that the majority of asthma in aluminium smelters is not attributed to irritant mechanisms as it is seen in workers without non-specific responsiveness.

Personal factors

The main personal factor that predisposes to asthma is atopy (a positive skin-prick test to a common environmental allergen met with in the ordinary way or the identification of specific IgE in similar circumstances). Atopic workers are at increased risk of developing sensitization to important causes of occupational asthma, including laboratory animals, biological detergents, platinum salts, green coffee beans, locusts and probably colophony. Exclusion of atopic workers (30–50% of potential recruits) has been attempted to control occupational asthma. The consequences of excluding atopics has been investigated in animal laboratory workers where 5.7 workers would have to be excluded from employment to prevent one case of occupational asthma and occupational asthma would still occur in 2% of non-atopic workers. There would be no reduction in occupational rhinitis or urticaria. The specificity of atopy is therefore insufficient to make exclusion of atopics a viable proposition in any but extreme circumstances. Indeed, the incidence of sensitization to laboratory animals has been reduced by 300% without excluding atopics, principally by reducing exposure (Botham et al., 1987). There are several other occupational sensitizing agents in which atopics are sensitized at the same rate as non-atopics. This particularly applies to isocyanates and wood dusts.

REFERENCES

Alanko K, Keskinen H, Bjorksten F, Ojanen S. (1978) Immediate-type hypersensitivity to reactive dyes. *Clin Allergy*, **8**, 25–31.

Aldrich FD, Strange AW, Geesaman RE. (1987) Smoking and ethylene diamine sensitization in an industrial population. *J Occup Med*, **29**, 311–14.

Ayars GH, Altman LC, Frazier CE, Chi EY. (1989) The toxicity of constituents of cedar and pine woods to pulmonary epithelium. *J Allergy Clin Immunol*, **83**, 610–18.

Baur X, Fruhmann G, Haug B, Rasche B, Reiher W, Weiss W. (1986) Role of Aspergillus amylase in bakers asthma. *Lancet*, **i**, 43.

Baur X, Fruhmann G. (1979) Papain-induced asthma: diagnosis by skin test, RAST and bronchial provocation test. *Clin Allergy*, **9**, 75–81.

Bernstein DI, Gallagher JS, D'Souza L, Bernstein IL. (1984) Heterogeneity of specific IgE responses in workers sensitized to acid anhydride compounds. *J Allergy Clin Immunol*, **74**, 794–801.

Blainey AD, Topping MD, Ollier S, Davies RJ. (1988) Respiratory symptoms in arable farmworkers: role of storage mites. *Thorax*, **43**, 697–702.

Botham PA, Davies GE, Teasdale EL. (1987) Allergy to laboratory animals: a prospective study of its incidence and the influence of atopy on its development. *Brit J Industr Med*, **44**, 627–32.

Bourne MS, Flindt MLH, Walker JM. (1979) Asthma due to industrial use of chloramine. *BMJ*, **ii**, 10–12.

Bright P, Burge PS, O'Hickey SP, Gannon PF, Robertson AS, Boran A. (1997) Occupational asthma due to chrome and nickel electroplating. *Thorax*, **52**, 28–32.

Bright P, Burge PS. (1995) Computer assisted interpretation of occupational peak flow plots; OASYS-N. *Eur Respir J*, **8**, 220S.

Bright P, Burge PS. (1996) The diagnosis of occupational asthma from serial measurements of lung function at and away from work. *Thorax*, **51**, 857–63.

Burge PS. (1982a) Non-specific hyperreactivity in workers exposed to toluene diisocyanate, diphenyl methane diisocyanate and colophony. *Eur J Respir Dis*, **63** (Suppl.123), S91–6.

Burge PS. (1982b) Occupational asthma in electronics workers caused by colophony fumes: follow-up of affected workers. *Thorax*, **37**, 348–53.

Burge PS. (1982c) Single and serial measurements of lung function in the diagnosis of occupational asthma. *Eur J Respir Dis*, **63** (Suppl.123), S47–59.

Burge PS. (1984) Occupational asthma, rhinitis and alveolitis due to colophony. *Clin Immunol Allergy*, **4**, 55–82.

Burge PS. (1987) Problems in the diagnosis of occupational asthma. *Brit J Dis Chest*, **81**, 105–15.

Burge PS, Edge G, O'Brien IM, Harries MG, Hawkins R, Pepys J. (1980) Occupational asthma in a research centre breeding locusts. *Clin Allergy*, **10**, 355–63.

Burge PS, Harries MG, Lam WK, O'Brien IM, Patchett P. (1985) Occupational asthma due to formaldehyde. *Thorax*, **40**, 255–60.

Burge PS, O'Brien IM, Harries MG, Pepys J. (1979) Occupational asthma due to inhaled carmine. *Clin Allergy*, **9**, 185–9.

Burge PS, O'Brien IM, Harries MG. (1979a) Peak flow rate records in the diagnosis of occupational asthma due to colophony. *Thorax*, **34**, 308–16.

Burge PS, O'Brien IM, Harries MG. (1979b) Peak flow rate records in the diagnosis of occupational asthma due to isocyanates. *Thorax*, **34**, 317–23.

Burge PS, Perks WH, O'Brien IM, *et al*. (1979) Occupational asthma in an electronics factory; a case control study to evaluate aetiological factors. *Thorax*, **34**, 300–7.

Burge PS, Richardson MN. (1994) Occupational asthma due to indirect exposure to lauryl dimethyl benzyl ammonium chloride used in a floor cleaner. *Thorax*, **49**, 842–3.

Calverley AE, Rees D, Dowdeswell RJ, Linnett PJ, Kielkowski D. (1995) Platinum salt sensitivity in refinery workers: incidence and effects of smoking and exposure. *Occup Environ Med*, **52**, 661–6.

Cannon J, Cullinan P, Newman Taylor AJ. (1995) Consequences of occupational asthma. *BMJ*, **311**, 602–3.

Carlesi G, Ferrea E, Melino C, Messineo A, Pacelli E. (1979) Aspects of occupational hygiene and epidemiology in a pharmaceutical company manufacturing amoxacillin. *Nuovi Ann Ig Microbiol*, **30**, 185–96.

Cartier A, Bernstein IL, Burge PS, *et al*. (1989) Guidelines for bronchoprovocation on the investigation of occupational asthma. *J Allergy Clin Immunol*, **84**, 823–9.

Cartier A, Grammer L, Malo J-L, *et al*. (1989) Specific serum antibodies against isocyanates: association with occupational asthma. *J Allergy Clin Immunol*, **84**, 507–14.

Cartier A, Malo J-L, Forest F, *et al*. (1984a) Occupational asthma in snow crab processing workers. *J Allergy Clin Immunol*, **74**, 261–9.

Cartier A, Pineau L, Malo J-L. (1984b) Monitoring of maximum expiratory peak flow rates and histamine inhalation tests in the investigation of occupational asthma. *Clin Allergy*, **14**, 193–6.

Cathcart M, Nicholson P, Roberts D, *et al*. (1997) Enzyme exposure, smoking and lung function in employees in the detergent industry over 20 years. Medical Subcommittee of the UK Soap and Detergent Industry Association. *Occup Med*, **47**, 473–8.

Chan-Yeung M. (1982) Immunologic and nonimmunologic mechanisms in asthma due to western red cedar (*Thuja plicata*). *J Allergy Clin Immunol*, **70**, 32–7.

Chan-Yeung M, MacLean L, Paggiaro PL. (1987) Follow-up study of 232 patients with occupational asthma caused by western red cedar (*Thuja plicata*). *J Allergy Clin Immunol*, **79**, 792–6.

Cornillon J, Touraine J-P, Lesterlin P, *et al*. (1976) Asthmatic manifestations in workers engaged in preparing nutritional proteins from oil (an allergy to *Candida tropicalis*?). *Rev Franc Allergol*, **16**, 17–23.

Cote J, Kennedy S, Chan-Yeung M. (1990) Sensitivity and specificity of PC20 and peak expiratory flow rate in cedar asthma. *J Allergy Clin Immunol*, **85**, 592–8.

Cuthbert OD, Brostoff J, Wraith DG, Brighton WD. (1979) Barn allergy, asthma and rhinitis due to storage mites. *Clin Allergy*, **9**, 229–36.

Darke CS, Knowelden J, Lacey J. (1976) Respiratory disease of workers harvesting grain. *Thorax*, **31**, 294–302.

Davies RJ. (1984) Respiratory hypersensitivity to diisocyanates. *Clin Allergy Immunol*, **4**, 103–24.

Davies RJ, Hendrick DJ, Pepys J. (1974) Asthma due to inhaled chemical agents: ampicillin,benzyl penicillin, 6-amino penicillanic acid and related substances. *Clin Allergy*, **4**, 227–47.

Deschamps D, Rosenberg N, Soler P, *et al.* (1992) Persistent asthma after accidental exposure to ethylene oxide. *Brit J Industr Med*, **49**, 523–5.

Desjardins A, Malo JL, L'Archeveque J, Cartier A, McCants M, Lehrer SB. (1995) Occupational IgE-mediated sensitization and asthma caused by clam and shrimp. *J Allergy Clin Immunol*, **96**, 608–17.

Dowaliby JM. (1992) The hoarse obstetrician – an occupational hazard. *Arch Otolaryngol Head Neck Surgery*, **118**, 343–4.

Droxzcz W, Kowalski L, Piotrowska A, Pietruszewska E. (1981) Allergy to fish in fish meal factory workers. *Int Arch Occup Environ Health*, **49**, 13–19.

Durham SR, Graneek BJ, Hawkins R, Newman Taylor AJ. (1987) The temporal relationship between increases in airway responsiveness to histamine and late asthmatic responses induced by occupational agents. *J Allergy Clin Immunol*, **79**, 398–406.

Fawcett IW, Newman Taylor AJ, Pepys J. (1977) Asthma due to inhaled chemical agents- epoxy resin systems containing phthalic acid anhydride, trimellitic acid anhydride and triethylene tetramine. *Clin Allergy*, **7**, 1–14.

Fishwick D, Fletcher AM, Pickering CAC, Niven RM, Faragher EB. (1992) Lung function, bronchial reactivity, atopic status, and dust exposure in Lancashire cotton mill operatives. *Am Rev Respir Dis*, **145**, 1103–8.

Fishwick D, Fletcher AM, Pickering CAC, Niven RM, Faragher EB. (1994) Respiratory symptoms and dust exposure in Lancashire cotton and man-made fiber mill operatives. *Am J Respir Crit Care Med*, **150**, 441–7.

Flindt ML. (1996) Biological miracles and misadventures: identification of sensitization and asthma in enzyme detergent workers. *Am J Industr Med*, **29**, 99–110.

Gaddie J, Legge J, Friend JAR, Reid TMS. (1980) Pulmonary hypersensitivity in prawn workers. *Lancet*, **ii**, 1350–3.

Gannon PF, Burge PS. (1993) The Shield scheme in the West Midlands Region, United Kingdom. Midland Thoracic Society Research Group. *Brit J Industr Med*, **50**, 791–6.

Gannon PF, Weir DC, Robertson AS, Burge PS. (1993) Health, employment, and financial outcomes in workers with occupational asthma. *Brit J Industr Med*, **50**, 491–6.

Gannon PFG, Bright P, Campbell M, O'Hickey SP, Burge PS. (1995) Occupational asthma due to glutaraldehyde and formaldehyde in endoscopy and X-ray departments. *Thorax*, **50**, 156–9.

Gannon PFG, Dickinson S, Hitchings D, Burge PS. (1993) Quality of self recorded peak expiratory flow. *Thorax*, **48**, 1062.

Gannon PFG, Newton DT, Belcher J, Pantin CF, Burge PS. (1996) Development of oasys-2: a system for the analysis of serial measurement of peak expiratory flow in workers with suspected occupational asthma. *Thorax*, **51**, 484–9.

Gannon PFG, Newton DT, Pantin CFA, Burge PS. (1998) The effect of the number of peak expiratory flow readings per day on the estimation of diurnal variation. *Thorax*, **53**, 790–2.

Gheysens B, Auwerx J, van den Eekhout A, Demedts M. (1985) Cobalt-induced bronchial asthma in diamond polishers. *Chest*, **88**, 740–4.

Harries MG, Lacey J, Tee TD, Cayley GR, Newman Taylor AJ. (1985) *Didymella exitialis* and late summer asthma. *Lancet*, **i**, 1063–6.

Houba R, Heederik DJ, Doekes G, van Run PE. (1996) Exposure–sensitization relationship for alpha-amylase allergens in the baking industry. *Am J Respir & Crit Care Med*, **154**, 130–6.

Hunt LW, Fransway AF, Reed CE, *et al.* (1995) An epidemic of occupational allergy to latex involving health care workers. *J Occup Environ Med*, **37**, 1204–9.

Iversen M, Korsgaard J, Hallas T, Dahl R. (1990) Mite allergy and exposure to storage mites and house dust mites in farmers. *Clin Exp Allergy*, **20**, 211–19.

Juniper CP, How MJ, Goodwin BFJ, Kinshott AK. (1977) *Bacillus subtilis* enzymes: a 7 year clinical, epidemiological and immunological study of an industrial allergen. *J Soc Occup Med*, **27**, 3–12.

Kanerva L, Vaheri E. (1993) Occupational allergic rhinitis in Finland. *Int Arch Occup Environ Health*, **64**, 565–8.

Keskinen H, Alanko K, Saarinen L. (1978) Occupational asthma in Finland. *Clin Allergy*, **8**, 569–79.

Keskinen H, Kalliomaki P-L, Alanko K. (1980) Occupational asthma due to stainless steel welding fumes. *Clin Allergy*, **10**, 151–9.

Kongerud J, Samuelsen SO. (1991) A longitudinal study of respiratory symptoms in aluminium potroom workers. *Am Rev Respir Dis*, **144**, 10–16.

Kongerud J, Soyseth V, Burge PS. (1992) Serial measurements of peak expiratory flow and responsiveness to methacholine in the diagnosis of aluminium potroom asthma. *Thorax*, **47**, 292–7.

Lam S, Chan-Yeung M. (1980) Ethylene-diamine induced asthma. *Am Rev Respir Dis*, **121**, 151–5.

Lander F, Jepsen JR, Gravesen S. (1988) Allergic alveolitis and late asthmatic reaction due to molds in the tobacco industry. *Allergy*, **43**, 74–6.

Lankatilake KN, Uragoda CG. (1993) Respiratory function in chilli grinders. *Occup Med*, **43**, 139–42.

Lavaud F, Perdu D, Prevost A, Vallerand H, Cossart C, Passemard F. (1994) Baker's asthma related to soybean lecithin exposure. *Allergy*, **49**, 159–62.

Lemiere C, Desjardins A, Lehrer S, Malo J-L. (1996a) Occupational asthma to lobster and shrimp. *Allergy*, **51**, 272–3.

Lemiere C, Gautrin D, Trudeau C, *et al.* (1996b) Fever and leucocytosis accompanying asthmatic reactions due to occupational agents: frequency and associated factors. *Eur Respir J*, **9**, 517–23.

Liss GM, Tarlo SM. (1991) Peak expiratory flow rates in possible occupational asthma. *Chest*, **100**, 63–9.

Lozewicz S, Asoufi BK, Hawkins R, Newman Taylor AJ. (1987) Outcome of asthma induced by isocyanates. *Brit J Dis Chest*, **81**, 14–22.

Lozewicz S, Davison AG, Hopkirk A, *et al.* (1985) Occupational asthma due to methyl methacrylate and cyanoacrylates. *Thorax*, **40**, 836–9.

Machado L, Zetterstrom O, Fagerberg E. (1979) Occupational allergy in nurses to a bulk laxative. *Allergy*, **34**, 51–5.

Maestrelli P, Saetta M, Mapp C, Fabbri LM. (1997) Mechanisms of occupational asthma. *Clin Exp Allergy*, **27** (Suppl 1), S47–54.

Malo JL, Cartier A, Doepner M, Nieboer E, Evans S, Dolovich J. (1982) Occupational asthma caused by nickel sulphate. *Clin Allergy*, **69**, 55–9.

Malo JL, Cartier A, Ghezzo H, Lafrance M, McCants M, Lehrer SB. (1988) Patterns of improvement in spirometry, bronchial hyperresponsiveness, and specific IgE antibody levels after cessation of exposure in occupational asthma caused by snow-crab processing. *Am Rev Respir Dis*, **138**, 807–12.

Malo JL, Cartier A. (1988) Occupational asthma in workers of a pharmaceutical company processing spiramycin. *Thorax*, **43**, 371–7.

Malo JL, Cote J, Cartier A, Boulet LP, L'Archeveque J, Chan-Yeung M. (1993) How many times per day should peak expiratory flow rates be assessed when investigating occupational asthma? *Thorax*, **48**, 1211–17.

Meredith SK, McDonald JC. (1994) Work-related respiratory disease in the United Kingdom, 1989-1992: report of the SWORD project. *Occup Med*, **44**, 183–9.

Meredith SK, Nordman H. (1996) Occupational asthma: measures of frequency from four countries. *Thorax*, **51**, 435–40.

Moller M, Kayma M, Vieluf D, Paschke A, Steinhart H. (1998) Determination and characterisation of cross-reacting allergens in latex, avocado, banana and kiwi fruit. *Allergy*, **53**, 289–96.

Moscato G, Godnic-Cvar J, Maestrelli P, Malo J-L, Burge PS, Coifman R. (1995) Statement on self monitoring of peak expiratory flows in the investigation of occupational asthma. *Eur Respir J*, **8**, 1605–10.

Murdoch RD, Pepys J, Hughes EG. (1986) IgE antibody responses to platinum group metals: a large scale refinery survey. *Brit J Industr Med*, **43**, 37–43.

Musk AW, Venables KM, Crook B, *et al*. (1989) Respiratory symptoms, lung function, and sensitization to flour in a British bakery. *Brit J Industr Med*, **46**, 636–42.

Nagorka R, Rosskamp E, Seidel K. (1990) Air conditioning- assessment of humidification units. *Off Gesundh-Wes*, **52**, 168–73.

Newman Taylor AJ, Venables KM, Durham SR, Graneek BJ, Topping MD. (1987) Acid anhydrides and asthma. *Int Archs Appl Immun*, **82**, 435–9.

Newman Taylor AJ, Venables KM. (1989) Asthma related to occupation of spouse. *Practitioner*, **233**, 809–10.

Newman Taylor AJ. (1982) Laboratory animal allergy. *Eur J Respir Dis*, **63** (Suppl 123), S60–4.

Nieboer E, Evans SL, Dolovich J. (1984) Occupational asthma from nickel sensitivity. ii. Factors influencing the interaction of Ni^{2+}, HSA and serum antibodies with nickel related specificity. *Brit J Industr Med*, **41**, 56–63.

Paisley DPG. (1969) Isocyanate hazard from wire insulation; an old hazard in a new guise. *Brit J Industr Med*, **26**, 79–81.

Pepys J, Pickering CAC. (1972) Asthma due to inhaled chemical fumes – aminoethylethanolamine in aluminium soldering flux. *Clin Allergy*, **2**, 197–204.

Perrin B, Lagier F, L'Archeveque J, *et al*. (1992) Occupational asthma: validity of monitoring of peak expiratory flow rates and non-allergic bronchial responsiveness as compared to specific inhalation challenge. *Eur Respir J*, **5**, 40–8.

Quirce S, Contreras G, Dybuncio A, Chan-Yeung M. (1995) Peak expiratory flow monitoring is not a reliable method for establishing the diagnosis of occupational asthma. *Am J Respir Crit Care Med*, **152**, 1100–2.

Reijula K, Haahtela T, Klaukka T, Rantanen J. (1996) Incidence of occupational asthma and persistent asthma in young adults has increased in Finland. *Chest*, **110**, 58–61.

Reilly MJ, Rosenman KD, Watt FC, *et al*. (1994) Surveillance for occupational asthma – Michigan and New Jersey, 1988–1992. *MMWR CDC Surveillance Summaries*, **43**, 9–17.

Robertson AS, Weir DC, Burge PS. (1988) Occupational asthma due to oil mists. *Thorax*, **43**, 200–5.

Ross DJ, Keynes HL, McDonald JC. (1997) SWORD '96: surveillance of work-related and occupational respiratory disease in the UK. *Occup Med*, **47**, 377–81.

Ross DJ, McDonald JC. (1998) Health and employment after a diagnosis of occupational asthma: a descriptive study. *Occup Med*, **48**, 219–25.

Ross DJ, Sallie BA, McDonald JC. (1995) SWORD '94: surveillance of work-related and occupational respiratory disease in the UK. *Occup Med*, **45**, 175–8.

Saetta M, Maestrelli P, Di Stefano A, *et al*. (1992) Effect of cessation of exposure to toluene diisocyanate (TDI) on bronchial mucosa of subjects with TDI-induced asthma. *Am Rev Respir Dis*, **145**, 169–74.

Saetta M, Maestrelli P, Turato G, *et al*. (1995) Airway wall remodeling after cessation of exposure to isocyanates in sensitized asthmatic subjects. *Am J Respir Crit Care Med*, **151**, 489–94.

Shirakawa T, Kusaka Y, Fujimura N, *et al*. (1989) Occupational asthma from cobalt sensitivity in workers exposed to hard metal dust. *Chest*, **95**, 29–37.

Slovak AJM. (1981) Occupational asthma caused by a plastics blowing agent, azodicarbonamide. *Thorax*, **36**, 906–9.

Soyseth V, Kongerud J, Aalen OO, Botten G, Boe J. (1995) Bronchial responsiveness decreases in relocated aluminum potroom workers compared with workers who continue their potroom exposure. *Int Arch Occup Environ Health*, **67**, 53–7.

Soyseth V, Kongerud J. (1992) Prevalence of respiratory disorders among aluminium potroom workers in relation to exposure to fluoride. *Brit J Industr Med*, **49**, 125–30.

Tee RD, Cullinan P, Welch J, Burge PS, Newman Taylor AJ. (1998) Specific IgE to isocyanates: A useful diagnostic role in occupational asthma. *J Allergy Clin Immunol*, **101**, 7109–15.

Thelin A, Tegler O, Rylander R. (1984) Lung reactions during poultry handling related to dust and bacterial endotoxin levels. *Eur J Respir Dis*, **65**, 266–71.

Thiel H. (1983) Baker's asthma: Epidemiological and clinical findings- needs for prospective studies. In: Kerr JW, Ganderton MA, eds. *Proceedings of invited symposia, 11th International Congress of Allergology and Clinical Immunology*. London: Macmillan, 429–33.

Tomaszunas S, Weclawik Z, Lewinski M. (1988) Allergic reactions to cuttlefish in deep-sea fishermen. *Lancet*, **1**, 1116.

Topping MD, Henderson RTS, Luczynska M, Woodmass A. (1982) Castor bean allergy among workers in the felt industry. *Allergy*, **37**, 603–8.

Topping MD, Scarisbrick DA, Luczynska CM, Clarke EC, Seaton A. (1985) Clinical and immunological reactions to *Aspergillus niger* among workers at a biotechnology plant. *Brit J Industr Med*, **42**, 312–18.

Uragoda CG. (1984) Asthma and other symptoms in cinnamon workers. *Brit J Industr Med*, **41**, 224–7.

Vandenplas O, Delwiche JP, Evrard G, *et al.* (1995) Prevalence of occupational asthma due to latex among hospital personnel. *Am J Respir Crit Care Med*, **151**, 54–60.

van Hage-Hamsten M, Johansson SGO, Zetterstrom O. (1987) Predominance of mite allergy over allergy to pollens and animal danders in a farming population. *Clin Allergy*, **17**, 417–23.

Venables KM, Dally MB, Nunn AJ, *et al.* (1989) Smoking and occupational allergy in workers in a platinum refinery. *BMJ*, **299**, 939–42.

Venables KM, Topping MD, Nunn AJ, Howe W, Newman Taylor AJ. (1987) Immunologic and functional consequences of chemical (tetrachlorphthalic anhydride)-induced asthma after four years of avoidance of exposure. *J Allergy Clin Immunol*, **80**, 212–18.

Virtanen T, Zeiler T, Rautiainen J, *et al.* (1996) Immune reactivity of cow-asthmatic dairy farmers to the major allergen of cow (BDA20) and to other cow-derived proteins. The use of purified BDA20 increases the performance of diagnostic tests in respiratory cow allergy. *Clin Exp Allergy*, **26**, 188–96.

Waclawski ER, McAlpine LG, Thomson NC. (1989) Occupational asthma in nurses due to chlorhexidine and alcohol aerosols. *BMJ*, **298**, 929–30.

Weir DC, Robertson AS, Jones S, Burge PS. (1989) Occupational asthma due to soft corrosive soldering fluxes containing zinc chloride and ammonium chloride. *Thorax*, **44**, 220–3.

Zetterstrom O, Osterman K, Machado L, Johansson SGO. (1981) Another smoking hazard: raised serum IgE concentration and increased risk of occupational allergy. *BMJ*, **283**, 1215–17.

11

β-Agonists: mode of action and place in management

ANNE E. TATTERSFIELD

THE β-RECEPTOR

The effects of β-agonists are mediated through the β-adrenoceptor (Fig. 11.1), a G protein coupled receptor containing 418 amino acids with seven transmembrane spanning domains (Strader *et al.*, 1989). β_1- and β_2-receptors were initially identified on the basis of tissue selectivity to a range of agonists (Lands *et al.*, 1967). Since then three β-adrenoceptors, β_1, β_2 and β_3-receptors, have been cloned and characterized (Frielle *et al.*, 1987; Emorine *et al.*, 1989; Strader *et al.*, 1989) and there are putative claims for a β_4-receptor in the heart (Molenaar *et al.*, 1997). Receptor binding studies show that β-receptors are widely distributed in the lungs, with the highest density being found in airway epithelium and alveoli (Carstairs *et al.*, 1985); around 70% are of the β_2-receptor subtype, the remainder being β_1-receptors. The receptors on airway and vascular smooth muscle are β_2-receptors whereas both β_1- and β_2-receptors are found on submucosal glands and alveoli (Barnes, 1995). The number of β-receptors in the lungs appears to be normal in people with mild asthma according to positron emission tomography studies (Qing *et al.*, 1997) and they may even be increased in patients dying from asthma (Bai *et al.*, 1992).

Site-directed mutagenesis studies show that β-agonists bind to residues on the third, fifth and sixth transmembrane domains of the β-receptor situated deep within the cell membrane as shown in Fig. 11.1 (Strader *et al.*, 1989; Green *et al.*, 1993; Barnes 1995). There is also evidence for an exosite on the fourth transmembrane domain where part of the salmeterol molecule anchors allowing it to stimulate the receptor repetitively (Green *et al.*, 1996). The

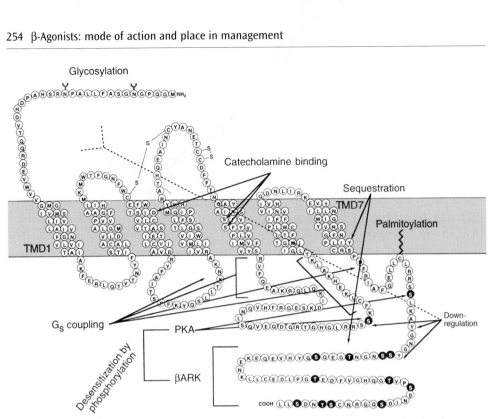

Figure 11.1 *Schematic representation of a human β₂-adrenoceptor. The figure shows the sites that are important for agonist binding, Gₛ protein coupling and regulation by protein kinase A (PKA) and β-adrenoceptor kinase (βARK). (Modified from Liggett and Green, 1997. Reproduced with permission.)*

intracellular third loop and 'tail' of the β-adrenoceptor contains phosphorylation sites that affect downregulation (Bouvier *et al.*, 1988).

Nine single base polymorphisms in the coding region of the β₂-adrenoceptor gene on chromosome 5q have been identified, though only four of these cause amino-acid substitutions – at codons 16, 27, 34 and 167 (Reihsaus *et al.*, 1993). The two most common polymorphisms involve substitutions of glycine for arginine at codon 16 and glutamine for glutamic acid at codon 27. In a general population study in Nottingham, UK, 37% and 23% of subjects were homozygous for the Gly 16 and Glu 27 polymorphisms, respectively (Dewar *et al.*, 1998). There is linkage disequilibrium between polymorphisms at codons 16 and 27, i.e. they are more likely to occur together, and this causes difficulties when trying to determine the functional effects of the individual polymorphisms (see p. 263).

β-RECEPTOR ACTIVATION

Binding of a β-agonist to the active binding sites on the β-adrenoceptor causes conformational changes to the associated stimulatory G protein (Gₛ), thereby releasing GDP and allowing GTP to bind to the α subunit of Gₛ (Fig. 11.2) The α subunit of Gₛ then dissociates from the β-receptor and activates adenylate cyclase, which catalyzes the conversion of ATP to the second messenger, cyclic 3′,5′-AMP (Barnes 1995; Dessauer *et al.*, 1996). Cyclic AMP in turn mediates a number of effects through activation of protein kinase A (PKA), an enzyme with several actions that reduce intracellular calcium concentrations as shown in Fig. 11.2. This causes smooth muscle relaxation and inhibition of mediator release from inflammatory

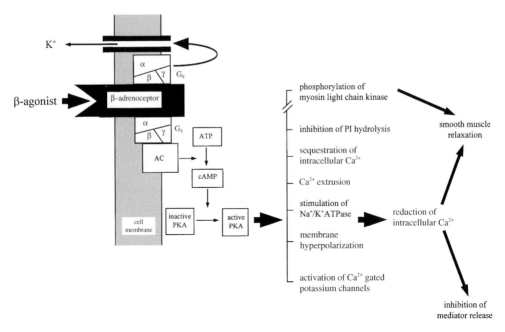

Figure 11.2   *Schematic representation of the signalling pathway following stimulation of the β-receptor, which causes coupling to the G_s protein and stimulation of adenylate cyclase (AC). This causes increased accumulation of cyclic-AMP (cAMP) and protein kinase A (PKA) and a fall in intracellular calcium. The most important cellular effects for asthma are smooth muscle relaxation and inhibition of mediator release from inflammatory cells. For other effects, see text.*

cells (Torphy and Hall, 1994; Knox and Tattersfield, 1995). Most of the effects of β-agonists are mediated via cyclic AMP and activation of protein kinase A, but some, such as the opening of maxi K^+ channels, can also occur due to a direct effect of the G_s α subunit (Kume *et al.*, 1994).

Protein kinase A is also able to phosphorylate and activate the cyclic AMP response element binding protein, a transcription factor known as CREB. By binding to the cyclic AMP response element (CRE) on the promoter region of target genes, CREB is able to cause gene transcription, including transcription of the β-receptor gene (Barnes, 1995). Thus stimulation by a β-agonist may increase $β_2$-receptor expression transiently, though this is not maintained. CREB also interacts with other transcription factors within the nucleus, including some that are associated with inflammation, such as activating protein (AP 1) and nuclear factor κB (NFκB).

REGULATION OF β-RECEPTOR NUMBERS AND ACTIVITY

The number of β-adrenoceptors in the airways depends on the rates at which they are synthesized and degraded; their function also depends on the extent to which they are coupled to the catalytic unit. Both receptor numbers and function are modified by β-agonists and by various other factors, of which cytokines and corticosteroids are particularly relevant to asthma. The pro-inflammatory cytokine, interleukin 1β has been shown to attenuate β-receptor responsiveness by uncoupling the receptor from its catalytic unit (Koto *et al.*, 1996), possibly by the induction of COX-2, the inducible form of cyclooxygenase, and release of inhibitory prostanoids (Pang *et al.*, 1998). Corticosteroids have a number of effects *in vitro* which may increase or decrease the response to a β-agonist. They are able to increase β-receptor numbers by inhibiting downregulation of β-receptors (Mak *et al.*, 1995b) and by increasing β-receptor gene transcription (Mak *et al.*, 1995a; Baraniuk *et al.*, 1997). The activity of CREB can, however, be inhibited by glucocorticoid transcription factors (Adcock *et al.*, 1995), thus providing a possible mechanism whereby glucocorticoids might reduce the efficacy of a β-agonist.

Effect of β-agonist exposure

With repeated or continuous exposure to a β-agonist there is a reduction in the response, a phenomenon known as desensitization or tolerance. Several mechanisms appear to underlie the development of tolerance to β-agonists.

1 *Receptor uncoupling.* Exposure to a β-agonist causes phosphorylation of sites on the third intracellular loop and tail of the β-adrenoceptor causing the β-receptor to become uncoupled from its G_s protein and catalytic unit (*see* Fig. 11.1). At least two kinases, the cyclic AMP-dependent protein kinase A and the G protein dependent β-adrenergic receptor kinase (βARK), are involved (Lefkowitz *et al.*, 1990) and protein kinase G may also contribute (Barnes, 1995). PKA is activated by fairly low concentrations of β-agonist, as seen with therapeutic drug doses, whereas activation of βARK requires higher concentrations of agonist and a cofactor, β-arrestin. βARK causes homologous β-receptor desensitization, i.e. to β-agonists only, whereas PKA causes heterologous desensitization so that the response to other agonists that use the same catalytic unit, e.g. forskolin, is reduced. Receptor uncoupling occurs within minutes and is rapidly reversible
2 *Sequestration of receptors.* Exposure to β-agonists may also cause β-receptors to be internalized within the cell, thereby causing desensitization. The receptors are sequestered temporarily into vesicles and can then be recycled to the cell surface. This also can occur within minutes and is again reversible.
3 *Downregulation.* With longer term exposure to β-agonists, β-receptors may be internalized and degraded and not then available for recycling. Receptor numbers may also be lower as a result of a reduction in β-receptor mRNA following continuous exposure (Hadcock and Malbon, 1988). Polymorphisms at codons 16 and 27 affect β-adrenoceptor downregulation *in vitro*, with receptors that have the Gly 16 polymorphism showing increased downregulation and those with the Glu 27 polymorphism being protected against downregulation (Green *et al.*, 1995).

PHARMACOKINETICS OF β-AGONISTS

Catecholamines

Catecholamines are well absorbed from the buccal mucosa and lung but almost completely conjugated and inactivated following ingestion. They have a relatively short half-life, being removed by two active uptake mechanisms and metabolized by two widely distributed enzymes, catechol-*O*-methyl transferase (COMT) and monoamine oxidase (MAO).

The action of adrenaline and noradrenaline, but not isoprenaline, is terminated by uptake into sympathetic nerve terminals, known as Uptake 1, which is inhibited by amphetamine, cocaine and imipramine. Catecholamines including isoprenaline are taken into non-neuronal tissue such as smooth muscle cells where metabolic degradation occurs, by a process, known as Uptake 2, which is inhibited by corticosteroids.

The main metabolic pathway for catecholamines is 3-O-methylation of the catechol nucleus by COMT and cleavage of the sympathomimetic amine between the α-carbon atom and the amine group by MAO. Although COMT is generally more important, MAO is clearly making a significant contribution, as dangerous hypertension can occur in patients on monoamine oxidase inhibitors following administration of tyramine-containing food or drugs such as ephedrine which release noradrenaline from sympathetic nerve endings. The metabolic products of catecholamines are excreted in the urine.

Non-catecholamines

Salbutamol is well absorbed from the buccal mucosa and lung and in steady-state studies roughly half was unchanged and half converted to the sulphate conjugate during first pass metabolism (Morgan et al., 1986). Oral absorption of terbutaline may be more variable but most of the absorbed drug is conjugated. The drugs are largely excreted in urine unchanged or as inactive conjugates. The longer-acting β_2-agonists formoterol fumarate and salmeterol xinafoate are well absorbed from the lung and gut. Following oral administration formoterol is largely metabolized to the glucoronide, which is mainly excreted in urine. Oral salmeterol is hydroxylated in the liver and eliminated predominantly in faeces (Dollery, 1999).

Non-catecholamines have a longer half-life than catecholamines because they are not taken up by either uptake mechanisms, and are resistant to COMT and usually to deamination by MAO.

Most of the systemic effects of inhaled β-agonists in current use are a consequence of absorption from the lungs. Peak drug levels in blood and marked systemic effects are seen within minutes following inhalation of high doses of β-agonists (Collier et al., 1980; Bennett and Tattersfield, 1997; Lecaillon et al., 1999). Studies using oral charcoal suggest that two-thirds of the systemic effects from high doses of salmeterol inhaled from a metered dose inhaler result from drug absorbed from the lung (Bennett et al., 1999).

DIFFERENCES BETWEEN β-AGONISTS

Partial or full agonists

Some β_2-selective agonists, such as salmeterol and to a lesser extent salbutamol and terbutaline, are partial agonists in vitro compared to isoprenaline, fenoterol and formoterol which are full agonists. Being a partial agonist could be important for two reasons. First the bronchodilator response to a partial agonist would be smaller than that to a full agonist if there were no spare receptors and assuming bronchodilatation was limited by the extent of airway smooth muscle relaxation. There is, however, no evidence that the maximal airway response to any of the drugs with partial agonist activity is reduced in vivo relative to that seen with the full agonists (Barnes and Pride 1983; Wong et al., 1990). The second reason is that a partial agonist must also be a partial antagonist since by occupying receptors it reduces access to drugs with fuller agonist activity. Salmeterol, for example, as a partial agonist with a long duration of action could limit the efficacy of salbutamol, a fuller agonist, if this was given during an acute attack of asthma. Salmeterol has not, however, inhibited the maximum airway response achieved following inhaled salbutamol in studies of patients with stable asthma (Smyth et al., 1993; Grove and Lipworth, 1995). This is reassuring, although an interaction in acute asthma – the situation where such an effect is most likely to occur – has not been studied.

Speed of onset and duration of action

Most β-agonists have a rapid onset of action following inhalation, achieving somewhere around 70% of maximum bronchodilatation within 5 minutes. Salmeterol has a slower onset of action taking 15 to 20 minutes to achieve 70% maximum bronchodilatation (van Noord *et al.*, 1996; Palmqvist *et al.*, 1997). The slower onset with salmeterol is attributed to its greater lipophilicity which makes it more soluble in the cell membrane lipid bilayer and thus less available to the receptor.

The duration of action of all β-agonists increases with increasing dose. β-Agonists can nevertheless be divided into three broad groups according to their duration of action following inhalation of conventional doses:

- the catecholamines, isoprenaline and rimiterol, which have a very short action of one to two hours;
- those conventionally described as short-acting such as salbutamol and terbutaline which are active for three to six hours; fenoterol may have a slightly shorter action;
- the long-acting β-agonists salmeterol and formoterol which cause bronchodilatation for at least 12 hours.

Although both salmeterol and formoterol are lipophilic and hence taken up into the lipid cell membrane, the mechanisms underlying their long duration of action may differ. Salmeterol is a long molecule and site-directed mutagenesis studies suggest that it anchors to an exosite on the fourth transmembrane domain of the β-receptor (Green *et al.*, 1996) although this has been disputed (Teschemacher and Lemoine, 1999). Formoterol is thought to remain in the cell wall from which it diffuses slowly to stimulate the β-receptor over a prolonged period (Anderson, 1993).

Bronchial selectivity

All β-agonists currently used to treat asthma are β_2-selective *in vitro* compared to isoprenaline. A functional measure of bronchial selectivity can be obtained *in vivo* by comparing the airway response to a β-agonist (β_2 effect) with the heart rate response (β_1 and β_2 effects). Bronchial selectivity will be affected by factors other than the drug's β_2-selectivity such as homeostatic mechanisms and pharmacokinetic factors, but it reflects the selectivity of β-agonists as used in clinical practice. Such studies suggest that salbutamol, terbutaline, formoterol and salmeterol have broadly similar bronchial selectivity and that fenoterol has slightly less (Löfdahl and Svedmyr, 1989; Wong *et al.*, 1990; Bremner *et al.*, 1993; Bennett and Tattersfield, 1997).

CHIRALITY OF β-AGONISTS

Like many drugs, β-agonists are administered as racemic mixtures consisting of two stereoisomers (or enantiomers) only one of which, the *R*-isomer is pharmacologically active (Ind, 1997). The *S*-isomer was assumed to be inactive until animal studies suggested that it might have deleterious effects. Metabolism is stereoselective, with the *S*-isomer being cleared more slowly than the active isomer (Fawcett and Taylor, 1999). This raised the possibility that a deleterious effect from the *S*-isomer might be responsible for the rebound increase in bronchial responsiveness seen in clinical studies when the bronchodilator effect of β-agonists wears off. This hypothesis was difficult to test until the individual isomers were available for use in man, but some results have now been published for salbutamol. Two relatively small studies found no evidence that the *S*-isomer of salbutamol caused adverse effects or that the racemic mixture was less beneficial than the *R*-isomer administered in half the dose (Cockcroft and Swystun, 1997; Lipworth *et al.*, 1997). In a larger parallel group study, patients taking racemic salbutamol showed a slightly smaller bronchodilator response than those taking the *R*-isomer on entry and after 4 weeks treatment but whether this was due to differences between groups or between isomers is not clear (Nelson *et al.*, 1998).

CLINICAL PHARMACOLOGY OF β-AGONISTS

This section describes the pharmacological actions of β-agonists that are relevant to asthma (*see* Table 11.1).

Airways

β-Agonists have several actions that may affect airway function. The extent to which each contributes to the airway response is uncertain and is likely to differ in different circumstances. The main actions are:

1 *Smooth muscle relaxation.* β_2-Agonists are described as functional antagonists as they antagonize the effects of a wide variety of bronchoconstrictor agents on airway smooth muscle *in vitro* and *in vivo*.
2 *Inhibition of mediator release from inflammatory cells.* β-Agonists inhibit the release of histamine from sensitized human lungs (Assem and Schild, 1969), basophils (Marone *et al.*, 1979) and mast cells (Peters *et al.*, 1982) and they inhibit cytokine gene expression in T lymphocytes (Borger *et al.*, 1998). They also inhibit the increase in various circulating mediators that occur in response to antigen challenge in patients with asthma (Howarth *et al.*, 1985).
3 *Inhibition of cholinergic neurotransmission.* β-Agonists inhibit cholinergic neurotransmission *in vitro* (Skoogh, 1983). This suggests a possible mechanism to explain how

Table 11.1 *Distribution and function of β-adrenergic subtypes that may be relevant to patients with asthma*

Tissue	Receptor	Response
Airways	β_2	Bronchodilatation, reduction in mediator release from mast cells, increased mucus production, increased ciliary activity
Heart	β_1 / β_2 ? β_4	Tachycardia, inotropic action
Blood vessels	β_2	Dilatation, fall in blood pressure, compensatory reflex increase in heart rate
Uterus	β_2	Relaxation
Metabolic	β_2 / β_3	Increase in glucose, insulin, lactate, pyruvate, non-esterified fatty acids, glycerol and ketone bodies; decrease in potassium, phosphate, calcium and magnesium; increase in oxygen uptake, carbon dioxide production and ventilation
Muscle	β_2	Tremor

β-blocking drugs cause bronchoconstriction in patients with asthma, in view of the paucity of sympathetic nerves in the vicinity of airway smooth muscle (Barnes, 1989).

4   *Reduced vascular permeability.* Although β-agonists can reduce permeability and oedema in response to mediators such as histamine and leukotrienes in animals, this is not a consistent finding (Chung *et al.*, 1990) and the relevance of these observations to therapeutic doses of β-agonists in asthma is uncertain.

5   *Changes to mucociliary clearance and function.* Mucociliary clearance is increased with β-agonists probably as a result of increased ciliary beat frequency and increased production of periciliary cytosol (Wanner *et al.*, 1996). There is some evidence *in vitro* to suggest that salmeterol may protect against cell damage from *Pseudomonas aeruginosa* infection of the respiratory mucosa (Dowling *et al.*, 1997).

β$_2$-Agonists cause bronchodilatation in patients with airflow obstruction. Most normal patients also respond to a β$_2$-agonist with an increase in airway conductance or flow rates from a partial flow volume curve; however, measurements such as the FEV$_1$ which involve a full inflation do not usually change, owing to the overriding effects of inflation on airway and parenchymal hysteresis (Pride *et al.*, 1991).

β$_2$-Agonists also cause marked protection against all non-specific constrictor stimuli such as histamine, methacholine, eucapnic hyperventilation and exercise in patients with asthma. For example, a single large dose of an inhaled β$_2$-agonist usually causes an acute shift in the dose–response curve to histamine or methacholine, such that two to four more doubling doses of stimulus can be given before the same degree of bronchoconstriction occurs (Tattersfield, 1987). When given prior to an allergen challenge, all β$_2$-agonists inhibit the early response to allergen. The late response is inhibited by the long-acting β$_2$-agonists and by high doses of the shorter-acting β-agonists (Twentyman *et al.*, 1990, 1991; Wong *et al.*, 1992). It was thought initially that the inhibitory effect of the long-acting β$_2$-agonists was due to an antiinflammatory action but it now seems more likely that it is due to their longer bronchodilator action, causing more prolonged functional antagonism (Wong *et al.*, 1992).

Cardiac effects

β-Agonists cause tachycardia due to stimulation of cardiac β$_1$- and β$_2$-receptors and secondary compensatory effects following β$_2$-mediated vasodilatation. When autonomic dysfunction prevents compensatory changes, as in quadriplegic patients, β$_2$-agonists cause a large fall in systemic vascular resistance and blood pressure despite an increase in cardiac output (Pingleton *et al.*, 1982). Tachycardia and palpitations occur less often with β$_2$-selective agonists particularly when given by the inhaled route but they can occur with systemic therapy and with higher inhaled doses (Wong *et al.*, 1990; Bennett and Tattersfield, 1997) as shown in Fig. 11.3. The extent to which β-agonists may precipitate dysrhythmias is more controversial (see below). β-agonists cause a small fall in pulmonary artery pressure in patients with asthma (Wagner *et al.*, 1978).

Arterial oxygen tension and carbon dioxide production

By increasing cardiac output and hence increasing mixed venous oxygen tension, β-agonists may cause arterial oxygen tension (PaO_2) to rise; PaO_2 quite often falls following a β-agonist, however, as a result of pulmonary vasodilatation causing increased perfusion of poorly ventilated areas. Blood flow to areas with a low ventilation/perfusion ratio doubled following

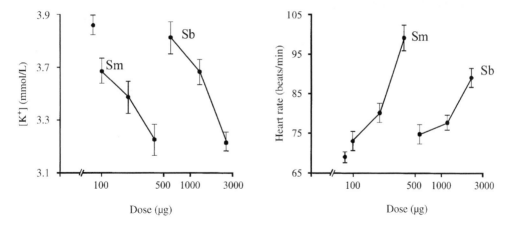

Figure 11.3   *Dose–response curves showing mean maximum changes in heart rate and serum potassium concentration with increasing doses of inhaled salmeterol (Sm) and salbutamol (Sb) in healthy persons. There was little change in either measure with recommended doses but the relatively steep dose–response curve indicates that both drugs have only a modest therapeutic window. (From Bennett and Tattersfield, 1997, with permission from BMJ publishers.)*

isoprenaline in inert gas studies (Wagner *et al.*, 1978). The fall in PaO_2 is usually small, around 0.5 kPa (3–4 mmHg), although occasional patients show larger changes.

High doses of β_2-agonists increase carbon dioxide production and oxygen consumption and thus increase ventilatory requirements. The increase in ventilation is probably due to several factors, including an increase in tremor, which increases metabolism, and an increase in cardiac output, which increases carbon dioxide excretion (Tattersfield and Wilding, 1993). In a study in normal individuals, 1200 µg inhaled salbutamol increased ventilation by 25% (Amoroso *et al.*, 1993) and, although tolerance developed with regular treatment (Wilson *et al.*, 1993), an increased ventilatory requirement could be an important negative effect for patients with limited capacity to increase their ventilation.

Metabolic changes

β_2-Agonists cause a wide range of metabolic changes (Harvey *et al.*, 1981) but these rarely cause problems apart from the fall in serum potassium. The fall has been up to 0.9 mmol/L with conventional single doses of β-agonist by the inhaled or parenteral route (Scheinin *et al.*, 1987), though larger changes are seen in some patients with higher doses (Wong *et al.*, 1990; Bennett and Tattersfield, 1997) *see* Fig. 11.3. The extent to which these acute changes are sustained with long-term treatment is uncertain. Ketoacidosis has been precipitated by β-agonists in diabetic patients (Leslie and Coats, 1977).

Other adverse effects

A fine tremor can be a nuisance with β-agonists particularly when given orally or in high doses by nebulizer; it tends to decrease with prolonged treatment as tolerance develops. Cramp occurs occasionally with β-agonists and headaches may occur with higher doses.

TOLERANCE TO β-AGONISTS

With regular use patients might be expected to develop tolerance to the effects of β-agonists as a clinical corollary of the β-receptor desensitization and downregulation seen with continuous exposure to a β-agonist *in vitro*. Some early retrospective evidence had suggested that this might occur in patients taking extremely high doses of isoprenaline, up to an inhaler a day (van Metre, 1969; Reisman, 1970) and the idea gained impetus as a possible explanation for the epidemic of asthma deaths in the 1960s. This stimulated a large number of studies, the results of which can be summarized as follows:

- *Effects on inflammatory cells.* There is evidence of functional desensitization of human lung mast cells *in vitro* (Chong *et al.*, 1995) and lymphocytes *ex vivo* (Hauck *et al.*, 1990) with prolonged exposure to a β-agonist. The study by Hauck *et al.* (1990) was undertaken in patients undergoing lung resection who inhaled terbutaline prior to surgery. In contrast to the findings in lymphocytes, there was no downregulation of β_2-receptors in human lung tissue. Care is needed therefore in extrapolating changes in β-receptor numbers from one tissue to another.
- *Tolerance to their systemic effects.* Following regular treatment many studies have shown a reduction in the tremor, heart rate, metabolic and ventilatory response to a β-agonist in asthmatic and non-asthmatic people (Larrson *et al.*, 1977; Harvey *et al.*, 1981; Lipworth *et al.*, 1989; Wilson *et al.*, 1993).
- *Tolerance to their bronchodilator effect.* Most early studies in patients with asthma did not show a reduced bronchodilator response to the short-acting β-agonists following regular β-agonist treatment (Tattersfield, 1985) and this appeared to contrast with the findings in normals (Holgate *et al.*, 1977). Some recent studies have shown some reduction in the bronchodilator response, particularly to formoterol (Yates *et al.*, 1995; Tan *et al.*, 1997). In the year-long study of regular formoterol (FACET) there was a small early reduction in the bronchodilatation seen with formoterol but the response then remained stable for the rest of the year (Pauwels *et al.*, 1997). Whether there is a true difference between different β-agonists in their ability to produce bronchodilator tolerance is not clear, though it is possible that full agonists such as formoterol are more likely to show such an effect. The FACET study shows that most of the bronchodilator effect of formoterol is maintained long term, however.
- *Tolerance to their bronchoprotective effects.* The protective effect of β-agonists against constrictor stimuli is reduced following regular treatment with both the short-acting and long-acting β_2-agonists. The loss of protection has been documented with histamine, methacholine, AMP, antigen and exercise (Vathenen *et al.*, 1988; Cheung *et al.*, 1992; O'Connor *et al.*, 1992; Cockcroft *et al.*, 1993; Wahedna *et al.*, 1993; Nelson *et al.*, 1998) and is presumed to occur with all constrictor stimuli.
- *Rebound increase in bronchial responsiveness.* A rebound increase in bronchial responsiveness has been seen 12 to 59 hours after cessation of treatment with a short-acting β_2-agonist in several studies (Kraan *et al.*, 1985; Vathenen *et al.*, 1988; Cockcroft *et al.*, 1993, 1995; Wahedna *et al.*, 1993). This is likely to be a consequence of β-receptor desensitization or downregulation causing a reduced response to, and protection afforded by, endogenous sympathetic drive once the bronchodilator effect of the β-agonist has worn off. In some studies the increase in bronchial responsiveness has been associated with a fall in FEV_1 (van Arsdel *et al.*, 1978; Trembath *et al.*, 1979; Harvey and Tattersfield, 1982; Wahedna *et al.*, 1993). This rebound effect has not been seen following salmeterol or formoterol, possibly because their effect wanes more gradually, allowing the β-receptor more time to recover.

Given that susceptibility to β-receptor downregulation *in vitro* is determined by β-receptor polymorphisms, it was anticipated that patients with the Gly 16 polymorphism would show more tolerance to β-agonists when taken regularly and those with the Glu 27 polymorphism would show less tolerance (see p. 257), but there is limited evidence for this as yet. In one study, patients with the Gly 16 polymorphism showed a greater reduction in the bronchodilator response to formoterol following regular treatment as anticipated (Tan *et al.*, 1997). However, in a further study, change in bronchial responsiveness to methacholine following regular terbutaline and formoterol was unrelated to either polymorphism (Lipworth *et al.*, 1999). Data from the Sears study (Sears *et al.*, 1990) have now been analysed in relation to β_2-receptor polymorphisms. Although the asthma deterioration seen with regular fenoterol overall showed no relationship to β-receptor polymorphisms, the increase in bronchial responsiveness to methacholine was less in patients with the Gly 16 polymorphism and the increase in evening peak flow was less in those with the Glu 27 polymorphism (Hancox *et al.*, 1998); both findings are the opposite of those expected from the studies *in vitro*.

CLINICAL STUDIES OF INHALED β-AGONISTS

The selective β_2-agonists work rapidly when given by inhalation and this route of administration allows higher doses to be deposited in the airways with less systemic absorption and fewer adverse effects. The intravenous route may be used for acute severe asthma if it responds poorly to nebulized β-agonists. The use of β-agonists administered by the oral, subcutaneous and intramuscular routes are discussed briefly at the end of the chapter.

The short-acting β-agonists have a different role in the management of asthma from the long-acting β-agonists and the two are considered separately. The balance of efficacy and adverse effects from β-agonists varies according to the indications for their use and are summarized for the different indications below.

SHORT-ACTING INHALED β-AGONISTS

There are four potential indications for the shorter-acting β-agonists such as salbutamol and terbutaline in the treatment of asthma: to treat acute asthma; for symptomatic relief; to prevent bronchoconstriction, e.g. exercise-induced asthma; and as regular treatment.

Acute severe asthma

High doses of short-acting β-agonists are one of the mainstays of treatment for acute severe asthma. Most guidelines recommend that they be given by a nebulizer in the first instance and most patients respond to the combination of nebulized β-agonists, oxygen and oral or intravenous corticosteroids. When given in recommended doses few patients complain of adverse effects from nebulized β-agonists although the same doses given to patients when stable not infrequently produce tremor and palpitations. There is some uncertainty about the optimum dose in acute asthma, which will produce maximum bronchodilatation with minimal systemic effects. An excessive dose of β-agonists is likely to increase metabolism and carbon dioxide production and thus increase ventilatory requirements (Amoroso *et al.*, 1993). In practice an initial dose of 5 mg salbutamol or 10 mg terbutaline four-hourly is satisfactory for most patients, reducing to half the dose once the patient starts to improve. Dysrhythmias and significant hypokalaemia are potential serious adverse effects but both are rare with recommended doses and the benefits of β-agonists in acute asthma far outweigh the risks. Nevertheless patients having high doses of β-agonists, particularly when taken in conjunction with corticosteroids and theophylline, should have their serum potassium monitored.

Many studies have found that β-agonists are at least as effective when given by nebulizer as by the intravenous route (Salmeron et al., 1994). Others have found a faster increase in peak flow with intravenous β-agonists although the doses used usually cause an appreciably greater increase in heart rate. In a study of 76 patients the mean difference in heart rate four hours after allocation to intravenous or nebulized β-agonist was 18 beats per minute (Cheong et al., 1988). Because intravenous β-agonists are more likely to cause adverse effects, they should be reserved for patients not responding to nebulized treatment.

For relief of symptoms

β_2-agonists are widely used for occasional relief of symptoms. They are extremely effective for this purpose and when taken in conventional doses of one or two puffs from an inhaler they rarely cause adverse effects. The benefit very clearly outweighs any adverse effects in this situation.

To prevent bronchoconstriction

The short-acting β_2-agonists are widely used to prevent exercise-induced asthma and occasionally to prevent asthma that is anticipated in certain situations, e.g. going out on a cold, windy day or prior to exposure to allergen. The short-acting β-agonists are very effective in this situation although they are likely to be less effective when taken regularly (Cockcroft et al., 1993, 1995). There is a potential danger that patients might use a β-agonist instead of trying to avoid an allergen to which they are sensitive but there is little evidence to suggest that this happens in practice. Again the benefits of using short-acting β-agonists as preventative treatment far outweigh any occasional risk or adverse effect. It is also preferable that patients use a β-agonist and take part in exercise rather than avoid activities that might cause bronchoconstriction.

As regular treatment

Although many patients take β-agonists regularly this is the indication for which there is least evidence of efficacy and most evidence of risk.

EFFICACY

It was widely assumed until the last few years that because β_2-agonists were clearly effective when given for acute attacks of asthma, their use on a regular basis must also be beneficial. This view was challenged in 1990 when Sears et al. reported the results of a 6-month cross-over study comparing regular fenoterol (400 μg qid) with placebo in patients with asthma. Using a composite predetermined hierarchical score they found that more patients were worse during the fenoterol period, with lower FEV_1 and morning peak flow rates, more symptoms, increased steroid use and shorter time to relapse (Sears et al., 1990). Since then a further nine studies at least have compared the effect of treating asthma with regular salbutamol or placebo for periods ranging from 2 to 52 weeks. Of the ten studies, two showed some deterioration with the β-agonist compared with placebo in terms of asthma control (Sears et al., 1990;

Taylor *et al.*, 1998), three showed no difference (Pearlman *et al.*, 1992; D'Alonzo *et al.*, 1994; Drazen *et al.*, 1996) and five showed some benefit from regular salbutamol for some end points (Chapman *et al.*, 1994; Juniper *et al.*, 1995; Apter *et al.*, 1996; Leblanc *et al.*, 1996; Hancox *et al.*, 1999), though one study was only 2 weeks long (Chapman *et al.*, 1994) and the study looking at quality of life concluded that the differences were clinically unimportant (Juniper *et al.*, 1995). All the differences that have been seen between placebo and short-acting β-agonists in the different studies have been small and could easily be explained by differences in methodology and/or in duration of treatment.

In a different approach to the same question we randomized patients taking high doses of β-agonist to maintaining the high dose or replacing it with placebo, but allowing all patients to take a β-agonist as needed (Harrison *et al.*, 1999). Patients randomized to placebo were able to reduce the dose of β-agonist by 80% (Fig. 11.4) without loss of asthma control but also with no improvement although they were slightly more responsive to β-agonists.

Some studies have compared short-acting β-agonists with other medication. Treatment with regular salbutamol for 4 weeks proved to be less effective than nedocromil in one study (Wasserman *et al.*, 1995) and regular terbutaline was considerably less effective than inhaled budesonide for symptom control, morning peak flow rate and need for supplemental β-agonists in both children (van Essen-Zandvliet *et al.*, 1992) and adults (Haahtela *et al.*, 1991). In Haahtela's study (1991) almost half the adults treated with regular terbutaline withdrew during the two-year study or had to add theophylline to their treatment.

Taking all these studies together there appears to be little benefit in taking a short-acting β-agonist regularly. It seems sensible to encourage patients to take their β-agonist as and when required, on the grounds that the β-agonist might then be more effective when needed.

SAFETY

Despite the millions of puffs of β_2-agonist that are inhaled everyday, the incidence of documented side-effects from inhaled β_2-agonists is extremely low. The main problems reported are tremor, headache, palpitations, flushing and occasionally cramp. Hypokalaemia may also occur.

The main concern with β-agonists relates to their possible role in the epidemics of asthma deaths in the 1960s (Inman and Adelstein, 1969; Stolley, 1972) and subsequently in New Zealand (Jackson *et al.*, 1982). The 1960s' epidemic was associated with increased use of a non-selective β-agonist, isoprenaline, and the New Zealand epidemic with the less β_2-selective β-agonist, fenoterol. Both drugs were marketed in doses that were high and which caused more systemic effects than comparable doses of β_2-selective drugs such as salbutamol (Warrell *et al.*, 1970; Crane *et al.*, 1989a; Wong *et al.*, 1990; Bremner *et al.*, 1993). In the 1960s there was

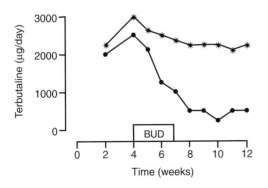

Figure 11.4 *Change in β-agonist use in asthmatic patients previously taking high doses of β-agonist regularly, after randomization to placebo (●) or to continue with a β-agonist (✳). Both groups were allowed β-agonists for relief medication. Patients randomized to placebo were able to reduce the dose of β-agonist by 80% without loss of asthma control (data not shown). (From Harrison et al., 1999, with permission from BMJ publishers.) BUD, budesonide.*

a temporal association between the increase in asthma deaths and increased sales of high-dose isoprenaline (*see* Fig. 11.5) and a geographical association with countries that had the high-dose formulations (Stolley, 1972). Three case–control studies in New Zealand suggested that patients dying from asthma were more likely to have received fenoterol than salbutamol (Crane *et al.*, 1989b; Pearce *et al.*, 1990; Granger *et al.*, 1991) though whether the relation was related to an adverse effect of fenoterol or to the selective use of fenoterol in patients with more severe asthma is still debated. Further non-epidemic data from Saskatchewan (Spitzer *et al.*, 1992) showed a dose–response relation between β-agonist usage and life-threatening attacks of asthma, but this may merely reflect the fact that patients with more severe asthma are likely to take more β-agonists and also more likely to die. Such an explanation does not however explain why there were epidemics of asthma deaths in countries marketing high-dose β-agonist preparations.

Serious adverse effects are clearly very rare with the currently used shorter-acting β-agonists but they could nevertheless be important. For example, if β-agonists caused a fatal outcome in 1 in 8000 patients using the drug regularly it would never be detected in a prospective trial but would account for half of the UK asthma deaths in those under the age 55. It seems unlikely that the association of both epidemics with the use of high doses of relatively unselective β-agonists is coincidental and more probable that the β-agonists were causally related to the 1960s epidemic and, in part at least, to the more recent epidemic in New Zealand.

If β-agonists were responsible for the epidemics of asthma deaths and possibly for some deaths at other times, what are the underlying mechanisms? Several suggestions have been made with three main hypotheses:

- *Excess reliance on β-agonists.* It has been argued that because β-agonists give good symptomatic relief, patients might rely too heavily on their β-agonists and take insufficient prophylactic treatment. Apart from oral steroids the additional treatment available in the 1960s was not very effective, consisting mainly of theophylline preparations. Nor does this hypothesis explain why New Zealand alone should have run into a second epidemic in the 1970s. Inadequate and/or inappropriate treatment undoubtedly underlies many asthma deaths but it does not explain why the epidemics occurred.

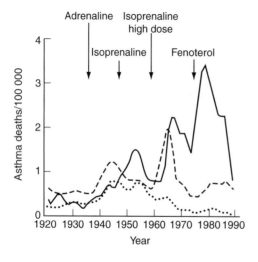

Figure 11.5 *Change in asthma mortality (age 5–34) since 1920 in three countries, one of which (the Netherlands) did not have high-dose preparations of isoprenaline. The figure demonstrates the changes in mortality in relation to the introduction of high-dose preparations of isoprenaline in the UK and New Zealand and fenoterol in New Zealand and the lack of epidemics in the Netherlands. (From Blauw and Westendorp, 1995, with permission from* The Lancet.*)*

- *Tolerance to β-agonists.* Tolerance may cause a reduction in the bronchodilator response to a β-agonist or a loss of protection against constrictor stimuli (see p. 262). Patients who had been taking their β-agonist regularly would be more vulnerable to bronchoconstrictor stimuli such as allergens or cold air, as their β-agonist inhaler would be less effective in countering these stimuli. The rebound increase in bronchial responsiveness seen when the bronchodilator effect has worn off is not usually large but it may be accompanied by a reduction in airway calibre and it may be important for an occasional patient, and could contribute very rarely to a severe or even fatal attack of asthma.

- *Dysrhythmias.* Both selective and non-selective β-agonists have caused myocardial necrosis, coronary steal and death from ventricular tachydysrhythmias when given to animals in high doses (Rona *et al.*, 1959; Todd *et al.*, 1985) or, when combined with theophylline, in lower doses comparable to those given to patients (Joseph *et al.*, 1981; Nicklas *et al.*, 1984). The dysrhythmic effects of β-agonists are more pronounced in the presence of hypoxaemia (Bremner *et al.*, 1992; Kiely *et al.*, 1995). Trying to determine whether β-agonists have caused a dysrhythmia or cardiac toxicity in patients who die from asthma is difficult as death usually occurs outside hospital. The finding of widespread mucus plugging of the airways at autopsy does not exclude a dysrhythmia as the final event.

  Several prospective studies have looked at the cardiac effects of β-agonists given alone or in combination with methylxanthines and roughly half have shown no increase in cardiac dysrhythmias whilst half have found a significant increase, albeit of clinically unimportant dysrhythmias (Wong and Tattersfield, 1993). Most studies excluded patients with cardiac problems and most were small and considerably underpowered to detect what must at most be a very rare event. Adverse cardiac effects during treatment with a β-agonist are well described, and it would be surprising perhaps if β-agonists, particularly when taken in high doses, didn't occasionally cause cardiac problems. This is more likely in patients with underlying heart disease or with hypokalaemia or hypoxaemia as a result of their asthma or other treatment.

BALANCE OF SAFETY AND EFFICACY

It is difficult to recommend the regular use of short-acting β-agonists in view of their limited efficacy even in the most favourable long-term study. Although their overall safety record is good there are concerns about the safety of high dose, less selective β-agonists and occasional patients are likely to be vulnerable to lower doses of more selective agents. It is also clear that many patients on high doses can reduce the dose of β-agonist without deterioration in their asthma.

Role of short-acting β-agonists

Inhaled short-acting β-agonists continue to play an extremely important role in acute severe asthma, for symptom relief and to prevent bronchoconstriction, particularly exercise-induced asthma. There is little evidence to justify their being prescribed on a regular basis given that efficacy has been difficult to demonstrate and there are some questions about safety, although the risk of serious problems is small.

LONG-ACTING β-AGONISTS

The longer-acting β-agonists salmeterol and formoterol have a different role from the short-acting β-agonists in the management of asthma. Both are normally given on a regular twice-daily basis and most studies have looked at their use when given in this way.

Comparison with placebo and shorter-acting β-agonists

A large number of clinical studies have compared regular treatment with salmeterol or formoterol with placebo or regular short-acting β-agonists. The findings in adults have been more consistent than those in children and are discussed first. The controlled prospective studies in adults lasting for four weeks or more are shown in Table 11.2.

When compared with placebo, salmeterol and formoterol have shown sustained bronchodilatation and a reduction in symptoms in adults (see references in Table 11.2) and an improvement in asthma-specific quality of life (Juniper *et al.*, 1995, 1999). A 6-month cross-over study, based on the Sears' study of fenoterol (1990) but allowing patients to adjust their inhaled steroid dose, found that salmeterol 50 µg bd was associated with a reduction in inhaled steroid use and improved asthma control (Wilding *et al.*, 1997). There was a reduction in symptoms and bronchodilator use and an increase in FEV_1 and PEF compared to placebo. In a large multicentre study treatment with 24 µg formoterol twice-daily for 6 months was associated with reduced symptoms and bronchodilator use and an increase in peak flow rate compared with placebo (van der Molen *et al.*, 1997).

Because the long-acting β-agonists have not reduced airway inflammation in most studies, as judged by measurement of inflammatory cells in bronchoalveolar lavage (Gardiner *et al.*, 1994), there was concern that they may mask asthma and that this would lead to more severe exacerbations. Most studies of long-acting β-agonists have not been designed to look at their

Table 11.2 *Controlled studies of four weeks' duration or more in adults in which the clinical response to salmeterol or formoterol has been compared with the response to placebo or a short-acting β-agonist*

First author, date	No. of patients (no. receiving long-acting β-agonist)		Duration (weeks)		bd dose (µg)	Control drug
Salmeterol						
Dahl, 1991	692	(520)	4		12.5, 50, 100	P
Jones, 1994	427	(282)	6		50	P
Boyd, 1995	119	(55)	12		100	P
Pearlman, 1992	234	(78)	12		42	P + Sb 180 µg qid
D'Alonzo, 1994	257	(84)	12		42	P + Sb 180 µg qid
Juniper, 1995	140	(46)	12		50	P + Sb 200 µg qid
Britton, 1992	667	(334)	12		50	Sb 200 µg bd
Lundback, 1993	388	(190)	12		50	Sb 400 µg qid
Castle, 1993	25 180	(14 113)	16		50	Sb 200 µg qid
Leblanc, 1996*	367	(367)	4		50	P + Sb 400 µg qid
Rutten van Molken, 1995	120	(53)	6		50	Sb 400 µg qid
Faurschou, 1996	190	(96)	6		100	Sb 400 µg qid
Wilding, 1997*	89	(89)	52	(26)▲	50	P
Taylor, 1998	157	(157)	78	(26)▲	50	P + Sb 400 µg qid
Formoterol						
Wallin, 1990	16*		4		24	Sb 400 µg bd
Kesten, 1991	145	(73)	12		12	Sb 200 µg qid
Arvidsson, 1991	18	(10)	52		12	Sb 200 µg bd
Midgren, 1992	35	(19)	4		24**	Sb 400 µg bd
Pauwels, 1997	852	(425)	52		12	placebo

Sb, salbutamol; P, placebo; *, cross-over study; **, could take more as necessary; ▲, duration of long-lasting β-agonist treatment.

effect on exacerbations and have had insufficient power to do so. A recent, large, year-long study designed to look specifically at exacerbations showed a reduction in both mild and severe exacerbations when formoterol was given to patients taking both low and high doses of the inhaled steroid budesonide (Fig. 11.6) (Pauwels *et al.*, 1997). The severity and duration of exacerbations when they occurred were similar in all treatment groups whether or not patients were taking formoterol (Tattersfield *et al.*, 1999a). In a large post-marketing surveillance study of 25 180 patients, fewer patients randomized to salmeterol had to withdraw because of asthma exacerbations compared with patients taking salbutamol (2.91 vs. 3.79%), but there was no placebo group for comparison (Castle, 1993). In a recent cross-over study in which patients inhaled salbutamol, salmeterol or placebo for 6 months the exacerbation rate was reduced by salmeterol with no difference in rates between salbutamol and placebo (Fig. 11.7) although the duration of major exacerbations was greater with salbutamol (Taylor *et al.*, 1998).

When salmeterol and formoterol have been compared with regular shorter-acting β-agonists (invariably salbutamol to date), similar conclusions can be drawn (*see* Table 11.2). The long-acting β-agonists provide sustained bronchodilatation over 24 hours, daytime and night-time symptoms are reduced and quality of life is improved (Juniper *et al.*, 1995). In two studies showing a detailed profile of FEV_1 over 12 hours the bronchodilator response to salmeterol was unchanged after treatment for 3 months and treatment was associated with a reduction in symptoms (Pearlman *et al.*, 1992; D'Alonzo *et al.*, 1994).

In all but two of the studies detailed in Table 11.2, patients were taking an inhaled corticosteroid on entry into the study. Most of the patients in the studies of Pearlman *et al.*

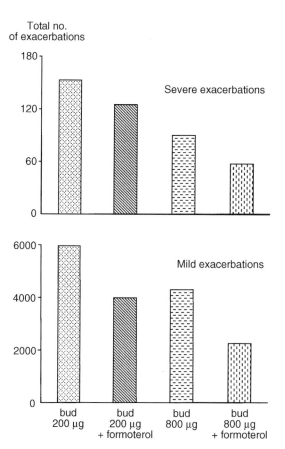

Figure 11.6 *FACET. Total number of severe and mild exacerbation rates in one year amongst patients randomized to receive budesonide at 100 or 400 µg bd with and without formoterol at 12 µg bd. (Data redrawn from Pauwels et al, 1997.)*

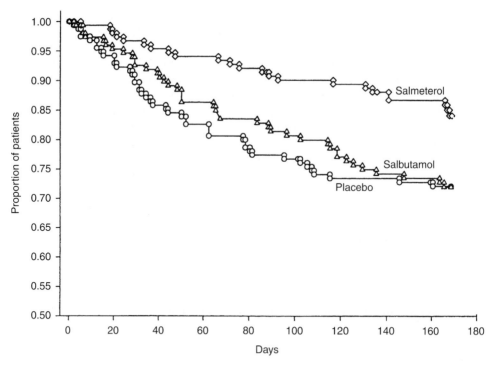

Figure 11.7 *Kaplan Meier plot showing the proportion of patients who remained free of an exacerbation when taking salmeterol, salbutamol and placebo for 6 months in a randomized cross-over study. The difference between salmeterol and salbutamol is notable. (From Taylor et al., 1998, with permission from BMJ publishers.)*

(1992) and D'Alonzo *et al.* (1994) were steroid-naïve, however, and the response to salmeterol was said to be similar irrespective of whether the patients were taking an inhaled corticosteroid or not.

The findings in studies of children have been less impressive. Salmeterol caused some bronchodilatation initially in a 4-month study in 40 asthmatic children taking an inhaled corticosteroid but the difference from placebo was not significant after the first week (Meijer *et al.*, 1995). When compared with regular salbutamol in steroid-naïve children with mild asthma there was an improvement in bronchial responsiveness with salmeterol over the 4 months but no difference in lung function or symptoms (Verberne *et al.*, 1996). The children in these two studies had relatively mild asthma and this may possibly explain the relatively small effects seen with salmeterol.

Comparison with inhaled corticosteroids

Two year-long studies in corticosteroid-naïve children with mild asthma compared the effect of twice-daily treatment with salmeterol 50 μg and beclomethasone dipropionate 200 μg and both studies found better asthma control and fewer exacerbations with the inhaled corticosteroid (Verberne *et al.*, 1996; Simons *et al.*, 1997). There appeared to be some benefit from salmeterol in the study by Simons *et al.* although neither study had a placebo limb for comparison. Again the response to a long-acting β-agonist appeared to be less than would have been expected in adults although there are no published data on the relative effects of the long-acting β-agonists compared with an inhaled corticosteroid in steroid-naïve adults.

Three studies have looked at the effect of adding salmeterol to an inhaled corticosteroid compared with an increased dose of inhaled corticosteroid in adults. Two large, parallel group studies in patients with symptomatic asthma compared the effect of adding salmeterol (50 µg bd) with increasing the dose of beclomethasone diproprionate, from 200 to 500 µg twice-daily (Greening *et al.*, 1994), or from 500 to 1000 µg twice-daily (Woolcock *et al.*, 1996). Over the 6 months of the study, peak flow rate and day and night-time symptoms improved to a greater extent in the salmeterol group in both studies, with no difference between groups in the number of exacerbations. A third group receiving salmeterol at 100 µg bd in the study by Woolcock *et al.* showed similar efficacy to the group on salmeterol at 50 µg bd. The findings were similar in a more recent study which compared the addition of salmeterol to doubling the dose of fluticasone in patients taking 100 µg or 250 µg fluticasone twice-daily (van Noord *et al.*, 1999).

Comparison with other bronchodilators

Salmeterol at 50 µg bd provided better symptom control and fewer side-effects than a combination of theophylline at 300 mg and ketotifen at 1 mg bd (Muir *et al.*, 1992), and better asthma control (improved peak flow and reduction in symptoms) than theophylline alone following individual dose titration of theophylline (Fjellbirkeland *et al.*, 1994).

Nocturnal and exercise-induced asthma

It was expected that the long-acting β-agonists would be helpful in nocturnal asthma and this has been seen with both salmeterol and formoterol in most of the larger studies detailed in Table 11.2. A study looking specifically at nocturnal asthma showed an improvement in evening and morning peak flow and some reduction in the nocturnal fall in peak flow with salmeterol at 50 or 100 µg bd for 2 weeks compared with placebo (Fitzpatrick *et al.*, 1990). There was no difference between the two doses of salmeterol though sleep architecture only improved significantly with the 50 µg bd dose. In another study the overnight fall in FEV_1 was less following formoterol 12 µg compared to salbutamol 200 µg (Maesen *et al.*, 1990).

When given as a single dose both salmeterol and formoterol have caused a reduction in exercise-induced bronchoconstriction over 12 hours (Kemp *et al.*, 1994; Nelson *et al.*, 1998b). The protective effect was attenuated, however, following regular salmeterol at 50 µg bd for 4 weeks (Nelson *et al.*, 1998b). Single doses of salmeterol and salbutamol had no effect on exercise capacity in asthmatic men (Robertson *et al.*, 1994).

Safety of long-acting β-agonists

The adverse effects reported with the long-acting β-agonists are largely those expected of a β-agonist – tremor, headache, cramps and palpitations. The frequency of these side-effects with salmeterol at 50 µg bd or formoterol at 12 µg bd has generally been low. In three out of four studies comparing 50 µg and 100 µg twice-daily, the higher dose of salmeterol caused more adverse effects than the lower, particularly as regards tremor and palpitations, and with no additional benefit (Fitzpatrick *et al.*, 1990; Palmer *et al.*, 1992; Boyd *et al.*, 1995; Woolcock *et al.*, 1996). There is less information on the relative effect of regular treatment with different doses of formoterol although a recent study in patients with mild-to-moderate asthma showed near maximum benefit from 6 µg bd compared with 12 and 24 µg twice daily (Schreurs *et al.*, 1996).

Some specific safety issues with the long-acting β-agonists require comment.

BRONCHOCONSTRICTION

Bronchoconstriction can occur following inhalation of salmeterol by metered dose inhaler and although not common it can be severe (Wilkinson *et al.*, 1992; Shaheen *et al.*, 1994). It is probably caused by the propellant and appears to be more likely in patients whose asthma is deteriorating or poorly controlled. It has not been described with formoterol probably because formoterol is mainly marketed as a dry powder preparation and because bronchodilatation occurs more rapidly with formoterol and is thus able to counteract the bronchoconstriction.

PARTIAL AGONISM

Although salmeterol is a partial agonist there is no evidence to date to suggest that this is a clinical problem (see p. 258).

SYSTEMIC ACTIVITY

Both formoterol and salmeterol show marked β_2-selectivity *in vitro* and when given in recommended doses cardiovascular effects are generally minimal. In dose–response studies normal people show a marked increase in heart rate and QTc interval and a fall in serum potassium (a β_2-mediated effect) with higher doses of both drugs indicating that they have a relatively modest therapeutic window (Bennett and Tattersfield, 1997; Totterman *et al.*, 1998; Guhan *et al.*, 2000). These studies suggest that both drugs have been marketed at a relatively high dose and highlight the propensity of inhaled long-acting β-agonists to cause systemic effects if taken in doses above those recommended. Two of the studies were carried out in fit people and there is some evidence that systemic effects may be less in asthmatic patients. Nevertheless, larger effects may occur in the occasional patient with a vulnerable myocardium and/or other risk factors.

The duration of systemic effects may be less with formoterol than salmeterol though with high doses there is evidence of some systemic activity 8 hours after administration with both drugs, though more so with salmeterol (Guhan *et al.*, 1998).

TOLERANCE TO THE LONG-ACTING β-AGONISTS

The protection afforded by salmeterol and formoterol against bronchoconstrictor challenge such as exercise and methacholine is reduced with their continued use (Cheung *et al.*, 1992; Nelson *et al.*, 1998) as with all β-agonists. There is also some evidence of tolerance to the bronchodilating effects of formoterol (Tan *et al.*, 1997). The clinical relevance of tolerance can be deduced from the FACET study where the bronchodilator effect of formoterol fell slightly during the first few days of treatment but thereafter was maintained throughout the year-long study (Pauwels *et al.*, 1997). Furthermore exacerbations were reduced and those that did occur were not made worse by use of formoterol. The study by Taylor *et al.* (1998) suggests that the same is true for salmeterol. There is no evidence of a rebound bronchoconstrictor effect after regular treatment with the long-acting β-agonists which may be related to the more gradual offset of action of these drugs compared to the shorter-acting β-agonists.

Balance of efficacy and safety

The long-acting β-agonists are clearly efficacious and have invariably been better than regular use of short-acting β-agonists for all clinical end points. Why there should be this difference is less clear but may relate to the fact that even when given regularly the response to a short-acting β-agonist is not maintained for six hours (Pearlman *et al.*, 1992; D'Alonzo *et al.*, 1994). The long-acting β-agonists are generally well tolerated and adverse effects are rarely a problem with doses of 50 μg salmeterol and 12 μg formoterol. The drugs only have a modest therapeutic window, however, and adverse effects are more likely with higher doses. There is some tolerance to their effects with regular use but long-term studies show continued efficacy.

Role of long-acting β-agonists

Inhaled long-acting β-agonists are currently recommended for regular use at step 3 of the asthma guidelines and this is supported by the continued benefit seen in long-term studies. There is some evidence to suggest that for patients not controlled on a low dose of an inhaled corticosteroid the addition of a long-acting β-agonist is more likely to improve symptoms (Greening *et al.*, 1994; Woolcock *et al.*, 1996) whereas an increased dose of inhaled corticosteroid may be better at preventing exacerbations (Pauwels *et al.*, 1997).

Because formoterol has a rapid onset of action the question of whether it could be used as relief medication has arisen and is currently being studied. Although higher doses will carry a risk of more adverse effects this would also be true of alternative treatments such as the shorter-acting β-agonists. In a recent study comparing formoterol at 4.5 μg and terbutaline at 500 μg for relief medication there was a reduction in exacerbations in the formoterol group and no evidence of increased adverse effects (Tattersfield *et al.*, 1999b). This suggests that formoterol could be preferable to terbutaline as relief medication.

β-AGONISTS ADMINISTERED BY OTHER ROUTES

Oral β-agonists

There are few published studies of the efficacy and safety of regular treatment with oral β-agonists in adults. When studied acutely, oral β-agonists cause more systemic and adverse effects with less benefit than when given by inhalation (Larsson and Svedmyr, 1977) and it is assumed that this adverse balance is maintained with regular treatment. In a recent study, healthy individuals still had a marked tachycardia (13 beats/min) twelve hours after finishing a week's course of oral salbutamol at 8 mg twice-daily (Thompson Coon *et al.*, 1999). The protective effect of oral β-agonists against exercise-induced bronchoconstriction appears to be lost with regular use, as with β-agonists given by other routes (Gibson *et al.*, 1978).

Bambuterol, a terbutaline carbamate prodrug, was designed to reduce the systemic adverse effects associated with oral β-agonists. It is protected against first-pass metabolism following oral absorption and has high affinity for lung tissue. It has a long half-life (20 h) and is given once daily. Both the 10 and 20 mg doses of bambuterol are effective bronchodilators (Persson *et al.*, 1995) but how they compare with inhaled long-acting β-agonists is not clear.

In general the oral β-agonists have been superseded by the long-acting inhaled β-agonists and their role in the management of asthma is limited, at least in countries where long-acting inhaled β-agonists are available.

Intravenous , intramuscular and subcutaneous β-agonists

β-Agonists may be given intravenously for acute severe asthma not responding well to nebulized β-agonists (*see* Chapter 15) and to prevent premature labour. Prolonged intravenous treatment has been associated with focal myocardial necrosis and pulmonary oedema (Clesham, 1994).

β-Agonists such as salbutamol and terbutaline can be given by the subcutaneous and intramuscular routes and this may be helpful when access via other routes is difficult. Patients prone to sudden acute attacks of asthma can be given a β-agonist, usually terbutaline, for subcutaneous self-administration in the event of a severe attack. Patients will normally need to be assessed soon afterwards by a doctor and it is important that the patient understands this.

Long-term subcutaneous β-agonists given by a pump or by regular injections have also been tried in patients with brittle or chronic severe asthma, with apparent benefit in brittle asthma. Subcutaneous nodules and abscesses have been reported at the site of the infusion, also cramps and tremor, though infrequently (Ayres, 1992). Raised creatine kinase levels are thought to reflect increased muscle activity (Sykes et al., 1991). Although continuing efficacy for long-term subcutaneous terbutaline is claimed, patients with brittle asthma are difficult to assess and many physicians continue to be sceptical in the absence of any formal assessment of their effectiveness.

THE FUTURE

β-Agonists continue to have an extremely important role in the management of asthma. The short-acting β-agonists are the first line treatment for acute attacks of asthma whether mild or severe and they are also used to prevent bronchoconstriction, particularly exercise-induced asthma. The introduction of the long-acting β-agonists has extended the role of β-agonists since, unlike the short-acting β-agonists, they are clearly beneficial when taken as regular medication and the benefit is maintained long-term. Salmeterol and formoterol have some pharmacological differences and these are likely to be exploited in the next few years. It is likely that formoterol, because of its rapid onset of action and ability to reduce exacerbations, will have a role as relief medication. Administering a long-acting β-agonist in the same inhaler as a corticosteroid is also being pursued in the expectation that compliance will be improved.

REFERENCES

Adcock IM, Peters MJ, Brown CR, Stevens DA, Barnes PJ. (1995) High concentrations of β-adrenergic agonists inhibit DNS binding of glucorticoids in human lung *in vitro*. *Biochem Soc Trans*, **23**, 217S.

Amoroso P, Wilson SR, Moxham J, Ponte J. (1993) Acute effects of inhaled salbutamol on the metabolic rate of normal subjects. *Thorax*, **48**, 882–5.

Anderson GP. (1993) Formoterol: pharmacology, molecular basis of agonism, and mechanism of long duration of highly potent and selective β$_2$-adrenoceptor agonist bronchodilator. *Life Sciences*, **52**, 2145–60.

Apter AJ, Reisine ST, Willard A, *et al.* (1996) The effect of inhaled albuterol in moderate to severe asthma. *J Allergy Clin Immunol*, **98**, 295–301.

Arvidsson P, Larsson S, Lofdahl C-G, Melande B, Svedmyr N, Wahlander L. (1991) Inhaled formoterol during one year in asthma: a comparison with salbutamol. *Eur Respir J*, **4**, 1168–73.

Assem ESK, Schild HO. (1969) Inhibition by sympathomimetic amines of histamine release induced by antigen in passively sensitized human lung. *Nature*, **224**, 1028–9.

Ayres J. (1992) Continuous subcutaneous bronchodilators in brittle asthma. *Br J Hosp Med*, **47**, 569–71.

Bai TR, Mak JCW, Barnes PJ. (1992) A comparison of β-adrenergic receptors and *in vitro* relaxant responses to isoproterenol in asthmatic airway smooth muscle. *Am J Respir Cell Mol Biol*, **6**, 647–51.

Baraniuk JN, Mushtaq A, Brody D, *et al*. (1997) Glucocorticoids induce $β_2$-adrenergic receptor function in human nasal mucosa. *Am J Respir Crit Care Med*, **155**, 704–10.

Barnes PJ. (1989) Muscarinic receptor subtypes: implications for lung disease. *Thorax*, **44**, 161–7.

Barnes PJ. (1995) Beta-adrenergic receptors and their regulation *Am J Respir Crit Care Med*, **152**, 838–60.

Barnes PJ, Pride NB. (1983) Dose–response curves to inhaled β-adrenoceptor agonists in normal and asthmatic subjects. *Br J Clin Pharmacol*, **15**, 677–82.

Bennett JA, Harrison TW, Tattersfield AE. (1999) The contribution of the swallowed fraction of an inhaled dose of salmeterol to its systemic effects. *Eur Respir J*, **13**, 445–8.

Bennett JA, Tattersfield AE. (1997) Time course and relative dose potency of systemic effects from salmeterol and salbutamol in healthy subjects. *Thorax*, **52**, 458–64.

Blauw GJ, Westendorp RGJ. (1995) Asthma deaths in New Zealand; whodunnit? *Lancet*, **345**, 2–3.

Borger P, Hoekstra Y, Esselink MR, *et al*. (1998) β-Adrenoceptor-mediated inhibition of IFN-γ, IL-3, and GM-CSF mRNA accumulation in activated human T lymphocytes is solely mediated by the $β_2$-adrenoceptor subtype. *Am J Respir Cell Mol Biol*, **19**, 400–7.

Bouvier M, Mausdorff WP, De Blasi A, *et al*. (1988) Removal of phosphorylation sites from the $β_2$-adrenergic receptor delays onset of agonist-promoted desensitisation. *Nature*, **333**, 370–3.

Boyd G, on behalf of a UK Study group. (1995) Salmeterol xinafoate in asthmatic patients under consideration for maintenance oral corticosteroid therapy. *Eur Respir J*, **8**, 1494–8.

Bremner P, Burgess CD, Crane J, *et al*. (1992) Cardiovascular effects of fenoterol under conditions of hypoxaemia. *Thorax*, **47**, 814–7.

Bremner P, Woodman K, Burgess C, *et al*. (1993) A comparison of the cardiovascular and metabolic effects of formoterol, salbutamol and fenoterol. *Eur Respir J*, **6**, 204–10.

Britton MG, Earnshaw JS, Palmer JB.D. (1992) A twelve month comparison of salmeterol with salbutamol in asthmatic patients. *Eur Respir J*, **5**, 1062–7.

Carstairs JR, Nimmo AJ, Barnes PJ. (1985) Autoradiographic visualization of beta-adrenoceptor subtypes in human lung. *Am Rev Respir Dis*, **132**, 541–7.

Castle W, Fuller R, Hall J, Palmer J. (1993) Serevent nationwide surveillance study: comparison of salmeterol with salbutamol in patients who require regular bronchodilator treatment. *BMJ*, **306**, 1034–7.

Chapman KR, Kesten S, Szalai JP. (1994) Regular vs. as-needed inhaled salbutamol in asthma control. *Lancet*, **343**, 1379–82.

Cheong B, Reynolds SR, Ward MJ. (1988) Intravenous β-agonist in severe acute asthma. *BMJ*, **297**, 448–50.

Cheung D, Timmers MK, Zwinderman AH, Bel EH, Dijkman JH, Sterk PJ. (1992) Long term effects of a long acting $β_2$-adrenoceptor agonist, salmeterol, on airway hyperresponsiveness in patients with mild asthma. *N Engl J Med*, **327**, 1198–203.

Chong LK, Morice AH, Yeo WW, Schleimer RP, Peachell PT. (1995) Functional desensitization of β-agonist responses in human lung mast cells. *Am J Respir Cell Mol Biol*, **13**, 540–6.

Chung KF, Rogers DF, Barnes PJ, Evans TW. (1990) The role of increased airway microvascular permeability and plasma exudation in asthma. *Eur Respir J*, **3**, 329–37.

Clesham GJ. (1994) β-Adrenergic agonists and pulmonary oedema in preterm labour. *BMJ*, **308**, 260–2.

Cockcroft DW, McParland CP, Britto SA, Swystun VA, Rutherford BC. (1993) Regular inhaled salbutamol and airway responsiveness to allergen. *Lancet*, **342**, 833–7.

Cockcroft DW, O'Byrne PM, Swystun VA, Bhagat R. (1995) Regular use of inhaled albuterol and the allergen-induced late asthmatic response. *J Allergy Clin Immunol*, **96**, 44–9.

Cockcroft DW, Swystun VA. (1997) Effect of single doses of *S*-salbutamol, *R*-salbutamol, racemic salbutamol, and placebo on the airway response to methacholine. *Thorax*, **52**, 845–8.

Collier JG, Dobbs RJ, Williams I. (1980) Salbutamol aerosol causes a tachycardia due to the inhaled rather than the swallowed fraction. *Br J Clin Pharmacol*, **9**, 273–4.

Crane J, Burgess C, Beasley R. (1989a) Cardiovascular and hypokalaemic effects of inhaled salbutamol, fenoterol, and isoprenaline. *Thorax*, **44**, 136–40.

Crane J, Pearce N, Flatt A, *et al*. (1989b) Prescribed fenoterol and death from asthma in New Zealand, 1981–83; case–control study. *Lancet*, **1**, 917.

Dahl R, Earnshaw JS, Palmer JBD. (1991) Salmeterol: a four week study of a long acting β-adrenoceptor agonist for the treatment of reversible airways disease. *Eur Respir J*, **4**, 1178–84.

D'Alonzo GE, Nathan RA, Henochowicz S, Morris RJ, Ratner P, Rennard SI. (1994) Salmeterol xinafoate as maintenance therapy compared with albuterol in patients with asthma. *J Am Med Assoc*, **271**, 1412–16.

Dessauer CW, Posner BA, Gilman AG. (1996) Visualizing signal transduction: receptors, G-proteins, and adenylate cyclases. *Clin Sci*, **91**, 527–37.

Dewar JC, Wheatley AP, Venn A, Morrison JFJ, Britton J, Hall IP. (1998) β₂-Adrenoceptor polymorphisms are in linkage disequilibrium, but are not associated with asthma in an adult population. *Clin Exp Allergy*, **28**, 442–8.

Dollery C. (1999) Formoterol (fumerate). In: Dollery C, ed. *Therapeutic drugs*. Edinburgh: Churchill Livingstone, Vol 1, F155–8.

Dowling RB, Rayner CFJ, Rutman A, *et al*. (1997) Effect of salmeterol on *Pseudomonas aeruginosa* infection of respiratory mucosa. *Am J Respir Crit Care Med*, **155**, 327–36.

Drazen JM, Israel E, Boushey HA, for the National Heart, Lung, and Blood Institute's Asthma Clinical Research Network. (1996) Comparison of regularly scheduled with as-needed use of albuterol in mild asthma. *N Engl J Med*, **335**, 841–7.

Emorine LJ, Marullo S, Briend-Sutren MM, *et al*. (1989) Molecular characterisation and the human β₃-adrenergic receptor. *Science*, **245**, 1118–21.

Faurschou P, Steffensen I, Jacques L, on behalf of a European Respiratory Study Group. (1996) Effect of addition of inhaled salmeterol to the treatment of moderate-to-severe asthmatics uncontrolled on high-dose inhaled steroids. *Eur Respir J*, **9**, 1885–90.

Fawcett JP, Taylor DR. (1999) β₂-Agonist enantiomers: is there a glitch with the chiral switch? *Eur Respir J*, **13**, 1223–4.

Fitzpatrick MF, Mackay T, Driver H, Douglas NJ. (1990) Salmeterol in nocturnal asthma: a double blind, placebo controlled trial of a long acting inhaled β₂-agonist. *BMJ*, **301**, 1365–8.

Fjellbirkeland L, Gulsvik A, Palmer JBD. (1994) The efficacy and tolerability of inhaled salmeterol and individually dose-titrated, sustained-release theophylline in patients with reversible airways disease. *Respir Med*, **88**, 599–607.

Frielle T, Collins S, Daniel KW, Capron MG, Lefkowitz RJ, Kobilka BK. (1987) Cloning of the cDNA for the β₁-adrenergic receptor. *Proc Nat Acad Sci USA*, **84**, 7920–4.

Gardiner PV, Ward C, Booth H, Allison A, Hendrick DJ, Walters EH. (1994) Effect of eight weeks of treatment with salmeterol on bronchoalveolar lavage inflammatory indices in asthmatics. *Am J Respir Crit Care Med*, **150**, 1006–11.

Gibson GJ, Greenacre JK, Konig P, Connolly ME, Pride NB. (1978) Use of exercise challenge to investigate possible tolerance to β-adrenoceptor stimulation in asthma. *Br J Dis Chest*, **72**, 199–206.

Granger J, Woodman K, Pearce N, *et al*. (1991) Prescribed fenoterol and death from asthma in New Zealand, 1981–87: a further case–control study. *Thorax*, **46**, 105.

Green SA, Cole G, Jacinto M, Innis M, Liggett SB. (1993) A polymorphism of the human β₂-adrenergic receptor within the fourth transmembrane domain alters ligand binding and functional properties of the receptor. *J Biol Chem*, **268**, 23116–21.

Green SA, Spasoff AP, Coleman RA, Johnson M, Liggett SB. (1996) Sustained activation of a G protein coupled receptor via 'anchored' agonist binding. Molecular localization of the salmeterol exosite within the β₂-adrenergic receptor. *J Biol Chem*, **271**, 24029–35.

Green SA, Turki J, Bejarano P, Hall LP, Liggett SB. (1995) Influence of β₂-adrenergic receptor genotypes on signal transduction in human airway smooth muscle cells. *Am J Respir Cell Mol Biol*, **13**, 25–33.

Greening AP, Ind PW, Northfield M, Shaw G. (1994) Added salmeterol versus higher-dose corticosteroid in asthma patients with symptoms on existing inhaled corticosteroid. *Lancet*, **344**, 219–24.

Grove A, Lipworth BJ. (1995) Bronchodilator subsensitivity to salbutamol after twice daily salmeterol in asthmatic patients. *Lancet*, **346**, 201–6.

Guhan AR, Cooper S, Oborne J, Lewis S, Bennett J, Tattersfield AE. (2000) Systemic effects of formoterol and salmeterol – a dose–response study in healthy subjects. *Thorax*, (in press).

Haahtela T, Järvinen M, Kava T, *et al*. (1991) Comparison of a β_2-agonist, terbutaline, with an inhaled corticosteroid, budesonide, in newly detected asthma. *N Engl J Med*, **325**, 388–92.

Hadcock JR, Malbon CC. (1988) Down-regulation of β-adrenergic receptors: agonist-induced reduction in receptor mRNA levels. *Proc Natl Acad Sci USA*, **85**, 5021–5.

Hancox RJ, Sears MR, Taylor DR. (1998) Polymorphism of the β_2-adrenoceptor and the response to long-term β_2-agonist therapy in asthma. *Eur Respir J*, **11**, 589–93.

Hancox RJ, Cowan JO, Flannery EM, *et al*. (1999) Randomised trial of an inhaled β_2-agonist, inhaled corticosteroid and their combination in the treatment of asthma. *Thorax*, **54**, 482–7.

Harrison TW, Oborne J, Wilding PJ, Tattersfield AE. (1999) Randomised placebo controlled trial of β-agonist dose reduction in asthma. *Thorax*, **54**, 98–102.

Harvey JE, Baldwin CJ, Wood PJ, Alberti KGMM, Tattersfield AE. (1981) Airway and metabolic responsiveness to intravenous salbutamol in asthma – effect of regular inhaled salbutamol. *Clin Sci*, **60**, 579–85.

Harvey JE, Tattersfield AE. (1982) Airway response to salbutamol: effect of regular salbutamol inhalation in normal, atopic and asthmatic subjects. *Thorax*, **37**, 280–7.

Holgate ST, Baldwin CJ, Tattersfield AE. (1977) β-Adrenergic agonist resistance in normal human airways. *Lancet*, **2**, 375–7.

Howarth PH, Durham SR, Lee TH, Kay AB, Church MK, Holgate ST. (1985) Influence of albuterol, cromolyn sodium and ipratropium bromide on the airway and circulating mediator responses to allergen bronchial provocation in asthma. *Am Rev Respir Dis*, **132**, 986–92.

Hauck RW, Böhm M, Gengenbach S, Sunder-Plassmann L, Gruhmann G, Erdmann E. (1990) β_2-adrenoceptors in human lung and peripheral mononuclear leukocytes of untreated and terbutaline-treated patients. *Chest*, **98**, 376–81.

Ind PW. (1997) Salbutamol enantiomers: early clinical evidence in humans. *Thorax*, **52**, 839–40.

Inman WHW, Adelstein AM. (1969) Rise and fall of asthma mortality in England and Wales in relation to use of pressurised aerosols. *Lancet*, **ii**, 279–85.

Jackson RT, Beaglehole R, Rea HH, Sutherland DC. (1982) Mortality from asthma: a new epidemic in New Zealand. *BMJ*, **285**, 771–4.

Jones KP. (1994) Salmeterol xinafoate in the treatment of mild to moderate asthma in primary care. *Thorax*, **49**, 971–5.

Joseph X, Whiteburst VE, Bloom S, Balazs T. (1981) Enhancement of cardiotoxic effects of beta-adrenergic bronchodilators by aminophylline in experimental animals. *Fund Appl Toxicol*, **1**, 443–7.

Juniper EF, Johnston PR, Borkhoff CM, Guyatt GH, Boulet, L-P, Haukioja A. (1995) Quality of life in asthma clinical trials: comparison of salmeterol and salbutamol. *Am J Respir Crit Care Med*, **151**, 66–70.

Juniper EF, Svensson K, O'Byrne PM, *et al*. (1999) Asthma quality of life during one year of treatment with budesonide with or without formoterol. *Eur Respir J*, **14**(5), 1038–43.

Kemp JP, Dockhorn RJ, Busse WW, Bleecker ER, van As A. (1994) Prolonged effect of inhaled salmeterol against exercise-induced bronchospasm. *Am J Respir Crit Care Med*, **150**, 1612–15.

Kesten S, Chapman KR, Broder I, *et al*. (1991) A three-month comparison of twice daily inhaled formoterol versus four times daily inhaled albuterol in the management of stable asthma. *Am Rev Respir Disease*, **144**, 622–5.

Kiely DG, Cargill RI, Lipworth BJ. (1995) Cardiopulmonary interactions of salbutamol and hypoxaemia in healthy young volunteers. *Br J Clin Pharmacol*, **40**, 313–8.

Knox AJ, Tattersfield AE. (1995) Airway smooth muscle relaxation. *Thorax*, **50**, 894–901.

Koto H, Mak JC, Haddad EB, *et al*. (1996) Mechanism of impaired β-adrenoceptor induced airway relaxation by interleukin 1β *in vivo* in the rat. *J Clin Invest*, **98**, 1780–7.

Kraan J, Koeter GH, van der Mark ThW, Sluiter H, de Vries K. (1985) Changes in bronchial hyperreactivity induced by 4 weeks of treatment with antiasthmatic drugs in patients with allergic asthma: a comparison between budesonide and terbutaline. *J Allergy Clin Immunol*, **76**, 628–36.

Kume H, Hall IP, Washabau RJ, Takagi K, Kotlikoff MI. (1994) β-Adrenergic agonists regulate K(Ca) channels in airway smooth muscle by cAMP-dependent and -independent mechanisms. *J Clin Invest*, **93**, 371–9.

Lands AM, Arnold A, McAuliff JP, *et al*. (1967) Differentiation of receptor systems activated by sympathomimetic amines. *Nature*, **214**, 597–8.

Larsson S, Svedmyr N. (1977) Bronchodilating effect and side effects of β₂-adrenoceptor stimulants by different modes of administration (tablets, metered aerosol, and combinations thereof). *Am Rev Respir Dis*, **116**, 861–9.

Larsson S, Svedmyr N, Thiringer G. (1977) Lack of bronchial beta adrenoceptor resistance in asthmatics during long-term treatment with terbutaline. *J Allergy Clin Immunol*, **59**, 93–100.

Leblanc P, Knight A, Kreisman H, Borkhoff CM, Johnston PR. (1996) A placebo-controlled, crossover comparison of salmeterol and salbutamol in patients with asthma. *Am J Respir Crit Care Med*, **154**, 324–8.

Lecaillon JB, Kaiser G, Palmisano M, Morgan J, Della Cioppa, G. (1999) Pharmacokinetics and tolerability of formoterol in healthy volunteers after a single high dose of Foradil dry powder inhalation via aerolizer™. *Eur J Clin Pharmacol*, **55**, 131–8.

Lefkowitz RJ, Hausdorff WP, Caron MG. (1990) Role of phosphorylation in desensitization of the β-adrenoceptor. *Trends Pharmacol Sci*, **11**, 190–4.

Leslie D, Coats PM. (1997) Salbutamol-induced diabetic ketoacidosis. *BMJ*, **2**, 768.

Liggett SB, Green SA. (1997) Molecular biology of the Beta₂-adrenergic receptor: focus on interactions of agonist with receptor. In: Pauwels R, O'Byrne PM, eds. *Beta₂-agonists in asthma treatment*. New York: Marcel Dekker, 19–34.

Lipworth BJ, Struthers AD, McDevitt DG. (1989) Tachyphylaxis to systemic but not to airway responses during prolonged therapy with high dose inhaled salbutamol in asthmatics. *Am Rev Respir Dis*, **140**, 586–92.

Lipworth BJ, Hall IP, Aziz I, Tan KS, Wheatley A. (1999) β₂-Adrenoceptor polymorphism and bronchoprotective sensitivity with regular short- and long-acting β₂-agonist therapy. *Clin Sci*, **96**, 253–9.

Lipworth BJ, Clark DJ, Koch P, Arbeeny C. (1997) Pharmacokinetics and extrapulmonary β₂ adrenoceptor activity of nebulised racemic salbutamol and its *R* and *S* isomers in healthy volunteers. *Thorax*, **52**, 849–52.

Löfdahl, C-G, Svedmyr N. (1989) Formoterol fumarate, a new β₂-adrenoceptor agonist. *Allergy*, **44**, 264–71.

Lundback B, Rawlinson DW, Palmer JBD. (1993) Twelve month comparison of salmeterol and salbutamol as dry powder formulations in asthmatic patients. *Thorax*, **48**, 148–53.

Maesen FPV, Smeets JJ, Gubbelmans HLL, Zweers PGMA. (1990) Formoterol in the treatment of nocturnal asthma. *Chest*, **98**, 866–70.

Mak JCW, Nishikawa M, Barnes PJ. (1995a) Glucocorticosteroids increase β₂-adrenergic receptor transcription in human lung. *Am J Physiol*, **268**, L41–L46.

Mak JCW, Nishikawa M, Shirasaki H, Miyayasu K, Barnes PJ. (1995b) Protective effects of a glucocorticoid on downregulation of pulmonary β₂-adrenergic receptors in vivo. *J Clin Invest*, **96**, 99–106.

Marone G, Kagey-Sobotka A, Lichtenstein LM. (1979) Effects of arachidonic acid and its metabolites on antigen-induced histamine release from human basophils *in vitro*. *J Immunol*, **123**, 1669–77.

Meijer GG, Postma DS, Mulder PG.H, van Aalderen MC. (1995) Long-term circadian effects of salmeterol in asthmatic children treated with inhaled corticosteroids. *Am J Respir Crit Care Med*, **152**, 1887–92.

Midgren B, Melander B, Persson G. (1992) Formoterol, a new long acting β_2-agonist, inhaled twice daily, in stable asthmatic subjects. *Chest*, **101**, 1019–22.

Molenaar P, Sarsevo D, Kaumann AJ. (1997) Proposal for the interaction of non-conventional partial agonists and catecholamines with the putative β_4-adrenoceptor in mammalian heart. *Clin and Exp Pharmacol Physiol*, **24**, 647–56.

Morgan DJ, Paull JD, Richmond BH, Wilson-Evered E, Ziccone SP. (1986) Pharmacokinetics of intravenous and oral salbutamol and its sulphate conjugate. *Br J Clin Pharmacol*, **22**, 587–93.

Muir JF, Bertin L, Georges D, for the French Multicentre Study Group. (1992) Salmeterol versus slow-release theophylline combined with ketotifen in nocturnal asthma: a multicentre trial. *Eur Respir J*, **5**, 1197–200.

Nelson HS, Bensch G, Pleskow WW, *et al*. (1998a) Improved bronchodilation with levalbuterol compared with racemic albuterol in patients with asthma. *J Allergy Clin Immunol*, **102**, 943–52.

Nelson JA, Strauss L, Skowronski M, Ciufo R, Novak R, McFadden ER. (1998b) Effect of long-term salmeterol treatment on exercise-induced asthma. *N Engl J Med*, **339**, 141–6.

Nicklas RA, Whitehurst VE, Donohoe RF, Balazs T. (1984) Concomitant use of beta-adrenergic agonists and methylxanthines. *J Allergy Clin Immunol*, **73**, 20–4.

O'Connor BJ, Aikman SL, Barnes PJ. (1992) Tolerance to the nonbronchodilator effects of inhaled β_2-agonists in asthma. *N Engl J Med*, **327**, 1204–8.

Palmer JB.D, Stuart AM, Shepherd GL, Viskum K. (1992) Inhaled salmeterol in the treatment of patients with moderate to severe reversible obstructive airways disease – a 3-month comparison of the efficacy and safety of twice-daily salmeterol (100 µg) with salmeterol (50 µg). *Respir Med*, **86**, 409–17.

Palmqvist M, Persson G, Lazer L, Rosenborg J, Larsson P, Lötvall J. (1997) Inhaled dry-powder formoterol and salmeterol in asthmatic patients: onset of action, duration of effect and potency. *Eur Respir J*, **10**, 2484–9.

Pang L, Holland E, Knox AJ. (1998) Role of cyclo-oxygenase-2 induction in interkeukin-1β induced attenuation of cultured human airway smooth muscle cell cyclic AMP generation in response to isoprenaline. *Br J Pharmacol*, **125**, 1320–8.

Pauwels RA, Löfdahl C-G, Postma DS, Tattersfield AE, O'Byrne P, Barnes PJ, Ullman A, for the Formoterol and Corticosteroids Establishing Therapy (FACET) International Study Group. (1997) Effect of inhaled formoterol and budesonide on exacerbations of asthma. *N Engl J Med*, **337**, 1405–11.

Pearce N, Grainger J, Atkinson M, *et al*. (1990) Case control study of prescribed fenoterol and death from asthma in New Zealand, 1977–81. *Thorax*, **45**, 170–5.

Pearlman DS, Chervinski P, LaForce C, *et al*. (1992) A comparison of salmeterol with albuterol in the treatment of mild-to-moderate asthma. *N Engl J Med*, **327**, 1420–5.

Persson G, Baas A, Knight A, Larsen B, Olsson H (1995) One month treatment with the once daily oral β_2-agonist bambuterol in asthmatic patients. *Eur Respir J*, **8**, 34–9.

Peters SP, Schulman ES, Schleimer RP, Macglashan DW, Newball HH, Lichtenstein LM. (1982) Dispersed human lung mast cells. Pharmacological aspects and comparison with human lung tissue fragments. *Am Rev Respir Dis*, **126**, 1034–9.

Pingleton SK, Schwartz O, Szymanski D, Epstein M. (1982) Hypotension associated with terbutaline therapy in acute quadriplegia. *Am Rev Respir Dis*, **126**, 723–5.

Pride NB, Ingram RH, Lim TK. (1991) Interaction between parenchyma and airways in chronic obstructive pulmonary disease and in asthma. *Am Rev Respir Dis*, **143**, 1446–9.

Qing F, Rahman SU, Rhodes CG, *et al*. (1997) Pulmonary and cardiac β-adrenoceptor density *in vivo* in asthmatic subjects. *Am J Respir Crit Care Med*, **155**, 1130–4.

Reihsaus E, Innis M, MacIntyre N, Liggett SB. (1993) Mutations in the gene encoding for the β_2-adrenergic receptor in normal and asthmatic subjects. American *J Respir Cell Mol Biol*, **8**, 334–9.

Reisman RE. (1970) Asthma induced by adrenergic aerosols. *J Allergy*, **46**, 162–77.

Robertson W, Simkins J, O'Hickey SP, Freeman S, Cayton RM. (1994) Does single dose salmeterol affect exercise capacity in asthmatic men? *Eur Respir J*, **7**, 1978–84.

Rona G, Chappel CI, Balazs T, Gaudry R. (1959) An infarct-like myocardial lesion and other toxic manifestations produced by isoproterenol in the rat. *Arch Pathol*, **67**, 443–5.

Rutten-van Mölken MPMH, Custers F, Vandoorslaer EKA, *et al*. (1995) Comparison of performance of four instruments in evaluating the effects of salmeterol on asthma quality of life. *Eur Respir J*, **8**, 888–98.

Salmeron S, Brochard L, Mal H, *et al*. (1994) Nebulized versus intravenous albuterol in hypercapnic acute asthma. *Am J Respir Crit Care Med*, **149**, 1466–70.

Scheinin M, Koulu M, Laurikainen E, Allonen H. (1987) Hypokalaemia and other non-bronchial effects of inhaled fenoterol and salbutamol: a placebo-controlled dose–response study in healthy volunteers. *Br J Clin Pharmacol*, **24**, 645–53.

Schreurs AJ.M, Sinninghe Damsté HEJ, de Graaff CS, Greefhorst APM. (1996) A dose–response study with formoterol Tubuhaler® as maintenance therapy in asthmatic patients. *Eur Respir J*, **9**, 1678–83.

Sears MR, Taylor DR, Print CG, *et al*. (1990) Regular inhaled β-agonist treatment in bronchial asthma. *Lancet*, **336**, 1391–6.

Shaheen MZ, Ayres JG, Benincasa C. (1994) Incidence of acute decreases in peak expiratory flow following the use of metered dose inhalers in asthmatic patients. *Eur Respir J*, **7**, 2160–4.

Simons FER and the Canadian Beclomethasone Diproprionate – Salmeterol Xinafoate Study Group. (1997) A comparison of beclomethasone, salmeterol, and placebo in children with asthma. *N Engl J Med*, **337**, 1659–65.

Skoogh BE. (1983) Transmission through airway ganglia. *Eur J Respir Dis*, **64** (131), 159–70.

Smyth ET, Pavord ID, Wong CS, Wisniewski AF, Williams J, Tattersfield AE. (1993) Interaction and dose equivalence of salbutamol and salmeterol in patients with asthma. *BMJ*, **306**, 543–5.

Spitzer WO, Suissa S, Ernst P, *et al*. (1992) The use of β-agonists and the risk of death and near death from asthma. *N Engl J Med*, **326**, 501.

Stolley PD. (1972) Asthma mortality: why the United States was spared an epidemic of deaths due to asthma. *Am Rev Respir Dis*, **105**, 883–90.

Strader CD, Sigal IS, Dixon AF. (1989) Mapping the functional domains of the β-adrenergic receptor. *Am J Respir Cell Mol Biol*, **1**, 81–6.

Sykes AP, Lawson N, Finnegan JA, Ayres JG. (1991) Creatine kinase activity in patients with brittle asthma treated with long term subcutaneous terbutaline. *Thorax*, **46**, 580–3.

Tan S, Hall IP, Dewar J, Dow E, Lipworth B. (1997) Association between β₂-adrenoceptor polymorphism and susceptibility to bronchodilator desensitisation in moderately severe stable asthmatics. *Lancet*, **350**, 995–9.

Tattersfield AE. (1985) Tolerance to β-agonists. *Bull Eur Physiopathol Respir (Clin Respir Physiol)*, **21**, 1S–5S.

Tattersfield AE. (1987) Effect of beta agonists and anticholinergic drugs on bronchial reactivity. *Am Rev Respir Dis*, **136**, S64–S68.

Tattersfield AE, Wilding P. (1993) β-agonists and ventilation. *Thorax*, **48**, 877–8.

Tattersfield AE, Postma DS, Barnes PJ, *et al*. (1999a) Exacerbations of asthma – a descriptive study of 425 severe exacerbations. *Am J Respir Crit Care Med*, **160**, 594–9.

Tattersfield AE, Löfdahl, C-G, Postma DS, *et al*. (1999b) On demand treatment comparison of formoterol and terbutaline in moderate asthma. *Eur Respir J*, **14**, 45.

Taylor DR, Town GI, Herbison GP, *et al*. (1998) Asthma control during long term treatment with regular inhaled salbutamol and salmeterol. *Thorax*, **53**, 744–52.

Teschemacher A, Lemoine H. (1999) Kinetic analysis of drug–receptor interactions of long acting β₂-sympathomimetics in isolated receptor membranes: evidence against prolonged effects of salmeterol and formoterol on receptor-coupled adenyl cyclase. *Pharmacol Exp Therap*, **288**, 1084–92.

Thompson Coon J, Johnson S, Harrison T, Tattersfield A. (1999) Effect of adding prednisolone to regular β-agonists on the systemic response to inhaled salbutamol. *Am J Respir Crit Care Med*, **159**, A635.

Todd GL, Baroldi G, Pieper GM, Clayton FC, Eliot RS. (1985) Experimental catecholamine-induced myocardial necrosis. I. Morphology, quantification and regional distribution of acute contraction band lesions. *J Mol Cell Cardiol*, **17**, 317–38.

Torphy TJ, Hall IP. (1994) Cyclic AMP and the control of airways smooth muscle tone. In: Raeburn D, Giembycz MA, eds. *Airways smooth muscle: biochemical control of contraction and relaxation*. Basel: Birkhauser Verlag, 215–33.

Tötterman KJ, Huhti L, Sutinen E, Backman R, Pietinalho A, Falck M, Larsson P, Selroos O. (1998) Tolerability to high doses of formoterol and terbutaline via Turbuhaler® for 3 days in stable asthmatic patients. *Eur Respir J*, **12**, 573–9.

Trembath PW, Greenacre JK, Anderson M, *et al.* (1979) Comparison of four weeks' treatment with fenoterol and terbutaline aerosols in adult asthmatics. *J Allergy Clin Immunol*, **63**, 395–400.

Twentyman OP, Finnerty JP, Harris A, Palmer J, Holgate ST. (1990) Protection against allergen-induced asthma by salmeterol. *Lancet*, **336**, 1338–42.

Twentyman OP, Finnerty JP, Holgate ST. (1991) The inhibitory effect of nebulized albuterol on the early and late asthmatic reactions and increase in airway responsiveness provoked by inhaled allergen in asthma. *Am Rev Respir Dis*, **144**, 782–7.

van Arsdel PP, Schaffrin RM, Rosenblatt J, Sprenkle AC, Altman LC. (1978) Evaluation of oral fenoterol in chronic asthmatic patients. *Chest*, **73**, 997–8.

van der Molen T, Postma DS, Turner MO, *et al.*, on behalf of The Netherlands and Canadian formoterol study investigators. (1997) Effect of the long acting β-agonist formoterol in asthmatic patients using inhaled corticosteroid. *Thorax*, **52**, 535–9.

van Essen-Zandvliet EE, Hughes MD, Waalkens HJ, Duiverman EJ, Pocock SJ, Kerrebijn KF, The Dutch Chronic Non-Specific Lung Disease Study Group. (1992) Effects of 22 months of treatment with inhaled corticosteroids and/or β₂-agonists on lung function, airway responsiveness, and symptoms in children with asthma. *Am Rev Respir Dis*, **146**, 547–54.

van Metre TE. (1969) Adverse effects of inhalation of excessive amounts of nebulised isoproterenol in status asthmaticus. *J Allergy*, **43**, 101–13.

van Noord JA, Smeets JJ, Raaijmakers JAM, Bommer AM, Maesen FPV. (1996) Salmeterol versus formoterol in patients with moderately severe asthma: onset and duration of action. *Eur Respir J*, **9**, 1684–8.

van Noord JA, Schreurs AJM, Mol SJM, Mulder PGH. (1999) Addition of salmeterol versus doubling the dose of fluticasone propionate in patients with mild to moderate asthma. *Thorax*, **54**, 207–12.

Vathenen AS, Knox AJ, Higgins BG, Britton JR, Tattersfield AE. (1988) Rebound increase in bronchial responsiveness after treatment with inhaled terbutaline. *Lancet*, **i**, 554–8.

Verberne AAPH, Hop WCJ, Creyghton FBM, *et al.* (1996) Airway responsiveness after a single dose of salmeterol and during four months of treatment in children with asthma. *J Allergy Clin Immunol*, **97**, 938–46.

Wagner PD, Dantzker DR, Iacovoni VE, Tomlin WC, West JB. (1978) Ventilation–perfusion inequality in asymptomatic asthma. *Am Rev Respir Dis*, **118**, 511–25.

Wahedna I, Wong CS, Wisniewski AFZ, Pavord ID, Tattersfield AE. (1993) Asthma control during and after cessation of regular β₂-agonist treatment. *Am Rev Respir Dis*, 148, 707–12.

Wallin A, Melander B, Rosenhall L, Sandström T, Wåhlander L. (1990) Formoterol, a new long acting β₂-agonist for inhalation twice daily, compared with salbutamol in the treatment of asthma. *Thorax*, **45**, 259–61.

Wanner A, Salathé M, O'Riordan TC. (1996) Mucociliary clearance in the airways. *Am J Respir Crit Care Med*, **154**, 1868–902.

Warrell DA, Robertson DG, Newton Howes J, *et al.* (1970) Comparison of cardiorespiratory effects of isoprenaline and salbutamol in patients with bronchial asthma. *BMJ*, **i**, 65–70.

Wasserman SI, Furukawa CT, Henochowicz SI, *et al.* (1995) Asthma symptoms and airway hyperresponsiveness are lower during treatment with nedocromil sodium than during treatment with regular inhaled albuterol. *J Allergy Clin Immunol*, **95**, 541–7.

Wilding P, Clark M, Thompson Coon J, *et al.* (1997) Effect of long term treatment with salmeterol on asthma control. *BMJ*, **314**, 1441–6.

Wilkinson JR.W, Roberts JA, Bradding P, Holgate ST, Howarth PH. (1992) Paradoxical bronchoconstriction in asthmatic patients after salmeterol by metered dose inhaler. *BMJ*, **305**, 931–2.

Wilson SR, Amoroso P, Moxham J, Ponte J. (1993) Modification of the thermogenic effect of acutely inhaled salbutamol by chronic inhalation in normal subjects. *Thorax*, **48**, 886–9.

Wong BJ, Dolovich J, Ramsdale EH, *et al.* (1992) Formoterol compared with beclomethasone and placebo on allergen-induced asthmatic responses. *Am Rev Respir Dis*, **146**, 1156–60.

Wong CS, Pavord ID, Williams J, Britton JR, Tattersfield AE. (1990) Bronchodilator, cardiovascular, and hypokalaemic effects of fenoterol, salbutamol, and terbutaline in asthma. *Lancet*, **336**, 1396–9.

Wong CS, Tattersfield AE. (1993) The long term effects of β-receptor agonist therapy in relation to morbidity and mortality. In: Beasley R, Pearce NE, eds. *The role of β-receptor agonist therapy in asthma mortality*. Boca Raton, FL: CRC Press, 201–22.

Woolcock A, Lundbak B, Ringdal OLN, Jacques LA. (1996) Comparison of addition of salmeterol to inhaled steroids in asthmatic patients. *Am Rev Respir Dis*, **153**, 1481–8.

Yates DH, Sussman HS, Shaw MJ, Barnes PJ, Chung KF. (1995) Regular formoterol treatment in mild asthma. *Am J Respir Crit Care Med*, **152**, 1170–4.

12

Non-steroidal prophylactic agents: mode of action and place in management

NEIL C. THOMSON

INTRODUCTION

Inhaled and oral corticosteroids are the most effective antiinflammatory drugs currently available for the treatment of asthma. Non-steroidal prophylactic drugs also have an important role in asthma management. These drugs can be used as alternative therapies to low-dose inhaled corticosteroids, as add-on treatment to patients in whom asthma control is inadequate despite inhaled corticosteroids, or as oral-steroid sparing agents.

CROMONES

Sodium cromoglycate was the first prophylactic non-steroidal drug licensed for the treatment of chronic asthma. It is a derivative of chromone-2-carboxylic acid and has a flexible hydrophilic structure with a bicyclic ring system (Fig. 12.1). Nedocromil sodium, which was introduced in the 1980s as a prophylactic agent in adult asthma, is the disodium salt of pyranoquinolone dicarboxylic acid, and unlike sodium cromoglycate, it is a rigid hydrophobic molecule with a tricyclic ring system (Fig. 12.1; Gonzalez and Brogden, 1987).

Mode of action

The modes of action of sodium cromoglycate or nedocromil sodium have not been clearly established. Recently, it has been reported that both drugs act as non-specific chloride channel blockers in a large range of cell types (Norris and Alton, 1996) and through this mode of action these compounds may reduce alterations in cell volume and function.

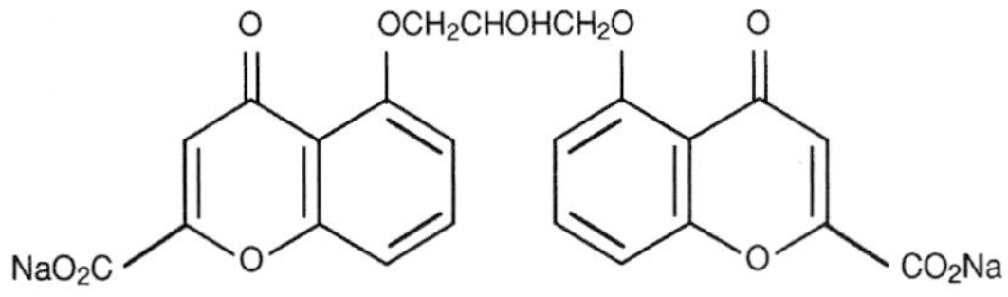

Figure 12.1 *Chemical structure of sodium cromoglycate and nedocromil sodium.*

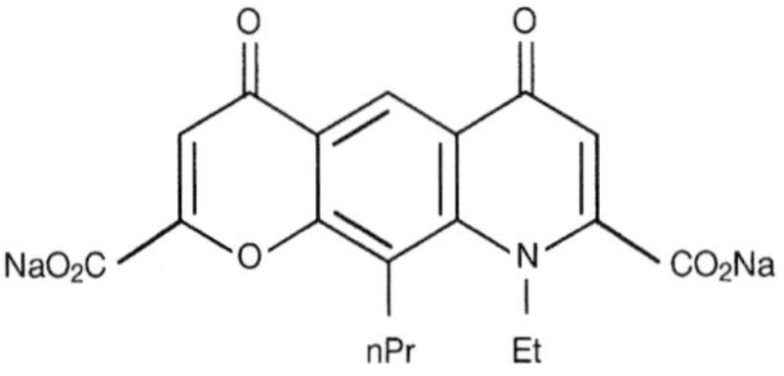

Both drugs have effects on a variety of different inflammatory cell types (Thomson, 1989; Barnes *et al.*, 1995; Norris and Alton, 1996). Sodium cromoglycate inhibits degranulation of mast cells triggered by immunological and non-immunological stimuli. Pretreatment of eosinophils and neutrophils with sodium cromoglycate inhibits certain cell responses such as complement (C3b) and IgG (Fc) receptor expression and cytotoxicity against schistosomula (Kay *et al.*, 1987). Sodium cromoglycate also has inhibitory effects *in vitro* on alveolar macrophage function. Similarly, the inhibitory effects of nedocromil sodium *in vitro* have been demonstrated in a variety of different inflammatory cells. Nedocromil sodium can inhibit anti-human IgE histamine release from mast cells obtained by bronchoalveolar lavage and it has been shown to be more active against these mast cells than against parenchymal-derived mast cells. The drug has also been shown to produce a dose-dependent inhibition of human eosinophil and neutrophil cell activation and to have inhibitory effects on alveolar macrophage function. Ozone-induced cytokine release from human epithelial cells is attenuated by nedocromil sodium. The platelets of patients with aspirin-induced asthma demonstrate increased cytotoxicity against schistosomula in the presence of aspirin and other non-steroidal antiinflammatory drugs. This response is not found in platelets from normal individuals or non-aspirin-sensitive asthmatic patients. Nedocromil sodium inhibits the cytotoxic response to aspirin, whereas sodium cromoglycate demonstrates markedly reduced potency in this system (Joseph *et al.*, 1988). In animal models, nedocromil sodium has been shown to inhibit cellular influx of eosinophils and neutrophils into the airways and to reduce microvascular leakage. Thus these drugs possess properties that may reduce some components of airway inflammation in asthma.

In vitro studies of human inflammatory cells and *in vivo* studies in experimental animals have demonstrated that nedocromil sodium has either similar or slightly greater potency than sodium cromoglycate (*see* Thomson, 1989). The main exception to this finding is the markedly enhanced potency of nedocromil sodium, as compared to sodium cromoglycate, in preventing activation by aspirin of platelets from aspirin-sensitive asthmatic patients (Joseph *et al.*, 1993). The clinical relevance of this observation is uncertain.

Both sodium cromoglycate and nedocromil sodium may have inhibitory effects on sensory nerve endings in the lung, thus preventing the release of tachykinins. In dogs, pretreatment with sodium cromoglycate or nedocromil sodium inhibits reflex bronchoconstriction induced by the sensory nerve stimulus capsaicin. In humans, these drugs inhibit the broncho-constrictor effect to neuropeptides, such as bradykinin, and to sulphur dioxide, both of which are thought to act on sensory nerve endings.

CLINICAL EVIDENCE FOR ANTIINFLAMMATORY ACTIONS

Clinical evidence for an antiinflammatory effect of sodium cromoglycate is based on studies in humans in whom chronic treatment has been shown to reduce significantly the percentage of eosinophils in bronchial alveolar lavage specimens following four weeks of treatment (Diaz et al., 1984). Recently, an open study of 12 weeks of treatment with inhaled sodium cromoglycate reported a reduction in the numbers of eosinophils, mast cells and T lymphocytes and in the expression of adhesion molecules in bronchial biopsy specimens from nine patients with atopic asthma (Hoshino and Nakamura, 1997). A double-blind, placebo-controlled trial compared nedocromil sodium treatment with regular salbutamol for a period of 16 weeks in patients with mild-to-moderate asthma (Manolitsas et al., 1995). The change in bronchial biopsy eosinophil counts was reduced in the nedocromil sodium treatment group as compared to an increase in the salbutamol treatment group, but neither change was significantly different from the placebo group.

Clinical studies

BRONCHIAL CHALLENGE

Pretreatment with sodium cromoglycate has been shown to reduce bronchoconstriction following allergen challenge and after non-allergic stimuli such as exercise in both children and adults (see Holgate, 1996a). Sodium cromoglycate can inhibit allergen-induced early and late asthmatic responses and the increase in histamine reactivity that is associated with late asthmatic responses. The seasonal increase in non-allergic bronchial reactivity can be prevented by sodium cromoglycate treatment. The results of studies examining the effects of sodium cromoglycate therapy on non-seasonal bronchial hyperreactivity have produced conflicting results; any reduction in bronchial reactivity is likely to be very small.

Nedocromil sodium also attenuates the bronchoconstrictor response induced by exercise (Fig. 12.2; Roberts and Thomson, 1985), cold air and the early and late response to allergen (see Thomson, 1989; Barnes et al., 1995). The increase in histamine reactivity that occurs during the pollen season in pollen-sensitive patients can be attenuated by nedocromil sodium (Dorward et al., 1986). It has no acute inhibitory effect on methacholine or leukotriene D_4-induced bronchoconstriction but continuous treatment over several weeks can produce small reductions in non-seasonal bronchial reactivity (Svendsen et al., 1989; Bel et al., 1990).

Comparison of sodium cromoglycate and nedocromil sodium

In a small number of bronchial challenge studies nedocromil sodium has been compared with sodium cromoglycate. The interpretation of these studies is difficult owing to the absence of dose–response data for each drug. Konig et al. (1987) demonstrated that nedocromil sodium (4 mg from an MDI (metered dose inhaler)) and sodium cromoglycate (20 mg from a spinhaler) inhibited exercise-induced asthma to a similar degree 20 min after administration whereas at 2 h only sodium cromoglycate was still effective. Both drugs have been found to protect against bradykinin and cold air-induced bronchoconstriction to a similar degree. Nedocromil sodium is slightly more effective than sodium cromoglycate in protecting against bronchospasm induced by adenosine (Phillips et al., 1989) or sodium metabisulphite.

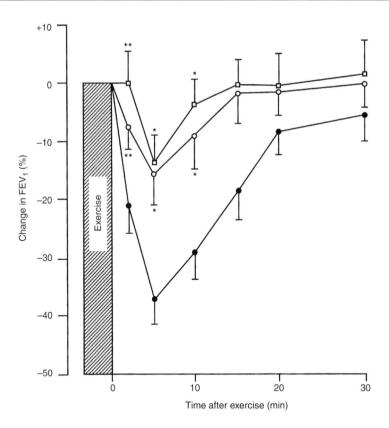

Figure 12.2 *Effect of pretreatment with nedocromil sodium (□, 2 mg; or ○, 4 mg) or placebo (●) on the percentage fall in FEV₁ after exercise in nine adult asthmatic patients. *, P < 0.05; **, P < 0.01. (Reproduced from Roberts and Thomson, 1985 with permission.)*

CLINICAL ASTHMA

Comparison with placebo

In both paediatric and adult asthma, treatment with inhaled sodium cromoglycate has been shown to improve asthma control (Brompton Hospital/Medical Research Council Collaborative Trial, 1972; Eigen *et al.*, 1987; *see* Carlsen and Larsson, 1996). A recent study, however, questioned the efficacy of sodium cromoglycate in children with asthma below the age of 4 years (Tasche *et al.*, 1997). In older children it has been shown to be as effective as regular theophylline treatment and its use is associated with significantly fewer side-effects. Both atopic and non-atopic asthmatic patients have been shown to respond to sodium cromoglycate treatment. Studies comparing nedocromil sodium with placebo have demonstrated efficacy in both children and adult asthmatic patients (Edwards and Stevens, 1993; *see* Holgate, 1996b). Patients with moderate asthma, currently receiving treatment with inhaled or oral bronchodilators responded best to the introduction of nedocromil sodium (Edwards and Stevens, 1993).

Comparison with inhaled steroids

Most studies suggest that the improvements in asthma control resulting from sodium cromoglycate or nedocromil sodium treatment are either equivalent or more commonly slightly less than those produced by inhaled beclomethasone in a dose of 400 μg daily

(Svendsen *et al.*, 1989; Bel *et al.*, 1990; Faurschou *et al.*, 1994). The differences in results among studies may be explained in part by the dose of sodium cromoglycate or nedocromil sodium administered, e.g. nedocromil sodium 8 mg or 16 mg daily, and the severity of asthma. In one recent study, sodium cromoglycate 10 mg (four times a day) was demonstrated to be equally as effective as inhaled beclomethasone 400 μg daily in patients with mild adult asthma (Faurschou *et al.*, 1994). Several studies suggest that nedocromil sodium can partially replace inhaled corticosteroids therapy. In these trials, during the run-in period, the dose of inhaled corticosteroid was reduced to the 'minimum effective dose' (Lal *et al.*, 1984; Fyans *et al.*, 1986). In the study by Lal *et al.* (1984), the introduction of nedocromil sodium compared to placebo produced significant reductions in daytime asthma, cough and additional daytime bronchodilator use. In the study by Fyans *et al.* (1986), a further reduction in inhaled corticosteroid dose was made after 2–3 weeks of treatment with nedocromil sodium; improvements in daytime asthma and bronchodilator use were seen in the nedocromil sodium group when compared to the placebo group. Nedocromil sodium cannot, however, completely replace inhaled corticosteroids when the steroid is withdrawn over a period of a few weeks (Ruffin *et al.*, 1987).

The addition of inhaled nedocromil sodium to asthmatic patients with symptoms poorly controlled by high dose (>1000 μg) inhaled corticosteroids has been reported to produce small improvements in symptom scores, peak flow readings and bronchodilator use (Svendsen and Jorgensen, 1991).

Oral corticosteroids sparing effects
In a study reported by Golden and Bateman (1988), the total corticosteroid reduction in the nedocromil sodium-treated group (2.5 mg) was not significantly different from that in the placebo-treated group (3 mg). In contrast to this result, Boulet *et al.* (1990) reported a small but significant oral steroid-sparing action of nedocromil sodium.

Comparison of sodium cromoglycate and nedocromil sodium
A small number of clinical trials in adult asthma have compared these two cromones and in most studies the therapeutic effects were found to be comparable (Boldy and Ayres, 1993; Schwartz *et al.*, 1996).

Adverse effects
Sodium cromoglycate is a safe drug and uncommonly causes side-effects. Very occasionally it can cause acute bronchoconstriction in a sensitive individual and some patients may notice slight cough or irritation of the throat following inhalation. Occasional complaints of nausea and headaches have been reported. Nedocromil sodium has not been associated with any severe side-effects. The main side-effects reported include a distinctive bitter taste, headache and nausea.

Place in management

Sodium cromoglycate was first introduced as a prophylactic anti-asthma treatment over 25 years ago and nedocromil sodium first became available in the 1980s. Both drugs have been shown to be effective in children and adults with asthma and are well tolerated. Most studies suggest that the improvements in asthma control resulting from sodium cromoglycate or nedocromil sodium treatment are less than those produced by inhaled beclomethasone in a dose of 400 μg daily. The need for three or four times daily dosing is a major disadvantage when compared to twice or even once daily dosing with inhaled steroids. The value of these drugs as 'add-on' therapy is not clearly defined. The effects of nedocromil sodium on the partial replacement of oral corticosteroids are conflicting, suggesting that any oral corticosteroid sparing effect is likely to be very small.

POSITION IN GUIDELINES

First-line prophylactic therapy
The National Institutes of Health (1997) expert panel report on the Guidelines for the Diagnosis and Management of Asthma suggest that sodium cromoglycate or nedocromil sodium may be considered as initial prophylactic therapy for children and as preventative treatment prior to exercise or unavoidable exposure to known allergens. The report emphasizes that safety is the primary advantage of these drugs. The British Guidelines on Asthma Management (1997) recommend the cromones as alternative antiinflammatory agents to low-dose inhaled steroids for patients whose asthma is not controlled with the occasional use of a relief bronchodilator (step 2).

Add-on therapy in mild-to-moderate asthma
The British Guidelines on Asthma Management (1997) recommend that both inhaled sodium cromoglycate and nedocromil sodium can be used as additional therapy at steps 3 and 4 of the guidelines. The cromones are less effective than other add-on therapies such as long-acting inhaled β_2-agonists. In clinical practice these drugs are rarely prescribed as 'add-on' therapy.

Chronic severe asthma
The cromones are not generally found to be effective in this group of patients.

LEUKOTRIENE SYNTHESIS INHIBITORS AND RECEPTOR ANTAGONISTS

Over the last 15 years a number of drugs have been developed that can block the effects of leukotrienes on the lungs. One group, the 5-lipoxygenase inhibitors, prevent the production of the leukotrienes whereas another group, the leukotriene receptor antagonists, block their effects at the receptor level. In recent years a number of these drugs have been launched in different countries throughout the world. The oral 5-lipoxygenase inhibitor zileuton is available in the USA. Montelukast, pranlukast and zafirlukast are orally-active leukotriene receptor antagonists that are licensed in several countries for the treatment of asthma. Zafirlukast and pranlukast are administered twice daily and montelukast is administered once daily at bedtime. This review will concentrate principally on the pharmacological properties of zileuton, zafirlukast and montelukast.

Mode of action

Leukotrienes are inflammatory mediators that play a role in the pathogenesis of asthma (*see* Chapter 6). There are several different cysteinyl leukotrienes, C_4, D_4 and E_4, which contribute to the bronchoconstriction, mucus secretion, eosinophil recruitment and oedema formation found in asthma. Several cells involved in airway inflammation in asthma, including eosinophils and mast cells can produce large quantities of the leukotrienes. The cysteinyl leukotrienes are formed in the cell walls from arachidonic acid by the 5-lipoxygenase pathway.

DRUGS ACTING ON THE 5-LIPOXYGENASE PATHWAY
The effects of the leukotrienes can be blocked in two ways (Fig. 12.3).

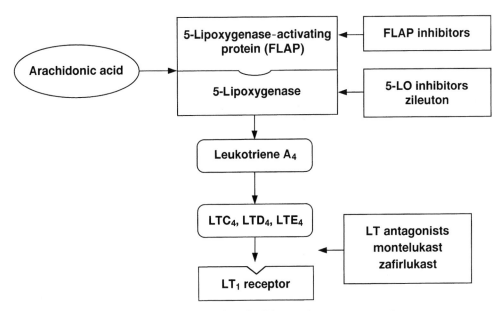

Figure 12.3 *Sites of action of leukotriene synthesis inhibitors and receptor antagonists.*

Inhibition of synthesis

The main approach to preventing the synthesis of the leukotrienes is by blocking their production with drugs that inhibit either 5-lipoxygenase or 5-lipoxygenase-activating protein (FLAP). The 5-lipoxygenase inhibitors block the enzyme directly whereas the FLAP inhibitors prevent it binding with FLAP on the nuclear membrane. Zileuton is an example of a direct 5-lipoxygenase inhibitor that is available for clinical use. FLAP inhibitors are currently under evaluation but to date no compound has been licensed for use in asthma. In addition to inhibiting the production of the cysteinyl leukotrienes the 5-lipoxygenase inhibitors also prevent the formation of leukotriene B_4 and other 5-lipoxygenase products. The clinical significance of the additional effects of 5-lipoxygenase inhibitors compared to leukotriene receptor antagonists is uncertain. Interestingly, naturally occurring mutations in the 5-lipoxygenase gene may confer a poor clinical response to zileuton (Drazen *et al.*, 1997).

Leukotriene receptor antagonists

There are two subtypes of cysteinyl leukotriene (Cys-LT) receptors termed the Cys-LT1 receptor and the Cys-LT2 receptor. In human airway smooth muscle, leukotrienes C_4, D_4 and E_4 all act on the Cys-LT1 receptor. Leukotriene receptor antagonists such as zafirlukast, pranlukast and montelukast all act at the Cys-LT1 receptor. On the other hand, Cys-LT2 receptors are present in pulmonary vascular tissue and are not thought to be involved in the pathogenesis of asthma.

CLINICAL EVIDENCE FOR ANTIINFLAMMATORY ACTIONS

In asthma, both 5-lipoxygenase inhibitors and leukotriene receptor antagonists should have inhibitory effects on the pro-inflammatory actions of the leukotrienes. In support of this hypothesis, the 5-lipoxygenase inhibitor, zileuton, decreases nocturnal bronchoalveolar lavage and blood eosinophil counts in patients with nocturnal asthma (Wenzel *et al.*, 1995) and the influx of eosinophils following segmental allergen challenge (Kane *et al.*, 1996). Compared with placebo, the leukotriene receptor antagonist montelukast decreases peripheral blood and induced sputum eosinophil counts induced by allergen challenge (Pizzichini *et al.*, 1999). The leukotriene receptor antagonist zafirlukast, when administered at a dose of 20 mg twice daily for one week, significantly reduces bronchoalveolar lavage lymphocyte and basophil counts but not eosinophil influx 48 hours following segmental allergen challenge (Calhoun *et al.* 1998). A further study with zafirlukast using a similar protocol but administered at a dose of 160 mg twice daily, which is a higher dose than currently recommended, reduced eosinophil influx 48 hours following segmental allergen challenge (Calhoun *et al.*, 1997). Furthermore, chronic treatment with zileuton and the leukotriene receptor antagonists reduced circulating blood eosinophil counts (Liu *et al.*, 1996; Reiss *et al.*, 1998). A number of studies have found that zileuton suppresses urinary leukotriene E_4 excretion (Hui *et al.*, 1991; Israel *et al.*, 1993a,b).

Clinical studies

BRONCHIAL CHALLENGE

Both 5-lipoxygenase inhibitors and leukotriene receptor antagonists are reported to attenuate the bronchoconstrictor response to a number of trigger factors including allergen, exercise, cold air and aspirin (Chung, 1995; McGill and Busse, 1996; Ind, 1996). In addition, a single dose of zileuton attenuates bronchial reactivity to histamine and to ultrasonically nebulized distilled water (Dekhuijzen *et al.*, 1997).

Allergen-induced asthma

A single dose of 800 mg zileuton, the 5-lipoxygenase inhibitor, had no effect on the early or late response to allergen. The leukotriene receptor antagonist zafirlukast, administered in a single oral dose 2 hours before allergen challenge, inhibited the early response by 80% and the late response by 50% (Taylor *et al.*, 1991). Similar results to those obtained with zafirlukast have been reported with the leukotriene receptor antagonist montelukast.

Exercise-induced asthma

The leukotriene receptor antagonists zafirlukast and montelukast both attenuate exercise-induced asthma in both children and adults (Finnerty *et al.*, 1992; Kemp *et al.*, 1998; Leff *et al.*, 1998; Turpin *et al.*, 1998). The mean maximal percentage fall in FEV_1 after exercise following a single dose of zafirlukast was 22% compared with 36% after placebo (Finnerty *et al.*, 1992). Following 3 months' treatment with montelukast, the maximal fall in FEV_1 after exercise was 22% compared with 32% after placebo (Leff *et al.*, 1998). The results remained consistent throughout the study and tolerance did not develop. In one study of patients with mild asthma not receiving inhaled corticosteroid therapy, inhaled salmeterol but not montelukast showed an attenuation of bronchoprotection after 4 and 8 weeks of treatment (Turpin *et al.*, 1998). Acute and long-term treatment with zileuton has been shown to decrease the response to isocapnic hyperventilation (Fischer *et al.*, 1995).

Aspirin-induced asthma

Aspirin-sensitive asthma is associated with elevated formation of the cysteinyl leukotrienes. Interestingly, the response to aspirin challenge in these patients is very effectively inhibited by both 5-lipoxygenase inhibitors and leukotriene receptor antagonists (Chung, 1995). One week's treatment with zileuton not only prevented the fall in FEV_1 after aspirin challenge but blocked nasal, gastrointestinal and dermal symptoms (Israel *et al.*, 1993a). Zileuton also caused a decrease in urinary leukotriene E_4 at baseline and after aspirin challenge.

BASELINE LUNG FUNCTION

The observation that 5-lipoxygenase inhibitors and leukotriene receptor antagonists produce a mild bronchodilation in patients with airflow obstruction suggests that leukotrienes released within the airways contribute to the bronchoconstriction of asthma. In a group of 139 asthmatic patients whose baseline FEV_1 values were approximately 60% of predicted, a single 600 mg dose of zileuton increased mean FEV_1 values by 14.6% at 1 hour, which was significantly greater than the change with placebo (Israel *et al.*, 1993b). Further improvements in FEV_1 values occurred during the following 4 weeks of chronic dosing with zileuton. A single 40 mg oral dose of zafirlukast produced a small bronchodilator effect, increasing the mean FEV_1 value by 8% (Hui and Barnes, 1991). In this study the increase in FEV_1 after nebulized salbutamol and zafirlukast was 26% compared with 18% after nebulized salbutamol and placebo. Although this finding suggests that the bronchodilator effect of β_2-agonists and leukotriene receptor antagonists is additive, further dose–response studies are indicated.

CLINICAL ASTHMA

Comparison with placebo

Three large multicentre trials using the 5-lipoxygenase inhibitor, zileuton, in mild-to-moderate chronic asthma have shown evidence of efficacy (Israel *et al.*, 1993b, 1996; Liu *et al.*, 1996; Table 12.1). The duration of the trials was 4, 13 and 26 weeks respectively and each employed a double-blind, parallel group, placebo-controlled study design. Zileuton was shown to improve daily symptoms of asthma, night waking and peak expiratory flow measurements, and to reduce the use of rescue inhaled β_2-agonists and the number of exacerbations of asthma requiring corticosteroids (Fig. 12.4).

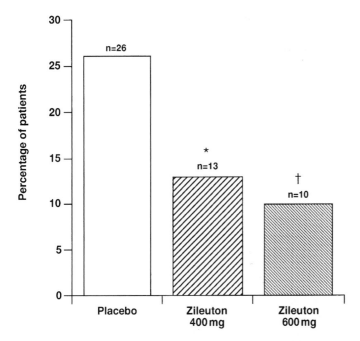

Figure 12.4 *Percentage of patients in each study group requiring at least one course of corticosteroid treatment during the 6-month trial. *, P < 0.05, 400 mg zileuton group versus placebo group; †, P < 0.001, 600 mg zileuton group versus placebo group. (Reproduced from Liu et al., 1996.)*

Table 12.1 *Effect of 5-lipoxygenase inhibitors and leukotriene receptor antagonists compared to placebo in mild-to-moderate chronic asthma*

Drug	Dose (daily)	Duration (weeks)	Number of patients	Design	Results: symptoms, β-agonist use	Peak expiratory flow	Exacerbation rate	Reference
Zileuton	1.6 g or 2.4 g	4	139	PC	↓	↑	Not assessed	Israel *et al.*, 1993
	1.6 g or 2.4 g	13	401	PG, PC	↓ (quality of life ↑)	↑	↓	Israel *et al.*, 1996
	1.6 g or 2.4 g	26	373	PG, PC	↓	↑	Not assessed	Liu *et al.*, 1996
Zafirlukast	10 mg, 20 mg or 40 mg	6	266	PG, PC	↓	↑	Not assessed	Spector *et al.*, 1994
Montelukast	10 mg	12	681	PG, PC	↓ (quality of life ↑)	↑	↓	Reiss *et al.*, 1998

Abbreviations: PC, placebo controlled; PG, parallel group.

Similar results have been obtained with leukotriene receptor antagonists, such as zafirlukast and montelukast (Spector *et al.*, 1994; Suissa *et al.*, 1997; Reiss *et al.*, 1998; Table 12.1). In a 6-week trial of zafirlukast, significant improvements in symptoms and lung function were seen in the highest dose group (40 mg daily) (Spector *et al.*, 1994). Treatment with zafirlukast in a dose of 40 mg daily for 3 months was also found to reduce the rate of exacerbation of asthma (Suissa *et al.*, 1997). In a group of 681 adult patients with chronic stable asthma, 23% of whom were receiving inhaled corticosteroids, montelukast, compared with placebo, significantly improved asthma control (FEV_1, morning and evening peak expiratory flow, asthma symptoms and exacerbation rates) during a 3-month treatment period (Reiss *et al.*, 1998). Montelukast has also been shown to improve asthma control in 6 to 14-year-old children with chronic asthma (Knorr *et al.*, 1998). In general the 5-lipoxygenase inhibitors and leukotriene receptor antagonists appear to produce similar clinical effects, although to date there have been no comparative studies.

In aspirin-sensitive asthma, chronic dosing with montelukast for 4 weeks (Dahlen *et al.*, 1997) or with zileuton for 6 weeks (Dahlen *et al.*, 1998) has been shown to improve asthma control over that achieved with medium-to-high doses of inhaled corticosteroids.

Comparison with inhaled corticosteroids

To date, there is little published data comparing inhaled corticosteroid therapy. Preliminary studies suggest that the clinical efficacy of montelukast and zafirlukast is slightly less than seen with low doses of inhaled corticosteroids (equivalent to 400 µg daily of beclomethasone) (Laitinen *et al.*, 1997; Busse *et al.*, 1999; Malmstrom *et al.*, 1999). A multicentre randomized controlled trial of zafirlukast (20 mg twice daily) compared with inhaled fluticasone (100 µg twice daily) found that the improvement in pulmonary function and symptom control was greater in the inhaled corticosteroid group over a 3-month period in patients with persistent asthma who were not using inhaled corticosteroids at the start of the study (Kalberg *et al.*, 1998). In a group of 895 adult patients with chronic stable asthma, montelukast at 10 mg once daily, compared with inhaled beclomethasone at 200 µg twice daily, significantly increased mean FEV_1 values by 7.5% compared with 13.3% after the inhaled corticosteroid during a 3-month treatment period (Malmstrom *et al.*, 1999).

In a randomized, placebo-controlled, parallel group trial of 642 adult asthmatic patients not adequately controlled on inhaled beclomethasone (400 µg daily), the addition of montelukast resulted in an improvement in FEV_1 of 5.43% compared with 1.04% for inhaled corticosteroids alone (Laviolette *et al.*, 1999).

Comparison with add-on therapies

A randomized controlled trial of inhaled salmeterol (50 µg twice daily) compared to zafirlukast (20 mg twice daily) found that the long-acting inhaled β_2-agonists were more effective in terms of improving pulmonary function and symptom control in a group of 301 patients aged above 12 years with persistent asthma (Busse *et al.*, 1999). The majority of patients in this study were receiving inhaled corticosteroids.

ADVERSE EFFECTS

In clinical trials the 5-lipoxygenase inhibitor zileuton and the leukotriene receptor antagonists zafirlukast and montelukast have been well tolerated. Zileuton has been associated with rises in liver enzymes that return to normal on stopping administration of the drug (Israel *et al.*, 1993b, 1996). The incidence of zileuton-induced hepatitis is approximately 3%. In the USA, the Food and Drug Administration (FDA) recommends that liver function tests be monitored every two weeks during the first year of treatment. The main side-effects reported with the use of zafirlukast include headache, gastritis and pharyngitis, although these occurred with similar frequency in the placebo group (Spector *et al.*, 1994). In clinical trials with montelukast, abdominal pain, dyspepsia and headaches were reported in $\geq 2\%$ of patients although the incidence was not significantly different from those receiving placebo (US data sheet for montelukast, 1998).

The administration of the leukotriene receptor antagonist zafirlukast has been associated with the emergence of the Churg–Strauss syndrome. Six patients developed the Churg–Strauss syndrome while taking zafirlukast (Josefson, 1997) and further cases have reported with the use of both zafirlukast (Wechsier *et al.*, 1998) and montelukast. In each case the patient was on a reducing dose of oral corticosteroids for asthma. There is no proof of a causal relationship between the Churg–Strauss syndrome and these drugs. It is possible that the reduction in oral steroid dose by these patients resulted in the manifestations of the syndrome. Nevertheless, it would be advisable that patients with chronic oral steroid-dependent asthma who are receiving a leukotriene receptor antagonist are monitored carefully, with regular checks of the eosinophil count.

Place in management

In asthma, the 5-lipoxygenase inhibitors and the leukotriene receptor antagonists have been shown to have a mild bronchodilator effect in patients with airflow obstruction and to attenuate bronchoconstriction induced by exercise, allergen and aspirin. There is also some evidence to indicate that they have antiinflammatory actions. Several therapeutic studies in mild-to-moderate asthma have shown evidence of efficacy. A theoretical advantage of the oral formulation of these drugs, and for some agents, the infrequent dose scheduling, is improved concordance with therapy. In addition, systemic administration of therapy may also improve co-existing disease such as allergic rhinitis. In clinical trials, the 5-lipoxygenase inhibitor, zileuton, and the leukotriene receptor antagonists, zafirlukast and montelukast, have been well tolerated. The main adverse effect is hepatitis, which is associated with the administration of zileuton.

In clinical trials, the clinical effectiveness of the 5-lipoxygenase inhibitors and the leukotriene receptor antagonists appears to be quite variable between individuals. To date, there are few known predictors of response to therapy, although naturally occurring mutations in the 5-lipoxygenase gene may confer a poor clinical response to zileuton. The involvement of leukotrienes in aspirin-induced asthma and the beneficial effect of these agents in clinical trials would suggest that these patients would respond particularly well to treatment with anti-leukotrienes.

POSITION IN GUIDELINES

The place of the 5-lipoxygenase inhibitors and the leukotriene receptor antagonists in asthma management guidelines has not been clearly established.

(a) First-line prophylactic therapy

The National Institutes of Health (1997) expert panel report on the Guidelines for the Diagnosis and Management of Asthma recommends that leukotriene receptor antagonists or zileuton may be considered as alternative therapy to low doses of inhaled corticosteroids or the cromones in mild persistent asthma in patients ≥ 12 years of age. The British Guidelines on Asthma Management (1997) made no recommendations about their use. Both guidelines stress the need for data from comparative studies against established therapies.

(b) Add-on therapy in mild-to-moderate asthma

In the UK, the leukotriene receptor antagonist montelukast is licensed for the treatment of asthma as an add-on therapy in adults and children ($\geq$6 years) with chronic mild-to-moderate asthma who are inadequately controlled with inhaled steroids, and also as a prophylactic agent against exercise-induced asthma. Further clinical studies are required to compare the efficacy and side-effect profile of anti-leukotrienes such as montelukast with other add-on therapies such as long-acting inhaled β_2-agonists and oral theophyllines.

(c) Chronic severe asthma

The role of the 5-lipoxygenase inhibitors and the leukotriene receptor antagonists in chronic severe asthma is unknown. Nevertheless, it is likely that these drugs will be tried in more severe patients. It should be noted that the administration of zafirlukast, though not montelukast, has been associated with the emergence of the Churg–Strauss syndrome. Although there is no evidence to indicate that this was a cause and effect relationship, it would be advisable to carefully monitor patients with chronic oral steroid-dependent asthma, who are prescribed a leukotriene receptor antagonist, for features of the Churg–Strauss syndrome.

In conclusion the 5-lipoxygenase inhibitors and the leukotriene receptor antagonists are a completely new class of drug for the treatment of asthma. Further studies are required to clarify their position in the asthma management guidelines.

OTHER MEDIATOR SYNTHESIS INHIBITORS AND RECEPTOR ANTAGONISTS

In addition to the leukotrienes, a large number of other inflammatory mediators including histamine, platelet activating factor (PAF) and various cyclo-oxygenase products may be involved in the pathogenesis of asthma. To date, drugs developed as synthesis inhibitors or receptor antagonists of these mediators have been rather disappointing in the control of asthma. A number of studies are currently underway to assess the efficacy of inhibitors of other putative mediators of asthma, including interleukin-1β, interleukin-4 and interleukin-5.

Histamine receptor antagonists

MODE OF ACTION

Non-sedating antihistamines, such as astemizole, azelastine, cetirizine, loratadine and terfenadine, act as histamine $(H)_1$-receptor antagonists. A number of these compounds possess additional pharmacological properties. For example, *in vitro* studies have shown that cetirizine inhibits eosinophil chemotaxis (Walsh, 1994) and loratadine inhibits leukotriene release (Temple and McCluskey, 1988). Ketotifen inhibits mediator release *in vitro* from mast cells and possibly from other inflammatory cells and reverses β-adrenergic tachyphylaxis. The exact mode of action of ketotifen *in vivo* is unclear, although the main pharmacological effects are likely to be due to H_1-receptor antagonism (Craps, 1985; Grant *et al.*, 1990).

CLINICAL STUDIES

Antihistamines have been shown to attenuate the early and late response to allergen, although the combination of H_1-receptor antagonists, loratadine and the leukotriene receptor antagonist, zafirlukast was more effective than either drug alone (Roquet *et al.*, 1997). H_1-receptor antagonists also inhibit exercise-induced asthma. In clinical trials in chronic asthma, cetirizine and terfenadine have been shown to cause small reductions in symptoms and in the use of rescue inhaled β_2-agonists. Azelastine was shown to slightly reduce the need for inhaled corticosteroids (Busse *et al.*, 1996). Ketotifen has been found to be of little value in the treatment of asthma (Grant *et al.*, 1990). On starting therapy, drowsiness occurs in 15 to 20% of patients, but this effect usually disappears.

PLACE IN MANAGEMENT

Antihistamines have a weak anti-asthma activity in mild asthma. This action may be of value in the treatment of patients suffering from both seasonal allergic rhinitis and asthma. In the absence of comparative studies against established therapies it remains unclear whether there is a role for H_1-receptor antagonists in chronic asthma.

Platelet activating factor receptor antagonists

Several platelet activating factor (PAF) receptor antagonists have been developed (WEB 2086, UK 74505, modipafant), but these drugs have proven ineffective in preventing allergen-induced bronchoconstriction or in the treatment of chronic asthma (Kuitert, *et al.*, 1995). Recently, a more potent PAF antagonist, SR 27417A, has been found to have a modest inhibitory effect on the late asthmatic response to allergen (Evans *et al.*, 1997). It seems unlikely that PAF antagonists will have a place in asthma treatment.

Cyclo-oxygenase and thromboxane synthesis inhibitors

MODE OF ACTION

There are two types of cyclo-oxygenases: COX1 generates endogenous prostanoids and COX2 is involved in prostanoid production in inflammatory diseases including asthma (Demoly *et al.*, 1997). Drugs such as indomethacin or flurbiprofen are non-specific cyclo-oxygenase inhibitors, although they block COX1 to a greater extent than COX2. Recently, selective COX2 inhibitors have been developed. Thromboxane synthesis inhibitors and receptor antagonists prevent the production or effects of thromboxanes, respectively.

CLINICAL STUDIES

Evidence for the influence of cyclo-oxygenase inhibitors on the early and late asthmatic response to allergen is conflicting. Thromboxane synthesis inhibitors and receptor antagonists have shown little activity in challenge studies or in chronic asthma.

PLACE IN MANAGEMENT

In conclusion, there is no convincing evidence that chronic treatment with these groups of drugs has a role in asthma treatment.

OTHER NON-STEROIDAL PROPHYLACTIC AGENTS

Other groups of drugs have been assessed for their ability to act as non-steroidal prophylactic agents or as long-term control medications in asthma including long-acting β_2-agonists (*see* Chapter 11), methylxanthines and immunosuppressive drugs.

Methylxanthines

This section will review the possible role of methylxanthines as antiinflammatory agents in asthma. Detailed reviews of the other properties of the theophyllines have been published elsewhere (Weinberger and Hendeles, 1996).

MODE OF ACTION

Although the molecular mechanism of action of methylxanthines has not been fully established, the non-selective inhibition of phosphodiesterases in airway smooth muscle and inflammatory cells is almost certainly important. Phosphodiesterases form seven families of isoenzymes (types I to VII) with distinct tissue distributions and with subtypes of phosphodiesterase within each family (Dent and Giembycz, 1996). Inhibition of cAMP phosphodiesterase types III and IV in airway smooth muscle causes relaxation of resting and precontracted bronchi. Type IV isoenzyme predominates in many inflammatory cells including eosinophils and T lymphocytes. The antiinflammatory effects of theophylline *in vitro* are thought to be due principally to its inhibition of the type IV isoenzyme in inflammatory cells. Studies *in vitro* have demonstrated that theophylline inhibits the activation and the release of inflammatory mediators from a variety of cells implicated in the pathogenesis of asthma, including eosinophils and T lymphocytes (Barnes and Pauwels,1994; Dent and Giembycz, 1996). In addition, *in vivo* animal studies have shown that pretreatment with theophylline reduces eosinophil recruitment induced by allergen challenge.

CLINICAL EVIDENCE FOR ANTIINFLAMMATORY ACTION

Recent clinical studies have provided indirect evidence for antiinflammatory actions of theophylline in asthma. Several different clinical models have been used to assess the effects of theophylline on airway inflammation:

- Late asthmatic response (LAR) to allergen. Several studies have reported that the LAR to allergen, which is associated with increased airway inflammation, is reduced by theophylline (Sullivan *et al.*, 1994). A randomized placebo-controlled parallel group study undertaken in mild asthma patients demonstrated that 6 weeks of treatment with theophylline attenuated the LAR to allergen. Furthermore, bronchial biopsies performed 24 hours after the allergen challenge showed a significant reduction in the number of EG2-positive activated eosinophils in the theophylline-treated group. Interestingly this effect occurred at low plasma concentrations of theophylline (<10 mg/L).
- Nocturnal asthma. In a group of 8 patients with nocturnal asthma two weeks treatment with theophylline was found to suppress alveolar macrophage leukotriene B_4 production and decrease bronchoalveolar lavage neutrophil numbers (Kraft *et al.*, 1996). These cellular effects were associated with improvements in overnight lung function.
- Theophylline withdrawal. A controlled trial of theophylline withdrawal in 27 patients with severe chronic asthma who were maintained on high doses of inhaled steroids (mean dose >1500 mcg daily) caused a small but significant increase in nocturnal asthma symptoms and a fall in peak flow rates (Kidney *et al.*, 1995). These changes in clinical outcome measurements were accompanied by a fall in peripheral blood activated helper T lymphocytes (CD4+/CD25+) and activated suppressor T lymphocytes (CD8+/HLA/DR+) in those patients with a plasma theophylline level of >5 mg/L (n = 20). Bronchial biopsies were performed in eight of these patients and the changes mirrored those seen in the blood

with an increase in CD4+ and CD8+ T lymphocytes in the airways. The inverse relationship between blood and airway T lymphocyte populations suggest that theophylline may influence the influx of T-cells into the airways.

- Chronic theophylline treatment. The effects of 6 weeks' treatment with oral theophylline on clinical outcome measures and cells in bronchial biopsies were performed in 26 mild atopic asthmatic patients (Finnerty et al., 1996). Patients were randomized to either placebo (n = 11) or theophylline (n = 15). Nine of the placebo group and 12 of the theophylline patients completed the study. The mean (SD) plasma concentrations for theophylline was 10.9 (6.0) mg/L. There was a small but significant decrease in the change in mean (SD) nocturnal asthma symptom score during theophylline treatment [0.18 (0.30)] compared to the placebo treatment period [0.36 (0.42)]. Daytime symptom scores and β_2-agonist inhaler use did not differ between the theophylline and placebo treatment groups. A decrease in epithelial CD8+ T lymphocytes and interleukin-4 expression on submucosal cells was seen in biopsies from the theophylline-treated group compared with placebo. There was a trend for a reduction in the expression of the cytokine interleukin-5 on submucosal cells but this change was not statistically significant. The number of mast cells and eosinophils identified by the cell-specific markers, tryptase and eosinophilic cationic protein respectively, were unaltered by theophylline.

PLACE IN MANAGEMENT

When taken together the above clinical studies demonstrate that oral theophylline has inhibitory effects in certain components of the inflammatory response in asthma and that the effects occur at low plasma concentrations ($\leq$11 mg/L). Nevertheless, the clinical effects noted in these studies were generally small. Thus the relative importance of the antiinflammatory properties of theophyllines when compared with their bronchodilator actions in the clinical efficacy of these drugs remains uncertain.

POSITION IN GUIDELINES

First-line prophylactic therapy
The National Institutes of Health (1997) expert panel report on the Guidelines for the Diagnosis and Management of Asthma suggests that methylxanthines may be considered as alternative to either inhaled steroids or cromones as long-term control medications in adults and children over 5 years old. The British Guidelines on Asthma Management (1997) do not recommend the use of theophylline as a first-line antiinflammatory agent.

Add-on therapy in mild-to-moderate asthma
Current guidelines recommend theophylline as an additional treatment to inhaled β_2-agonists and high-dose inhaled steroids (beclomethasone or budesonide, 800–2000 mcg daily or fluticasone, 400–800 mcg daily) for patients whose asthma is not controlled. The British Guidelines on Asthma Management (1997) recommend that theophylline is also considered as an additional treatment option for a 'minority of patients' on low-dose inhaled steroids (beclomethasone or budesonide, 100–400 mcg daily or fluticasone, 50–200 mcg).

Chronic severe asthma
Chronic oral steroid-dependent asthmatic patients may also benefit from the addition of oral theophylline (Nassif et al., 1981).

Immunosuppressive agents

The oral steroid-sparing action of various immunosuppressive drugs including methotrexate, gold and cyclosporin has been investigated in chronic asthma (Hill and Tattersfield, 1995; Corrigan, 1998).

MODE OF ACTION

The mode of action of these drugs in asthma is uncertain. The immunosuppressive and antiinflammatory properties that are likely to be relevant to asthma are the ability of these drugs to inhibit T lymphocyte activation and mediator release from inflammatory cells such as mast cells (Corrigan, 1998).

CLINICAL STUDIES

Methotrexate: A small, oral steroid-sparing effect of methotrexate therapy in asthma has been reported in four out of seven double-blind trials (*see* Hill and Tattersfield, 1995*)*. Methotrexate was administered by the oral or intramuscular route in doses ranging from 15 to 30 mg per week. It took several months before the clinical benefits of methotrexate were seen and these did not persist following the cessation of treatment. Serious side-effects can occur, including liver damage and pulmonary fibrosis and there are a few reports of fatal opportunistic pulmonary infections.

Gold: Two controlled clinical trials with oral gold (3 mg twice daily) have shown reductions in oral steroid dosage. In one study a reduction of 4 mg of prednisolone was achieved over 26 weeks compared with 0.3 mg in those receiving placebo (Nierop *et al.*, 1992). In the other study, 60% of patients reduced the daily steroid dose by at least 50% compared with 32% in the placebo group (Bernstein *et al.*, 1996). The main side-effects of oral gold therapy are exacerbation of pre-existing eczema and gastrointestinal problems. More serious toxic effects include proteinuria, blood dyscrasias and pulmonary fibrosis.

Cyclosporin: Three controlled studies have examined the steroid-sparing activity of cyclosporin. In the first study over 36 weeks the median prednisolone dose fell by 7.5 mg compared with 2.5 mg in those receiving placebo (Lock *et al.*, 1996). A second study failed to confirm this finding (Nizankowska *et al.*, 1995). A further study showed improvement of asthma control following the introduction of cyclosporin in oral steroid-dependent asthmatic patients whose oral steroid dose was kept constant throughout the study (Alexander *et al.*, 1992). Side-effects included increased blood pressure, reduced renal function and hypertrichosis.

Other immunosuppressive drugs: Several small studies have failed to show that azathioprine, hydroxychloroquine or colchicine has any oral steroid-sparing action in asthma.

PLACE IN MANAGEMENT

Immunosuppressive drugs such as methotrexate, gold and cyclosporin have a limited role in the management of chronic oral steroid-dependent asthma because of their poor efficacy and potential to produce severe side-effects. These drugs should only be considered for use in those patients requiring a dose of prednisolone in excess of 10 mg daily for a period of one year or longer. In each patient the side-effects of oral steroids must be balanced against the potential toxic effects from immunosuppressive therapy. The value of these agents for the treatment of steroid-resistant asthma is unknown.

REFERENCES

Alexander AG, Barnes NC, Kay AB. (1992). Trial of cyclosporin in corticosteroid-dependent chronic severe asthma. *Lancet*, **339**, 324–8.

Barnes PJ, Pauwels RA. (1994) Theophylline in the management of asthma: time for reappraisal? *Eur Respir J*, **7**, 579–91.

Barnes PJ, Holgate ST, Laitinin LA, *et al.* (1995) Asthma mechanisms, determinants of severity and treatment: the role of nedocromil sodium. *Clin Exp Allergy*, **25**, 771–87.

Bel EH, Timmers MC, Hermans J, *et al.* (1990) The long-term effects of nedocromil sodium and beclomethasone dipropionate on bronchial responsiveness to methacholine in nonatopic asthmatic subjects. *Am Rev Respir Dis*, **141**, 21–8.

Bernstein IL, Bernstein DI, Dubb JW, Faiferman I, Wallin B. (1996). A placebo-controlled multicenter study of auranofin in the treatment of patients with corticosteroid-dependent asthma. Auranofin Multicenter Drug Trial. *J Allergy Clin Immunol*, **98**, 317–24.

Boldy DAR, Ayres JG. (1993) Nedocromil sodium and sodium cromoglycate in patients aged over 50 years with asthma. *Respir Med*, **87**, 517–23.

Boulet L-P, Cartier A, Cockcroft DW, *et al.* (1990) Tolerance to reduction of oral steroid dosage in severely asthmatic patients receiving nedocromil sodium. *Respir Med*, **84**, 317–23.

British Guidelines on Asthma Management: 1995 review and position statement. (1997) *Thorax*, **52**, S1–S21.

Brompton Hospital/Medical Research Council Collaborative Trial. (1972) Long term study of disodium cromoglycate in the treatment of severe extrinsic or intrinsic bronchial asthma in adults. *BMJ*, **4**, 383–8.

Busse WW, Middleton E, Storms W, *et al.* (1996) Corticosteroid-sparing effect of azelastine in the management of bronchial asthma. *Am J Respir Crit Care Med*, **153**, 122–7.

Busse W, Nelson H, Wolfe J, *et al.* (1999) Comparison of inhaled salmeterol and oral zafirlukast in patients with asthma. *J Allergy Clin Immunol*, **103**, 1075–80.

Calhoun WJ, Williams KL, Simonson SG. *et al.* (1997) Effect of zafirlukast (Accolate) on airway inflammation after segmental allergen challenge in patients with mild asthma. *Am J Repir Crit Care Med*, **155**, A662.

Calhoun WJ, Lavins BJ, Minkwitz MC, *et al.* (1998) Effect of zafirlukast (Accolate) on cellular mediators of inflammation. Bronchoalveolar lavage fluid findings after segmental allergen challenge. *Am J Repir Crit Care Med*, **157**, 1381–9.

Carlsen K-H, Larsson K. (1996) The efficacy of inhaled disodium cromoglycate and glucocorticoids. *Clin Exper Allergy*, **26**, Suppl 4, 8–17.

Chung KF. (1995) Leukotriene receptor antagonists and biosynthesis inhibitors: potential breakthrough in asthma therapy. *Eur Respir J*, **6**, 1203–13.

Corrigan CL. (1998) Immunomodulators In: Barnes PJ, Rodger IW, Thomson NC, eds. *Asthma basic mechanisms and clinical management*. London: Academic Press, 783–94.

Craps LP. (1985) Immunologic and therapeutic aspects of ketotifen. *J Allergy Clin Immunol*, **76**, 389–93.

Dahlen SE, Malmstrom K, Kuna P, *et al.* (1997) Improvement of asthma in aspirin-intolerant patients by montelukast (MK-0476) a potent and specific CYSLT1 receptor antagonist: correlations with patient's baseline characteristics. *Eur Respir J*, **10**, Suppl 25, 419s.

Dahlen B, Nizankowska E, Szczeklik A, *et al.* (1998) Benefits from adding the 5-lipoxygenase inhibitor zileuton to conventional therapy in aspirin-intolerant asthmatics. *Am J Repir Crit Care Med*, **157**, 1187–94.

Dekhuijzen PNR, Bootsma GP, Wieldres PLNL, *et al.* (1997) Effects of a single-dose zileuton on bronchial hyperresponsiveness in asthmatic patients treated with inhaled corticosteroids. *Eur Respir J*, **10**, 2749–53.

Demoly P, Jaffuel D, Lequeux N, *et al*. (1997). Prostaglandin H synthase 1 and 2 immunoreactivities in bronchial mucosa of asthmatics. *Am J Respir Crit Care Med*, **155**, 670–5.

Dent G, Giembycz MA. (1996) Phosphodiesterase inhibitors: Lily the Pink's medicinal compound for asthma? *Thorax*, **51**, 647–9.

Diaz P, Galleguillos FR, Gonazelez MC. *et al*. (1984) Bronchoalveolar lavage in asthma: the effect of sodium cromoglycate (Cromolyn) on leucocyte counts. *J Allergy Clinic Immunol*, **74**, 41–8.

Dorward AJ, Roberts JA, Thomson NC. (1986) Effect of nedocromil sodium on histamine airway responsiveness in grass-pollen sensitive asthmatics during the pollen season. *Clin Allergy*, **16**, 309–15.

Drazen JM, Yandava C, Pillari A, *et al*. (1997) Relationship between 5-LO gene promotor mutations and lung function response to 5-LO inhibition. *Am J Repir Crit Care Med*, **155**, A257.

Edwards AM, Stevens MT. (1993) The clinical efficacy of inhaled nedocromil sodium (Tilade) in the treatment of asthma. *Eur Respir J*, **6**, 35–41.

Eigen H, Reid JJ, Dahl R, *et al*. (1987) Evaluation of the addition of cromolyn sodium to bronchodilator maintenance therapy in the long-term management of asthma. *J Allergy Clin Immunol*, **80**, 612–21.

Evans DJ, Barnes PJ, Cluzel M, *et al*. (1997). Effects of a potent platelet-activating factor antagonist, SR27417A, on allergen-induced asthmatic responses. *Am J Respir Crit Care Med*, **156**, 11–16.

Faurschou P, Bing J, Edman G, *et al*. (1994) Comparison between sodium cromoglycate MDI: metered dose inhaler and beclomethasone diproprionate MDI in treatment of adult patients with mild to moderate bronchial asthma. A double-blind, double dummy randomized, parallel-group study. *Allergy*, **49**, 656–60.

Finnerty JP, Wood-Baker R, Thomson H, *et al*. (1992) Role of leukotrienes in exercise-induced asthma. Inhibitory effect of ICI-204-219, a potent leukotriene D4 antagonist. *Am Rev Respir Dis*, **145**, 746–9.

Finnerty JP, Lee C, Wilson S, *et al*. (1996) Effects of theophylline on inflammatory cells and cytokines in asthmatic subjects: a placebo-controlled parallel group study. *Eur Respir J*, **9**, 1672–7.

Fischer AR, McFadden CA, Frantz R, *et al*. (1995) Effect of chronic 5-lipoxygenase inhibition on airway hyperresponsiveness in asthmatic subjects. *Am J Respir Crit Care Med*, **152**, 1203–7.

Fyans PG, Chatterjee PC, Chatterjee SS. (1986) A trial comparing nedocromil sodium (TILADE) and placebo in the management of bronchial asthma. *Clin Allergy*, **16**, 505–11.

Golden JG, Bateman ED. (1988) Does nedocromil sodium have a steroid sparing effect in adult asthmatic patients requiring maintenance oral corticosteroids? *Thorax*, **43**, 982–6.

Gonzalez JP, Brogden RN. (1987) Nedocromil sodium. A preliminary review of its pharmacodynamic and pharmacokinetic properties and therapeutic efficacy in the treatment of reversible obstructive airways disease. *Drugs*, **34**, 560–77.

Grant SM, Goa KL, Fitton A, *et al*. (1990) Ketotifen. A review of its pharmacodynamic and pharmacokinetic properties, and therapeutic use in asthma and allergic disorders. *Drugs*, **40**, 412–48.

Hill JM, Tattersfield AE. (1995) Corticosteroid sparing agents in asthma. *Thorax*, **50**, 577–82.

Holgate ST. (1996a) Inhaled sodium cromoglycate. *Respir Med*, **90**, 387–90.

Holgate ST. (1996b) The efficacy and therapeutic position of nedocromil sodium. *Respir Med*, **90**, 391–4.

Hoshino M, Nakamura Y. (1997) The effects of inhaled sodium cromoglycate on cellular infiltration into the bronchial mucosa and the expression of adhesion molecules in asthmatics. *Eur Respir J*, **10**, 858–65.

Hui KP, Barnes NC. (1991) Lung function improvement in asthma with a cysteinyl-leukotriene receptor antagonist. *Lancet*, **337**, 1062–3.

Ind PW. (1996) Anti-leukotriene intervention: is there adequate information for clinical use in asthma? *Respir Med*, **90**, 575–86.

Israel E, Cohn J, Dube L, Drazen JM. (1996) Effect of treatment with zileuton, a 5-lipoxygenase inhibitor, in patients with asthma. A randomised controlled trial. Zileuton Clinical Trial Group. *JAMA*, **275**, 931–6.

Israel E, Fischer AR, Rosenberg, MA, *et al*. (1993a) The pivotal role of 5-lipoxygenase products in the reaction of aspirin-sensitive asthmatics to aspirin. *Am Rev Respir Dis*, **148**, 1447–51.

Israel E, Rubin P, Kemp J, *et al.* (1993b) The effect of inhibition of 5-lipoxygenases by zileuton in mild to moderate asthma. *Ann Intern Med*, **119**, 1059–66.

Josefson D. (1997). Asthma drug linked with Churg–Strauss syndrome. *BMJ*, **315**, 330.

Joseph M, Tsicopoulos A, Tonnel AB, *et al.* (1993) Modulation of nedocromil sodium of immunologic and nonimmunologic activation of monocytes, macrophages and platelets, *J Allergy Clin Immunol*, **92**, 165–70.

Kane GC, Dube LM, Lancaster J, *et al.* (1996) A controlled trial of the effects of the 5-lipoxygenase inhibitor, zileuton, on lung inflammation produced by segmental antigen challenge in human beings. *J Allergy Clin Immunol*, **97**, 646–54.

Kay AB, Walsh GM, Davis S, *et al.* (1987) Disodium cromoglycate inhibits activation of human inflammatory cells *in vitro*. *J Allergy Clin Immunol*, **80**, 1–8.

Kemp JP, Dockhorn RJ, Shapiro GG, *et al.* (1998) Montelukast once daily inhibits exercise-induced bronchoconstriction in 6- to 14-year-old children with asthma. *J Pediatr*, **133,** 424–8.

Kidney J, Dominguez M, Taylor PM, *et al.* (1995) Immunomodulation by theophylline in asthma-demonstration by withdrawal of therapy. *Am J Respir Crit Care Med*, **151**, 1907–14.

Knorr B, Matz J, Bernstein JA, *et al*, (1998) Montelukast for chronic asthma in 6- to 14-year-old children. *JAMA*, **279**, 1181–6.

Konig P, Hordvik NL, Kreutz BS. (1987) The preventive effect and duration of action of nedocromil sodium and cromolyn sodium on exercise-induced asthma (EIA) in adults. *J Allergy Clin Immunol*, **79**, 64–8.

Kraft M, Torvik JA, Trudeau JB, *et al.* (1996) Theophylline: potential anti-inflammatory effects in nocturnal asthma. *J Allergy Clin Immunol*, **97**, 1242–6.

Kuitert LM, Angus RM, Barnes NC, *et al.* (1995) Effect of a novel potent platelet activating antagonist, Modipafant, in clinical asthma. *Am J Respir Crit Care Med*, **151**, 1331–5.

Laitinen LA, Naya IP, Binks S, Harris A. (1997) Comparative efficacy of zafirlukast and low dose steroids in asthmatics on prn β_2-agonists. *Eur Respir J*, **10** (Suppl 25), 419–20S.

Lal S, Malhotra S, Gribben D, Hodder D. (1984) Nedocromil sodium: a new drug for the management of bronchial asthma. *Thorax*, **39**, 809–12.

Laviolette M, Malmstrom K, Lu S, *et al.* (1999) Montelukast added to inhaled beclomethasone in the treatment of asthma. *Am J Respir Crit Care Med*, **160**, 1862–8.

Leff JA, Busse WW, Pearlman D, *et al.* (1998) Montelukast, a leukotriene-receptor antagonist, for the treatment of mild asthma and exercise-induced bronchoconstriction. *N Engl J Med*, **339**, 147–52.

Liu MC, Dube LM, Lancaster J. (1996) Acute and chronic effects of a 5-lipoxygenase inhibitor in asthma: a 6-month randomized trial. Zileuton Study Group. *J Allergy Clin Immunol*, **98**, 859–71.

Lock SH, Kay AB, Barnes NC. (1996). Double-blind, placebo-controlled study of cyclosporin A as a corticosteroid-sparing agent in corticosteroid-dependent asthma. *Am J Respir Crit Care Med*, **153**, 509–14.

Manolitsas ND, Wang JH, Devalia JL. (1995) Regular albuterol, nedocromil sodium and bronchial inflammation in asthma. *Am J Repir Crit Care Med*, **151**, 1925–30.

McGill KA, Busse WW. (1996) Zileuton. *Lancet*, **348**, 519–24.

Malmstrom K, Rodriquez-Gomez G, Guerra J, *et al.* (1999). Oral montelukast, inhaled beclomethasone and placebo for chronic asthma. *Ann Int Med*, **130**, 487–95.

Nassif EG, Weinberger M, Thompson R, Huntely W. (1981) The value of maintenance theophylline in steroid-dependent asthma. *N Engl J Med*, **304**, 71–5.

National Institutes of Health. (1997) Highlights of the Expert Panel Report II: Guidelines for the Diagnosis and Management of Asthma. Bethesda, MD: US Department of Health and Human Services Publication.

Nierop G, Gijzel WP, Bel EH, Zwinderman AH, Dijkman JH. (1992) Auranofin in the treatment of steroid dependent asthma: a double blind study. *Thorax*, **47**, 349–54.

Nizankowska E, Soja J, Pinis G, *et al.* (1995) Treatment of steroid-dependent bronchial asthma with cyclosporin. *Eur Respir J*, **8**, 1091–9.

Norris AA, Alton EWFW. (1996) Chloride transport and the actions of sodium cromoglycate and nedocromil sodium in asthma. *Clin Exp Allergy*, **26**, 250–3.

Phillips GD, Scott VL, Richards R, Holgate ST. (1989) Effect of nedocromil sodium and sodium cromoglycate against bronchoconstriction induced by inhaled adenosine 5′-monophosphate. *Eur Respir J*, **2**, 210–17.

Pizzichini E, Leff JA, Reiss TF, *et al.* (1999) Montelukast reduces airway eosinophilic inflammation in asthma: a randomized controlled trial. *Eur Respir J*, **14**, 12–18.

Reiss TF, Chervinsky P, Dockhorn RJ, *et al.* (1998) Montelukast, a once-daily leukotriene receptor agonist, in the treatment of chronic asthma. *Arch Intern Med*, **158**, 1213–20.

Roberts JA, Thomson NC. (1985) Attenuation of exercise-induced asthma by pre-treatment with nedocromil sodium and minocromil. *Clin Allergy*, **15**, 377–81.

Roquet A, Dahlen B, Kumlin M, *et al.* (1997) Combined antagonism of leukotrienes and histamine produces predominant inhibition of allergen-induced early and late phase airway obstruction in asthmatics. *Am J Respir Crit Care Med*, **155**, 1856–63.

Ruffin RE, Alpers JH, Pain MCF, *et al.* (1987) The efficacy of nedocromil sodium (TILADE) in asthma. *Aust NZ J Med*, **17**, 557–61.

Schwartz HJ, Blumenthal M, Brady R, *et al.* (1996) A comparative study of the clinical efficacy of nedocromil sodium and placebo. How does cromolyn sodium compare as an active control treatment? *Chest*, **109**, 945–52.

Spector SL, Smith LJ, Glass M. (1994) Accolate Trialist Group. Effects of 6 weeks of therapy with oral doses of ICI 204,219, a leukotriene D4 receptor antagonist, in subjects with bronchial asthma. *Am J Respir Crit Care Med*, **150**, 618–23.

Suissa S, Dennis R, Ernst P, *et al.* (1997) Effectiveness of the leukotriene receptor antagonist zafirlukast for mild-to-moderate asthma. A randomised, double-blind, placebo-controlled trial. *Ann Inter Med*, **126**, 177–83.

Sullivan P, Bekir S, Jaffar Z, *et al.* (1994) Anti-inflammatory effects of low-dose theophylline in atopic asthma. *Lancet*, **343**, 1006–8.

Svendsen UG, Frolund L, Madsen F, Nielson NH. (1989) A comparison of the effects of nedocromil sodium and beclomethasone dipropionate on pulmonary function, symptoms, and bronchial responsiveness in patients with asthma. *J Allergy Clin Immunol*, **84**, 224–31.

Svendsen UG, Jorgensen H. (1991) Inhaled nedocromil sodium as additional treatment to high dose inhaled corticosteroids in the management of bronchial asthma. *Eur Respir J*, **4**, 992–9.

Tasche MJA, van der Wouden JC, Uijen JHJM, *et al.* (1997) Randomised placebo-controlled trial of inhaled sodium cromoglycate in 1–4-year-old children with moderate asthma. *Lancet*, **350**, 1060–4.

Taylor IK, O'Shaughnessy KM, Fuller RW, *et al.* (1991) Effect of cysteinyl-leukotriene receptor antagonist ICI 204,219 on allergen-induced bronchoconstriction and airway hyperreactivity in atopic subjects. *Lancet*, **337**, 690–4.

Temple DM, McCluskey M. (1988) Loratadine, an antihistamine, blocks antigen and ionophore-induced leukotriene release from human lung, *in vitro*. *Prostaglandins*, **35**, 549–54.

Thomson NC. (1989) Nedocromil sodium: an overview. *Respir Med*, **83**, 269–76.

Turpin JA, Edelman JM, DeLucca PT, *et al.* (1998) Chronic administration of montelukast (MK-476) is superior to inhaled salmeterol in the prevention of exercised-induced bronchoconstriction (EIB). *Am J Respir Crit Care Med*, **157**, A456.

Walsh GM. (1994) The anti-inflammatory effects of cetirizine. *Clin Exp Allergy*, **24**, 81–5.

Wechsler ME, Garpestad E, Flier SR, *et al.* (1998) Pulmonary infiltrates, eosinophilia, and cardiomyopathy following corticosteroid withdrawal in patients with asthma receiving zafirlukast. *JAMA*, **279**, 455–7.

Weinberger M, Hendeles L. (1996) Theophylline in asthma. *N Engl J Med*, **334**, 1380–8.

Wenzel SE, Trudeau JB, Kaminsky DA, *et al.* (1995) Effect of 5-lipoxgenase inhibition on the bronchoconstriction and airway inflammation in nocturnal asthma. *Am J Repir Crit Care Med*, **152**, 897–905.

13

Corticosteroids: mode of action and place in management

PETER J. BARNES

INTRODUCTION

Corticosteroids are the most effective therapy currently available for asthma, and improvement with corticosteroids is one of the hallmarks of asthma. Inhaled corticosteroids have revolutionized asthma treatment and have become the mainstay of therapy for patients with chronic disease. We now have a much better understanding of the molecular mechanisms whereby corticosteroids suppress inflammation in asthma and this has led to changes in the way corticosteroids are used and may point the way to the development of more specific therapies in the future. This chapter discusses current understanding of the mechanism of action of corticosteroids and how they are used in the management of asthma.

MOLECULAR MECHANISMS

Corticosteroids are a highly effective antiinflammatory therapy in asthma and the molecular mechanisms involved in suppression of airway inflammation in asthma are now better understood. Corticosteroids are effective in asthma because they block many of the inflammatory pathways that are abnormally activated in asthma and they have a wide spectrum of antiinflammatory actions.

Glucocorticoid receptors

Corticosteroids bind to a single class of glucocorticoid receptors (GRs) that are localized to the cytoplasm of target cells. Corticosteroids bind at the C-terminal end of the receptor, whereas the N-terminal end of the receptor is involved in gene transcription. Between these domains is the DNA-binding domain which has two finger-like projections formed by a zinc molecule bound to four cysteine residues that bind to the DNA double helix. The inactive GR is bound to a protein complex that includes two molecules of 90 kDa heat shock protein (hsp90) and various other proteins which act as a 'molecular chaperone' preventing the unoccupied GR from moving into the nuclear compartment. Once corticosteroids bind to GRs, conformational changes in the receptor structure result in dissociation of these molecules, thereby exposing nuclear localization signals on GRs which then results in rapid nuclear localization of the activated GR–corticosteroid complex and its binding to DNA (Fig. 13.1). Two GR molecules bind to DNA as a dimer, resulting in changed transcription. Recently a splice variant of GR, termed GR-β, has been identified that does not bind corticosteroids, but binds to DNA and may therefore interfere with the action of corticosteroids.

Effects on gene transcription

Corticosteroids produce their effect on responsive cells by activating GRs to directly or indirectly regulate the transcription of certain target genes. The number of genes per cell *directly* regulated by corticosteroids is estimated to lie between 10 and 100, but many genes are

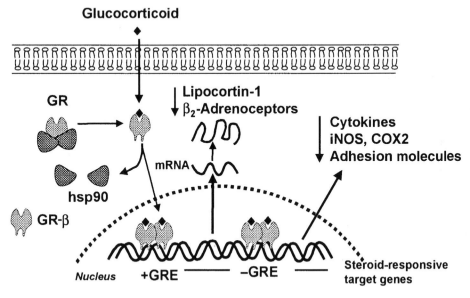

Figure 13.1 *Classical model of glucocorticoid action. The glucocorticoid enters the cell and binds to a cytoplasmic glucocorticoid receptor (GR) that is complexed with two molecules of a 90 kDa heat shock protein (hsp90). GR translocates to the nucleus where, as a dimer, it binds to a recognition sequence, the glucocorticoid response element (GRE) on the 5'-upstream promoter sequence of corticosteroid-responsive genes. GREs may increase transcription and nGREs (negative glucocorticoid response element) may decrease transcription, resulting in increased or decreased mRNA and protein synthesis. An isoform of GR, GR-β, binds to DNA but is not activated by corticosteroids.*

indirectly regulated through an interaction with other transcription factors. GR dimers bind to DNA at consensus sites termed glucocorticoid response elements (GREs) in the 5′-upstream promoter region of steroid responsive genes. This interaction changes the rate of transcription, resulting in either induction or repression of the gene. The consensus sequence for GRE binding is the palindromic 15 base-pair sequence GGTACAnnnTGTTCT (where n is any nucleotide). Crystallographic studies indicate that the zinc finger binding to DNA occurs within the major groove of DNA with one finger of each receptor in the homodimer interacting with one half of the DNA palindrome. Interaction of the activated GR homodimer with GRE usually increases transcription, resulting in increased protein synthesis. GRs may increase transcription by interacting with a large co-activator molecule, CREB-binding protein (CBP), which is bound at the start site of transcription and switches on RNA polymerase.

However, in controlling inflammation, the major effect of corticosteroids is to inhibit the synthesis of inflammatory proteins, such as cytokines. This was originally believed to be through interaction of GRs with a negative GRE, resulting in repression of transcription. However, such negative GREs have rarely been demonstrated. GRs may also affect protein synthesis by altering the stability of mRNA, through effects on ribonucleases that break down mRNA.

Interaction with transcription factors

Activated GRs may bind directly with several other activated transcription factors as a protein–protein interaction. This could be an important determinant of corticosteroid responsiveness and is a key mechanism whereby corticosteroids switch off inflammatory genes. Most of the inflammatory genes that are activated in asthma do not appear to have GREs in their promoter regions yet are repressed by corticosteroids. There is increasing evidence that this may be due to a direct interaction between the activated GR and transcription factors that regulate the expression of genes that code for inflammatory proteins, such as cytokines, inflammatory enzymes, adhesion molecules and inflammatory receptors. These 'inflammatory' transcription factors include activator protein-1 (AP-1) and nuclear factor-κB (NF-κB) which may regulate many of the inflammatory genes that are switched on in asthmatic airways (Fig. 13.2).

Effects on chromatin structure

There is increasing evidence that corticosteroids may have effects on the chromatin structure. DNA in chromosomes is wound around histone molecules in the form of nucleosomes. Several transcription factors interact with large co-activator molecules, such as CBP and the related molecule p300, which bind to the basal transcription factor apparatus. Several transcription factors have now been shown to bind directly to CBP, including AP-1, NF-κB and GR. Since binding sites on this molecule may be limited, this may result in competition between transcription factors for the limited binding sites available, so that there is an indirect rather than a direct protein–protein interaction (Fig. 13.3). At a microscopic level chromatin may become dense or opaque due to the winding or unwinding of DNA around the histone core. CBP and p300 have histone acetylation activity which is activated by the binding of transcription factors, such as AP-1 and NF-κB. Acetylation of histone residues results in unwinding of DNA coiled around the histone core, thus opening up the chromatin structure, which allows transcription factors to bind more readily, thereby increasing transcription. Repression of genes reverses this process by histone deacetylation which increases the winding of DNA round histone residues, resulting in dense chromatin structure

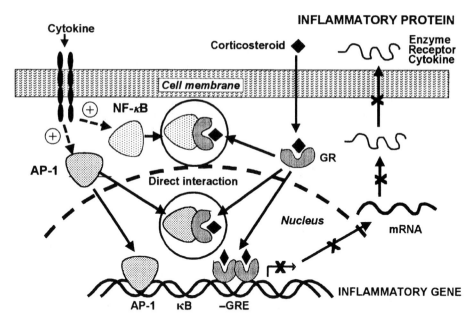

Figure 13.2 *Direct interaction between the transcription factors, activator protein-1 (AP-1) and nuclear factor-kappa B (NF-κB) and the glucocorticoid receptor (GR), may result in mutual repression. In this way corticosteroids may counteract the chronic inflammatory effects of cytokines that activate these transcription factors.*

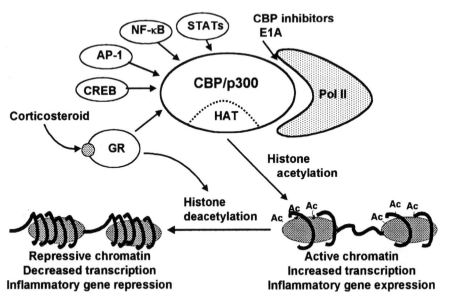

Figure 13.3 *Effect of corticosteroids on chromatin structure. Transcription factors, such as STATs, AP-1 and NF-κB bind to co-activator molecules, such as CREB-binding protein (CBP) or p300, which have intrinsic histone acetyltransferase (HAT) activity, resulting in acetylation (Ac) of histone residues. This leads to unwinding of DNA and allows increased binding of transcription factors, resulting in increased gene transcription. Glucocorticoid receptors (GRs) after activation by corticosteroids bind to a glucocorticoid receptor co-activator that is bound to CBP. This results in deacetylation of histone, with increased coiling of DNA around histone, thus preventing transcription factor binding leading to gene repression.*

and reduced access of transcription factors to their binding sites, thereby leading to repressed transcription of inflammatory genes. Activated GRs may bind to several transcription corepressor molecules that associate with proteins that have histone deacetylase activity, resulting in deacetylation of histone, increased winding of DNA around histone residues and thus reduced access of transcription factors to their binding sites and therefore repression of inflammatory genes.

Target genes in inflammation control

Corticosteroids may control inflammation by inhibiting many aspects of the inflammatory process through increasing the transcription of antiinflammatory genes and decreasing the transcription of inflammatory genes (Table 13.1).

ANTIINFLAMMATORY PROTEINS

Corticosteroids may suppress inflammation by increasing the synthesis of antiinflammatory proteins. For example, corticosteroids increase the synthesis of lipocortin-1, a 37 kDa protein that has an inhibitory effect on phospholipase A_2 (PLA$_2$), and therefore may inhibit the production of lipid mediators. Corticosteroids induce the formation of lipocortin-1 in several cells and recombinant lipocortin-1 has acute antiinflammatory properties. However, lipocortin-1 does not appear to be increased by inhaled corticosteroid treatment in asthma. Corticosteroids increase the expression of other potentially antiinflammatory proteins, such as interleukin (IL)-1 receptor antagonist (which inhibits the binding of IL-1 to its receptor), secretory leukoprotease inhibitor (which inhibits proteases, such as tryptase), neutral endopeptidase (which degrades bronchoactive peptides such as kinins), CC-10 (an immunomodulatory protein), an inhibitor of NF-κB (IκB-α) and IL-10 (an antiinflammatory cytokine).

Table 13.1 *Effect of corticosteroids on gene transcription*

Increased transcription
Lipocortin-1 (phospholipase A_2 inhibitor)
β_2-Adrenoceptor
Secretory leucocyte inhibitory protein
Clara cell protein (CC10)
IL-1 receptor antagonist
IL-1R2 (decoy receptor)
IκB-α (inhibitor of NF-κB)

Decreased transcription
Cytokines:
    IL-1, IL-2, IL-3, IL-4, IL-5, IL-6, IL-11, IL-12, IL-13, TNFα, GM-CSF, SCF
Chemokines:
    IL-8, RANTES, MIP-1α, MCP-1, MCP-3, MCP-4, eotaxin
Inducible nitric oxide synthase (iNOS)
Inducible cyclo-oxygenase (COX-2)
Cytosolic phospholipase A_2 (cPLA$_2$)
Endothelin-1
NK$_1$-receptors, NK$_2$-receptors
Adhesion molecules (ICAM-1, E-selectin)

β₂-ADRENOCEPTORS

Corticosteroids increase the expression of β_2-adrenoceptors by increasing the rate of transcription and the human β_2-receptor gene has three potential GREs. Corticosteroids double the rate of β_2-receptor gene transcription in human lung *in vitro*, resulting in increased expression of β_2-receptors. This may be relevant in asthma as corticosteroids may prevent downregulation of β-receptors in response to prolonged treatment with β_2-agonists. In rats corticosteroids prevent downregulation and reduce transcription of β_2-receptors in response to chronic β-agonist exposure.

CYTOKINES

The inhibitory effect of corticosteroids on cytokine synthesis is likely to be of particular importance in the control of inflammation in asthma. Corticosteroids inhibit the transcription of many cytokines and chemokines that are relevant in asthma (Table 13.1). These inhibitory effects are due, at least in part, to an inhibitory effect on the transcription factors that regulate induction of these cytokine genes, including AP-1 and NF-κB. For example, eotaxin which is important in selective attraction of eosinophils from the circulation into the airways is regulated in part by NF-κB and its expression in airway epithelial cells is inhibited by corticosteroids. Many transcription factors are likely to be involved in the regulation of inflammatory genes in asthma in addition to AP-1 and NF-κB. IL-4 and IL-5 expression in T lymphocytes plays a critical role in allergic inflammation, but NF-κB does not play a role, whereas the transcription factor of activated T-cells (NF-AT) is important. AP-1 is a component of the NF-AT transcription complex, so that corticosteroids inhibit IL-5, at least in part, by inhibiting the AP-1 component of NF-AT.

There may be marked differences in the response of different cells and of different cytokines to the inhibitory action of corticosteroids and this may be dependent on the relative abundance of transcription factors within different cell types. Thus in alveolar macrophages and peripheral blood monocytes GM-CSF secretion is more potently inhibited by corticosteroids than IL-1β or IL-6 secretion.

INFLAMMATORY ENZYMES

Nitric oxide synthase (NOS) may be induced by pro-inflammatory cytokines, resulting in nitric oxide (NO) production. Nitric oxide may amplify asthmatic inflammation and contribute to epithelial shedding and airway hyperresponsiveness through the formation of peroxynitrite. The induction of the inducible form of NOS (iNOS) is inhibited by corticosteroids. In cultured human pulmonary epithelial cells, pro-inflammatory cytokines result in increased expression of iNOS and increased NO formation, due to increased transcription of the iNOS gene, and this is inhibited by corticosteroids acting through inhibition of NF-κB. Corticosteroids inhibit the synthesis of several other inflammatory mediators implicated in asthma through an inhibitory effect on the induction of enzymes such as cyclo-oxygenase-2 and cytosolic phospholipase A_2.

Corticosteroids also inhibit the synthesis of endothelin-1 in lung and airway epithelial cells and this effect may also be via inhibition of transcription factors that regulate its expression.

INFLAMMATORY RECEPTORS

Corticosteroids also decrease the transcription of genes coding for certain receptors. Thus the gene for the NK₁-receptor, which mediates the inflammatory effects of tachykinins in the airways, has an increased expression in asthma and is inhibited by corticosteroids, probably via an inhibitory effect on AP-1. Corticosteroids also inhibit the transcription of the neurokinin NK_2-receptor which mediates the bronchoconstrictor effects of tachykinins.

ADHESION MOLECULES

Adhesion molecules play a key role in the trafficking of inflammatory cells to sites of inflammation. The expression of many adhesion molecules on endothelial cells is induced by cytokines and corticosteroids may lead indirectly to a reduced expression via their inhibitory effects on cytokines, such as IL-1β and TNF-α. Corticosteroids may also have a direct inhibitory effect on the expression of adhesion molecules, such as ICAM-1 and E-selectin, at the level of gene transcription. ICAM-1 expression in bronchial epithelial cell lines and monocytes is inhibited by corticosteroids.

APOPTOSIS

Corticosteroids markedly reduce the survival of certain inflammatory cells, such as eosinophils. Eosinophil survival is dependent on the presence of certain cytokines, such as IL-5 and GM-CSF. Exposure to corticosteroids blocks the effects of these cytokines and leads to programmed cell death or apoptosis, although the corticosteroid-sensitive molecular pathways have not yet been defined.

Effects on cell function

Corticosteroids may have direct inhibitory actions on several inflammatory cells and structural cells that are implicated in asthma (Fig. 13.4).

MACROPHAGES

Corticosteroids inhibit the release of inflammatory mediators and cytokines from alveolar macrophages *in vitro*. Inhaled corticosteroids reduce the secretion of chemokines and pro-

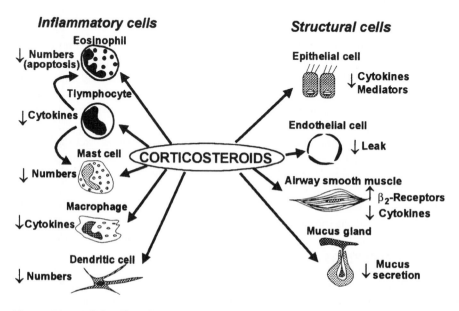

Figure 13.4 *Cellular effect of corticosteroids.*

inflammatory cytokines from alveolar macrophages from asthmatic patients, whereas the secretion of IL-10 is increased.

EOSINOPHILS

Corticosteroids have a direct inhibitory effect on mediator release from eosinophils, although they are only weakly effective in inhibiting secretion of reactive oxygen species and eosinophil basic proteins. More importantly corticosteroids induce apoptosis by inhibiting the prolonged survival due to IL-3, IL-5 and GM-CSF, resulting in an increased number of apoptotic eosinophils in induced sputum of asthmatic patients. One of the best described actions of corticosteroids in asthma is a reduction in circulating eosinophils, which may reflect an action on eosinophil production in the bone marrow.

T LYMPHOCYTES

T helper 2 lymphocytes (Th2) play an important orchestrating role in asthma through the release of cytokines such as IL-4 and IL-5 and may be important targets for corticosteroids in asthma therapy.

MAST CELLS

While corticosteroids do not appear to have a direct inhibitory effect on mediator release from lung mast cells, chronic corticosteroid treatment is associated with a marked reduction in mucosal mast cell number. This may be linked to a reduction in IL-3 and stem cell factor (SCF) production, which are necessary for mast cell expression at mucosal surfaces. Mast cells also secrete various cytokines (TNF-α, IL-4, IL-5, IL-6, IL-8), and this secretion may also be inhibited by corticosteroids.

DENDRITIC CELLS

Dendritic cells in the epithelium of the respiratory tract appear to play a critical role in antigen presentation in the lung as they have the capacity to take up allergen, process it into peptides and present it via major histocompatibility complex molecules on the cell surface for presentation to uncommitted T lymphocytes. In experimental animals, the number of dendritic cells is markedly reduced by systemic and inhaled corticosteroids, thus dampening the immune response in the airways.

NEUTROPHILS

Neutrophils, which are not prominent in the biopsies of asthmatic patients, are not sensitive to the effects of corticosteroids. Indeed, systemic corticosteroids increase peripheral neutrophil counts which may reflect an increased survival time due to an inhibitory action of neutrophil apoptosis (in complete contrast to the increased apoptosis seen in eosinophils).

ENDOTHELIAL CELLS

Glucocorticoid-receptor gene expression in the airways is most prominent in endothelial cells of the bronchial circulation and airway epithelial cells. Corticosteroids do not appear to directly inhibit the expression of adhesion molecules, although they may inhibit cell adhesion indirectly by suppression of cytokines involved in the regulation of adhesion molecule expression. Corticosteroids may have an inhibitory action on airway microvascular leak induced by inflammatory mediators. This appears to be a direct effect on postcapillary venular epithelial cells. The mechanism for this antipermeability effect has not been fully elucidated, but there is evidence that synthesis of a 100 kDa protein distinct from lipocortin-1, termed vasocortin, may be involved. Although there have been no direct measurements of the effects of corticosteroids on airway microvascular leakage in asthmatic airways, regular treatment with inhaled corticosteroids decreases the elevated plasma proteins found in bronchoalveolar lavage fluid of patients with stable asthma.

EPITHELIAL CELLS

Epithelial cells may be an important source of many inflammatory mediators in asthmatic airways and may drive and amplify the inflammatory response in the airways through the secretion of pro-inflammatory cytokines, chemokines and inflammatory peptides. Airway epithelium may be one of the most important targets for inhaled corticosteroids in asthma (Fig. 13.5). Inhaled corticosteroids inhibit the increased expression of many inflammatory proteins in airway epithelial cells. An example is iNOS which has an increased expression in airway epithelial and inflammatory cells in asthma and is reduced by inhaled corticosteroids. This is reflected by a reduction in the elevated levels of exhaled NO in asthma after inhaled corticosteroids.

MUCUS SECRETION

Corticosteroids inhibit mucus secretion in airways and this may be a direct action of corticosteroids on submucosal gland cells. Corticosteroids may also inhibit the expression of mucin genes, such as MUC2 and MUC5AC. In addition there are indirect inhibitory effects due to the reduction in inflammatory mediators that stimulate increased mucus secretion.

EFFECTS ON ASTHMATIC INFLAMMATION

Corticosteroids are remarkably effective in controlling the inflammation in asthmatic airways and it is likely that they have multiple cellular effects. Biopsy studies in patients with asthma

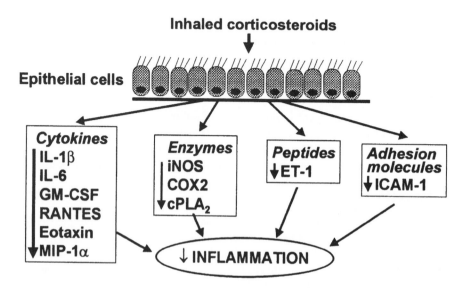

Figure 13.5 *Inhaled corticosteroids may inhibit the transcription of several 'inflammatory' genes in airway epithelial cells and thus reduce inflammation in the airway wall. For abbreviations, see text.*

have now confirmed that inhaled corticosteroids reduce the number and activation of inflammatory cells in the airway mucosa and in bronchoalveolar lavage. These effects may be due to inhibition of cytokine synthesis in inflammatory and structural cells and suppression of adhesion molecules. The disrupted epithelium is restored and the ciliated-to-goblet cell ratio is normalized after three months of therapy with inhaled corticosteroids. There is also some evidence for a reduction in the thickness of the basement membrane, although in asthmatic patients taking inhaled corticosteroids for over 10 years the characteristic thickening of the basement membrane was still present.

Effects on airway hyperresponsiveness

By reducing airway inflammation, inhaled corticosteroids consistently reduce airway hyperresponsiveness in asthmatic adults and children. Chronic treatment with inhaled corticosteroids reduces responsiveness to histamine, cholinergic agonists, allergen (early and late responses), exercise, fog, cold air, bradykinin, adenosine and irritants (such as sulphur dioxide and metabisulphite). The reduction in airway hyperresponsiveness takes place over several weeks and may not be maximal until several months of therapy. The magnitude of reduction is variable between patients and is in the order of one to two doubling dilutions for most challenges and often fails to return to the normal range. This may reflect suppression of the inflammation but persistence of structural changes that cannot be reversed by corticosteroids. Inhaled corticosteroids not only make the airways less sensitive to spasmogens, but they also limit the maximal airway narrowing in response to spasmogens.

CLINICAL EFFICACY OF INHALED CORTICOSTEROIDS

Inhaled corticosteroids are very effective in controlling asthma symptoms in asthmatic patients of all ages and severity (Table 13.2). Inhaled corticosteroids improve the quality of life of patients with asthma and allow many patients to lead normal lives, improve lung function, reduce the frequency of exacerbations and may prevent irreversible airway changes. They were first introduced to reduce the requirement for oral corticosteroids in patients with severe asthma and many studies have confirmed that the majority of patients can be weaned off oral corticosteroids.

Table 13.2   *Effects of inhaled corticosteroids in asthma*

- Control symptoms
- Improve quality of life
- Improve lung function
- Prevent exacerbations
- Reduce mortality (probably)
- Prevent irreversible airway changes
- Alter natural history of asthma?

Studies in adults

As experience has been gained with inhaled corticosteroids they have been introduced in patients with milder asthma, with the recognition that inflammation is present even in patients with mild asthma. Inhaled antiinflammatory drugs have now become first-line therapy in any patient who needs to use a β_2-agonist inhaler more than once a day and this is reflected in national and international guidelines for the management of chronic asthma. In patients with newly diagnosed asthma, inhaled corticosteroids (budesonide 600 µg twice daily) reduced symptoms and β_2-agonist inhaler usage and improved peak expiratory flows. These effects persisted over the two years of the study, whereas in a parallel group treated with inhaled β_2-agonists alone there was no significant change in symptoms or lung function. In another study, patients with mild asthma treated with a low dose of inhaled corticosteroid (budesonide 400 µg daily) showed less symptoms and a progressive improvement in lung function over several months and many patients became completely asymptomatic. There was also a significant reduction in the number of exacerbations. Although the effects of inhaled corticosteroids on airway hyperresponsiveness may take several months to reach a plateau, the reduction in asthma symptoms occurs more rapidly.

High-dose inhaled corticosteroids have now been introduced for the control of more severe asthma. This markedly reduces the need for maintenance oral corticosteroids and has revolutionized the management of more severe and unstable asthma. Inhaled corticosteroids are the treatment of choice in nocturnal asthma, which is a manifestation of inflamed airways, reducing night-time awakening and reducing the diurnal variation in airway function.

High doses of inhaled corticosteroids may also substitute for a course of oral steroids in controlling acute exacerbations of asthma. High-dose fluticasone propionate (2000 µg daily) was as effective as a course of oral prednisolone in controlling acute exacerbations of asthma in general practice.

Inhaled corticosteroids effectively control asthmatic inflammation but must be taken regularly. When inhaled corticosteroids are discontinued there is usually a gradual increase in symptoms and airway responsiveness back to pretreatment values, although in patients with mild asthma who have been treated with inhaled corticosteroids for a long time symptoms may not recur in some of them.

Studies in children

Inhaled corticosteroids are equally effective in children. In an extensive study of children aged 7–17 years there was a significant improvement in symptoms, peak flow variability and lung function compared with a regularly inhaled β_2-agonist which was maintained over the 22 months of the study, but asthma deteriorated when the inhaled corticosteroids were withdrawn. There was a high proportion of drop-outs (45%) in the group treated with inhaled β_2-agonist alone.

Inhaled corticosteroids are more effective than a long-acting β_2-agonist in controlling asthma in children and they are also effective in younger children. Nebulized budesonide reduces the need for oral corticosteroids and also improves lung function in children under the age of three. Inhaled corticosteroids given via a large volume spacer improve asthma symptoms and reduce the number of exacerbations in preschool children and in infants.

Dose–response studies

Surprisingly, the dose–response curve for the clinical efficacy of inhaled corticosteroids is relatively flat and, while all studies have demonstrated a clinical benefit of inhaled corticosteroids, it has been difficult to demonstrate differences between doses, with most benefit obtained at the lowest doses used. This is in contrast to the steeper dose–response for systemic effects, implying that while there is little clinical benefit from increasing doses of inhaled corticosteroids the risk of adverse effects is increased. However, the dose–response effect of inhaled corticosteroids may depend on the parameters measured and, while it is difficult to discern a dose–response when traditional lung function parameters are measured, there may be a dose–response effect in prevention of asthma exacerbations. Thus, in a recent study there was a significantly greater effect of budesonide at 800 μg daily compared with 200 μg daily in preventing severe and mild asthma exacerbations. Normally, a four-fold or greater difference in dose has been required to detect a statistically significant (but often small) difference in effect on commonly measured outcomes such as symptoms, PEF, use of rescue β_2-agonist and lung function and even such large differences in dose are not always associated with significant differences in response. These findings suggest that pulmonary function tests or symptoms may have a rather low sensitivity in the assessment of the effects of inhaled corticosteroids. This is obviously important for the interpretation of clinical comparisons between different inhaled corticosteroids or inhalers. It is also important to consider the type of patient included in clinical studies. Patients with relatively mild asthma may have relatively little room for improvement with inhaled corticosteroids, so that maximal improvement is obtained with relatively low doses. Patients with more severe asthma or with unstable asthma may have more room for improvement and may therefore show a greater response to increasing doses, but it is often difficult to include such patients in controlled clinical trials.

More studies are needed to assess whether other outcome measures such as airway hyperresponsiveness or more direct measurements of inflammation, such as sputum eosinophils or exhaled nitric oxide, may be more sensitive than traditional outcome measures such as symptoms or lung function tests.

Prevention of irreversible airway changes

Some patients with asthma develop an element of irreversible airflow obstruction, but the pathophysiological basis of these changes is not yet understood. It is likely that they are the result of chronic airway inflammation and that they may be prevented by treatment with inhaled corticosteroids. There is some evidence that the annual decline in lung function may be slowed by the introduction of inhaled corticosteroids. Increasing evidence also suggests that delay in starting inhaled corticosteroids may result in less overall improvement in lung function in both adults and children. These studies suggest that introduction of inhaled corticosteroids at the time of diagnosis is likely to have the greatest impact. Several large studies are now underway to assess the benefit of very early introduction of inhaled corticosteroids in children and adults. So far there is no evidence that early use of inhaled corticosteroids is curative, and even when inhaled corticosteroids are introduced at the time of diagnosis, symptoms and lung function revert to pretreatment levels when corticosteroids are withdrawn.

Reduction in mortality

Inhaled corticosteroids may reduce the mortality from asthma but prospective studies are almost impossible to conduct. In a retrospective review of the risk of mortality and prescribed anti-asthma medication, there was a significant apparent protection provided by regular inhaled beclomethasone diproprionate (BDP) therapy (adjusted odds ratio of 0.1), although numbers were small.

Comparison between inhaled corticosteroids

Several inhaled corticosteroids are currently prescribable in asthma, although their availability varies between countries. There have been relatively few studies comparing efficacy of the different inhaled corticosteroids, and it is important to take into account the delivery system and the type of patient under investigation when such comparisons are made. Because of the relatively flat dose–response curve for the clinical parameters normally used in comparing doses of inhaled corticosteroids, it may be difficult to see differences in efficacy of inhaled corticosteroids and most comparisons have concentrated on differences in systemic effects at equally efficacious doses, although it has often proved difficult to establish true clinical efficacy. In the United Kingdom, BDP, budesonide and fluticasone proprionate (FP) are available, whereas in the United States, BDP, flunisolide, triamcinolone, FP and budesonide are available. There are few studies comparing different doses of inhaled corticosteroids in asthmatic patients. Budesonide has been compared with BDP and in adults and children appears to have comparable anti-asthma effects at equal doses, whereas FP appears to be approximately twice as potent as BDP and budesonide. There do appear to be some differences between inhaled corticosteroids in terms of their systemic effects at comparable anti-asthma doses, however.

CLINICAL USE OF INHALED CORTICOSTEROIDS

Inhaled corticosteroids are now recommended as first-line therapy for all patients with persistent symptoms. Inhaled corticosteroids should be started in any patient who needs to use a β_2-agonist inhaler for symptom control more than once daily (or possibly three times weekly). It is conventional to start with a low dose of inhaled corticosteroid and to increase the dose until asthma control is achieved. However, this may take time and a preferable approach is to start with a dose of corticosteroids in the middle of the dose range (400 μg twice daily) to establish control of asthma more rapidly. Once control is achieved (defined as normal or best possible lung function and infrequent need to use an inhaled β_2-agonist), the dose of inhaled corticosteroid should be reduced in a stepwise manner to the lowest dose needed for optimal control. It may take as long as three months to reach a plateau in response and any changes in dose should be made at intervals of three months or more. This strategy ('start high – go low') is emphasized in the most recent USA and UK guidelines. When daily doses of ≥800 μg daily are needed a large volume spacer device should be used with a metered dose inhaler and mouth-washing with a dry powder inhaler in order to reduce local and systemic side-effects. Inhaled corticosteroids are usually give as a twice-daily dose in order to increase compliance. When asthma is more unstable four times daily dosage is preferable. For patients who require ≤400 μg daily, once daily dosing appears to be as effective as twice daily dosing, at least for budesonide.

The dose of inhaled corticosteroid should be increased to 2000 μg daily if necessary, but higher doses may result in systemic effects and it may be preferable to add a low dose of oral corticosteroid, as higher doses of inhaled corticosteroids are expensive and have a high incidence of local side-effects. Nebulized budesonide has been advocated in order to give an increased dose of inhaled corticosteroid and to reduce the requirement for oral corticosteroids, but this treatment is expensive and may achieve its effects largely via systemic absorption.

Additional bronchodilators

Conventional advice was to increase the dose of inhaled corticosteroids if asthma was not controlled, on the assumption that there was residual inflammation of the airways. However it is now apparent that the dose–response effect of inhaled corticosteroids is relatively flat, so that there is little improvement in lung function after doubling the dose of inhaled corticosteroids. An alternative strategy is to add some other type of prophylactic drug. In patients in general practice who were not controlled on BDP 200 μg twice daily, addition of salmeterol at 50 μg twice daily was more effective than increasing the dose of inhaled corticosteroid to 500 μg twice daily, in terms of lung function improvement, use of rescue β_2-agonist use and symptom control. This surprising result was confirmed in a more severe group of patients who were not controlled on 800–1000 μg BDP daily. Similar results have been found with another long-acting inhaled β_2-agonist formoterol, which in addition reduced the frequency of mild and severe asthma exacerbations. Recent studies have also shown that addition of low doses of theophylline (giving plasma concentrations of <10 mg/L) were more effective than doubling the dose of inhaled budesonide, either in mild or severe asthma. Similar data are now emerging with anti-leukotrienes. The reason why these alternative treatments are more effective than higher doses of inhaled corticosteroids remains to be elucidated, but does suggest that there is a reversible component of asthma that may not be steroid-sensitive inflammation. It is possible that this may be an abnormality in airway smooth muscle itself (as a result of remodelling), oedematous swelling of the airway or production of cysteinyl-leukotrienes that is not sensitive to inhibition by inhaled corticosteroids.

Cost-effectiveness

Although inhaled corticosteroids may be more expensive than short-acting inhaled β_2-agonists, they are the most cost-effective way of controlling asthma, as reducing the frequency of asthma attacks will save on total costs. Inhaled corticosteroids also improve the quality of life of patients with asthma and allow many patients a normal lifestyle, thus saving costs indirectly.

Corticosteroid-sparing therapy

In patients who have serious side-effects with maintenance corticosteroid therapy there are several treatments which have been shown to reduce the requirement for oral corticosteroids. These treatments are commonly termed corticosteroid-sparing, although this misleading description could be applied to any additional asthma therapy (including bronchodilators). The amount of corticosteroid-sparing with these therapies is not impressive.

Several immunosuppressive agents have been shown to have corticosteroid effects, including methotrexate, oral gold and cyclosporin A. These therapies all have side-effects that may be more troublesome than those of oral corticosteroids, and are therefore only indicated as an additional therapy to reduce the requirement of oral corticosteroids. None of these treatments is very effective, but there are occasional patients who appear to show a good response. Because of side-effects these treatments cannot be considered as a way to reduce the requirement for inhaled corticosteroids. Several other therapies, including azathioprine, dapsone and hydroxychloroquine have not been found to be beneficial. The macrolide antibiotic troleandomycin is also reported to have corticosteroid-sparing effects, but this is only seen with methylprednisolone and is related to reduced metabolism of this corticosteroid, so that there is little therapeutic gain.

PHARMACOKINETICS

The pharmacokinetics of inhaled corticosteroids is important in determining the concentration of drug reaching target cells in the airways and in the fraction of drug reaching the systemic circulation and therefore causing side-effects. Beneficial properties in an inhaled corticosteroid are a high topical potency, a low systemic bioavailability of the swallowed portion of the dose and rapid metabolic clearance of any corticosteroid reaching the systemic circulation. After inhalation a large proportion of the inhaled dose (80–90%) is deposited on the oropharynx and is then swallowed and therefore available for absorption via the liver into the systemic circulation (Fig. 13.6). This fraction is markedly reduced by using a large volume spacer device with a metered dose inhaler (MDI) or by mouth-washing and discarding the washing with dry powder inhalers. Between 10 and 20% of inhaled drug enters the respiratory tract, where it is deposited in the airways and this fraction is available for absorption into the systemic circulation. Most of the early studies on the distribution of inhaled corticosteroids were conducted in healthy volunteers, and it is not certain what effect inflammatory disease, airway obstruction, age of the patient or concomitant medication may have had on the disposition of the inhaled dose. There may be important differences in the metabolism of different inhaled corticosteroids. BDP is metabolized to its more active metabolite beclomethasone monopropionate in many tissues including lung, but there is no information about its absorption or metabolism of this metabolite in humans. Flunisolide and budesonide are subject to extensive first-pass metabolism in the liver so that less reaches the systemic circulation. Little is known about the distribution of triamcinolone. FP is almost completely metabolized by first-pass metabolism, which reduces systemic effects.

When inhaled corticosteroids were first introduced it was recommended that they should be given four times daily, but several studies have now demonstrated that twice daily administration gives comparable control, although four times daily administration may be preferable in patients with more severe asthma. However, patients may find it difficult to comply with such frequent administration unless they have troublesome symptoms. For patients with mild asthma who require ≤400 mg daily, once daily therapy may be sufficient.

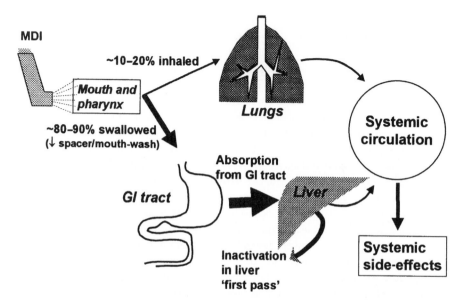

Figure 13.6 *Pharmacokinetics of inhaled corticosteroids. MDI, metered dose inhaler.*

SIDE-EFFECTS OF INHALED CORTICOSTEROIDS

The efficacy of inhaled corticosteroids is now established in short- and long-term studies in adults and children, but there are still concerns about side-effects, particularly in children and when high inhaled doses are needed. Several side-effects have been recognized (Table 13.3).

Table 13.3 *Side-effects of inhaled corticosteroids*

Local side-effects
Dysphonia
Oropharyngeal candidiasis
Cough

Systemic side-effects
Adrenal suppression
Growth suppression
Bruising
Osteoporosis
Cataracts
Glaucoma
Metabolic abnormalities (glucose, insulin, triglycerides)
Psychiatric disturbances

Local side-effects

Side-effects due to the local deposition of the inhaled corticosteroids in the oropharynx may occur with inhaled corticosteroids, but the frequency of complaints depends on the dose and frequency of administration and on the delivery system used.

DYSPHONIA

The commonest complaint is hoarseness of the voice (dysphonia) which may occur in over 50% of patients using an MDI. Dysphonia is not appreciably reduced by using spacers, but may be less with dry powder devices. Dysphonia may be due to myopathy of laryngeal muscles and is reversible when treatment is withdrawn. For most patients it is not troublesome but may be disabling in singers and lecturers.

OROPHARYNGEAL CANDIDIASIS

Oropharyngeal candidiasis (thrush) may be a problem in some patients, particularly in the elderly, with concomitant oral corticosteroids and more than twice daily administration. Large volume spacer devices protect against this local side-effect by reducing the dose of inhaled corticosteroid that deposits in the oropharynx.

OTHER LOCAL COMPLICATIONS

There is no evidence that inhaled corticosteroids, even in high doses, increase the frequency of infections, including tuberculosis, in the lower respiratory tract. There is no evidence for atrophy of the airway epithelium and even after 10 years of treatment with inhaled corticosteroids there is no evidence for any structural changes in the epithelium. Cough and throat irritation, sometimes accompanied by reflex bronchoconstriction, may occur when inhaled corticosteroids are given via an MDI. These symptoms are likely to be due to surfactants in pressurized aerosols, as they disappear after switching to a dry powder corticosteroid inhaler device.

Systemic side-effects

The efficacy of inhaled corticosteroids in the control of asthma is undisputed, but there are concerns about systemic effects of inhaled corticosteroids, particularly as they are likely to be used over long periods and in children of all ages. The safety of inhaled corticosteroids has been extensively investigated since their introduction 30 years ago. One of the major problems is to decide whether a measurable systemic effect has any significant clinical consequence and this necessitates careful long-term follow-up studies. As biochemical markers of systemic corticosteroid effects become more sensitive, then such effects may be seen more often, but this does not mean that they are clinically relevant. There are several case reports of adverse systemic effects of inhaled corticosteroids, and these may be idiosyncratic reactions, which may be due to abnormal pharmacokinetic handling of the inhaled corticosteroid. The systemic effect of an inhaled corticosteroid will depend on several factors, including the dose delivered to the patient, the site of delivery (gastrointestinal tract and lung), the delivery system used and individual differences in the patient's response to the corticosteroid.

EFFECT OF DELIVERY SYSTEMS

The systemic effect of an inhaled corticosteroid is dependent on the amount of drug absorbed into the systemic circulation. Approximately 90% of the inhaled dose from an MDI deposits in the oropharynx and is swallowed and subsequently absorbed from the gastrointestinal tract. Use of a large volume spacer device markedly reduces the oropharyngeal deposition, and therefore the systemic effects of inhaled corticosteroids, although this is less important when oral bioavailability is minimal, as with FP. For dry powder inhalers similar reductions in systemic effects may be achieved with mouth-washing and discarding the fluid. All patients using a daily dose of ≥800 µg of an inhaled corticosteroid should therefore use either a spacer or mouth-washing to reduce systemic absorption. Approximately 10% of an MDI enters the lung and this fraction (which presumably exerts the therapeutic effect) may be absorbed into the systemic circulation. As the fraction of inhaled corticosteroid deposited in the oropharynx is reduced, the proportion of the inhaled dose entering the lungs is increased. More efficient delivery to the lungs is therefore accompanied by increased systemic absorption, but this is offset by a reduction in the dose needed for optimal control of airway inflammation. For example, a multiple dry powder delivery system, the Turbuhaler, delivers approximately twice as much corticosteroid to the lungs as other devices, and therefore has increased systemic effects. However this is compensated for by the fact that only half the dose is required.

HYPOTHALAMIC–PITUITARY–ADRENAL AXIS

Corticosteroids may cause hypothalamic–pituitary–adrenal (HPA) axis suppression by reducing adrenocorticotrophin (ACTH) production, which reduces cortisol secretion by the adrenal gland. The degree of HPA suppression is dependent on dose, duration, frequency and timing of corticosteroid administration. There is no evidence that cortisol responses to the stress of an asthma exacerbation or insulin-induced hypoglycaemia are impaired, even with high doses of inhaled corticosteroids. However, measurement of HPA axis function provides evidence for systemic effects of an inhaled corticosteroid. Basal adrenal cortisol secretion may be measured by a morning plasma cortisol, 24 h urinary cortisol or by plasma cortisol profile over 24 h. Other tests measure the HPA response following stimulation with tetracosactrin (which measures adrenal reserve) or stimulation with metyrapone and insulin (which measures the response to stress).

There are many studies of HPA axis function in asthmatic patients taking inhaled corticosteroids, but the results are inconsistent as the studies have often been uncontrolled and patients have also been taking courses of oral corticosteroids (which may affect the HPA axis for weeks). BDP, budesonide and FP at high doses by conventional MDI (>1600 µg daily) give a dose-related decrease in morning serum cortisol levels and 24 h urinary cortisol, although values still lie well within the normal range. However, when a large volume spacer is used, doses of 2000 µg daily of BDP or budesonide have little effect on 24 h urinary cortisol excretion. Stimulation tests of HPA axis function similarly show no consistent effects of doses of 1500 µg or less of inhaled corticosteroid. At high doses (>1500 µg daily) budesonide and FP have less effect than BDP on HPA axis function. In children, no suppression of urinary cortisol is seen with doses of BDP of 800 µg or less. In studies where plasma cortisol has been measured at frequent intervals there was a significant reduction in cortisol peaks with doses of inhaled BDP as low as 400 µg daily, although this does not appear to be dose-related in the range 400–1000 µg. The clinical significance of these effects is not certain, however.

Overall, those studies which are not confounded by concomitant treatment with oral corticosteroids have consistently shown that there are no significant suppressive effects on HPA axis function at doses of ≤1500 µg in adults and ≤400 µg in children.

EFFECTS ON BONE METABOLISM

Corticosteroids lead to a reduction in bone mass by direct effects on bone formation and resorption, indirectly by suppression of the pituitary–gonadal and HPA axes, effects on intestinal calcium absorption, renal tubular calcium reabsorption and secondary hyperparathyroidism. The effects of oral corticosteroids on osteoporosis and increased risk of vertebral and rib fractures are well known, but there are no reports suggesting that long-term treatment with inhaled corticosteroids is associated with an increased risk of fractures. Bone densitometry has been used to assess the effect of inhaled corticosteroids on bone mass. Although there is evidence that bone density is less in patients taking high-dose inhaled corticosteroids, interpretation is confounded by the fact that these patients are also taking intermittent courses of oral corticosteroids.

Changes in bone mass occur very slowly and several biochemical indices have been used to assess the short-term effects of inhaled corticosteroids on bone metabolism. Bone formation has been measured by plasma concentrations of bone-specific alkaline phosphatase, serum osteocalcin or procollagen peptides. Bone resorption may be assessed by urinary hydroxyproline after a 12-hour fast, urinary calcium excretion and pyridinium cross-link excretion. It is important to consider the age, diet, time of day and physical activity of the patient in interpreting any abnormalities. It is also necessary to choose appropriate control groups, as asthma itself may have an effect on some of the measurements, such as osteocalcin. Inhaled corticosteroids, even at doses up to 2000 µg daily, have no significant effect on calcium excretion, but acute and reversible dose-related suppression of serum osteocalcin has been reported with BDP and budesonide when given by conventional MDI in several studies. Budesonide consistently has less effect than BDP at equivalent doses, and only BDP increases urinary hydroxyproline at high doses. With a large volume spacer, even doses of 2000 µg daily of either BDP or budesonide are without effect on plasma osteocalcin concentrations, however. Urinary pyridinium and deoxypyridinoline cross-links, which are a more accurate and stable measurement of bone and collagen degradation, are not increased with inhaled corticosteroids (BDP at >1000 µg daily), even with intermittent courses of oral corticosteroids.

It is important to monitor changes in markers of bone formation as well as bone degradation, as the net effect on bone turnover is important.

There has been particular concern about the effect of inhaled corticosteroids on bone metabolism in growing children. A very low dose of oral corticosteroids (prednisolone at 2.5 mg) causes significant changes in serum osteocalcin and urinary hydroxyproline excretion, whereas daily BDP and budesonide at doses up to 800 μg daily have no effect. It is important to recognize that the changes in biochemical indices of bone metabolism are less than those seen even with low doses of oral corticosteroids. This suggests that even high doses of inhaled corticosteroids, particularly when used with a spacer device, are unlikely to have any long-term effect on bone structure. Careful long-term follow-up studies in patients with asthma are needed.

There is no evidence that inhaled corticosteroids increase the frequency of fractures. Long-term treatment with high-dose inhaled corticosteroids has not been associated with any consistent change in bone density. Indeed, in elderly patients there may be an increase in bone density due to increased mobility.

EFFECTS ON CONNECTIVE TISSUE

Oral and topical corticosteroids cause thinning of the skin, telangiectases and easy bruising, probably as a result of loss of extracellular ground substance within the dermis, due to an inhibitory effect on dermal fibroblasts. There are reports of increased skin bruising and purpura in patients using high doses of inhaled BDP, but the amount of intermittent oral corticosteroids in these patients is not known. Easy bruising in association with inhaled corticosteroids is more frequent in elderly patients and there are no reports of this problem in children. Long-term prospective studies with objective measurements of skin thickness are needed using different inhaled corticosteroids.

OCULAR EFFECTS

Long-term treatment with oral corticosteroids increases the risk of posterior subcapsular cataracts and there are several case reports describing cataracts in individual patients taking inhaled corticosteroids. In a recent cross-sectional study in patients aged 5–25 years taking either inhaled BDP or budesonide, no cataracts were found on slit-lamp examination, even in patients taking 2000 μg daily for over 10 years. However, epidemiological studies have identified an increased risk of cataracts in patients taking high-dose inhaled steroids over prolonged periods. A slight increase in the risk of glaucoma in patients taking very high doses of inhaled corticosteroids has also been identified.

GROWTH

There has been particular concern that inhaled corticosteroids may cause stunting of growth and several studies have addressed this issue. Asthma itself (as with other chronic diseases) may have an effect on the growth pattern and has been associated with delayed onset of puberty and deceleration of growth velocity that is more pronounced with more severe disease. However, asthmatic children appear to grow for longer, so that their final height is normal. The effect of asthma on growth makes it difficult to assess the effects of inhaled corticosteroids on growth in cross-sectional studies, particularly as courses of oral corticosteroids are a confounding factor. Longitudinal studies have demonstrated that there is no significant effect of inhaled corticosteroids on statural growth in doses of up to 800 μg daily and for up to 5 years of treatment. A meta-analysis of 21 studies, including over 800 children, showed no effect of inhaled BDP on statural height, even with higher doses and long duration of therapy. In a large study of asthmatics treated with inhaled corticosteroids during childhood there was no difference in statural height compared with normal children.

Short-term growth measurements (knemometry) have demonstrated that even a low dose of an oral corticosteroid (prednisolone at 2.5 mg) is sufficient to give complete suppression of lower leg growth. However, inhaled budesonide up to 400 μg is without effect, although some suppression is seen with 800 μg and with 400 μg BDP. The relationship between knemometry measurements and final height is uncertain considering low doses of oral corticosteroid that have no effect on final height cause profound suppression.

METABOLIC EFFECTS

Several metabolic effects have been reported after inhaled corticosteroids, but there is no evidence that these are clinically relevant at therapeutic doses. In adults, fasting glucose and insulin are unchanged after doses of BDP up to 2000 μg daily and in children with inhaled budesonide up to 800 μg daily. In normal individuals, high-dose inhaled BDP may slightly increase resistance to insulin. However, in patients with poorly controlled asthma, high doses of BDP and budesonide paradoxically decrease insulin resistance and improve glucose tolerance, suggesting that the disease itself may lead to abnormalities in carbohydrate metabolism. Neither BDP at 2000 μg daily in adults nor budesonide at 800 μg daily in children have any effect on plasma cholesterol or triglyceride levels.

HAEMATOLOGICAL EFFECTS

Inhaled corticosteroids may reduce the numbers of circulating eosinophils in asthmatic patients, possibly due to an effect on local cytokine generation in the airways. Inhaled corticosteroids may cause a small increase in circulating neutrophil counts.

CENTRAL NERVOUS SYSTEM EFFECTS

There are various reports of psychiatric disturbance, including emotional lability, euphoria, depression, aggressiveness and insomnia, after inhaled corticosteroids. Only eight such patients have so far been reported, suggesting that this is very infrequent and a causal link with inhaled corticosteroids has usually not been established.

SAFETY IN PREGNANCY

Based on extensive clinical experience, inhaled corticosteroids appear to be safe in pregnancy, although no controlled studies have been performed. There is no evidence for any adverse effects of inhaled corticosteroids on the pregnancy, the delivery, or on the foetus. It is important to recognize that poorly controlled asthma may increase the incidence of perinatal mortality and retard intra-uterine growth, so that more effective control of asthma with inhaled corticosteroids may reduce these problems.

SYSTEMIC CORTICOSTEROIDS

Oral or intravenous corticosteroids may be indicated in several situations. Prednisolone, rather than prednisone, is the preferred oral corticosteroid, as prednisone has to be converted in the liver to the active prednisolone. In pregnant patients prednisone may be preferable as it is not converted to prednisolone in the foetal liver, thus diminishing the exposure of the foetus to corticosteroids. Enteric-coated preparations of prednisolone are used to reduce side-effects (particularly gastric side-effects) and give delayed and reduced peak plasma concentrations, although the bioavailability and therapeutic efficacy of these preparations are similar to uncoated tablets. Prednisolone and prednisone are preferable to dexamethasone, betamethasone or triamcinolone, which have longer plasma half-lives and therefore an increased frequency of adverse effects.

Short courses of oral corticosteroids (30–40 mg prednisolone daily for 1–2 weeks or until the peak flow values return to best attainable) are indicated for exacerbations of asthma, and the dose may be tailed off over 1 week once the exacerbation is resolved. The tail-off period is not strictly necessary, but some patients find it reassuring.

Maintenance oral corticosteroids are only needed in a small proportion of asthmatic patients with the most severe asthma that cannot be controlled with maximal doses of inhaled corticosteroids (2000 µg daily) and additional bronchodilators. The minimal dose of oral corticosteroid needed for control should be used and reductions in the dose should be made slowly in patients who have been on oral corticosteroids for long periods (e.g. by 2.5 mg per month for doses down to 10 mg daily and thereafter by 1 mg per month). Oral corticosteroids are usually given as a single morning dose, as this coincides with the peak diurnal concentrations and thus reduces the risk of adverse effects. There is some evidence that administration in the afternoon may be optimal for some patients who have severe nocturnal asthma. Alternate day administration may also reduce adverse effects, but control of asthma may not be as good on the day when the oral dose is omitted in some patients.

Intramuscular triamcinolone acetonide (80 mg monthly) has been advocated in patients with severe asthma as an alternative to oral corticosteroids. This may be considered in patients in whom compliance is a particular problem, but the major concern is the high frequency of proximal myopathy associated with this fluorinated corticosteroid. Some patients who do not respond well to prednisolone are reported to respond to oral betamethasone, presumably because of pharmacokinetic handling problems with prednisolone.

Acute severe asthma

Intravenous hydrocortisone is given in acute severe asthma. The recommended dose is 200 mg i.v. While the value of corticosteroids in acute severe asthma has been questioned, others have found that they speed the resolution of attacks. There is no apparent advantage in giving very high doses of intravenous corticosteroids (such as methylprednisolone at 1 g). Indeed, intravenous corticosteroids have occasionally been associated with an acute severe myopathy. In a recent study no difference in recovery from acute severe asthma was seen whether i.v. hydrocortisone in doses of 50, 200 or 500 mg 6-hourly were used, and another placebo-controlled study showed no beneficial effect at all of i.v. corticosteroids. Intravenous corticosteroids are indicated in acute asthma if lung function is <30% predicted and in whom there is no significant improvement with nebulized β_2-agonist. Intravenous therapy is usually given until a satisfactory response is obtained and then oral prednisolone may be substituted. Oral prednisolone (40–60 mg) has a similar effect to i.v. hydrocortisone and is easier to administer. Oral prednisolone is the preferred treatment for acute severe asthma, providing there are no contraindications to oral therapy.

CORTICOSTEROID-RESISTANT ASTHMA

Although glucocorticoids are highly effective in the control of asthma and other chronic inflammatory or immune diseases, a small proportion of patients with asthma fail to respond even to high doses of oral corticosteroids. Resistance to the therapeutic effects of corticosteroids is also recognized in other inflammatory and immune diseases, including rheumatoid arthritis and inflammatory bowel disease. Corticosteroid-resistant patients, although uncommon, present considerable management problems. Recently, new insights into the mechanisms whereby corticosteroids suppress chronic inflammation have shed new light on the molecular basis of corticosteroid-resistant asthma.

Corticosteroid-resistant asthma is defined as a failure to improve FEV_1 or peak expiratory flow by >15% after treatment with oral prednisolone at 30–40 mg daily for 2 weeks, providing the oral steroid is taken (verified by plasma prednisolone level or a reduction in early morning cortisol level). These patients are not Addisonian and they do not suffer from the abnormalities in sex hormones that are described in the very rare familial glucocorticoid resistance. Plasma cortisol and adrenal suppression in response to exogenous cortisol is normal in these patients, so they suffer from side-effects of corticosteroids.

Complete corticosteroid resistance in asthma is very rare, with a prevalence of <1 : 1000 asthmatic patients. Much more common is a reduced responsiveness to corticosteroids, so that large inhaled or oral doses are needed to control asthma adequately (corticosteroid-dependent asthma). It is likely that there is a range of responsiveness to corticosteroids and that corticosteroid resistance is at one extreme of this range.

It is important to establish that the patient has asthma, rather than chronic obstructive pulmonary disease (COPD), 'pseudoasthma' (a hysterical conversion syndrome involving vocal cord dysfunction), left ventricular failure or cystic fibrosis which do not respond to corticosteroids. Asthmatic patients are characterized by a variability in peak expiratory flow and, in particular, a diurnal variability of >15% and episodic symptoms. It is also important to identify provoking factors (allergens, drugs, psychological problems) that may increase the severity of asthma and its resistance to therapy. Biopsy studies have demonstrated the typical eosinophilic inflammation of asthma in these patients.

Mechanisms of corticosteroid resistance

There may be several mechanisms for resistance to the effects of glucocorticoids. Certain cytokines (particularly IL-2, IL-4 and IL-13) may induce a reduction in affinity of GRs in inflammatory cells such as T lymphocytes, resulting in local resistance to the antiinflammatory actions of corticosteroids. Another mechanism is an increased activation of the transcription factor AP-1 by inflammatory cytokines, so that AP-1 may consume activated GRs and thus reduce their availability for suppression of inflammation at inflamed sites (Fig. 13.7). There is an increased expression of c-Fos, one of the components of AP-1. The reasons for this excessive activation of AP-1 by activating enzymes is currently unknown, but may be genetically determined.

FUTURE DIRECTIONS

Inhaled corticosteroids are now used as first-line therapy for the treatment of persistent asthma in adults and children in many countries, as they are the most effective treatments for asthma currently available. The recent trend to start with a relatively high dose of inhaled corticosteroids in order to achieve more rapid control of asthma, before the dose is reduced to the minimum needed to maintain control, may lead to lower overall maintenance doses. While many patients, particularly with more severe asthma, remain undertreated, there is also a danger of overtreatment and many patients with mild asthma who may require very low

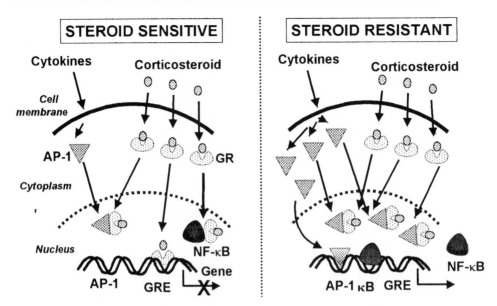

Figure 13.7 *Proposed mechanism of primary corticosteroid resistance in asthma. Increased activation of activator protein-1 (AP-1) results in the consumption of glucocorticoid receptors (GRs), thus preventing the antiinflammatory action of corticosteroids, either through binding to GREs or through inhibition of NF-κB.*

doses of inhaled corticosteroids are inappropriately treated with high doses. It is essential that inhaled corticosteroids are slowly reduced to the minimal dose required to control asthma. An important clinical development is the recognition that asthma is better controlled by addition of an alternative class of treatment (long-acting inhaled β_2-agonists, low-dose theophylline, anti-leukotrienes) than on increasing the dose of inhaled steroid. However, there may be some patients who are better treated with a higher dose of inhaled corticosteroid and at present it is not possible to identify such patients clinically. Improvement in techniques for the non-invasive monitoring of airway inflammation may be valuable in the future for assessing the requirement for inhaled corticosteroids.

New corticosteroids

Budesonide and FP have been important advances in inhaled corticosteroid therapy as they have reduced systemic effects because of greater first-pass hepatic metabolism than BDP. There are other inhaled corticosteroids in development, such as mometasone, which show a similar improved profile. However, all currently available corticosteroids are absorbed from the lungs into the systemic circulation and therefore inevitably have some systemic component. A class of steroids was developed that was metabolized in the lung, but such so-called 'soft' steroids, such as tipredane and butixocort, did not prove to be clinically effective, probably because they were metabolized too rapidly in the airways. Steroids that are metabolized by enzymes in the circulation may be the safest type to inhale and novel esterified corticosteroids are now in clinical development. However, it is still not certain whether the antiinflammatory effects of inhaled corticosteroids in asthma are mediated entirely by local antiinflammatory effects in the airways, and it is possible that there is a systemic component, for example on bone marrow eosinophil precursors. Furthermore, it is not clear whether inhaled corticosteroids are distributed from their point of deposition in the airways to more peripheral airways via the local circulation. If this is the case then corticosteroids that are degraded by enzymes in the circulation may not reach small airways which are known to be inflamed in asthma.

Understanding the molecular mechanisms of action of corticosteroids has led to the development of a new generation of corticosteroids. As discussed above, a major mechanism of the antiinflammatory effect of corticosteroids appears to be direct inhibition of transcription factors, such as NF-κB and AP-1, that are activated by pro-inflammatory cytokines (transrepression). By contrast the endocrine and metabolic effects of steroids that are responsible for the systemic side-effects of corticosteroids are likely to be mediated via DNA binding (transactivation). This has led to a search for novel corticosteroids that selectively transrepress, thus reducing the potential risk of systemic side-effects. As such corticosteroids bind to the same GRs, this seems at first to be an unlikely possibility, but while DNA binding involves a GR homodimer, interaction with transcription factors AP-1 and NF-κB involves only a single GR. A separation of transactivation and transrepression has been demonstrated using reporter gene constructs in transfected cells having selective mutations of the glucocorticoid receptor. Furthermore, some steroids, such as the antagonist RU486, have a greater transrepression than transactivation effect. Indeed, the topical steroids used in asthma therapy today, such as FP and budesonide, appear to have more potent transrepression than transactivation effects, which may account for their selection as potent antiinflammatory agents. Recently, a novel class of steroids has been described in which there is potent transrepression with relatively little transactivation. These 'dissociated' steroids, including RU24858 and RU40066, have antiinflammatory effects *in vivo*. This suggests that the development of steroids with a greater margin of safety is possible and may even lead to the development of oral steroids that do not have significant adverse effects.

New antiinflammatory drugs

There has been a concerted effort to find novel antiinflammatory drugs that might replace corticosteroids in the future. However, it has proved very difficult to find classes of drug that are as safe and efficacious as inhaled corticosteroids. More specific antiinflammatory drugs that selectively inhibit eosinophilic inflammation, such as anti-IL-5 drugs, chemokine receptor (CCR3) inhibitors and adhesion molecule blockers (such as VLA4 inhibitors) are currently in clinical development, but whether these more specific drugs will have the efficacy of corticosteroids is not yet known. Drugs that inhibit NF-κB are also in early development, but may prove to be too toxic for use in asthma. More generalized antiinflammatory drugs, such as phosphodiesterase 4 inhibitors, have proved to be disappointing because of side-effects and immunomodulators, such as cyclosporin A, lack clinical efficacy and a high degree of toxicity. It is likely that inhaled corticosteroids will remain the mainstay of asthma therapy for many years to come.

FURTHER READING

Molecular mechanisms

Barnes PJ. (1996) Mechanism of action of glucocorticoids in asthma. *Am J Respir Crit Care Med*, **154**, S21–7.

Barnes PJ. (1998) Antiinflammatory actions of glucocorticoids: molecular mechanisms. *Clin Sci*, **94**, 557–72.

Barnes PJ, Adcock IM. (1998) Transcription factors and asthma. *Eur Respir J*, **12**, 221–34.

Karin M. (1998) New twists in gene regulation by glucocorticoid receptor: is DNA binding dispensable? *Cell*, **93**, 487–90.

Reichardt HM, Schutz G. (1998) Glucocorticoid signalling – multiple variations of a common theme. *Mol Cell Endocrinol*, **146**, 1–6.

Schweibert LM, Stellato C, Schleimer RP. (1996) The epithelium as a target for glucocorticoid action in the treatment of asthma. *Am J Respir Crit Care Med*, **154**, S16–20.

Clinical efficacy

Barnes PJ. (1995) Inhaled glucocorticoids for asthma. *New Engl J Med*, **332**, 868–75.

Barnes PJ. (1998) Efficacy of inhaled corticosteroids in asthma. *J Allergy Clin Immunol*, **102**, 531–8.

Barnes PJ. (1998) Current issues for establishing inhaled corticosteroids as the antiinflammatory agents of choice in asthma. *J Allergy Clin Immunol*, **101**, S427–33.

Barnes PJ, Pedersen S, Busse WW. (1998) Efficacy and safety of inhaled corticosteroids: an update. *Am J Respir Crit Care Med*, **157**, S1–53.

Boushey HA. (1998) Effects of inhaled corticosteroids on the consequences of asthma. *J Allergy Clin Immunol*, **102**, S5–16.

Hill SJ, Tattersfield AE. (1995) Corticosteroid sparing agents in asthma. *Thorax*, **50**, 577–82.

O'Byrne PM, Pedersen S. (1998) Measuring efficacy and safety of different inhaled corticosteroid preparations. *J Allergy Clin Immunol*, **102**, 879–86.

Safety

Allen DB, Mullen M, Mullen B. (1994) A meta-analysis of the effects of oral and inhaled corticosteroids on growth. *J Allergy Clin Immunol*, **93**, 967–76.

Barnes PJ, Pedersen S, Busse WW. (1998) Efficacy and safety of inhaled corticosteroids: an update. *Am J Respir Crit Care Med*, **157**, S1–53.

Derendorf H, Hochhaus G, Meibohm B, Mollmann H, Barth J. (1998) Pharmacokinetics and pharmacodynamics of inhaled corticosteroids. *J Allergy Clin Immunol*, **101**, S440–6.

Efthimou J, Barnes PJ. (1998) Effect of inhaled corticosteroids on bone and growth. *Eur Respir J*, **11**, 1167–77.

Kamada AK, Szefler SJ, Martin RJ, *et al.* (1996) Issues in the use of inhaled steroids. *Am J Respir Crit Care Med*, **153**, 1739–48.

O'Byrne PM, Pedersen S. (1998) Measuring efficacy and safety of different inhaled corticosteroid preparations. *J Allergy Clin Immunol*, **102**, 879–86.

Simons FE. (1998) Benefits and risks of inhaled glucocorticoids in children with persistent asthma. *J Allergy Clin Immunol*, **102**, S77–84.

Toogood JH. (1998) Side effects of inhaled corticosteroids. *J Allergy Clin Immunol*, **102**, 705–13.

Corticosteroid resistance

Barnes PJ, Adcock IM. (1995) Steroid-resistant asthma. *Q J Med*, **88**, 455–68.

Barnes PJ, Greening AP, Crompton GK. (1995) Glucocorticoid resistance in asthma. *Am J Respir Crit Care Med*, **152**, 125S–140S.

Leung DY, de Castro M, Szefler SJ, Chrousos GP. (1998) Mechanisms of glucocorticoid-resistant asthma. *Ann N Y Acad Sci*, **840**, 735–46.

Szefler SJ, Leung DY. (1997) Glucocorticoid-resistant asthma: pathogenesis and clinical implications for management. *Eur Respir J*, **10**, 1640–7.

14

Devices for inhaling medications

STEPHEN P. NEWMAN

INTRODUCTION

Drug delivery by the aerosol route is often regarded as a twentieth century innovation, but in fact records of inhalation therapy can be found in the writings of most ancient cultures, notably those in China, India, Greece, Rome and the Middle East. These early therapies consisted of aromatic fumes and vapours derived either from natural plant essences or from burning organic materials. Hippocrates was probably the first person to describe an inhaler device, which was a crude clay pot for imbibing hot vapours. Some species of tobacco plant were being smoked in the sixteenth century as a remedy for lung diseases, and at one time tobacco smoke was hailed as a panacea, not only for the respiratory tract, but also as a form of systemic drug delivery.

The modern era of asthma therapy, and of asthma inhalers, dates from about 70 years ago, when the first reports were published of adrenaline given by aerosol using a hand-held squeeze-bulb nebulizer. Without doubt, the single most important development in inhalation technology was the pressurized metered dose inhaler (pMDI) introduced by 3M Riker Laboratories in 1956. The convenience of the pMDI was quickly recognized; yet this very popular device is not without its problems, and alternatives are sometimes preferable. There are a number of major driving forces which are leading to the development of new inhalers at that present time, namely: (a) the need for inhalers that patients can use easily and reliably, (b) the ban (for environmental reasons) upon chlorofluorocarbon (CFC) propellants, which will soon lead to the elimination of CFC-powered pMDIs, and (c) the recognition that inhalation devices are required not only for the treatment and prophylaxis of asthma, but also for other purposes, including the efficient and reproducible delivery of inhaled peptides and proteins. This chapter will review the types of inhalation device currently available and those likely to be available in the near future, concentrating upon the use of inhalers in the management of asthma. Recent technological developments that are helping to overcome the deficiencies and limitations of earlier systems will be highlighted.

PRESSURIZED METERED DOSE INHALERS (pMDIs)

Basic description

The pMDI (Fig. 14.1) has become the most widely used inhalation device in the treatment and prophylaxis of asthma (Newman, 1997). The original pMDIs contained the non-selective β-agonists isoprenaline and adrenaline, but these were superseded by short-acting selective β_2-adrenergic agents such as salbutamol and terbutaline sulphate, and later by long-acting β-agonists (salmeterol and formoterol). Delivery by pMDI of topical corticosteroids, including beclomethasone dipropionate, budesonide and fluticasone propionate followed subsequently, and inhaled corticosteroid therapy has become first-line therapy for asthma in many countries.

Until recently, all pMDIs were powered by chlorofluorocarbon (CFC) propellants, which are often known, sometimes erroneously, by the Dupont trade name 'Freon'. The most common formulation, at least in Europe, has involved a suspension of micronized polar drug particles in a mixture of two or three non-polar CFCs (CFC-11, CFC-12 and CFC-114), chosen to achieve the desired vapour pressure and spray characteristics. Of these three propellants, CFC-12 is the one mainly responsible for producing the high vapour pressure inside the canister, typically 300 to 500 kPa. The key component of the pMDI is the metering valve, which delivers an accurately known volume of CFCs (25 to 100 μL), containing the micronized drug (ranging from 12 μg to 5 mg for different drugs), at each valve actuation. A surfactant (usually sorbitan trioleate, oleic acid or lecithin) is also needed to reduce particle agglomeration and to lubricate the metering valve mechanism. The pMDI is filled either at low temperature, when the propellants can be handled in the liquid phase, or under pressure. Although the range of products delivered by pMDI has been widened to reflect the development of new drug substances and formulations, the basic design of the pMDI has changed remarkably little since its introduction 40 years ago.

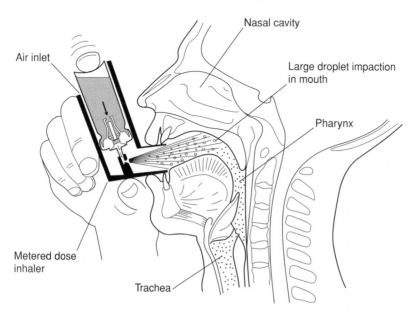

Figure 14.1 *Pressurized metered dose inhaler. (From Newman, 1997, with permission.)*

Spray formation is a complex process, involving fragmentation into droplets at the actuator orifice, an initial 'flashing' of some of the CFCs, and a slower evaporation of the remainder. The physics of aerosol formulation in pMDIs was recently described in detail by Clark (1996). The velocity of the spray at the actuator orifice may exceed 30 m/s and the initial droplet mass median diameter is typically >10 μm, although this velocity is rapidly lost owing to air resistance, and the propellant droplets shrink rapidly by evaporation.

Reformulation in hydrofluoroalkanes (HFAs)

Following the recognition that serious damage to the ozone layer in the stratosphere is being caused by the release of certain chemicals, primarily CFCs, international agreement has been reached to prohibit the use of these substances through the Montreal Protocol. Uniquely, the use of CFCs in inhalers for pulmonary drug delivery has been granted temporary 'essential use' exemption from this ban until satisfactory alternatives have been developed. The pharmaceutical industry has sought alternative substances that meet the exacting requirements of being inert, non-flammable, safe for human use, inexpensive and similar in thermodynamic properties to the CFCs. Two hydrofluoroalkane (HFA) propellants, HFA-134a (tetrafluoroethane) and HFA-227 (heptafluoropropane) appear to meet these requirements and pMDIs reformulated with one or other of these substances are being developed at the present time. However, the reformulation of pMDIs is not a simple matter, and there are many technical challenges (McDonald and Martin, 2000), requiring novel surfactants and other excipients, new valve materials, and new filling techniques.

It is intended that a seamless transition from CFC to HFA-based pMDIs should be made, in order to maintain patient and physician confidence (Smith, 1995). Nevertheless, the switch from CFC-based products will produce a major change in the therapy of most asthma patients, who will need to be made aware that their new inhalers may feel different in the hand, and may give a different sensation on the back of the throat compared with products with which they have been familiar (Partridge *et al.*, 1998). The complete transition to HFA products is inevitably a slow process, resulting not only from the need to overcome technical challenges, but also to conduct necessary safety assessments and clinical trials. Such is the importance given to the development of HFA-based pMDIs that the pharmaceutical industry has taken the unusual step of forming consortia which have collaborated on the toxicity testing of the new formulations. At the time of writing, very few HFA products have been marketed, but the switch from CFC to HFA products is expected to be complete in the early years of this century. It should be borne in mind, however, that while HFA propellants do not destroy ozone, they are 'greenhouse' gases (although less potent than CFCs), and there may be increasing demands for them to be banned in future years.

Deposition efficiency of pMDIs

Most pMDIs deliver only a small fraction of the drug dose to the required site of action in the lungs. This is a direct consequence of the rapid velocity and large size of the droplets in the spray, most of which simply impact on the back of the throat, and have been confirmed in many gamma scintigraphic studies of lung deposition (Newman, 1993, 1998). Even under the most favourable conditions, no more than about 20% of the dose from a CFC pMDI generally reaches the lungs with the majority deposited in the oropharynx (Fig. 14.2). High oropharyngeal deposition of glucocorticosteroids may contribute to both local and systemic side-effects (Barnes *et al.*, 1998). Formulations containing micronized drug suspended in HFA propellants appear to give broadly comparable amounts of drug in 'respirable' (<5 μm

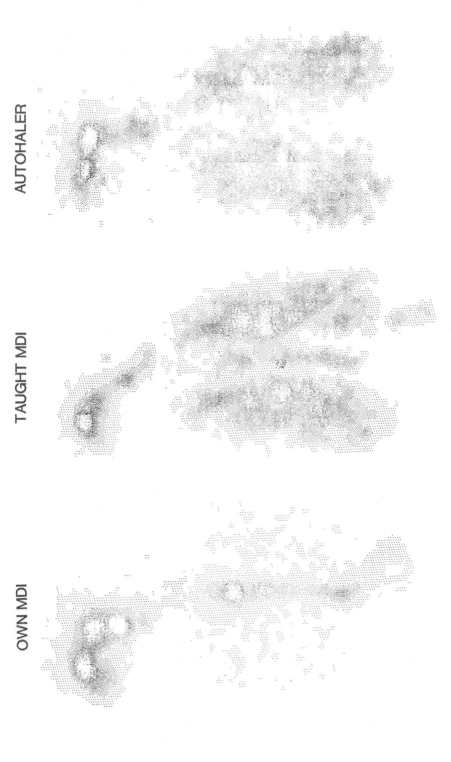

OWN MDI   TAUGHT MDI   AUTOHALER

Figure 14.2   *Deposition of drug from a pMDI in a patient with poor inhaler technique inhaled by patient's own pMDI technique, by taught (optimal) technique and by a breath-actuated pMDI (Autohaler). When the patient inhaled by his own technique, the pMDI was actuated after inhalation had been completed. (From Newman et al., 1991, with permission of BMJ Publishing Group.)*

diameter) particles as CFC formulations. Recent data suggest that some formulations of HFA pMDIs containing the drug as a solution may result in a very high yield of 'respirable' particles, so that a greater percentage of the drug dose is deposited in the lungs (Leach *et al.*, 1998). This prospect is an exciting one, as improved percentage drug delivery to the target site offers the potential opportunity for asthma control with a significantly reduced drug dose (Busse *et al.*, 1999), and with an improved safety profile (Thompson *et al.*, 1998). A novel formulation of hollow porous drug particles was shown recently to give more efficient and reproducible delivery of salbutamol by pMDI (Weers *et al.*, 2000).

The potency of β-agonists and topical corticosteroids is remarkable, considering both are effective when only about 10–20 µg (10 to 20% of a 100 µg metered dose) is spread over a large surface area of the lung mucosa, and long-acting β-agonists are effective in even smaller airway doses than this. It is essential to recognize that the efficacies of inhaled β-agonists, glucocorticosteroids and other inhaled medications derive essentially from the small inhaled fraction, given that the swallowed fraction of inhaled β-agonists and glucocorticosteroids from pMDIs is diluted in the bloodstream, and is metabolized and largely inactivated during passage through the liver, while sodium cromoglycate is not absorbed significantly from the gastrointestinal tract. β-Agonists are, of course, effective when given orally, but only in doses much higher than those given by pMDI. At least one β-agonist has been shown to produce bronchodilatation when sprayed into the nose, perhaps reflecting absorption via the nasal mucosa, but this route is rarely if ever used.

Correct and incorrect pMDI use

Because pMDIs generally have a low inherent delivery efficiency to the target site and the swallowed fraction of the dose is largely or totally ineffective, it is important to know how patients should inhale from pMDIs for maximal delivery to the lungs and optimal effect. Optimal inhaler technique for pMDIs has been defined from systematically varied inhalation techniques in either clinical efficacy studies or assessments of aerosol deposition in the lungs (Newman *et al.*, 1981).

These studies have arrived at a good consensus regarding correct pMDI technique (Table 14.1), and there have been moves to standardize manufacturers' instructions throughout the pharmaceutical industry. An inspired airstream which carries some of the aerosol into the lungs is the crucial feature. Thus the pMDI should be actuated during the course of inhalation; there may be a reduction in response if actuation occurs before inhalation, and a complete absence of drug deposition in the lungs and subsequent clinical response if actuation occurs after inhalation (Fig. 14.2). A slow steady inhalation (at about 30 L/min) seems necessary for optimal drug deposition (Newman *et al.*, 1982), and a breath-holding pause of 10 seconds is generally recommended. This inhalation technique is logical, since slow

Table 14.1 *Correct technique for using a pMDI*

1 Take the cap off the inhaler mouthpiece
2 Shake the inhaler
3 Hold the inhaler upright
4 Breathe out
5 Place the inhaler mouthpiece between the lips
6 Fire the inhaler while breathing in deeply and slowly
7 Continue to inhale until the lungs are full
8 Hold the breath while counting to 10
9 Breathe out

inhalation minimizes impaction of drug particles in the oropharynx, while breath-holding enables particles to sediment on to the airway surfaces under gravity. The inhalation should be deep, but need not begin at residual volume. Although derived chiefly from experimental work using bronchodilators, the optimal technique is believed to apply to all drug substances when given by pMDI, and also to all patients irrespective of their diagnosis or degree of airway obstruction.

The inhaler mouthpiece is usually held between closed lips. It has been suggested that the inhaler should be held away from the open mouth for optimal drug deposition (Dolovich *et al.*, 1981), but other authorities do not favour this approach for fear that it could introduce unnecessary errors by causing the patient to fire the pMDI on to the face rather than into the mouth. There is a theoretical advantage to be gained from a pause of several minutes between successive doses of bronchodilator, or between a dose of bronchodilator and a dose of glucocorticosteroid, in order that a first dose should open partially obstructed airways into which a second dose might penetrate, but the evidence that this helps in clinical practice is inconclusive.

Sadly, many patients cannot use pMDIs satisfactorily, and this has been demonstrated in numerous studies. The most important errors in pMDI technique appear to be: (i) poor co-ordination between actuating the pMDI and inhaling, particularly if this dysco-ordination is at the end of inhalation; this error takes an extreme form in the patient who actuates the pMDI and then blows out immediately, and (ii) the so-called 'cold-Freon' effect, where the patient stops inhaling completely, or inhales through the nose only, when the cold blast of propellant strikes the back of the throat (Crompton, 1982).

It is difficult to estimate the proportion of patients whose inhaler technique is seriously inadequate, but it has been estimated that as many as half of adult patients and a greater proportion of children are getting reduced benefit from using pMDIs because of poor technique. Correct instruction plus regular checking of technique are of paramount importance, as many patients who could once use a pMDI successfully can develop inefficient technique spontaneously. Bizarre errors in pMDI technique are occasionally reported, for instance failure to take the cap off the mouthpiece, or actuating the pMDI on to the outside of the chest. Such errors will obviously result in complete treatment failure, and this emphasizes the need for correct instruction. Other errors, such as fast inhalation (a very common fault), shallow inhalation, failure to breath-hold and actuating the pMDI more than once during a single inhalation, should be corrected, but they are unlikely to prevent at least some aerosol from reaching its target site.

Advantages and disadvantages of pMDIs

The design and formulation of the pMDI itself dictates its strengths and weaknesses. The pressurized formulation has resulted in a device that is inexpensive, portable, convenient and inconspicuous, and which generally contains at least 200 accurately metered doses that are immediately ready for use. These are very positive practical features, which explains the success and popularity of the pMDI over several decades.

Conversely, the pMDI suffers from a number of significant limitations, all of which have been alluded to in earlier sections of this chapter. First, many patients use the device incorrectly, often disastrously so. Second, most pMDIs still contain CFC propellants, which have been banned throughout the developed world. Third, pMDIs are generally inefficient in delivering drug to the lungs, with a high percentage of the dose being either wasted or delivered to sites where it may contribute to side-effects but not to the treatment of asthma. Taken together, these factors mean that the pMDI is far from perfect, and that there is a need for alternative types of aerosol delivery systems in the management of asthma.

pMDI AUXILIARY DEVICES

Breath-actuated pMDIs

Considering a major cause of pMDI misuse is poor co-ordination between firing the pMDI and inhaling, it is logical to think in terms of an inhaler that is actuated automatically, and which is triggered by the patient's inhalation. At the end of the 1980s, 3M Health Care introduced the Autohaler™, a compact device which contains a conventional pMDI canister. To operate the device, the priming lever is first lifted; this compresses a conical spring which pushes the canister downwards within the inhaler, but further movement of the canister is blocked when the valve ferrule comes into contact with a precision-moulded triggering mechanism. The inhaler is then in a state of equilibrium and no drug is released. However, when the patient inhales through the mouthpiece, a vane is pulled forward, the canister completes its downward motion, and the inhaler is actuated, in automatic synchrony with the patient's inhalation (Newman *et al.*, 1991). The mechanism is reset by lowering the priming lever. Operation of the device is virtually silent in contrast to an earlier device introduced by the same manufacturers almost 20 years earlier, and low inhaled flow rates that virtually any patient can attain are sufficient to trigger the inhaler. A scintigraphic study conducted in patients with severe co-ordination problems, showed that Autohaler™ can give drug deposition in the lungs and bronchodilator efficacy equivalent to those achieved by a correctly used 'press and breathe' pMDI (Fig. 14.2). The problem of poor co-ordination in children was solved by Autohaler™, but the device was unable to influence the problem of cold Freon droplets, which may cause younger children to stop inhaling or to inhale through the nose rather than through the mouth. A further breath-actuated pMDI device (Easibreathe™, Norton Health Care) works on broadly similar principles, and may be even easier to use as it is not necessary to lift a priming lever.

An even more sophisticated breath-actuated pMDI (SmartMist®, Aradigm) includes a microprocessor which monitors the patient's inhaler technique, and which will only actuate the pMDI when a predetermined combination of inhaled flow rate and cumulative inhaled volume has been achieved (Farr *et al.*, 1995). Indicator lights on the device are used to guide the patient to inhale slowly and steadily. The pMDI spray can thus be inhaled under very carefully controlled inhalation conditions, hence helping to reduce a major source of variability in drug delivery *in vivo*. Although perhaps somewhat expensive for day-to-day asthma therapy, devices such as the SmartMist® may have additional roles including controlling inhaler technique in clinical trials, and for delivering more expensive drug substances to the lungs in a controlled manner.

Novel actuators

Improvements to pMDI actuator technology may lead to significant benefits in inhaler therapy. A compact novel actuator (Spacehaler®, Celltech Medeva), which releases a much more slowly moving spray than that from a conventional pMDI, has recently been marketed. This device results in a marked reduction in oropharyngeal deposition of asthma drugs, while lung deposition is either unchanged or enhanced (Newman *et al.*, 1999). A similar improvement in drug delivery was provided by the Aerosol Drug Delivery System (ADDS, Sheffield Pharmaceuticals) (Newman *et al.*, 2000). In addition to improving drug targeting from pMDIs, such devices which produce slowly moving sprays may also make pMDIs easier to use, by reducing the likelihood of both co-ordination and 'cold Freon' problems.

Spacer devices

Over the last 20 years, a number of spacer tubes and mouthpiece extensions, as well as valved chambers and collapsible bags to contain the spray briefly before inhalation, have been developed. Some of these devices that are available commercially are shown in Fig. 14.3. Spacer devices may be divided into three broad types (Table 14.2): (i) simple 'tube spacer' extensions to the inhaler mouthpiece, (ii) 'holding chambers', which generally have a one-way inhalation valve at the mouthpiece, and (iii) 'reverse flow' devices, with the pMDI being fired in a direction

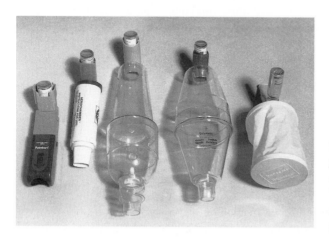

Figure 14.3 *Some spacer devices, from left to right: Inhalet tube, AeroChamber®, Nebuhaler®, Volumatic®, InspirEase®. (From Newman and Clark, 1992, with permission.)*

Table 14.2 *Some spacer devices used in inhaled asthma therapy, with their manufacturers and approximate volumes*

Device	Manufacturer	Volume (mL)
Tube spacers		
Inhalet tube	Astra Zeneca	80
Boehringer tube	Boehringer Ingelheim	50
Syncroner tube	Rhône–Poulenc Rorer (Aventis)	100
Azmacort tube	Rhône–Poulenc Rorer (Aventis)	110
Optimiser	Norton Health Care	50
Holding chambers		
Nebuhaler®	Astra	750
Volumatic®	Glaxo–Wellcome	750
Rondo®	Leiras	270
Aerochamber™	Monaghan	145
Babyhaler®	Glaxo–Wellcome	350
Fisonair®	Rhône–Poulenc Rorer (Aventis)	750
Inhacort spacer [a]	Boehringer Ingelheim	250
Babyspacer	Astra Zeneca	260
Nebuchamber® [b]	Astra Zeneca	250
Integra [a]	Glaxo–Wellcome	312
Reverse-flow devices		
Optihaler®	Respironics	70
InspirEase®	Schering–Plough	600
ACE	DHD Health care	170

[a] No one-way valve in mouthpiece; [b] metal spacer.

180 degrees from the mouth, either into a collapsible bag, or into small volume from which outside air is entrained (Newman and Newhouse, 1996). In addition to devices supplied by the pharmaceutical industry, everyday objects such as disposable coffee cups, empty bottles and paper or plastic bags have been used as spacers, often with satisfactory results.

Despite differences in design, spacers generally have a number of common properties and aims, from which beneficial changes in the pattern of aerosol deposition should result: (i) the spacer constitutes a volume into which the patient actuates the pMDI and from which the patient then inhales, without necessarily having to co-ordinate the two manoeuvres, (ii) given that the aerosol is generated at some distance from the mouth, problems with the 'cold Freon' effect should be less acute or even eliminated entirely, and (iii) when the aerosol reaches the patient it will be moving more slowly and will be contained in smaller droplets, compared to the spray from the standard pMDI.

The best known spacers in Europe are Nebuhaler® (Astra Zeneca) and Volumatic® (Glaxo–Wellcome). Other devices such as Aerochamber® (Monaghan) and InspirEase® (Schering–Plough) are used in North America. Nebuhaler® and Volumatic® are purpose-built chambers of approximately 750 mL in volume, intended for use with terbutaline or budesonide sprays, and salbutamol or beclomethasone dipropionate sprays, respectively. These two spacers contain one-way valves in the mouthpiece which will foil any patient who actuates the pMDI and who then exhales immediately; this will simply result in valve closure, leaving the aerosol contained within the device ready for inhalation.

Spacer devices inevitably lead to a reduction in oropharyngeal drug deposition, because a significant proportion of the 'non-respirable' fraction of the aerosol spray is deposited on the walls of the spacer itself. Lung deposition from spacers is generally either increased or is unchanged (Newman and Newhouse, 1996). The total body dose of drug may be reduced by over 80% for some spacer devices, while targeting of drug to the lungs is greatly improved. However, the fractionation of the dose between lungs, oropharynx and spacer is unique to each combination of spacer and drug formulation. Spacer devices may enable asthma to be controlled with a lower dose of drug than from a pMDI alone, resulting in a reduction in oropharyngeal side-effects from inhaled glucocorticosteroids, and a reduction in systemic drug delivery for a given therapeutic dose, with a consequent improvement in therapeutic ratio. Current British Thoracic Society guidelines recommend that all children and adults taking doses of beclomethasone dipropionate or budesonide ≥1000 µg per day, or fluticasone propionate ≥500 µg per day should take them through a large volume spacer device (British Asthma Guidelines Coordinating Committee, 1997).

Spacers have proved to be very versatile, as they can be fitted with a facemask to ensure satisfactory drug delivery in infants (Conner et al., 1989), and have proved to be viable lower cost alternatives to nebulizers for delivering high-dose bronchodilators to patients with severe acute asthma, and glucocorticosteroids to chronic asthmatics. They have also been used successfully as alternatives to nebulizers for delivering drugs to mechanically ventilated patients (Fuller et al., 1990). Spacers are easier to clean, more portable, less expensive and more convenient than nebulizers. While spacers may improve the efficacy of inhaled bronchodilators in patients with poor pMDI technique (Lee and Evans, 1987) it is likely that they will not confer any additional bronchodilatation in patients who can use pMDIs correctly, despite depositing a greater percentage of the drug dose in the lungs.

Correct and incorrect use of spacers

Although spacers often constitute a satisfactory solution for patients who have difficulty using pMDIs, it does not follow that the inhalation technique through the spacer is of no importance. *In vitro* studies on a number of devices have shown that the mass of drug contained within 'respirable' particles delivered from spacers is optimized by slow inhalation of single doses from the spacer (rather than firing multiple doses into the spacer and inhaling them all in a single breath) and minimizing the delay time between actuation of the dose into the spacer and starting to inhale (O'Callaghan *et al.*, 1993). In children, a series of tidal breaths, just sufficient to open the inhalation valve, were as effective as the manufacturers' recommended technique of slow, deep inhalation plus breath-holding for inhaling single doses from the Nebuhaler® device (Gleeson and Price, 1988).

Recent evidence has shown that plastic spacers are highly susceptible to the effects of static charge on their walls, which attract drug particles from the air to the walls of the spacer, causing them to deposit there and to be unavailable for inhalation (O'Callaghan *et al.*, 1993; Pierart *et al.*, 1999). New spacers taken straight out of their packaging may be highly charged, but washing a plastic spacer in soapy water, rinsing in clean water, and allowing the spacer to air-dry has a 'priming' effect that reduces static charge, and which consequently increases the dose that the patient receives. Previous use of spacers causes the walls of the spacer to become lined with a surfactant layer, and this also has a 'priming' function that reduces static charge effects. Metal spacers are not susceptible to static charge effects. In a recent scintigraphic study, we found that the amount of drug deposited in the lungs of asthmatic patients from Nebuhaler® and Volumatic® spacers was significantly enhanced if the spacer was primed by firing a number of placebo doses into the spacer to line the walls. In contrast, a metal spacer (Nebuchamber®), was equally efficient in terms of drug delivery to the lungs, whether or not it had been primed in advance (Kenyon *et al.*, 1998). The problems associated with static charge build-up on plastic spacers are complex, however, and remain incompletely understood at the present time.

DRY POWDER INHALERS (DPIs)

Single-dose DPIs

Following some early attempts to deliver antibiotic aerosols as dry powders in the 1940s, the first successful dry powder inhalers (DPIs) were developed almost 30 years ago. Initially these devices were single-dose units, containing the micronized drug mixed with larger glucose or lactose carrier particles in individual gelatine capsules to be loaded by the patient immediately before use. The best known single-dose powder inhalers are Rotahaler® (Glaxo–Wellcome), Spinhaler® (Rhône–Poulenc Rorer Aventis) and Cyclohaler/Aerolyser® (Pharmachemie/ Novartis). In Rotahaler®, the capsule is inserted into the end of the device and is broken into two halves by twisting the mouthpiece relative to the barrel. The powder falls into the body of the inhaler, and the patient has simply to inhale through the mouthpiece to disperse the powder and to deliver some of the micronized drug particles to the lungs. In Spinhaler®, the capsule is mounted in a rotor fitted with propeller blades, and is pierced by two needles. As the patient inhales, the rotor and capsule rotate, and powder is drawn out of the needle holes (Clark, 1995).

These DPIs have a marked advantage over pMDIs being breath-actuated; the patient's inhaled airstream is used to disperse drug powder and to draw a proportion of it into the lungs. During inhalation, the drug particles become separated from the surface of the carrier particles by shearing forces created in a turbulent airstream. In this way, co-ordination difficulties can be overcome, and single-dose DPIs were quickly recognized as satisfactory alternatives for patients unable to use a pMDI correctly. Further, they do not contain CFCs and hence problems with cold Freons are overcome and environmental objections are eliminated.

An obvious limitation of single-dose dry powder systems is the need to load a gelatine capsule prior to use, and this has led to the development of 'multiple unit-dose' DPIs, which contain a series of factory-metered doses, typically in blisters, and 'multidose' DPIs, in which individual doses are metered from a reservoir immediately prior to dosing. At the present time, relatively few of these devices have been marketed, but a bewildering array of possible novel multiple unit-dose and multidose DPIs has been described in the public domain (Table 14.3). Several of these have been reviewed in detail (Meeting Report, 1997).

Table 14.3 *Current dry powder inhalers, and some others under development which may be marketed in the future*

Device	Manufacturer	Notes
Single-dose DPIs (capsules, blisters)		
Spinhaler®	Rhône–Poulenc Rorer (Aventis)	C, P
Rotahaler®	Glaxo–Wellcome	C, P
FO2	Boehringer Ingelheim	C, P
Cyclohaler/Aerolyser®	Pharmachemie/Novartis	C, P
Turbospin	P, H and T	P
Omnihaler®	ML Labs (Innovata Biomed)	A, S
Innova	Inhale Therapeutics	A, S
Multiple unit-dose DPIs (capsules, blisters, cassette, cartridge etc.)		
Diskhaler®	Glaxo–Wellcome	C, P
Diskus (Accuhaler)™	Glaxo–Wellcome	C, P
Tape-based inhaler	3M Healthcare	A
Dynamic powder dispenser	Pfeiffer	A
Spiros™	Dura	A
Flowcaps	Hovione	P
Technohaler®	ML Labs (Innovata Biomed)	P
E-haler	Rhône–Poulenc Rorer (Aventis)	C, P
Multidose DPIs (metering from a powder reservoir)		
Turbuhaler®	Astra Zeneca	C, P
Easyhaler®	Orion	C, P
Taifun	Leiras	C, P
Clickhaler®	ML Labs (Innovata Biomed)	C, P
Pulvinal®	Chiesi	C, P
Ultrahaler®	Rhône–Poulenc Rorer (Aventis)	P, B
Jago inhaler	Skyepharma/Novartis	P
Prohaler	Valois	A
MAGhaler	Mundipharma/GGU	P, B
Cyclovent	Pharmachemie	P
AM-MDPI	Asta Medica	P
Miat-Haler	Miat SPA	P
Twisthaler™	Schering–Plough	P
Actif	Norton	P*

A, active powder dispersion; B, drug reservoir is a compacted powder block, not a free flowing powder; C, currently marketed (Spring 2000) in at least one country; P, passive powder dispersion (breath-actuation); P*, passive powder dispersion, but active powder metering; S, designed primarily for delivering drugs via the lungs to the systemic circulation.

Multiple unit-dose DPIs

The first multiple unit-dose DPI to be introduced was the Diskhaler® (Glaxo–Wellcome), consisting of small disks containing four or eight doses of drug, arranged in blisters around the periphery; this is sufficient drug for two days' therapy at conventional dosing levels. To use the inhaler, a flap is lifted through 90 degrees; this perforates a blister, and the drug substance falls into a small chamber adjacent to the mouthpiece, through which the patient immediately inhales.

This device has been largely superseded by the more practical Diskus™ (Glaxo–Wellcome), known as the Accuhaler™ in the UK, which contains 60 doses in sealed pockets on a strip, enough for one month's therapy (Prime et al., 1996). The device is primed by a slider which removes the cover to the next available pocket, and the patient inhales through the mouthpiece to disperse the powder. Each pocket contains sufficient powder to ensure that patients are able to sense the dose arriving at the back of the mouth. A dose counter tells the patient how many of the original 60 doses remain unused (Fig. 14.4a).

Two important benefits of multiple unit-dose systems are, first that the pockets may be precision filled in the factory to ensure a highly consistent dose throughout the lifetime of the

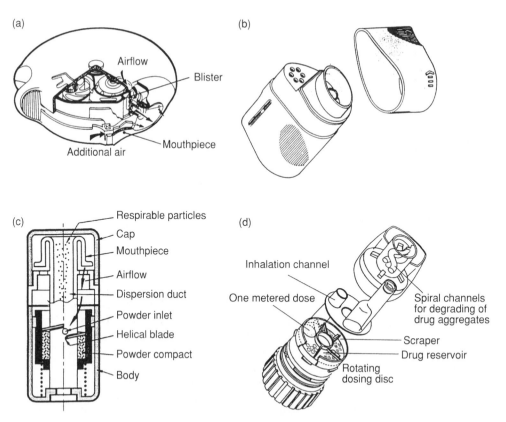

Figure 14.4   *Four dry powder inhalers: (a) Diskus™, (b) Taifun, (c) Ultrahaler, (d) Turbuhaler®. (From Prime et al., 1996, with permission; Pitcairn et al., 1995, with permission; Pitcairn et al., 1997, with permission; van Oort, 1995, reprinted with permission of Elsevier Science from In vitro testing of dry powder inhalers by M. van Oort, Aerosol Science and Technology, Vol 22, pp. 364–373, Copyright 1995 by the American Association for Aerosol Research.)*

device, and second that the contents of the pocket are totally protected from the effects of moisture in the environment up to the point of use by the patient.

Multidose DPIs

The first multidose DPI, in which individual doses are metered from a bulk powder reservoir, was the Turbuhaler® (Astra Zeneca) containing up to 200 doses of terbutaline sulphate or budesonide, and more recently formoterol and salbutamol (Wetterlin, 1988). The formulations for terbutaline sulphate and budesonide are unusual, as the powder consists entirely of drug, without additives of any kind. The drug substance, consisting of micronized drug particles that have been spheronized into loose agglomerates of approximate diameter 1 mm, occupies a storage reservoir immediately above the dosing disk, into which are set several series of small conical holes. When the base of the inhaler is twisted relative to the barrel, with the unit held vertically, a set of holes is filled with drug powder. When the patient inhales through the mouthpiece, some of the inhaled air passes through the dosing holes, carrying the drug powder. This is de-aggregated in the mouthpiece during passage through a pair of narrow spiral channels; de-aggregation takes place partly by turbulence and partly by a direct mechanical effect as the particles slide or roll against the walls of the channels. On the side of the inhaler there is an indicator which shows when no more than 20 doses remain. The inhaler contains a desiccant for some drugs, to protect the drug spheres against humidity, but the device must be stored with the mouthpiece cover securely in place. The Turbuhaler® has recently become the first multidose DPI to be launched in the USA (Fig. 14.4d).

Other multidose DPIs have used a range of mechanisms for metering drug from a reservoir, and for ensuring its dispersion in the patient's airstream. Several of these devices, including the Easyhaler® (Orion) and the Clickhaler® (ML Laboratories), resemble a pMDI in outward appearance. There have been concerns that the metering of powder in multidose DPIs may be too variable in some devices (Hindle and Byron, 1995), especially where it is required to meter very small powder volumes accurately. In an attempt to overcome this problem, the Ultrahaler® (Aventis Pharma) meters powder from a compacted block of drug and lactose using a helical blade to shave a dose precisely from the block (Fig. 14.4c). This results in a coefficient of variation (relative standard deviation) for a delivered dose of <10%. This device also contains a dose-ready window, through which patients can see the dose after it has been metered but before it has been inhaled, and a dose counter.

Drug delivery characteristics

The amount of drug contained within 'respirable' particles, and percentage of the drug dose reaching the lungs from DPIs varies markedly from device to device, and also according to both the characteristics of the powder formulation (Ganderton and Kassem, 1992) and the inhalation technique. Deposition of drug from DPIs has varied from 5% to more than 30% of the dose, but the efficiency of the system may depend as much upon the powder formulation as upon the device itself (Staniforth, 1995). Although early data suggested that the Turbuhaler® was similar to the pMDI in deposition efficiency, more recent studies (Thorsson et al., 1994, 1998) have shown that in comparative cross-over studies versus the pMDI, using optimal inhalation techniques for each device, the Turbuhaler® deposits twice as much drug in the lungs as the pMDI (typically 30% vs. 15% of the metered dose). As a consequence, a lower dose of asthma drug may be given in order to produce the required therapeutic effect (Bondesson et al., 1998). However, DPIs are not inevitably more efficient than pMDIs; for instance, data for the Diskhaler® suggests that it is approximately half as efficient as the corresponding pMDI at delivering drug to the lungs (Melchor et al., 1993).

A feature of breath-actuated DPIs is that yield of 'respirable' particles (<5 μm diameter) will generally be proportional to the airflow rate through the device. Consequently, efficient drug delivery from breath-actuated powder inhalers is likely to depend upon the patient's mode of inhalation, and in direct contrast to pMDIs, the key factor is rapid inhalation to de-aggregate drug/carrier complexes or large agglomerates of drug particles. In a study in asthmatic children, Pedersen (1986) found that rapid inhalation (71 to 130 L/min) and medium inhalation (60 to 80 L/min) through a Rotahaler® single-dose DPI gave better bronchodilator response than slow inhalation (36 to 50 L/min). The addition of breath holding and tilting the head did not augment the response produced by rapid or medium inhalation; hence it was possible to recommend a very simple inhalation method for this device. Fast inhalation through Spinhaler®-optimized lung deposition in a scintigraphic study (Newman *et al.*, 1994) and again, changes in breath-holding and in head-tilting made only minor contributions to the amount of drug reaching the lungs. In common with most other breath-actuated DPIs, lung deposition for the Turbuhaler® multidose DPI was optimized (mean 27%) with fast inhalation (60 L/min), compared with only 14% with slow inhalation (30 L/min) (Borgström *et al.*, 1994). For the Turbuhaler®, 60 L/min represents almost maximum effort for the patient owing to the relatively high resistance of this device to airflow.

It may appear paradoxical that most breath-actuated DPIs function optimally with fast inhalation. However, the increase in the probability of particle impaction in the oropharynx caused by fast inhalation is generally outweighed by the increased yield of finer particles that fast inhalation produces, and which ensure enhanced penetration of drug to the lungs. Not all breath-actuated DPIs are highly flow-rate dependent, however. Recent data have shown that the Taifun DPI (Leiras, Fig. 14.4b) deposits virtually the same amount of drug in the lungs with maximal and submaximal inspiratory effort (Pitcairn *et al.*, 2000).

Passive and active DPIs

All currently marketed DPIs are breath-actuated (or 'passive') devices, and clearly this is one of their major advantages. However, this is also a potential weakness, as patients usually have to inhale as hard as possible to disperse the powder with maximum efficiency. This may be a problem in asthmatic patients with acute wheeze or severe chronic breathing problems. Some novel DPIs use 'active' mechanisms other than the force of the patient's inhalation to disperse the powder (Table 14.3), including an internal source of compressed air (Dynamic Powder Dispenser, Pfeiffer) or a small battery-operated electric motor (Spiros®, Dura). In the Spiros device, the patient's inhalation triggers a battery-operated twin-blade impeller that blows the powder gently into the respiratory tract. The consequence of this mechanism is that fine particle dose measured *in vitro* and lung dose measured *in vivo* (Hill *et al.*, 1996) are virtually independent of inhalation flow rate, in marked contrast to the situation that generally applies with 'passive' systems. While none of these 'active' DPIs is currently marketed, their introduction will add an extra dimension to inhaler therapy.

NEBULIZERS

Roles for nebulizers

Although the nebulizer is the oldest genuine aerosol inhaler, it still retains its popularity and fulfils several important roles. Hand-held squeeze-bulb nebulizers originally introduced in the second half of the nineteenth century have been almost entirely superseded by 'jet' nebulizers powered by compressed air (generally from an electrically-operated compressor), or by ultrasonic nebulizers. Treatment by nebulizer is time-consuming, the equipment is bulky, relatively expensive and not always portable, and the contents can easily become contaminated. Nevertheless, nebulizers are useful for patients unable to use other devices successfully, and they may be the only type of inhaler suitable for infants. No specific inhalation technique is needed; the patient can simply inhale by relaxed tidal breathing. Nebulizers are a convenient way of delivering large doses of bronchodilators that may be required in the treatment of acute severe asthma or chronic severe asthma, although large-volume valved spacers may be an alternative, as discussed previously. Nebulizers have a great merit in terms of their flexibility, i.e. a spray can be made of virtually any drug substance and in virtually any dose, without the need for complex formulation work, and a nebulizer is likely to be the most practical way of delivering novel asthma therapies or drugs such as lignocaine and morphine in the setting of hospices. Suspensions of drug substances that are not water soluble, e.g. some corticosteroids, may be given successfully by nebulizer. A further advantage of nebulizers is that the droplet size can be adapted by appropriate selection and operation of nebulizers, thus offering the possibility to deliver droplets of a precisely known size that can be targeted to some specific site within the airways.

The use of nebulizers at home has become popular amongst patients, but the wisdom of this is sometimes challenged, and the increased use of home nebulizers has been termed an 'epidemic'. This reflects in part the inadequate instruction on the use of nebulizers that patients often receive, poor subsequent supervision of treatment, and misunderstanding by some patients of the limitations of nebulized bronchodilator therapy.

Jet nebulizers

Jet nebulizers (Fig. 14.5) function by the Bernoulli principle, by which compressed gas passing through a constriction (Venturi) undergoes a small reduction in pressure; this causes drug solution to be drawn up a feed tube from a reservoir and fragmented into droplets in the gas stream. These primary droplets may range in size up to 500 μm diameter, and hence are mostly far too large for inhalation. However, the largest primary droplets impact on 'baffles' within the nebulizer and are returned to the drug reservoir to be re-nebulized, and only the smallest droplets (ideally less than 5 μm diameter) are released from the mouthpiece. Consequently, the complete nebulization process takes several minutes. Many models of jet nebulizer are available

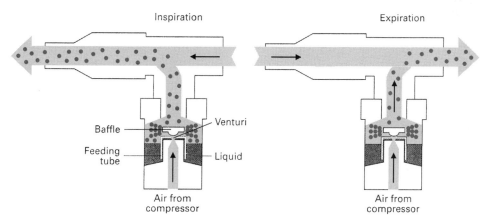

Figure 14.5 *A conventional jet nebulizer. (From O'Callaghan and Barry, 1997, with permission of BMJ Publishing Group.)*

with varying design features, including concentric liquid and gas feeds intended to minimize blockage by drug residue, or a flat liquid pick-up plate that enables the nebulizer to be tilted and to be used by patients in bed. Manual interrupters are sometimes used to synchronize aerosol generation with the patient's inspiration, hence avoiding the loss of aerosol that is generated during the exhalation phase of the breathing cycle. However, this results inevitably in increased nebulization times. Jet nebulizers can be used in conjunction with spacer devices (e.g. Miser, Medic-Aid) which 'store' aerosol generated during the exhalation phase of breathing, but such devices add significantly to the complexity and bulk of the system. Dosimetric nebulizers operate for a set period of time during inhalation, thus delivering a precisely known drug dose, and this facility is widely used in bronchial challenge testing.

There have been recent major advances in the design of jet nebulizers. The first of these was the introduction of 'open vent nebulizers' (e.g. Sidestream®, Medic-Aid), in which the negative pressure created at the Venturi is used to draw outside air into the nebulizer chamber through a vent in the top of the device, thus increasing the output of drug per unit time, and hence delivering the drug aerosol to the mouthpiece more quickly. 'Open vent' nebulizers can thus deliver a given amount of drug faster than conventional nebulizers, but are not necessarily more efficient since the losses during exhalation are the same as those in conventional devices.

A further advance in nebulizer design was the introduction of 'breath-assisted open-vent nebulizers' or 'active Venturi' nebulizers (e.g. Ventstream®, Medic-Aid; LC Plus, Pari®). During inspiration, a one-way inhalation valve situated on top of the device opens, allowing outside air to be drawn through the nebulizer as in the 'open-vent' devices (Fig. 14.6). However, during exhalation the valve closes, resulting in a greatly reduced generation of aerosol during the exhalation phase of breathing, so that aerosol lost from the nebulizer during exhalation is proportionately less than from a conventional device. The compressed airflows needed to operate 'breath-assisted open-vent' nebulizers are lower than those required by conventional nebulizer designs, so that compressors that are less powerful, lighter in weight and less expensive may be used. The principles by which these different designs of jet nebulizer function have recently been reviewed extensively (O'Callaghan and Barry, 1997).

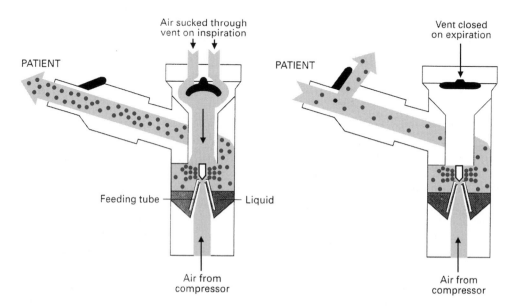

Figure 14.6 *A breath-assisted open-vent nebulizer, Pari LC Plus®. (From O'Callaghan and Barry, 1997, with permission of BMJ Publishing Group.)*

A very recent advance in jet nebulizer technology (Halo*Lite*®, Medic-Aid), which may signal a new trend in inhaler therapy, involves 'adaptive aerosol delivery', by which the patient's inhalation technique is continually monitored by a microprocessor chip. Aerosol is only released during the first part of the inhalation phase of the breathing cycle, and drug delivery is terminated when a precisely known amount of drug has been delivered. This approach permits much more controlled and reproducible aerosol delivery than that achieved by conventional jet nebulizers, co-ordinated with the patient's breathing pattern (Fig. 14.7). Potential benefits offered by this system include improved delivery efficiency, improved patient compliance and improved therapeutic response (Denyer, 1997).

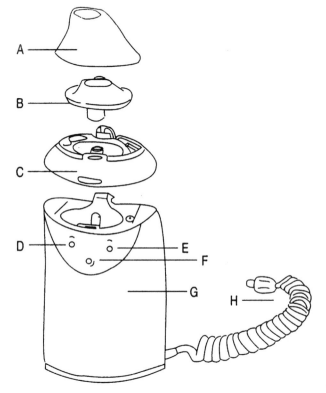

Figure 14.7 *HaloLite® adaptive aerosol delivery device (Medic-Aid Ltd). A, mouthpiece; B, baffle; C, medication chamber; D and E, selection buttons for drugs with differing doses; F, reset button; G, handpiece; H, air inlet tube. (From Denyer, 1997, with permission.)*

Ultrasonic nebulizers

Ultrasonic nebulizers function by principles quite different to those employed in jet nebulizers, the energy for spray formation being provided by a high frequency ultrasonic signal (usually in the 1 to 3 MHz range, but generally fixed for a given model) fed to a piezoelectric transducer (O'Callaghan and Barry, 1997). A fountain of droplets is then formed above a fluid reservoir, the largest of which again impact on baffles, to be returned to the fluid reservoir. The mean droplet size is inversely proportional to the two-thirds power of the acoustic frequency, and some models with frequencies rather less than 1 MHz may produce inappropriately large droplets (Sterk *et al.*, 1984). Some models vent aerosol continuously by means of a fan, while others only release aerosol in response to the patient's inhalation. In a further design of ultrasonic nebulizer, vibrations of a piezoelectric crystal are used to create peristalsis in the liquid feed tube, thus forcing the drug solution through an array of micron-sized holes at the mouthpiece (Omron U1, Omron Healthcare). Ultrasonic nebulizers are usually not powerful enough to nebulize suspensions of corticosteroid drugs successfully (Nikander, 1997), and may be unable to handle nebulizer formulations with unusually high viscosities or surface tensions. There is evidence that some drug molecules may be damaged by sonification in ultrasonic nebulizers.

Variations in output characteristics

While the use of a precise inhalation mode is important for a pMDI, but the choice of a specific brand of pMDI is much less so, the reverse tends to be the case for nebulizers. The patient and physician may choose from a wide range of commercially available nebulizer equipment which varies considerably in performance. The performance of currently available nebulizer systems has recently been reviewed (Clark, 1995; Smith *et al.*, 1995; Kendrick *et al.*, 1997). For instance, the droplet mass median diameter of the aerosol from jet nebulizers may vary from <3 μm to >10 μm, according to type of nebulizer and compressor used. A powerful compressor will produce a flow rate through a nebulizer of >10 L/min, while a weaker compressor may give a flow rate of <4 L/min; droplet size and nebulization time are both inversely proportional to compressed gas flow rate. Hence there is a need to match nebulizer and compressor in order to ensure optimal output characteristics (Clark, 1995). Jet nebulizers tend to have a smaller droplet size and a lower output rate than ultrasonic models (Sterk *et al.*, 1984), but this is not an invariable rule. Unfortunately, manufacturers' information on the output characteristics of nebulizers and on the flows and pressures generated by compressors is still sometimes scanty and inaccurate. British and European standards for nebulizer performance and testing have recently been proposed (Dennis, 1998). Guidance on appropriate selection of nebulizer equipment has recently been published. It is desirable that specific nebulizer/compressor combinations should be recommended for use with specific drug substances (Kendrick *et al.*, 1997).

An ideal nebulizer should have a high drug output, a short nebulization time to improve patient compliance, and a small droplet size for maximum delivery to the lungs (Fig. 14.8), although these requirements are to some degree mutually exclusive (Nikander, 1997). For any drug substance, a small (2 mL) volume fill will minimize nebulization time, while a larger (4 mL) fill will increase drug output, even if the additional 2 mL is comprised of diluent only; a compromise has thus to be reached regarding volume fill. Simple practical measures such as

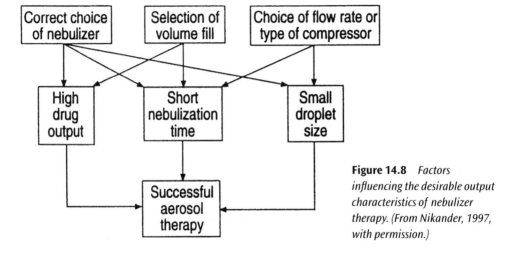

Figure 14.8 *Factors influencing the desirable output characteristics of nebulizer therapy. (From Nikander, 1997, with permission.)*

gently tapping the nebulizer to encourage recycling of droplets impacted on baffles can help to reduce the residual volume of drug retained in the nebulizer and to increase drug output.

The wide variations in performance that arise according to the type of nebulizer and its operating conditions are reflected in the results of radio-aerosol deposition studies. Deposition in the lungs may be optimized by nebulizer systems with a high yield of droplets smaller than 5 μm diameter (Johnson *et al.*, 1989). The percentage of the dose deposited in the lungs from a nebulizer may exceed 15% for some models, but may be less than 2% for others (Hardy *et al.*, 1993). The majority of the dose is retained within the nebulizer and tubing, and the drug becomes more concentrated in the nebulizer reservoir because of preferential evaporation of diluent. Oropharyngeal deposition may be high for nebulizers releasing few droplets smaller than 5 μm diameter. Current Guidelines from the British Thoracic Society recommend that nebulization times should be restricted to <10 minutes wherever possible, and that nebulizer systems should deliver at least 50% of the drug dose within 'respirable' droplets less than 5 μm diameter when operated optimally (Muers and Corris, 1997).

Inhalation modes from nebulizers

As discussed earlier, a major merit of nebulizers is that patients can inhale by relaxed tidal breathing, without recourse to any specific inhalation technique. Either a mouthpiece or facemask can be used, although significantly higher losses of aerosol in the upper airways are to be expected with the facemask. The use of a facemask provides effective delivery of nebulized aerosols to children and infants, but care must be taken to avoid the leakage of drug aerosol around the edges of the facemask.

Changes in total deposition in the lungs and in penetration of aerosol to the lung periphery can result from changes in the depth and speed of breathing, but these changes in inhalation technique do not seem to be very important to nebulizer therapy in clinical practice. Zainuddin *et al.* (1988) were unable to show increases in either lung deposition or in bronchodilator response by the additions of deep breathing, or of deep breathing plus breath-holding, to tidal breathing. There is often a tendency for deep breaths to be inhaled relatively rapidly, and since deep breathing and rapid breathing have opposite effects on aerosol deposition patterns, the overall affect of deep breathing manoeuvres may be small. Neither the addition of intermittent positive pressure breathing nor oral high frequency oscillation have been shown to clearly improve aerosol delivery to the lungs from nebulizers, and generally it seems difficult to improve on the effects obtained with nebulizers using relaxed tidal breathing.

Nebulized aerosol received by adult patients is generally inhaled in a mixture of air from two sources, i.e. air from the compressor or other compressed air source that has been used to generate the aerosol, and diluting air from the environment. In children with smaller tidal volumes, the contribution of diluting air will be reduced, and hence the child will receive a more concentrated aerosol cloud. In infants, the minute volume may be less than the nebulizer output rate, and hence the infant may not be able to inhale the entire delivered dose. However, the complex interactions associated with these so-called 'entrainment' phenomena remain incompletely understood (Collis *et al.*, 1990).

Clinical performance

While there are clear differences between nebulizer systems in terms of laboratory performance *in vitro* and aerosol deposition pattern, it has proved more difficult to demonstrate differences between nebulizers in terms of clinical response in asthmatic patients to a standard dose of bronchodilator. This probably reflects the large doses of bronchodilator that are conventionally and safely given by nebulizer, so that even a relatively inefficient nebulizer can deliver sufficient drug to the lungs for maximal clinical effect. For bronchodilator therapy, using conventional large doses of >1 mg, the choice of nebulizer is probably not of major clinical importance. For drugs other than bronchodilators, careful choice of nebulizer system may be more important; for instance, a haphazard choice of nebulizer for delivering suspensions of topical corticosteroids would be unwise, because a nebulizer that deposited most of the aerosol in the oropharynx might increase the incidence of local and systemic side-effects, but result in little clinical efficacy. For topical corticosteroids and for other substances such as antibiotic aerosols for treatment of respiratory tract infections, a nebulizer with a small droplet size (mass median diameter <5 μm) would be ideal, coupled to a powerful high-flow compressor for reduction of droplet size and nebulization time, although a powerful compressor has potential practical disadvantages in terms of increased weight, size, noise level and running costs.

SOFT MIST INHALERS

A major challenge in inhaler technology is currently to develop multiple unit-dose or multidose devices that do not use environmentally damaging propellants. The two categories of device so far considered in this chapter have been pMDIs formulated with HFA propellants, perhaps used in conjunction with spacer devices, and DPIs. However there is a third alternative: within the last few years, a new category of inhaler devices has been developed, and while none is currently marketed, it seems likely that they will eventually offer a viable alternative to pMDIs and to DPIs as portable devices for delivery of asthma medications. These are devices which deliver liquid sprays, but which are designed as compact multidose devices, operating either by forcing liquid through a narrow nozzle under pressure or by ultrasonic or electrohydrodynamic principles. Considering these devices release a much more slowly moving spray of droplets than that from pMDIs, and yet are not nebulizers in the conventional sense, the generic term 'soft mist inhalers (SMIs)' has been coined to describe them. A number of such devices have been described, and these are listed in Table 14.4.

Table 14.4 *Soft mist inhalers (multiple unit-dose or multidose spray systems)*

Device	Manufacturer	Operating principle
Respimat®	Boehringer	Energy stored in coiled spring forces liquid through nozzle
AERx™	Aradigm	Piston forces liquid through nozzle
Micro-spray pump	Pfeiffer	Internal compressed air supply aerosolizes liquid
Metered solution inhaler	Sheffield Pharmaceuticals	Ultrasonic nebulization
Piezoelectric inhaler	3M Healthcare	Ultrasonic pressure waves force liquid through nozzle
AeroDose™	Aerogen	Ultrasonics (vibrating orifice aerosol generator)
Piezoelectric actuator (PEA)	Bespak	Ultrasonics (vibrating orifice aerosol generator)
Touchmist	Technology Partnership	Ultrasonics (vibrating orifice aerosol generator)
Babtelle atomizer	Babtelle Pulmonary Therapeutics	Electrohydrodynamics

Respimat®

Arguably the best documented SMI at the present time is the Respimat® (Boehringer Ingelheim, Fig. 14.9). Formerly known as the BINEB®, this is a compact propellant-free device delivering up to 200 metered doses of drug solution formulated either in water or in ethanol (Zierenberg *et al.*, 1996). The device comprises a drug storage reservoir, surrounded by a helical spring. The energy needed to aerosolize the solution is stored in the coiled spring, when the lower part of the device is rotated. Simultaneously, the dosing chamber fills with a highly reproducible metered dose of drug, and when the energy stored in the coiled spring is released by pressing a button on the side of the device, the metered dose of drug is discharged through a sophisticated nozzle system. The nozzle includes two narrow channels (diameter 8 μm) set at an angle to one-another, such that they provide two jets of droplets that impact upon one-another just outside the device. This produces a dispersion of very fine droplets (mass median diameters <5 μm for aqueous-based formulations, and <3 μm for ethanol-based formulations). A filter system in the nozzle prevents clogging by drug residue. The velocity of the generated spray is only a fraction of that from a pMDI, and the time needed to generate the spray is about one second. It is considered that the lower spray velocity should better enable the patient to co-ordinate firing the spray with their inhalation.

Several recent scintigraphic studies have shown that the Respimat® delivers a significantly higher percentage of the drug dose into the lungs compared with a pMDI (Newman *et al.*, 1998), with a corresponding reduction in oropharyngeal deposition. In a three-way cross-over study in 10 healthy volunteers carried out to compare the deposition of 250 μg flunisolide from different inhaler devices (Newman *et al.*, 1996), a prototype Respimat® deposited a mean 39.7% of the dose in the lungs, compared with 15.3% for a pMDI, and 28.0% for a pMDI coupled to a cone-shaped spacer device. Oropharyngeal deposition was only 39.9% of the dose for the Respimat® compared with 66.9% for the pMDI, and 27.3% for the pMDI plus spacer. It was concluded that the Respimat® deposits an unusually high percentage of the dose in the lungs, and 'targets' the drug to the required site more effectively than a pMDI. The drug delivery characteristics broadly resemble those of a spacer device, and yet the Respimat® is much more compact and portable. The improved drug delivery to the target site with the

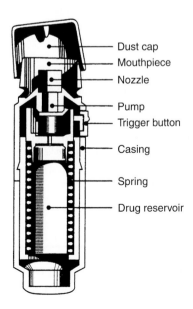

Dust cap
Mouthpiece
Nozzle

Pump
Trigger button

Casing

Spring

Drug reservoir

Figure 14.9   *Respimat® soft mist inhaler. (Fig. 4, 'Set-up of the BINEB®', from Zierenberg, Eicher, Dunne and Freund, 'Boehringer Ingelheim nebulizer BINEB®: a New Approach to Inhalation Therapy' In: Respiratory drug delivery V, edited by R.N. Dalby, P.R. Byron and S.J. Farr. Copyright 1996 by Interpharm Press, Inc. All rights reserved. Reprinted with permission.)*

Respimat offers the possibility that patients can be treated with a lower daily dose of inhaled corticosteroids, while maintaining the effectiveness of their therapy.

AERx™

The AERx™ device (Aradigm) is another SMI, but differs from the Respimat® in that doses are stored individually in blister packs rather than in a drug solution reservoir (Farr *et al.*, 1996). The doses are mounted on a strip which is wound through the device (rather like the individual doses in the Glaxo–Wellcome Diskus DPI), and hence the AERx™ can be considered a multiple unit-dose device. The use of individual dosing units permits very accurate filling of dosing units to be achieved under factory conditions, and overcomes potential sterility problems associated with multidose fluid reservoirs. Each dosing unit is connected to a single use nozzle comprising an array of precision drilled holes. The droplet size can be adjusted by altering the hole size in order to target drug to different parts of the lungs. The patient's inhalation technique is monitored by a microprocessor system within the device, and the inhaler is actuated when a pre-programmed combination of inhaled volume and inhaled flow rate is achieved. At this point, a piston system forces the individual drug doses out of the blister through the hole array. A scintigraphic study in healthy volunteers showed that a mean of 53.3% of the drug dose was deposited in the lungs, with remarkably little variability between individuals (coefficient of variation only 10.9%). The AERx™ device thus offers the possibility of delivering drugs very efficiently and very reproducibly to the lungs. The microprocessor technology also permits a 'lock and key' system, restricting users and preventing overuse.

Other soft mist inhalers

The performance of several other SMIs has been reviewed (Wolff and Niven, 1994). The Pfeiffer Micro-Pump Spray (Jäger-Waldau, 1994) uses compressed ambient air to force a metered dose of drug through a nozzle which includes a mixing chamber partly filled with polyurethane sponge. A mixture of compressed air and drug solution passing through the sponge pores causes the drug solution to be atomized. Since the device is operated by compressed air, the initial droplet velocity is high, and the device is less efficient at delivering drug to the lungs compared with Respimat® or AERx™, with only 8% of the dose reaching the lungs on average, although this could be increased to 13% when the device was used in conjunction with a spacer.

Several novel multidose SMIs operate on ultrasonic principles. In an earlier version of the Respimat® device, a metered dose of drug solution was allowed to fall on a piezoelectric crystal, and was nebulized within one second. This principle forms the basis of the Metered Solution Inhaler (Sheffield Pharmaceuticals, Inc.). Other prototype SMIs operating via ultrasonic technologies include the Breath-Actuated Piezoelectric Inhaler (3M Healthcare) in which ultrasonic pressure cycles are used to force drug solution through an array of micron-sized holes, the Piezoelectric Actuator (PEA, Bespak), and the AeroDose™ (Aerogen) in which the nozzle array itself is vibrated by an ultrasonic signal (De Young *et al.*, 1998). An SMI based upon electrohydrodynamic technologies was recently described (Zimlich *et al.*, 2000).

CONCLUDING REMARKS

It is currently an exciting time in the field of inhaler technology. The conventional pMDI continues to be popular, but it has well-recognized limitations. A new generation of asthma inhalers is emerging; these begin to make conventional pMDIs look rather haphazard, and spacers bulky and cumbersome. Further, it must be remembered that the pMDI is essentially a 1950s technology, and that the poor drug deposition characteristics of the CFC-based pMDI can now be improved upon dramatically by novel technologies. The improvements in drug deposition produced by some new inhalers are generally reflected in improved clinical performance or equivalent performance at a lower dose (Selroos *et al.*, 1996; Pauwels *et al.*, 1997). There are increasing trends towards improved targeting of drug to the required site (Howarth, 1997), which many new inhalers are able to achieve.

Given that new inhalers such as breath-actuated pMDIs and DPIs are as effective as the pMDI and are easier to use, there must be a strong argument for their use in preference to the pMDI unless inhalation technique is routinely checked. Unfortunately, many new devices are relatively expensive, but this may change as they gain wider acceptance. Spacers will continue to be used, although perhaps more as alternatives to nebulizers than as co-ordination aids. However, the cheapness of spacers should not be overlooked; once the spacer has been obtained, therapy via pMDI plus spacer is no more expensive than via pMDI alone. Lastly, there is likely to be a continuing need for nebulizers, not only for bronchodilator therapy, but also increasingly for a wide range of other aerosolized drugs. As the droplet size can be modified by choice of appropriate equipment, nebulizers have a potential role for targeting drug aerosol to specific lung regions.

The desirable objectives of new inhaler devices, in terms of both pharmaceutical and practical requirements, are listed in Table 14.5. It is unlikely that there will ever be an 'ideal' inhaler device, and certainly all current devices have both advantages and disadvantages. Pedersen (1996) has listed the key questions to consider when prescribing an inhaler as follows: (i) Which inhaler is the simplest and easiest to use optimally? (ii) Which inhaler most reproducibly delivers the highest percentage of the dose to the lungs? (iii) Which inhaler has the highest therapeutic ratio (best clinical effect for given systemic effect)? (iv) Which inhaler is preferred by patients? Hence, the development of a range of device categories (pMDIs, DPIs, SMIs and nebulizers) is valuable, helping to meet the requirements of various clinical situations and differing patient preferences.

Table 14.5 *Desirable objectives of new inhalers*

Pharmaceutical requirements
Similar or better performance compared with CFC-powered pMDI
Low variability in delivered and fine particle doses
Widely applicable to different drugs and dosages
Not affected by moisture or by static charge

Practical requirements
Multiple dose capability
Compact and lightweight
Easy to use correctly
High patient acceptability
'Dose sensing' capability (patient knows dose has been received)
Dose counter (patient knows when device is empty)
Mechanism to prevent overdosing
Robust
Cost-effective
Refillable

REFERENCES

Barnes PJ, Pedersen S, Busse WW. (1998) Efficacy and safety of inhaled corticosteroids: new developments. *Am J Respir Crit Care Med*, **157**, S1–S53.

Bondesson E, Friberg K, Soliman S, Löfdahl C-G. (1998) Safety and efficacy of a high cumulative dose of salbutamol inhaled via Turbuhaler® or via a pressurised metered dose inhaler in patients with asthma. *Respir Med*, **92**, 325–30.

Borgström L, Bondesson E, Morén F, Trofast E, Newman SP. (1994) Lung deposition of budesonide inhaled via Turbuhaler: a comparison with terbutaline sulphate in normal subjects. *Eur Respir J*, **7**, 69–73.

British Asthma Guidelines Coordinating Committee. (1997) British Guidelines on asthma management: 1995 review and position statement. *Thorax*, **52**, S1–S24.

Busse WW, Brazinsky S, Jacobson K, *et al.* (1999) Efficacy response of inhaled beclomethasone dipropionate in asthma is proportional to dose and is improved by formulation with a new propellant. *J Allergy Clin Immunol*, **104**, 1215–22.

Clark AR. (1995) Medical aerosol inhalers: past, present and future. *Aerosol Sci Tech*, **22**, 374–91.

Clark AR. (1996) MDIs: physics of aerosol formation. *J Aerosol Med*, **9** (Suppl. 1), S19–S26.

Collis GG, Cole CH, Le Souef PN. (1990) Dilution of nebulised aerosols by air entrainment in children. *Lancet*, **336**, 341–3.

Conner WT, Dolovich MB, Frame RA, Newhouse MT. (1989) Reliable salbutamol administration in 6- to 36-month-old children by means of a metered dose inhaler and Aerochamber® with mask. *Pediatr Pulmonol*, **6**, 263–7.

Crompton GK. (1982) Problems patients have using pressurised aerosol inhalers. *Eur J Respir Dis*, **63** (Suppl. 119), 57–65.

Dennis JH. (1998) A review of issues relating to nebuliser standards. *J Aerosol Med*, **11** (Supplement 1), S73–S79.

Denyer J. (1997) Adaptive aerosol delivery in practice. *Eur Respir Rev*, **7**, 388–9.

De Young L, Chambers F, Narayan S, Wu C. (1998) The AeroDose® multidose inhaler device: design and delivery characteristics. In: Dalby RN, Byron PR, Farr SJ, eds. *Respiratory drug delivery VI*. Buffalo Grove: Interpharm Press, 91–5.

Dolovich MB, Ruffin RE, Roberts R, Newhouse MT. (1981) Optimal delivery of aerosols from metered dose inhalers. *Chest*, **80** (Suppl.), 911–5.

Farr SJ, Rowe AM, Rubsamen R, Taylor G. (1995) Aerosol deposition in the human lung following administration from a microprocesor controlled metered dose inhaler. *Thorax*, **60**, 639–44.

Farr SJ, Schuster JA, Lloyd P, Lloyd LJ, Okikawa JK, Rubsamen RM. (1996) AERx™ development of a novel liquid aerosol delivery system: concept to clinic. In: Dalby RN, Byron PR, Farr SJ, eds. *Respiratory drug delivery V*. Buffalo Grove: Interpharm Press, 175–85.

Fuller HD, Dolovich MB, Posmituck G, Wong Pak W, Newhouse MT. (1990) Pressurized aerosol versus jet aerosol delivery to mechanically ventilated patients: comparison of dose to the lungs. *Am Rev Respir Dis*, **141**, 440–4.

Ganderton DJ, Kassem NM. (1992) Dry powder inhalers. In: Ganderton DJ, Jones T, eds. *Advances in Pharmaceutical Sciences*. London: Academic Press, 165–91.

Gleeson JGA, Price JF. (1988) Nebuhaler technique. *Br J Dis Chest*, **82**, 172–4.

Hardy JG, Newman SP, Knoch M. (1993) Lung deposition from four nebulisers. *Respir Med*, **87**, 461–5.

Hill M, Vaughan L, Dolovich M. (1996) Dose targeting for dry powder inhalers. In: Dalby RN, Byron PR, Farr SJ, eds. *Respiratory Drug Delivery V*. Buffalo Grove: Interpharm Press, 197–208.

Hindle M, Byron PR. (1995) Dose emissions from marketed dry powder inhalers. *Int J Pharm*, **116**, 169–77.

Howarth PH. (1997) What is the nature of asthma and where are the therapeutic targets? *Respir Med*, **91** (Suppl. A), 2–8.

Jäger-Waldau R. (1994) Feasibility of drug delivery to the respiratory tract by a mechanical micro spray pump. *J Aerosol Med, 7*, 147–54.

Johnson MA, Newman SP, Bloom RA, Talaee N, Clarke SW. (1989) Delivery of albuterol and ipratropium bromide from two nebulizer systems in chronic stable asthma. *Chest*, **96**, 1–10.

Kendrick AH, Smith EC, Wilson RSE. (1997) Selecting and using nebuliser equipment. *Thorax*, **52** (Suppl. 2), S92–S101.

Kenyon CJ, Thorsson L, Borgström L, Newman SP. (1998) The effects of static charge in spacer devices on glucocorticosteroid aerosol deposition in asthmatic patients. *Eur Respir J*, **11**, 606–10.

Leach CL, Davidson PJ, Boudreau RJ. (1998) Improved airway targeting with the CFC-free HFA-beclomethasone metered-dose inhaler compared with CFC-beclomethasone. *Eur Respir J*, **12**, 1346–53.

Lee H, Evans HE. (1987) Evaluation of inhalation aids of metered dose inhalers in asthmatic children. *Chest*, **91**, 366–9.

McDonald KJ, Martin GP. (2000) Transition to CFC-free metered dose inhalers: into the new millenium. *Int J Pharm*, **211**, 89–107.

Meeting Report (1997) Multi-dose dry-powder inhaler design: a game for many players. *Pharm J*, **259**, 134–5.

Melchor R, Biddiscombe MF, Mak VHF, Short MD, Spiro SG. (1993) Lung deposition patterns of directly labelled salbutamol in normal subjects and in patients with reversible airways obstruction. *Thorax*, **48**, 506–11.

Muers MF, Corris PA. (1997) Current best practice for nebuliser treatment. *Thorax*, **52** (Suppl. 2), S1–S17.

Newman SP. (1993) Scintigraphic assessment of therapeutic aerosols. *Crit Rev Ther Drug Carrier Syst*, **10**, 65–109.

Newman SP. (1997) New aerosol delivery systems. In: Barnes PJ, Grunstein MH, Leff AR, Woolcock AJ, eds. *Asthma*. Philadelphia: Lippincott-Raven, 1805–15.

Newman SP. (1998) Scintigraphic assessment of pulmonary delivery systems. *Pharm Tech*, **22** (June), 78–94.

Newman SP, Brown J, Steed KP, Reader SJ, Kladders H. (1998) Lung deposition of fenoterol and flunisolide delivered using a novel device for inhaled medications. *Chest*, **113**, 957–63.

Newman SP, Clarke SW. (1992) Inhalation devices and techniques. In: Clark TJH, Godfrey S, Lee TH, eds. *Asthma*, 3rd edn, London: Chapman & Hall Medical, 469–505.

Newman SP, Hirst PH, Bacon RE, *et al.* (2000) Pulmonary delivery of ergotamine tartrate using a new breath-actuated pressurized aerosol device, the Aerosol Drug Delivery System. In: Dalby RN, Byron PR, Farr SJ, Peart J, eds. *Respiratory Drug Delivery VII*. Raleigh: Serentec Press, 471–3.

Newman SP, Hollingworth A, Clark AR. (1994) Effect of different modes of inhalation on drug delivery from a dry powder inhaler. *Int J Pharm*, **102**, 127–32.

Newman SP, Newhouse MT. (1996) Effect of add-on devices for aerosol drug delivery: deposition studies and clinical aspects. *J Aerosol Med*, **9**, 55–70.

Newman SP, Pavia D, Clarke SW. (1981) How should a pressurised beta-adrenergic bronchodilator be inhaled? *Eur J Respir Dis*, **62**, 3–20.

Newman SP, Pavia D, Garland N, Clarke SW. (1982) Effects of various inhalation modes on the deposition of radioactive pressurised aerosols. *Eur J Respir Dis*, **63** (Suppl. 119), 57–65.

Newman SP, Steed KP, Reader SJ, Hooper G, Zierenberg B. (1996) Efficient delivery to the lungs of flunisolide aerosol from a new portable hand-held multidose nebulizer. *J Pharm Sci*, **85**, 960–4.

Newman SP, Steed KP, Hooper G, Jones JI, Upchurch FC. (1999) Improved targeting of beclomethasone dipropionate (250 µg metered dose inhaler) to the lungs of asthmatics with the Spacehaler®. *Respir Med*, **93**, 424–31.

Newman SP, Weisz AWB, Talaee N, Clarke SW. (1991) Improvement of drug delivery with a breath actuated pressurised aerosol for patients with poor inhaler technique. *Thorax*, **46**, 712–6.

Nikander K. (1997) Some technical, physicochemical and physiological aspects of nebulization of drugs. *Eur Respir Rev, 7*, 168–72.

O'Callaghan C, Barry PW. (1997) The science of nebulised drug delivery. *Thorax*, **52** (Suppl. 2), S31–S44.

O'Callaghan C, Lynch J, Cant M, Robertson C. (1993) Improvement in sodium cromoglycate delivery from a spacer device by use of an antistatic lining, immediate inhalation and avoiding multiple actuations of drug. *Thorax*, **48**, 603–6.

Partridge MR, Woodcock AA, Sheffer AL, Wanner A, Rubinfeld A. (1998) Chlorofluorocarbon-free inhalers: are we ready for the change? *Eur Respir J*, **11**, 1006–8.

Pauwels R, Newman SP, Borgström L. (1997) Airway deposition and airway effects of antiasthma drugs delivered from metered dose inhalers. *Eur Respir J*, **10**, 2127–38.

Pedersen S. (1986) How to use a Rotahaler®. *Arch Dis Child*, **61**, 11–4.

Pedersen S. (1996) Inhalers and nebulizers: which to choose and why? *Respir Med*, **90**, 69–77.

Pierart F, Wildhaber JH, Vrancken I, Devadason SG, Le Souef PN. (1999) Washing plastic spacers in household detergent reduces electrostatic charge and greatly improves delivery. *Eur Respir J*, **13**, 673–8.

Pitcairn GR, Lankinen T, Valkila E, Newman SP. (1995) Lung deposition of salbutamol from Leiras metered dose powder inhaler. *J Aerosol Med*, **8**, 307–11.

Pitcairn GR, Lim J, Hollingworth A, Newman SP. (1997) Scintigraphic assessment of drug delivery from the Ultrahaler® dry powder inhaler. *J Aerosol Med*, **10**, 295–306.

Pitcairn GR, Lankinen T, Seppala O-P, Newman SP. (2000) Pulmonary drug delivery from the Taifun dry powder inhaler is relatively independent of the patient's inspiratory effort. *J Aerosol Med*, (in press).

Prime D, Slater AL, Haywood PA, Smith IJ. (1996) Assessing dose delivery from the flixotide Diskus™ inhaler – a multi-dose powder inhaler. *Pharm Tech Eur,* **March**, 23–36.

Selroos O, Pietinalho A, Riska H. (1996) Delivery devices for inhaled asthma medication. *Clin Immunother*, **6**, 273–99.

Smith EC, Denyer J, Kendrick AH. (1995) Comparison of twenty three nebulizer/compressor combinations for domiciliary use. *Eur Respir J*, **8**, 1214–21.

Staniforth JN. (1995) Performance-modifying influences in dry powder inhalation systems. *Aerosol Sci Tech,* **22**, 346–53.

Sterk PJ, Plomp A, van der Vate JF, Quanjer PH. (1984) Physical properties of aerosols produced by several jet and ultrasonic nebulisers. *Bull Eur Physiopathol Respir,* **20**, 65–72.

Thompson PJ, Davies RJ, Young WF, Grossman AB, Donnell D. (1998) Safety of hydroalkane-134a beclomethasone dipropionate extrafine aerosol. *Respir Med*, **92** (Suppl. A), 33–9.

Thorsson L, Edsbäcker S, Conradson T-B. (1994) Lung deposition of budesonide from Turbuhaler is twice that from a pressurised metered dose inhaler p-MDI. *Eur Respir J*, **7**, 1839–44.

Thorsson L, Kenyon CJ, Newman SP, Borgström L. (1998) Lung deposition of budesonide in asthmatics: a comparison of different formulations. *Int J Pharm*, **168**, 119–27.

van Oort M. (1995) In vitro testing of dry powder inhalers. *Aerosol Sci Tech,* **22**, 364–73.

Weers JG, Tarara TE, Gill H, English BS, Dellamary LA. (2000) Homodispersion technology for HFA suspensions: particle engineering to reduce dosing variance. In: Dalby RN, Byron PR, Farr SJ, Peart J, eds. *Respiratory Drug Delivery VII*. Raleigh: Serentec Press, 91–7.

Wetterlin K. (1988) Turbuhaler®: a new powder inhaler for administration of drugs to the airways. *Pharm Res,* **5**, 506–8.

Wolff RK, Niven RW. (1994) Generation of aerosolized drugs. *J Aerosol Med*, **7**, 89–106.

Zainuddin BMZ, Tolfree SEJ, Short M, Spiro SG. (1988) Influence of breathing pattern on lung deposition and bronchodilator response to nebulised salbutamol in patients with stable asthma. *Thorax*, **43**, 987–91.

Zierenberg B, Eicher J, Dunne S, Freund B. (1996) Boehringer Ingelheim nebulizer BINEB®. A new approach to inhalation therapy. In: Dalby RN, Byron PR, Farr SJ, eds. *Respiratory drug delivery V*. Buffalo Grove: Interpharm Press, 187–93.

Zimlich WC, Ding JY, Busick DR, *et al.* (2000) The development of a novel electrohydrodynamic pulmonary drug delivery device. In: Dalby RN, Byron PR, Farr SJ, Peart J, eds. *Respiratory Drug Delivery VII*. Raleigh: Serentec Press, 241–6.

15

Management of asthma in adults

ANN J. WOOLCOCK

INTRODUCTION

This chapter discusses the management of chronic asthma in adults, with reference to the management of acute attacks where appropriate. The poor understanding of the natural history of asthma together with the lack of data from long-term controlled trials of different forms of treatment, means that there are no universally accepted methods of management. This has led to a variety of treatment practices, and patients often receive confusing information from doctors, nurses, pharmacists and asthma educators. Conflicting information about drugs and their side-effects exists in the literature. Furthermore, drugs that are widely used in one country appear to be not prescribed as often as in another (Kurosawa, 1994). To try to address this confusion, national asthma management plans were written in several countries (Woolcock et al., 1989; British Thoracic Society, 1990; Hargreave et al., 1990; US Department of Health and Human Services, 1991). These were followed by international and global plans (US Department of Health and Human Services, 1991; National Institutes of Health, 1995; Ait-Khaled and Enarson, 1996). The purpose of these plans is to provide a basis for a unified approach to management and, eventually, to allow self-management by the patient. Studies of the use of management plans suggest that not all components are well understood by physicians and compliance with the guidelines is low (Legoretta et al., 1998; Doerschug et al., 1999). Their effectiveness in improving the long-term outcome has still to be assessed.

In the absence of long-term data about outcomes, management plans have been written as 'consensus' documents. Most of them are extremely detailed and not easily used by busy doctors. The answers to specific questions frequently asked by doctors, such as when to use which drug, the appropriate doses and criteria for altering the doses, are only partially addressed. Furthermore, in the management plans the term 'asthma' is used to mean both the disease and the episodes of airway narrowing that causes symptoms, and this leads to confusion.

An approach to management is shown in a three-point management plan (Table 15.1). It is based on the National Asthma Campaign (1998) in Australia, and stresses reducing the

Table 15.1   *Three-part asthma management plan*

1. Assessment
    A. Severity
    B. Best achievable lung function
2. Intervention
    A. Drugs
    B. Avoidance of triggers/aggravators
    C. Lifestyle changes
3. Commitment
    A. Written 'action plan' for exacerbations
    B. Education of the patient and family
    C. Regular review

severity of the disease using both pharmacological and non-pharmacological measures. The emphasis is on the management of patients with severe, persistent asthma, but the principals are the same for all patients. Factors that trigger and aggravate the disease and are potentially able to be controlled are described. Commonly used drugs are described as first line of treatment while drugs with more specific applications are described as second line. Management of acute attacks is not described in detail. The management of patients with a poor response to conventional treatment is described separately and likely changes in treatment that will occur in coming years are discussed at the end of the chapter.

CLASSIFICATION OF ASTHMA

When a patient presents with symptoms of asthma the question is: 'Is it asthma?' If yes, then treatment with short-acting β-agonists (SABAs) plus or minus steroids is indicated. After recovery – hours, days or even weeks, when the acute symptoms are controlled, the important question to ask is: 'Is the airway function abnormal?' (*see* Fig. 15.1). There are three ways of doing this. First, spirometric function before and after a SABA; improvement of 15% in the forced expiratory volume in one second (FEV_1) is not only diagnostic of asthma but indicates abnormal airway function at that time. Second, if spirometric function is normal, a bronchial challenge test with a bronchoconstricting agent (methacholine or histamine) can be given. Alternatively, the third option is to monitor peak expiratory flow (PEF) values on waking for a week. The minimum value compared with the best value recorded after a SABA during that week (Reddel *et al.*, 1995). These tests are illustrated in Figs 15.2 and 15.3.

Persistent asthma

A patient with symptoms of asthma whose airway function is abnormal between attacks. The abnormal function can often be reversed with inhaled corticosteroids (ICS), especially if the treatment commences soon after the onset of symptoms of the disease.

Episodic asthma (often seasonal)

A patient whose airway function is normal between attacks (Laitinen *et al.*, 1985; Beasley *et al.*, 1989). Episodic asthma is more common in children than adults, but occurs in some

Management of asthma symptoms

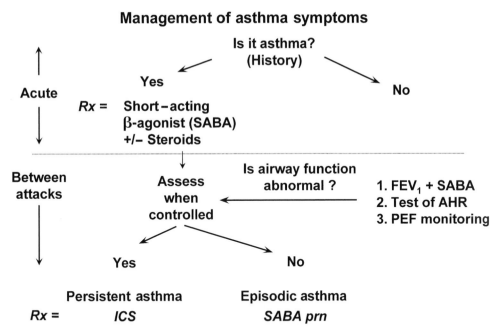

Figure 15.1 *This shows a theoretical simple algorithm for the management of asthma. When a patient presents with symptoms the question based mainly on history is: 'Is it asthma?' If the decision is yes, then the treatment is with short-acting β-agonist aerosols (SABA) plus or minus systemic steroids. If it is no, then other treatment for the symptoms is required. Once the acute symptoms are controlled, then the patient can be assessed. The most important question to ask is about the normality or not of the airway function. This can be done in three ways, one by spirometric function and giving a SABA. A 15% increase in forced expiratory volume in one second (FEV₁) is diagnostic of asthma and indicates that airway function at the time is abnormal. Similarly, a test of airway hyperresponsiveness (AHR) with methocholine or histamine can be undertaken and a fall in FEV₁ of 20% at 8 mg/ml or 4 μmol (dose) indicates AHR and therefore abnormal airway function. The third method is to monitor peak expiratory flow especially in the mornings. If any of these tests is abnormal then the patient can be considered to have persistent asthma and treatment, in the adult, with inhaled corticosteroids is indicated. If all these tests are normal then the patient can be considered to have episodic asthma and prescribed SABA prn. The response to bronchodilator and bronchoconstrictor is shown in Fig. 15.2 and peak flow monitoring is shown in Fig. 15.3.*

patients who are allergic to pollens and grain dusts during the season of exposure. Some patients, particularly children, have episodes of airway narrowing only during viral respiratory infections. The histological changes present during and between episodes of symptoms in patients with episodic asthma have not been reported.

Occupational asthma

A patient whose airways narrow in response to a specific substance to which the patient becomes 'sensitized' at the workplace. Usually it is episodic at first, but then becomes persistent. Occupational asthma is uncommon, but it is important to recognize patients with this disease at an early stage, because it is potentially reversible. The pathological changes appear to be the same as those seen in other forms of asthma (Saetta *et al.*, 1991).

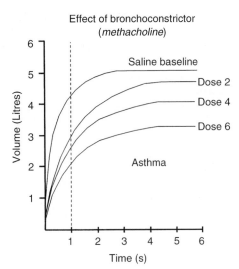

Figure 15.2 *This shows spirometric function with a bronchodilator with a response to a short-acting β-agonist on the left and a bronchoconstrictor on the right. The response of an asthmatic patient (40-year-old Caucasian male, 176 cm tall) before and after the β-agonist is shown compared with the response that might be seen in a normal person. On the right hand side the effect of methacholine in increasing doses on the FEV₁ from somebody with severe airway hyperresponsiveness is shown. The percent fall in the FEV₁ indicated by the dotted line is plotted against the dose or the concentration.*

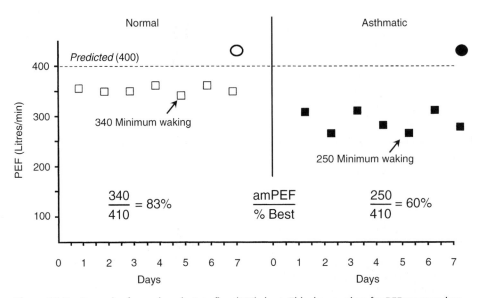

Figure 15.3 *Example of a peak expiratory flow (PEF) chart. This shows values for PEF measured on waking for seven days as indicated by the squares. The open squares are from a normal person and the filled ones are from an asthmatic patient (Caucasian female, 33 years old, 160 cm tall). The 'best' value is shown as circles representing post-bronchodilator PEF. These are obtained on day 7 in the clinic after a short-acting β-agonist. The predicted value is shown. The simplest way to indicate the severity of variability of lung function is to take the minimum value over 7 days and present it as a percentage of the best recent value after bronchodilator. Normal values are of 80% while 60% or less indicates severe airway abnormality.*

Asthma in remission

Routine lung function tests sometimes reveal adults without symptoms, but with well documented childhood asthma, who have had a small decrease in spirometric function, a mild degree of airway hyperresponsiveness (AHR) or an increased response to bronchodilator. There are no data on which to base a decision to treat such individuals, but it would seem important to monitor their airway function over time.

AIMS OF MANAGEMENT

1 To diagnose and classify the severity of the disease
2 To maintain 'tight' control of the disease with minimal exacerbations
3 To prevent the long-term decline in lung function
4 To minimize the side-effects of drugs

These aims are based on common sense and are an accepted part of asthma management plans but there have been no long-term trials to determine the best ways of achieving them. It is commonly thought not possible to control the disease, but complete control, based on the degree of AH, is possible as long as there is recognition by the doctor and the patient that the disease can be completely controlled in almost all patients and, the earlier that control is achieved after diagnosis, the better the outcome achieved. It is generally agreed that the aims of asthma management in the long term are largely related to prevention, yet prevention of the disease and of attacks is hardly ever mentioned in articles and book chapters relating to management, even though it is now well established that exposure to allergens is the most important risk factor for developing asthma (Sears *et al.*, 1989; Peat and Woolcock, 1991; Crater and Platts-Mills, 1998).

ASTHMA MANAGEMENT PLAN

Table 15.1 shows an example of a management plan. The plan stresses the assessment of the severity of asthma (when the patient is not having an attack) and indicates ways to reduce the severity of the disease.

Assessment

SEVERITY

There is no agreed 'gold standard' for defining the severity of asthma. Consensus guidelines suggest that a number of indicators including symptoms, frequency of bronchodilator use, history of medical attendances and peak expiratory flow measured on waking (amPEF), expressed as a percentage of the recent best, are needed. All other aspects of treatment depend on this assessment. The process of assessing severity includes confirmation of the diagnosis, classification of the nature and severity of the disease. Table 15.2 shows a guide to severity which includes symptoms, bronchodilator use over a 24-hour period, and amPEF expressed as a percentage of recent best. The symptoms are wheeze, chest tightness, breathlessness and cough, alone or in combination. The frequency of symptoms is important and, in particular, waking at night regularly with wheezing or coughing is a symptom of severe disease (Martin

Table 15.2 *Classification of asthma*

Symptoms of athma	Severe persistent	Moderate persistent	Mild persistent	Intermittent
Woken at night	>2×/week	1–2×/week	Rare	None
Bronchodilator (inhaled or oral)	>4×/day	2–4×/day	< 2×/day	With attacks
Seeks attention for acute symptoms	Monthly	2–3/month	Rarely	For attacks
amPEF (% recent best)	< 60	60–70	70–80	> 80

et al., 1990). Documenting SABA use helps in the assessment of severity when the patient has been advised to use SABA only for symptoms. The presence of daily symptoms, in spite of frequent SABA use, can indicate severe disease.

Measurement of amPEF is important for determining the severity of asthma and for continuing management. The minimum value for amPEF over a 7-day period, expressed as a percentage of the recent best (or even predicted) value, is a good indicator of the severity of the airway abnormality in most patients (Reddel *et al.*, 1995; Siersted *et al.*, 1994). Values above 80% are normal while values below 60% indicate severe disease as shown in Table 15.2. The PEF 'score' is illustrated in Fig. 15.3. This is a simple measurement compared with the standard PEF 'variability' calculation in most guidelines which is more cumbersome. In many guidelines the value of PEF and/or FEV_1 as a percentage of the predicted value is often used to classify severity. However, there is poor agreement between the two measurements (Sawyer *et al.*, 1998) and it is possible to have normal values for FEV_1 but severe disease on the basis of criteria in Table 15.2.

Most patients who have moderate or severe disease need to monitor amPEF while taking inhaled corticosteroids, especially at times when they are decreasing their doses or when they are experiencing more symptoms than usual. A week of readings, recorded both on waking and after a SABA use in the afternoons (Fig. 15.3) is enough to provide an initial assessment and accurate reflection of the situation, unless the patient is having, or has just had, a severe exacerbation.

When the amPEF is close to predicted and greater than 80% of the recent best and the symptoms are episodic, the patient can be regarded as having episodic or intermittent asthma. This can be confirmed by a provocation test with histamine or methacholine. Provocation with exercise or non-isotonic aerosols (Anderson *et al.*, 1994, 1996; du Toit *et al.*, 1997) can also be used but a negative test does not exclude the presence of AHR to histamine or methacholine. If the test is normal, the patient can be regarded as having episodic disease and be treated with SABA on demand. If AH is present, the patient should be regarded as having persistent disease. This can be mild, moderate or severe, depending on the history and amPEF values (Table 15.2).

BEST ACHIEVABLE LUNG FUNCTION

The best achievable values for PEF and spirometric function, forced vital capacity (FVC) and FEV_1, are needed as a guide to the long-term control of asthma. The best PEF value obtained is used to determine a 'target' range for PEF monitoring. The PEF that is 90% of the best is calculated, and this becomes the 'target' value for the patient to aim to achieve on waking. At the same time the 'best' spirometric value should be recorded at each clinic visit, while the patient is on prednisone. These serve as reference values for long-term management. If the patient has not achieved a PEF value close to the predicted value (obtained from the tables for age, sex, height and race) in a week of monitoring which includes the evening (p.m.) values after using a SABA, as shown in Fig. 15.3, it is possible that the best lung function has not been reached. In such a patient, a trial of oral steroids with PEF monitoring, should be undertaken. Usually 5 days of prednisone or prednisolone at 0.8 mg/kg body weight per day is enough, but if improvement is still occurring after 5 days, the medication can be continued for up to 10 days. The prednisone is then stopped and inhaled corticosteroids are continued. It is important to know if residual airflow limitation exists after this maximal therapy and also to determine the 'target' for the amPEF value.

Intervention

DRUGS

In patients with persistent disease, drug therapy is aimed at keeping the patient free from symptoms and the amPEF above 85% of the recent best. A suggested scheme for drugs, using the severity score as a guideline, is outlined in Table 15.3. The aim is to reduce the severity of the disease by treating the airway inflammation with inhaled corticosteroids (together with reducing exposure to triggers, treating aggravating-factors, removing causal factors and addressing lifestyle problems – see below).

In addition to these drugs, a number of others used in asthma management can be regarded as 'second line' and are dealt with later in this section (*see* Table 15.5).

Systemic steroids

These drugs are used to gain control in unstable patients, to find the best possible lung function (trial of steroids) and for exacerbations. Corticosteroids, when administered systemically, have similar actions to those described for topical steroids although their effect on small vessels in the airways is unknown. They take 4–6 hours to have an effect and will act on all the cells with steroid receptors.

Table 15.3   *Asthma management – medication (adults)*

Drug class	Name	Dose	Comment
Antiinflammatory			
Oral corticosteroid	Prednisone	1.0 mg/kg/day	Dose for exacerbation
Inhaled corticosteroid	Beclomethasone	0.4–2.0 mg/day	Dose depends on drug,
	Budesonide		form and device used
	Fluticasone		
Long-acting 'Controller'			
LA β_2-agonist-inhaled	Salmeterol	0.05 mg bd	
	Formoterol	0.12 mg bd	
(or) theophylline SR	Theodur	Dose variable	
	Nuelin		
(or) LA β_2-agonist tablets	Bambuterol	Dose variable	
Bronchodilator (quick relief)			
SABA	Salbutamol	1–2 puffs prn	Salbutamol sulphate also available
	Terbutaline		

LA = long-acting (12 hours); SABA = short-acting bronchodilator agonist (4–8 hours); SR = slow release. This list of drugs is reproduced from Fig. 10a of the Asthma Management and Prevention: Global Initiative for Asthma (du Toit *et al.*, 1997).

Clinical effects In the management plan, oral steroids are used as a trial to find the best lung function in patients whose PEF remains lower than the predicted value, and to treat severe exacerbations. In children it has been shown that a single dose (30 or 60 mg) of prednisone as well as nebulized bronchodilator, reduces the need for hospital admission (Storr *et al.*, 1987). Data showing this rapid effect have not been published for adults.

Side-effects These are well documented and described in the previous chapter. Bruising, osteoporosis, cataracts, hypertension, diabetes and Cushingoid features are the most important. These effects occur only with long-term use and are greatly reduced by changing the patient to inhaled corticosteroids. It takes many months to change patients to an inhaled form and care must be taken to implement all the other steps in the management plan at the same time.

Dose and administration For finding the best lung function, it is usual to use 0.8–1.0 mg/kg body weight per day in divided doses for 5–10 days (Fig. 15.4). For treatment of exacerbations, trial and error is needed to determine the symptoms and the amPEF values that herald deterioration of sufficient severity to need oral steroids, the dose of oral steroid needed to abort a severe attack can vary. Usually 25–50 mg, in divided doses for 1–2 days is sufficient. It is not necessary to reduce the dose slowly when it has been used for less than a week, unless experience shows that sudden withdrawal is associated with worsening asthma. The inhaled corticosteroids should not be stopped while the patient is on oral steroids.

A few patients, usually those who were on oral steroids before the advent of the inhaled forms, require some oral steroids to control symptoms. However, over a period of many months, sometimes years, it is possible to withdraw all oral steroids and replace them with the newer potent inhaled drugs.

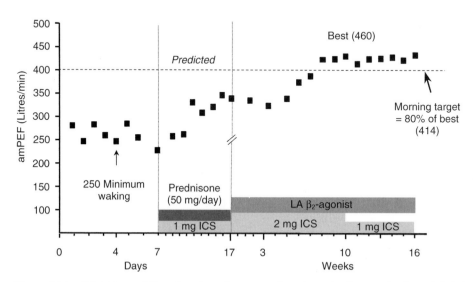

Figure 15.4 *This is the peak flow chart from the same patient shown in Fig. 15.3. On day 8, inhaled corticosteroids plus prednisone (50 mg/day) were added for 10 days and there was a progressive increase in the morning peak flow. After 10 days the prednisone was stopped, the dose of inhaled corticosteroids was increased and long-acting β-agonists were added. At 10 weeks the dose of inhaled corticosteroids was halved.*

Inhaled corticosteroids

The actions of inhaled corticosteroids have been described in Chapter 13. These drugs are effective because they have a number of actions (Barnes, 1998).

Fig. 15.4 shows the expected response of amPEF to ICS over time with treatment. Fig. 15.5 shows a diagram developed by Dr Soren Pedersen, representing the effects of ICS on symptoms, FEV₁, inflammatory markers, amPEF, and AH. The responses demonstrated represent the current 'gold standard' for asthma management in adults. No other drug class has been shown to affect all these modalities of airway function and, because of this, they remain the mandatory treatment if these outcomes are to be attained. There is controversy about the method of use, with a growing consensus for starting 'high' and reducing the dose once control is achieved, but the safest way of reducing has not been well defined, although reducing the dose by one inhalation every 10 weeks seems to work well. There is some controversy about the starting with high doses; Postma's group (van der Molen *et al.*, 1998) suggested that there is no real advantage to starting at high doses but this trial in primary care did not aim at getting prompt and full control.

The other area of controversy is when to use long-acting β-agonists (LABA). Increasing use of these drugs indicates that they are safe and are long-acting. When they are used with ICS they increase amPEF, decrease nocturnal symptoms and decrease exacerbations. As knowledge of asthma increases, it appears that in moderate and severe disease, the two drugs used together are likely to be beneficial (Barnes, 1998). The situation is not so clear with mild asthma where it is known that low doses of ICS can control asthma well and LABA may not be needed.

Fig. 15.6 shows the control achieved with 1.6 μg of budesonide in a group of patients in a recent trial (Reddel *et al.*, 1999). While the dose of budesonide was being decreased from 1.6 μg, the FEV₁ remained stable while the AH continued to improve.

Clinical effects When ICS are given acutely, they do not inhibit the early or late responses to allergen challenges. However, when given for several days they have some inhibitory effect on

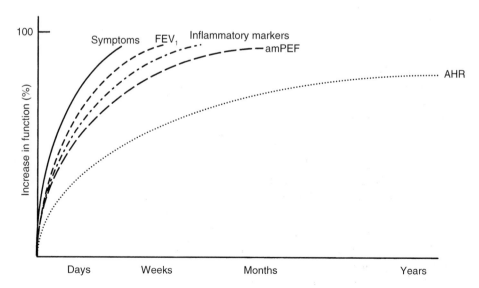

Figure 15.5 *A theoretical response to inhaled corticosteroids (ICS) when used in appropriate doses. The symptoms recover almost completely within days of beginning treatment. The forced expiratory volume in one second (FEV₁) recovers within two weeks, inflammatory markers at about the same time and the morning peak flow (amPEF) takes slightly longer and does not always reach the predicted value in all patients. Airway hyperresponsiveness (AHR) may take one to two years to completely return to normal.*

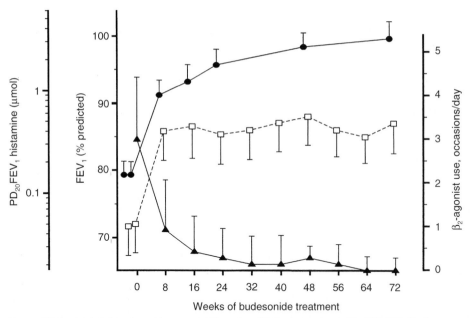

Figure 15.6 *A trial of budesonide use over 72 weeks with the improvement in FEV₁ (□), the improvement in airway hyperresponsiveness as a PD₂₀FEV₁ histamine (●) and the decrease in β-agonist use (▲). FEV₁ is at maximal level within 8 weeks of treatment and β-agonist use is virtually zero at 32 weeks of treatment, whereas the AHR is continuing to improve even at 72 weeks of treatment.*

these responses. In most patients, particularly those who have not taken the drugs previously, there is a dose-related effect in improving the severity of the disease as measured by symptoms, baseline lung function and amPEF. Improvement may take several weeks to become apparent to the patient and may continue for many months (Woolcock and Jenkins, 1991; Sont *et al.*, 1999; Prieto *et al.*, 1999). In some patients ICS appear to have little effect on AHR (Ryan *et al.*, 1985; Frankel *et al.*, 1990). It seems likely that the effectiveness of ICS depends on regular doses being taken after control is achieved by initial high doses.

The response to ICS appears to be dose related, but this is difficult to demonstrate because effects in AHR take months. The drugs are given twice daily, but in mild disease once daily treatment is possible (McFadden *et al.*, 1999). Although these drugs have now been in use for many years, there is little published about their long-term effectiveness in individual patients. Clinical experience suggests that relapse occurs in many patients when they are stopped (Gibson *et al.*, 1992; Haahtela, 1998). Finding the correct dose for maintenance treatment requires trial and error and the continuing use of diary cards to record symptoms and amPEF values.

Pharyngeal side-effects Some adult patients taking ICS experience dysphonia, the cause of which is unclear, and a smaller number develop thrush (Toogood *et al.*, 1980). These problems can be prevented by the use of a spacer device, (Toogood *et al.*, 1981, 1984) by reducing the number of inhalations (using high-strength aerosols) and by gargling after use. In some patients antifungal agents are needed to control the local symptoms.

Systemic side-effects The side-effects of ICS depend on the dose (Toogood, 1998). They are rarely seen in doses below 1.0 mg/day and are much less than those observed with the doses of oral steroids that are needed to maintain the same degree of control. Biochemical evidence of adrenal suppression rarely occurs on doses of less than 1.5 mg daily. When it is present, it is probably not medically important but indicates that enough drug is being absorbed to have a systemic effect. More important clinical effects are bruising, osteoporosis, and development of cataracts (Cumming *et al.*, 1997). All of these are likely to develop when these drugs are used in high dose for long periods, although there is no evidence that osteoporosis and cataracts occur in the absence of courses of oral steroids. The well-documented side-effects of steroids have caused patients, doctors and pharmacists to maintain an element of steroid phobia which is probably unjustified. Nevertheless, the long-term effects of these drugs has not been documented and it is prudent to continue to reduce the daily dose to the minimum that is needed to maintain control.

Dose and administration It is not possible to suggest doses of ICS for varying severity of disease because the drugs vary in potency and the formulation (aerosol or powder) and the delivery device used, all of which affect the dose prescribed. In general it makes sense to start with high doses and to reduce the dose as soon as the severity improves. Nebulized forms (available as budesonide) are used in some countries in patients with poor lung function, but the role of this form of the drug in adults is not established. Attention should be paid to teaching each patient how ICS work, how to use them and what to expect. This takes time, but is one of the most crucial elements of asthma management.

Refractoriness Steroid resistance rarely occurs and this is discussed below. To date refractoriness to ICS has not been described in the way that refractoriness to oral steroids appears to occur, but clinical experience suggests that some patients, who initially have good control, become more difficult to manage even when these drugs are used in high doses.

Long-acting β-agonists Long-acting β-agonists (LABA) are given in lower doses than the short-acting forms. They are more effective in controlling asthma than in relieving acute episodes of airway narrowing. By stimulating the β_2-receptor, these drugs increase cyclic AMP levels, which in turn increase cellular calcium leading to cell actions as described in Chapter 11. The main action of β-agonists in the airways is to relax (or prevent contraction) of smooth muscle cells. They also stabilize mast cells, preventing the provoked release of mediators. In this respect they are more potent than sodium cromoglycate (SCG). They act for 12 h (Arvidsson *et al.*, 1989; Ullman *et al.*, 1990) and, in the case of salmeterol, may have actions other than bronchodilation (Twentyman *et al.*, 1990). Their overall place in the management of patients with asthma is continuing to be defined. They have a stabilizing effect on the airways that allows the dose of ICS to be reduced (Wilding *et al.*, 1997). Salmeterol is more widely used than formoterol at present, and is best used in low doses (50 μg twice daily), higher doses are rarely more effective. These drugs need to be used with care and their actions carefully explained. Their greatest advantage is in preventing night-time symptoms and in improving the quality of sleep. The oral bronchodilator bambuterol is a prodrug which releases terbutaline over a 24-h period. In early studies it compares well with salmeterol in terms of nocturnal symptoms (Crompton *et al.*, 1999; Wallaert *et al.*, 1999).

Fig. 15.7 shows a diagram of the theoretical changes in FEV_1 over a 12-h period (10 p.m. to 10 a.m.). The advantages of LABA are that although less potent they significantly improve the control of asthma symptoms particularly at night (Douglas and Fitzpatrick, 1991). Side-effects do not appear to be a problem. Tachyphylaxis to bronchodilatation has not been demonstrated but there is tachyphylaxis to the protecting effects of salmeterol against stimuli such as exercise after the first few days of treatment (Cheung *et al.*, 1992).

The success of the LABA in controlling symptoms and the fact that a relatively fixed dose is used, creates an opportunity to make combination drugs. To date Seretide, a combination of salmeterol and fluticasone, has become available in some countries and it is expected that a combination of budesonide and formoterol will also be available soon. The data from Seretide suggest that the combination is a real advance for management because it allows patients to

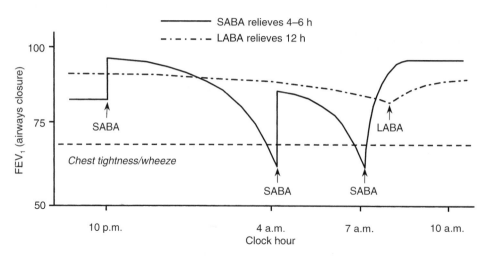

Figure 15.7 *A theoretical diagram of the FEV$_1$ during the night in somebody with uncontrolled asthma. With a short-acting β-agonist (SABA), quite good FEV$_1$ can be obtained when taken at bedtime (10 p.m.) but during the night there is a fall in FEV$_1$ to the point where chest tightness and wheezing occur, the patient wakes and takes more SABA which lasts even less time at this early time in the morning. The patient wakes at 7 a.m. again with tightness in the chest but improves with SABA. The dotted line shows what happens with a long-acting β-agonist (LABA) taken at 7 p.m. Although the FEV$_1$ may be only 90% of predicted it does not over the period of 12 hours fall to the point where there are any chest symptoms so that throughout the night the patient can sleep without being aroused by airways closure, in this case measured as the FEV$_1$.*

take just one puff, twice daily. Combination drugs may improve compliance (data not yet available) and it certainly makes therapeutic sense. The drugs may have complementary actions and recent studies show that LABA are able to activate the glucocorticoid receptor in human lung fibroblasts (Eickelberg *et al.*, 1999).

Theophylline

Fig. 15.8 shows an overall drug plan for asthma of varying severity; it also includes theophylline. This drug has many actions (Hendeles and Weinberger, 1983; Barnes and Pauwels, 1994). The mechanisms by which it bronchodilates are unknown, although it appears to increase intracellular cyclic AMP by a mechanism different from the β-agonists. It may also have some 'antiinflammatory' effects (Billing *et al.*, 1987), but the mechanisms are largely unknown. There is no place for theophylline as a second drug when a β-agonist has failed to control the disease. If the patient needs more than occasional β-agonist aerosols then ICS, not theophylline, is indicated.

Known effects Theophylline gives symptomatic relief to those with severe airway narrowing. A well-recognized group of patients, usually dependent on long-term or frequent short-term courses of oral steroids, need theophylline to control their symptoms. Many of these patients need doses above the usual level to keep the serum levels in the 'therapeutic' range. These patients apparently metabolize the drug differently. Its action in relieving symptoms is unknown. There are some patients who get immediate symptomatic relief from the drug and use it either intermittently or as a single dose at night.

Side-effects These are well-known for high doses and include: nausea, headache and hyperactivity in children. The drug can cause convulsions and cardiovascular arrhythmias if given in too high a dose (Skinner, 1990). The increasing awareness of side-effects of this drug has led to its decreasing use in some countries (Barnes and Pauwels, 1994). However, side-

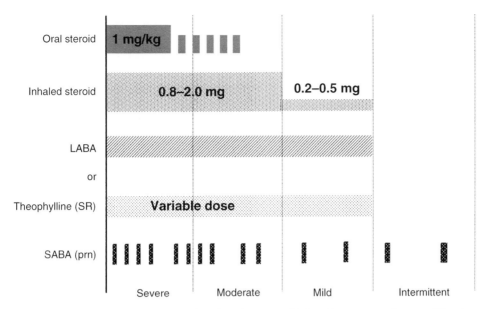

Figure 15.8 *This shows the treatment based on the GINA Guidelines for severe, moderate, mild and intermittent asthma. It shows oral steroids, inhaled steroids, long-acting β-agonists or theophylline (slow release) and short-acting β-agonists taken on a prn basis. The drugs in this figure can be considered the main drugs used in the treatment of adult asthma at the present time.*

effects can be avoided by using the drug in lower doses as an adjunct to other therapy, rather than as a primary bronchodilator. It is likely that the exact place of theophylline (which is cheap) will be defined in coming years and the side-effects largely avoided.

Dose and administration When used as a bronchodilator, particularly in treating severe attacks, doses are adjusted to keep the serum levels within the 'therapeutic' range, therefore avoiding toxicity. However, theophylline is rarely used for this purpose in most countries because of its side-effects. The slow-release forms are most effective in reducing large fluctuations in serum levels. In patients with severe disease, especially those requiring low doses of oral prednisone in addition to ICS, they appear to have a steroid-sparing effect and can be used in lower doses. The effort and expense of monitoring serum levels is not required for low-dose treatment. It is included in the drugs shown in Fig. 15.8 because some long-term users (usually poorly controlled) like it and it is has a place in populations that cannot afford LABA.

Short-acting β-agonists
Fig. 15.8 shows SABA to be used as required. Salbutamol and turbutaline bronchodilate for about 4–6 hours and are now called short-acting. However, the very short-acting drugs, such as isoprenaline, are now rarely used. Short-acting β-agonists are extensively used and are most effective when inhaled, but oral and intravenous forms are available. For reasons that are not understood, only the inhaled forms of β-agonists protect against provoked attacks such as exercise. Their duration of action as protectors rather than as bronchodilators is shorter (about 2 hours) and they are more effective protectors than sodium cromoglycate (SCG) (Church and Young, 1983; Howarth *et al.*, 1985).

The question as to whether salbutamol and terbutaline increase the severity of asthma when they are used regularly has not been resolved completely. In children, AHR was shown to increase when terbutaline was used alone in contrast to inhaled steroids which improved the severity (Kraan *et al.*, 1985; Kerrebijn *et al.*, 1987). A year-long study in New Zealand showed that four times a day use of fenoterol was associated with worsening control of asthma in 40 out of 64 patients who completed a trial (Sears *et al.*, 1990). However, the effects demonstrated by fenoterol may not apply to all β-agonists.

It is clear that when used alone, β-agonists do not improve the overall severity of asthma. Nevertheless, many people with episodic or mild disease use them to control symptoms and the severity of their asthma does not increase. Sales of salbutamol have been increasing worldwide in the last 20 years and there is little objective evidence that this drug has caused any problem.

Side-effects Tremor and slight tachycardia occur acutely and are well-known. These effects usually decrease with time and are rarely a problem unless the drugs are used to excess (Wong *et al.*, 1990). Attempts to demonstrate tachyphylaxis to the bronchodilating effects of salbutamol in asthmatic airways have been unsuccessful, although it may occur in non-asthmatics (Harvey and Tattersfield, 1982).

Dose and administration These drugs are usually given in the inhaled form with doses varying from 100–200 μg. Metered dose inhalers, nebulizing solutions and dry powder forms are available in addition to tablets and syrups. β-Agonists are used for making the diagnosis (if the FEV_1 increases by 15% within 10 minutes of an aerosol bronchodilator, this is diagnostic of asthma), for finding the 'best' lung function, for severe symptoms lasting more than 10 minutes and for reversing airway obstruction (e.g. when the PEF is less than 60–70% of the target PEF). Short-acting β-agonists are not needed on a regular basis except in those patients whose symptoms cannot be controlled by a combination of other drugs, including ICS and LABA.

Sodium cromoglycate and nedocromil sodium

Sodium cromoglycate (SCG) and nedocromil sodium (NS) are sometimes labelled as cromones. SCG has been available for nearly 30 years. It prevents airway narrowing induced

Table 15.4 *Indications for use of short-acting β-agonists*

- Acute severe attacks – these drugs may be life saving
- For diagnosis – does lung function improve within minutes?
- For assessment of severity – puffs per required plus best recent PEF
- For symptoms which are causing distress or anxiety
- Before exercise to prevent airway narrowing

Table 15.5 *Asthma medication in adults – Drugs for special purposes*

Class	Name	Comment
Cromones	Nedocromil sodium	These drugs are active for 4–6 hours
	Sodium cromoglycate	In long-term use, frequently prescribed as bd or tds
Leukotriene modifiers	Montelukast	Not all of these drugs are available in all countries
	Pranlukast	
	Zafirlukast	
	Zyleutin	
Antihistamine	Ketotifen	Not widely available
Steroid-sparing	Cyclosporin A	Doses depend on body weight, liver and renal
	Methotrexate	function and blood levels

by allergens, exercise, SO_2 and other irritants. It may have a small effect on airway inflammation, perhaps by preventing inflammation from worsening during the allergen season. Nedocromil sodium is more potent and has been developed for adults. It is effective in reducing cough in some patients and has a small effect on AHR.

Mechanisms of action   In spite of their widespread use and a large body of literature, little is known about how these drugs work. They stabilize isolated mucosal mast cells and reduce the release of mediators (Church and Young, 1983), but the extent to which they do this *in vivo* is not known. Recently NS has been shown to affect the chloride channel in cell membranes and it seems likely that their ability to antagonize the effects of osmotic changes in the airways may be related to this effect (Anderson *et al.*, 1994, 1996). It is likely that they act on other inflammatory cells and on afferent nerve endings, as well as on mast cells. *In vitro*, NS appears to be more potent in preventing mast cell degranulation than SCG, and it may be slightly more potent in preventing attacks.

Clinical effects   In the short term, the cromones prevent exercise-induced attacks in many adults and most children. The degree to which they inhibit the attacks is dose-related and is short-lived because the drugs are rapidly removed from the airways during exercise. Taken before an allergen challenge they prevent both early and late reactions (Booij-Noord *et al.*, 1971). They also inhibit the effects of other 'indirect' provoking stimuli such as SO_2. In this respect, NS is more effective than SCG.

In the long term, in patients with episodic asthma the cromones prevent seasonal 'spontaneous' exacerbations so that the episodes are prevented or decreased in adults and children. SCG has the reputation of being more effective in children, probably because episodic asthma is common in children. In one study a decrease in AHR has been observed while patients are taking SCG regularly (Hoag and McFadden, 1991). It appears that the drug must be given in adequate doses for at least 12 weeks. In patients already taking ICS, the response to SCG appears not to be as good as it is to inhaled steroids (Hoag and McFadden, 1991), but there is some evidence that NS improves the overall control of the disease in such patients (Boulet *et al.*, 1990). It has a clinical effect but not as good as 200 mg of beclomethasone dipropionate when both drugs are given twice daily (Svendsen *et al.*, 1989).

Side-effects   These drugs have virtually no side-effects. The dry powder form of SCG sometimes causes minor irritation and some patients complain that NS has an unpleasant taste.

Doses and administration   SCG is usually administered as 5 mg per puff and NS as 4 mg per puff from metered-dose aerosols, and two puffs are inhaled three or four times per day. SCG is also available as 20 mg spincaps and 20 mg nebulizer solution. These drugs can be used immediately prior to exposure to known triggers to prevent attacks.

For long-term use, they need to be given in an adequate dose and at regular intervals, initially four times a day. Once control is improved they are used three times a day. In adults with persistent disease the cromones seem to have little effect in controlling the disease in the long term.

Leukotriene modifying drugs

Listed in Table 15.5 are four available drugs: Zyleuton (a 5-lipoxygenase inhibitor) is available mainly in the USA and Pranlukast is available only in Japan. The other two are more widely available. Given once or twice daily, these drugs have been shown to improve symptoms and lung function during four to six months of therapy (Spector *et al.*, 1994; Knorr *et al.*, 1998; Nathan *et al.*, 1998; Reiss *et al.*, 1998; Kemp *et al.*, 1999; Lipworth, 1999; Malmstrom *et al.*, 1999). Although they are available in many countries, their place in treatment is not yet clear

(Smith, 1998). Because ICS do not affect the production of leukotrienes (O'Shaughnessy et al., 1993), these drugs may have an added effect when used with ICS. One trial compared ICS plus zafirlukast with ICS plus LABA and showed an added effect of zafirlukast on lung function but the effect was less than that of LABA (Busse et al., 1999). They are a potential advance in the control of asthma, especially in some forms of disease such as aspirin-sensitive asthma, but there have been few published papers that report results of long-term trials on the severity of the disease in terms of exacerbations and effects on AHR. It is established that montelukast and zafirlukast prevent the fall in FEV_1 produced by exercise and are effective for at least 12 hours and with long-term use. The blocking effect varies from patient to patient, probably indicating differing degrees of leukotriene release as a result of the exercise (Leff et al., 1998). The continuing debate about their place in treatment arises from the fact that comparisons with other drugs are not yet available so that their place in the drug plan shown in Fig. 15.8 is not yet established.

Zafirlukast and montelukast are not toxic to the liver but Churg–Strauss syndrome has been described with the use of these drugs (Drazen and Israel, 1998; Wenzel, 1998). This appears to have been related to the withdrawal of oral steroids in most but not all patients. It is of interest that this syndrome is appearing in patients prescribed other drugs including ICS (Wechsler and Drazen, 1999).

Antihistamines

In general, these drugs have no place in the treatment of asthma. However, the non-sedating antihistamines have few side-effects and are useful in those with other allergic problems that often accompany asthma, for example rhinitis, urticaria and allergic reactions to foods. A number of patients with seasonal exacerbations of asthma find that regular use of antihistamines during 'the season' controls their symptoms (Howarth, 1990).

Ketotifen is marketed as an antihistamine and is widely used (Grant et al., 1990; Kurasawa, 1994). There are no published trials that show that it is effective in reducing the severity of asthma in those with moderate and severe persistent disease, but it has some 'anti-inflammatory' properties in vitro. It is used in patients with mild disease and can reduce symptoms to the point where other drugs are not necessary.

Steroid-sparing agents

Some patients respond to steroids only in high doses. In some it is possible to reduce the oral steroid dose if a steroid-sparing drug is used.

Methotrexate is used commonly in the USA in patients who need high doses of oral steroids to control their asthma (Mullarkey et al., 1988, 1990; Shiner et al., 1990; Erzurum et al., 1991; Stewart et al., 1994). It has anti-inflammatory actions and in some patients can be used to reduce the dose of prednisone without causing too many side-effects. Discontinuing the methotrexate usually leads to a relapse. There has been no trial in patients who have first been treated with a strict management plan (as described above) that includes high doses of ICS. Overall its inconsistent effectiveness and its side-effects lead to the conclusion that it probably has little place except perhaps in the occasional patient who responds well and does not develop side-effects.

In one controlled trial of cylosporin (5 mg/kg/day) in steroid-dependent asthmatics (Alexander et al., 1992), the small improvements achieved seem to have been outweighed by the side-effects and cost. Anecdotal reports of its use have suggested it not to be a big advance, but as with methotrexate the occasional patient does well.

Gold salts, sometimes used for the treatment of arthritis, are used in some countries for the treatment of patients with severe asthma (Klaustermeyer et al., 1987). There has been no trial published of the effects on patients already enrolled in a management plan that maximizes the use of inhaled steroids and other measures aimed at reducing severity.

Other drugs

There has been recent interest in the use of macrolide antibiotics (Itkin and Menzel, 1970) in cases where chronic infection with *Chlamydia* pneumonia is playing a role, and formal trials are underway. There are many reports of attempts to use other antiinflammatory agents including colchicine (Schwartz *et al.*, 1990) and chloroquine (Charous, 1990). They are of research interest only at present and probably are not needed where the drugs described in the management plan are available and used effectively.

AVOIDANCE OF TRIGGERS/AGGRAVATORS

Physical factors

Factors that cause symptoms in patients with uncontrolled asthma include exercise, strong smells, cold air, changes in the weather, etc. They are usually easily identified by the patient. The effect of most can be minimized by appropriate use of SCG, NS or SABA aerosols before a known exposure, for example before exercise. However, these are short-term measures and control of the disease with ICS usually improves these symptoms.

Allergens

There is no doubt that aero-allergens are important triggers of attacks in most allergic asthmatics. There is also increasing evidence that asthma is caused by exposure to allergens (Sporik *et al.*, 1990), and that avoidance improves the severity of the disease (Murray and Ferguson, 1982; Platts-Mills *et al.*, 1982; Dorward *et al.*, 1988). Allergen exposure in the first years of life may be particularly important in causing severe disease in children. These, together with the fact that asthma rarely completely reverses once it becomes persistent, means that the most rational approach to asthma management is prevention (Peat, 1998). Allergen avoidance is important for families with a history of allergic disease. The allergens that are important throughout the world are dust, mites, moulds, pollens and animal proteins. Large amounts of these allergens can be found in house dust, particularly in carpets. House dust mites, both alive and dead, present the biggest problem. Present evidence suggests that most mattresses and pillows, apart from those in areas with very low humidity, harbour mites. It seems likely that allergens are constantly inhaled and lead to continuing inflammation of the airways. The most sensible solution for patients is to live in an environment that is as allergen-free as possible.

Rhinitis/sinusitis

It should be routine for the doctor to ask the patient about symptoms of rhinitis (nasal obstruction or sneezing), snoring and interrupted sleep, and about gastric reflux (heartburn). These problems, when treated, help the overall well-being of patients and cannot be ignored, though they may have only a small effect on the underlying severity of the asthma.

LIFESTYLE CHANGES

Recommendations for *reducing allergen levels* in houses are:

- The humidity in houses should be minimized by good ventilation. This is probably the most important measure (Nicolai *et al.*, 1998; Peat *et al.*, 1998).
- All bedding (mattress, pillow and doonas) that is not able to be washed regularly in hot water, should be encased in mite-proof covers, and bedding that can be washed regularly should be washed at 60°C. Sunlight is excellent and, whenever practical, bedding should be put in the sun which kills mites. Wall-to-wall carpet should be removed from the bedrooms where possible. It is almost impossible to make a house in a humid environment allergen-free while carpets remain. It should be explained to the patient that vacuum cleaning

removes no more than a small percentage of mites, which have legs designed to stick to carpet fibres. Furthermore, anti-mite sprays must be used frequently and in a quantity that penetrates the carpet completely.

- Sheep skins should be discarded or washed frequently with water at at least 60°C (Mahmic *et al.*, 1998).
- Clothes should be kept in cupboards and washed or dry-cleaned frequently.
- Cats should be removed completely. Cats kept outside the house remain an important source of allergen.

All patients should be encouraged to take *exercise*. Swimming appears to be particularly beneficial. Patients who have severe disease with panic attacks and hyperventilation benefit from swimming which helps to teach them to control their breathing rate. There are numerous studies that show the effectiveness of exercise in improving overall well-being (Svenonius *et al.*, 1983; Anderson, 1988). The acute symptoms of exercise-induced asthma can be prevented with SCG, NS or a SABA aerosol prior to the exercise (Woolley *et al.*, 1990; Anderson *et al.*, 1991).

Although there is little evidence that *increasing weight* makes asthma worse it may well limit the ability to stretch the airways. There is evidence that *obesity* is associated with a risk of adult-onset asthma (Camargo *et al.*, 1998).

Acupuncture, hypnosis, meditation, Chinese herbal medicine, garlic tablets and many other remedies are used frequently by patients with asthma. These measures are almost never successful in reducing the basic severity of the disease, but often the patient feels better. Patients should not be discouraged from using them but should also be encouraged to use their prescribed medication. β-blockers and aspirin are also important aggravators that must be constantly asked about.

Commitment

1 Written 'action plan' for exacerbations
   A written action plan is necessary for all patients, even if they have infrequent exacerbations. The general aim is to prevent a severe attack by increasing the dose of inhaled steroids or starting high dose oral steroids. There is no place for low doses of oral steroids in preventing attacks. A plan should be written and the patient should be able to recognize an impending attack, know which drugs to take and how to call for help.

2 Education of patient and family
   Controlled trials of educating patients with asthma in the absence of an agreed management plan leads to decreased severity or to improved control (Bailey *et al.*, 1990; Mayo *et al.*, 1990; Ringsberg *et al.*, 1990; Muhlhauser *et al.*, 1991; Wilson *et al.*, 1993; Kotses *et al.*, 1995). However, unless the patient, the family, and in the case of children, the teacher most involved with the child, understand the nature of asthma, the aims of treatment and the management plan, full control of the disease will not be achieved.

   Education takes time which may not be available to all doctors. This means that an education programme should be developed in association with hospitals where asthma is treated. Each doctor needs a kit which includes pictures of airways, drugs and a number of peak flow meters. The latter can be lent until it is decided whether the patient needs one permanently (score of 6 or more).

3 Regular review
   Asthma is a chronic disease which carries a number of long-term risks including: symptoms, altered lifestyle, the development of permanently abnormal lung function, the

side-effects of drugs and premature death. In those with moderate or severe persistent asthma, it almost never remits and this means continuing care. Regular visits to the doctor, at which the diaries are reviewed, are essential. At these visits a new score (hopefully lower) is calculated, the treatment changed, the action plan updated, drugs prescribed and education continued. Some patients improve rapidly, and others take much longer. In time, patients can take more responsibility for their own management, but in the first year of treatment, regular appointments, regardless of symptoms, must be made. Every patient with persistent asthma should have one doctor who is committed to her/his care for life.

TREATMENT OF ACUTE ATTACKS

If, in spite of the written plan, or because the plan was not used, the patient has a severe attack, the guidelines outlined by the British Thoracic Society (1997) or the Canadian Medical Association (Beveridge *et al.*, 1996) should be followed. The patient should be monitored with an ear oximeter and PEF measurements and oxygen given. The drugs needed are oral or intravenous steroids in adequate doses, nebulized bronchodilating drugs and, if the response is poor after several hours, parental bronchodilators, usually intravenous salbutamol. Intravenous aminophylline is rarely used now, but many patients respond well to it.

Short-acting β-agonists

Nebulized SABAs are usually used and often continued with anticholinergics. Recently McFadden *et al.* (1998) compared two dosage regimens of albuterol and found that the high-dose regimen increased lung function more rapidly and to a greater extent than the standard dose regimen.

Anticholinergics

The drugs ipratropium bromide and oxitropium are used to block the cholinergic receptors (Chapman, 1990). They are effective bronchodilators and are useful in patients with chronic obstructive pulmonary disease. They have a slower onset than the β-agonists. They are used in conjunction with β-agonists in the treatment of acute attacks, particularly in children. At present they have little role in long-term management of asthma, but they sometimes have a place in patients in whom constant use of SABA causes worsening control of the disease and who need a regular bronchodilator.

TREATMENT OF SEVERE PERSISTENT ASTHMA

In some patients, the management plan fails to reduce the severity of asthma. The reasons for this include severity and chronicity of the disease, diagnosis, lifestyle, lack of compliance or a combination. In this group of patients long-term commitment is needed and each step in the management plan should be implemented carefully. In addition, it is helpful to ask the following questions:

1   Does the patient have asthma? Sometimes a diagnosis is assumed in a patient who is hyperventilating, is simulating symptoms or who has bronchiectasis, cystic fibrosis or

smoking-related airflow limitation. A bronchial biopsy is usually diagnostic and can give helpful information.

2   Is the patient complying with drugs? Some patients deliberately avoid using the drugs, others forget or take them incorrectly. This may be difficult to determine, but often explains the lack of improvement. Objective studies of compliance show that the majority of patients fail to take their medications as prescribed (Horn *et al.*, 1990).

3   Have the relevant allergens and aggravators been removed/treated? In particular, does the patient snore or have severe gastro-oesophageal reflux? Treating rhinitis usually allows the patient to sleep better and treatment of severe snoring can be very helpful (Chan *et al.*, 1988).

4   Does the patient respond to high doses of prednisone using objective measures? If so, then adequate doses of inhalant plus oral pulse therapy are needed. If not, the diagnosis should be questioned. The patient may have chronic fixed airway obstruction and be incapable of improvement.

5   Is the environment a causal factor? If the patient knows that in a different house, region or country, asthma control is improved then a trial of living in a new environment is indicated.

6   Would a trial with cylosporin A or methotrexate help? A trial with one of these drugs is indicated if the management plan has been implemented and drugs complied with for at least a year. In addition, it should be demonstrated that steroid therapy is effective but needed in amounts that cause excessive side-effects before these potentially toxic agonists are used.

7   Does the patient have true steroid-resistant asthma? This condition is extremely rare and can only be recognized after the six previous points have been addressed. Such patients should be recognized and steroids kept at low doses while other treatments are used (Anonymous, 1996).

8   Does the patient have abnormal illness behaviour? Some patients have second gain from illness and will only respond to asthma management if they develop another illness. A variety of psychological problems occur in patients with severe persistent asthma and the help of a psychiatrist can be of great help.

LIKELY CHANGES TO MANAGEMENT

Asthma continues to be managed without the benefit of a systematic approach and without the results of long-term trials of treatment, in which the effect of specific management plans on the outcome of the disease are defined. Until such trials are done, it is unlikely that dramatic progress will be made. The following list outlines some of the likely changes to the overall approach to the management of asthma, based on results of recent studies and on the increasing use of management plans.

- More accurate assessment of severity and introduction of ICS in doses designed to gain control.
- It will become routine to attempt to lower the dose of ICS at regular intervals.
- The emphasis on the use of SABA, except in episodic disease, will decrease.
- Increasing use of LABA. Used in conjunction with ICS (and combined forms) LABAs may have a role in 'aborting' the disease if used soon after symptoms begin.
- Alternatives to metered-dose aerosols that rely on good patient co-ordination, such as dry powder dispensers and mini-nebulizers are being developed.
- New non-steroidal antiinflammatory medications are in development. It makes sense to

develop drugs that help to control the allergic reaction in the airways so that less cytokines are released and inflammation prevented.

- Self-management by each patient. This is already happening and will continue as management plans become widely introduced.
- More emphasis on non-pharmacological treatments. The role of controlling the patient's home environment, of swimming and exercise programmes and of relaxation, will be much more widely accepted. It is possible that some patients with mild, episodic asthma may benefit in the long term from minimal intervention with drugs.
- Large population studies of management plans to determine those treatments that lead to the best long-term outcome will be undertaken.
- As the cost of drugs increases, patients, doctors and governments will need to be assured that the drugs being used have definite effects to prevent or treat symptoms or to reduce the severity of the disease. Thus the introduction of protocols which will allow doctors to determine the exact number and doses of drugs needed to obtain predetermined outcomes, seems inevitable.

REFERENCES

Ait-Khaled N, Enarson D. (1996) Management of asthma in adults: a guide for low income countries. International Union Against Tuberculosis and Lung Disease. Paris.

Alexander AG, Barnes NC, Kay AB. (1992) Trial of cyclosporin in corticosteroid-dependent chronic severe asthma. *Lancet*, **339**(8789), 324–8.

Anderson SD, du Toit JI, Rodwell LT, Jenkins CR. (1994) Acute effect of sodium cromoglycate on airway narrowing induced by 4.5% saline aerosol. Outcome before and during treatment with aerosol corticosteroids in patients with asthma. *Chest*, **105**, 673–80.

Anderson SD, Rodwell LT, Daviskas E, Spring JF, du Toit J. (1996) The protective effect of nedocromil sodium and other drugs on airway narrowing provoked by hyperosmolar stimuli: a role for the airway epithelium? *J Allergy Clin Immunol*, **98** (Suppl 5): S124–34.

Anderson SD, Rodwell LT, du Toit J, Young IH. (1991) Duration of protection by inhaled salmeterol in exercise-induced asthma. *Chest*, **100**, 1254–60.

Anderson SD. (1988) Exercise-induced asthma: stimulus, mechanism and management. In: Barnes PJ, Rodgers IW, Thomson NC, eds. *Asthma: basic mechanisms and clinical management*. London: Academic Press, 503–22.

Anonymous. (1996) Corticosteroid action and resistance in asthma. *Am J Respir Crit Care Med*, **154** (2 pt 2), S1–79.

Arvidsson P, Larsson S, Lofdahl C-G, Melander B, Wahlander L, Svedmyr N. (1989) Formoterol, a new long-acting bronchodilator for inhalation. *Eur Respir J*, **2**, 325–30.

Bailey WC, Richards JMJ, Brooks CM, Soong S-J, Windsor RA, Manzella BA. (1990) A randomized trial to improve self-management practices of adults with asthma. *Arch Intern Med*, **150**(8), 1664–8.

Barnes PJ. (1998) Efficacy of inhaled corticosteroids in asthma. *J Allergy Clin Immunol*, **102**(4 Pt 1), 531–8.

Barnes PJ, Pauwels RA. (1994) Theophylline in the management of asthma: time for reappraisal? *Eur Respir J*, **7**(3), 579–91.

Beasley R, Roche WR, Roberts JA, Holgate ST. (1989) Cellular events in the bronchi in mild asthma and after bronchial provocation. *Am Rev Respir Dis*, **139**, 806–17.

Beveridge RC, Grunfeld AF, Hodder RV, Verbeek PR. (1996) Guidelines for the emergency management of asthma in adults. *Can Med Assoc J*, **155**(1), 25–37.

Billing B, Dahlqvist R, Hornblad Y, Leidman T, Skareke L, Ripe E. (1987) Theophylline in maintenance treatment of chronic asthma: concentration-dependent additional effect of beta 2 agonist therapy. *Eur J Respir Dis*, **70**, 35–43.

Booij-Noord H, Orie NGM, De Vries K. (1971) Immediate and late bronchial obstructive reactions to inhalation of house dust and protective effects of disodium cromoglycate and prednisolone. *J Allergy Clin Immunol*, **48**, 344–54.

Boulet LP, Cartier A, Cockcroft DW, *et al*. (1990) Tolerance to reduction of oral steroid dosage in severely asthmatic patients receiving nedocromil sodium. *Respir Med*, **84**(4), 317–23.

British Thoracic Society. (1990) Guidelines for the treatment of asthma. 1. Chronic persistent asthma. *BMJ*, **301**, 651–3.

British Thoracic Society. (1997) The British Guidelines on Asthma Management. 1995 Review and Position Statement. *Thorax*, **52**, S1–21.

Busse W, Nelson H, Wolfe J, Kalberg C, Yancey S, Rickard KA. (1999) Comparison of inhaled salmeterol and oral zafirlukast in patients with asthma. *J Allergy Clin Immunol*, **103**, 1075–80.

Camargo CAJ, Weiss ST, Zhang S, Willett WC, Speizer FE. (1998) Prospective study of body mass index and risk of adult-onset asthma. *Am J Respir Crit Care Med*, **157**(3), A47.

Chan CS, Woolcock AJ, Sullivan CE. (1988) Nocturnal asthma: role of snoring and obstructive sleep apnea. *Am Rev Respir Dis*, **137**, 1502–4.

Chapman KR. (1990) The role of anticholinergic bronchodilators in adult asthma and chronic obstructive pulmonary disease. *Lung*, **168** (Suppl), 295–303.

Charous BL. (1990) Open study of hydroxy chloroquine in the treatment of severe symptomatic or corticosteroid-dependent asthma. *Ann Allergy*, **65**, 53–8.

Cheung D, Timmers MC, Zwinderman AH, Bel EH, Dijkman JH, Sterk PJ. (1992) Long-term effects of a long-acting β_2-adrenoceptor agonist, salmeterol, on airway hyperresponsiveness in patients with mild asthma. *N Engl J Med*, **327**, 1198–203.

Church MK, Young KD. (1983) The characteristics of inhibition of histamine release from human lung fragments by sodium cromoglycate, salbutamol and chlorpromazine. *Br J Pharmacol*, **78**, 671–9.

Crater SE, Platts-Mills TA. (1998) Searching for the cause of the increase in asthma. *Curr Opin Pediatr*, **10**(6), 594–9.

Crompton GK, Ayres JG, Basran G, Schiraldi G, Brusasco V, Eivindson A. (1999) Comparison of oral bambuterol and inhaled salmeterol in patients with symptomatic asthma using inhaled corticosteroids. *Am J Respir Crit Care Med*, **159**, 824–8.

Cumming RG, Mitchell P, Leeder SR. (1997) Use of inhaled corticosteroids and the risk of cataracts. *N Engl J Med*, **337**(1), 8–14.

Doerschug KC, Peterson MW, Dayton CS, Kline JN. (1999) Asthma guidelines: an assessment of physician understanding and practice. *Am J Respir Crit Care Med*, **159**(6), 1735–41.

Dorward AJ, Colloff MJ, MacKay NS, McSharry C, Thomson NC. (1988) Effect of house dust mite avoidance measures on adult atopic asthma. *Thorax*, **43**, 98–102.

Douglas NJ, Fitzpatrick MF. (1991) Effects of salmeterol on nocturnal asthma. *Eur Respir Rev*, **1**(4), 293–6.

Drazen JM, Israel E. (1998) Should antileukotriene therapies be used instead of inhaled corticosteroids in asthma? Yes. *Am J Respir Crit Care Med*, **158**(6), 1697–8.

du Toit JI, Anderson SD, Jenkins CR, Woolcock AJ, Rodwell LT. (1997) Airway responsiveness in asthma: bronchial challenge with histamine and 4.5% sodium chloride before and after budesonide. *Allergy Asthma Proc*, **18**(1), 7–14.

Eickelberg O, Roth M, Rainer L, *et al*. (1999) Ligand-independent activation of the glucocorticoid receptor by β_2-adrenergic receptor agonists in primary human lung fibroblasts and vascular smooth muscle cells. *J Biol Chem*, **274**(2), 1005–10.

Erzurum SC, Leff JA, Cochran JE, *et al*. (1991) Lack of benefit of methotrexate in severe, steroid-dependent asthma. A double-blind, placebo-controlled study. *Ann Intern Med*, **114**, 353–60.

Frankel D, Latimer K, Ruffin R. (1990) Does bronchial hyperresponsiveness improve following hospitalisation for acute asthma? *Aust NZ J Med*, **20** (Suppl), 522.

Gibson PG, Wong BJO, Hepperle MJE, *et al*. (1992) A research method to induce and examine a mild exacerbation of asthma by withdrawal of inhaled corticosteroid. *Clin Exp Allergy*, **22**, 525–32.

Grant SM, Goa KL, Fitton A, Sorkin EM. (1990) Ketotifen: a review of its pharmacodynamics and pharmacokinetic properties, and therapeutic use in asthma and allergic disorders [Review]. *Drugs*, **40**, 412–48.

Haahtela T. (1998) The long-term influence of therapeutic interventions in asthma with emphasis on inhaled steroids and early disease. *Clin Exp Allergy*, **28** (Suppl 5), 133–40, 171–3.

Hargreave FE, Dolovich J, Newhouse MT. (1990) The assessment and treatment of asthma: a conference report. *J Allergy Clin Immunol*, **85**, 1098–111.

Harvey JE, Tattersfield AE. (1982) Airway response to salbutamol: effect of regular salbutamol inhalations in normal, atopic, and asthmatic subjects. *Thorax*, **37**, 280–7.

Hendeles L, Weinberger M. (1983) Theophylline: a 'state of the art' review. *Pharmacotherapy*, **3**, 2–44.

Hoag JE, McFadden ER. (1991) Long-term effect of cromolyn sodium on nonspecific bronchial hyperresponsiveness; a review. *Ann Allergy*, **66**, 53–63.

Horn CR, Clark TJH, Cochrane GM. (1990) Compliance with inhaled therapy and morbidity from asthma. *Respir Med*, **84**, 67–70.

Howarth PH. (1990) Histamine and asthma: an appraisal based on specific H1-receptor antagonism. *Clin Exp Allergy*, **20** (Suppl 2), 31–41.

Howarth PH, Durham SR, Lee TH, Kay AB, Church MK, Holgate ST. (1985) Influence of albuterol, cromolyn sodium and ipratropium bromide on the airway and circulating mediator responses to allergen bronchial provocation in asthma. *Am Rev Res Dis*, **132**, 986–92.

Itkin IH, Menzel ML. (1970) The use of macrolide antibiotic substances in the treatment of asthma. *J Allergy*, **45**, 146–9.

Kemp JP, Minkwitz MC, Bonuccelli C, Warren MS. (1999) Therapeutic effect of zafirludast as monotherapy in steroid-naïve patients with severe persistent asthma. *Chest*, **115**(2), 336–42.

Kerrebijn KF, van Essen-Zandvliet EEM, Neijens HJ. (1987) Effect of long-term treatment with inhaled glucocorticosteroids and beta-agonists on bronchial responsiveness in asthmatic children. *J Allergy Clin Immunol*, **79**, 653–9.

Klaustermeyer WB, Noritake DT, Kwong FK. (1987) Chrysotherapy in the treatment of corticosteroid-dependent asthma. *J Allergy Clin Immunol*, **79**, 720–5.

Knorr B, Matz J, Bernstein JA, *et al*. (1998) Montelukast for chronic asthma in 6- to14-year-old children. *JAMA*, **279**(15), 1181–6.

Kotses H, Bernstein IL, Bernstein DI, *et al*. (1995) A self-management program for adult asthma. Part 1, Development and evaluation. *J Allergy Clin Immunol*, **95**, 529–40.

Kraan J, Koeter GH, van der Mark TW, Sluiter HJ, De Vries K. (1985) Changes in bronchial hyperreactivity induced by 4 weeks of treatment with antiasthmatic drugs in patients with allergic asthma: a comparison between budesonide and terbutaline. *J Allergy Clin Immunol*, **76**(4), 628–36.

Kurosawa M. (1994) Anti-allergic drug use in Japan – the rationale and the clinical outcome. *Clin Exp Allergy*, **24**, 299–306.

Laitinen LA, Heino M, Laitinen A, Kava T, Haahtela T. (1985) Damage of the airway epithelium and bronchial reactivity in patients with asthma. *Am Rev Respir Dis*, **131**, 599–606.

Leff JA, Busse WW, Pearlman D, *et al*. (1998) Montelukast, a leukotriene-receptor antagonist, for the treatment of mild asthma and exercise-induced bronchoconstriction. *N Engl J Med*, **339**, 147–52.

Legorreta AP, Christian-Herman J, O'Connor RD, Hasan MM, Evans R, Leung KM. (1998) Compliance with national asthma management guidelines and specialty care: a health maintenance organization experience. *Arch Intern Med*, **158**(5), 457–64.

Lipworth BJ. (1999) Leukotriene-receptor antagonists. *Lancet*, **353**, 57–62.

Mahmic A, Tovey ER, Molloy CA, Young L. (1998) House dust mite allergen exposure in infancy. *Clin Exp Allergy*, **28**(12), 1487–92.

Malmstrom K, Rodriguez-Gomez G, Guerra J, *et al*. (1999) Oral montelukast, inhaled beclomethasone, and placebo for chronic asthma: a randomized controlled trial. *Ann Intern Med*, **130**(6), 487–95.

Martin RJ, Cicutto LC, Ballard RD. (1990) Factors related to the nocturnal worsening of asthma. *Am Rev Respir Dis*, **141**, 33–8.

Mayo PH, Richman J, Harris HW. (1990) Results of a program to reduce admissions for adult asthma. *Ann Intern Med*, **112**(11), 864–71.

McFadden ER, Casale TB, Edwards TB, *et al*. (1999) Administration of budesonide once daily by means of Turbuhaler to subjects with stable asthma. *J Allergy Clin Immunol*, **104**, 46–52.

McFadden ER Jr., Strauss L, Hejal R, Galan G, Dixon L. (1998) Comparison of two dosage regimens of albuterol in acute asthma. *Am J Med*, **105**(1), 12–17.

Muhlhauser I, Richter B, Kraut D, Weske G, Worth H, Berger M. (1991) Evaluation of a structured treatment and teaching programme on asthma. *J Intern Med*, **230**(2), 157–64.

Mullarkey MF, Blumenstein BA, Andrade WP, Bailey GA, Olason I, Wetzel CE. (1988) Methotrexate in the treatment of corticosteroid-dependent asthma. A double-blind crossover study. *N Engl J Med*, **318**, 603–7.

Mullarkey MF, Lammert JK, Blumenstein BA. (1990) Long-term methotrexate treatment in corticosteroid-dependent asthma. *Ann Intern Med*, **112**, 577–81.

Murray AM, Ferguson AC. (1982) Reduction of bronchial hyperreactivity during prolonged allergen avoidance (Letter). *Lancet*, **2**, 1212.

Nathan RA, Bernstein JA, Bielory L, *et al*. (1998) Zafirlukast improves asthma symptoms and quality of life in patients with moderate reversible airflow obstruction. *J Allergy Clin Immunol*, **102**, 935–42.

National Asthma Campaign. (1998) Asthma management handbook 1998. South Melbourne: National Asthma Campaign.

National Heart, Lung and Blood Institute. (1995) Global initiative for asthma. Global strategy for asthma management and prevention NHLBI/WHO workshop report. March 1993. Bethesda, MD: National Institutes of Health.

Nicolai T, Illi S, von Mutius E. (1998) Effect of dampness at home in childhood on bronchial hyperreactivity in adolescence. *Thorax*, **53**, 1035–40.

O'Shaughnessy KM, Wellings R, Gillies B, Fuller RW. (1993) Differential effects of fluticasone propionate on allergen-evoked bronchoconstriction and increased urinary leukotriene E4 excretion. *Am Rev Respir Dis*, **147**, 1472–6.

Peat J, Bjorksten B. (1998) Primary and secondary prevention of allergic asthma. *Eur Respir J*, **27**, 28S–34S.

Peat JK, Dickerson J, Li J. (1998) Effects of damp and mould in the home on respiratory health: a review of the literature. *Allergy*, **53**(2), 120–8.

Peat JK, Woolcock AJ. (1991) Sensitivity to common allergens: relation to respiratory symptoms and bronchial hyperresponsiveness in children from three different climatic areas of Australia. *Clin Exp Allergy*, **21**, 573–81.

Platts-Mills TAE, Tovey ER, Mitchell EB, Moszoro H, Nock P, Wilkins SR. (1982) Reduction of bronchial hyperreactivity during prolonged allergen avoidance. *Lancet*, **2**, 675–8.

Prieto L, Gutierrez V, Morales C. (1999) Maximal response plateau to methacholine as a reliable index for reducing inhaled budesonide in moderate asthma. *Eur Respir J*, **13**, 1236–44.

Reddel HK, Salome CM, Peat JK, Woolcock AJ. (1995) Which index of peak expiratory flow is most useful in the management of stable asthma? *Am J Resp Crit Care Med*, **151**(5), 1320–5.

Reddel HK, Ware SI, Marks GB, *et al*. (1999) Long-term back-titration of inhaled corticosteroids – the effect of starting dose. *Eur Respir J*, **14** (Suppl 30), 1S.

Reiss TF, Chervinsky P, Dockhorn RJ, Shingo S, Seidenberg B, Edwards TB. (1998) Montelukast, a once-daily leukotriene receptor antagonist, in the treatment of chronic asthma: a multicenter, randomized, double-blind trial. Montelukast Clinical Research Study Group. *Arch Intern Med*, **158**(11), 1213–20.

Ringsberg KC, Wiklund I, Wihelmsen L. (1990) Education of adult patients at an 'asthma school': effects on quality of life, knowledge and need for nursing. *Eur Respir J*, **3**(1), 33–7.

Ryan G, Latimer KM, Juniper EF, Roberts RS, Hargreave FE. (1985) Effect of beclomethasone dipropionate on bronchial responsiveness to histamine in controlled nonsteroid-dependent asthma. *J Allergy Clin Immunol*, **75**, 25–30.

Saetta M, Stefano AD, Rosina C, Thiene G, Fabbri LM. (1991) Quantitive structural analysis of peripheral airways and arteries in sudden fatal asthma. *Am Rev Respir Dis*, **143**, 138–43.

Sawyer G, Miles J, Lewis S, Fitzharris P, Pearce N, Beasley R. (1998) Classification of asthma severity: should the international guidelines be changed? *Clin Exp Allergy*, **28**(12), 1565–70.

Schwartz YA, Kivity S, Ilfeld DN, *et al.* (1990) A clinical and immunologic study of colchicine in asthma. *J Allergy Clin Immunol*, **85**(3), 578–82.

Sears MR, Herbison GP, Holdaway MD, Hewitt CJ, Flannery EM, Silva PA. (1989) The relative risks of sensitivity to grass pollen, house dust mite and cat dander in the development of childhood asthma. *Clin Exp Allergy*, **19**, 419–24.

Sears MR, Taylor DR, Print CG, *et al.* (1990) Regular inhaled beta-agonist treatment in bronchial asthma. *Lancet*, **336**, 1391–6.

Shiner RJ, Nunn AJ, Fan Chung K, Geddes DM. (1990) Randomised, double-blind, placebo-controlled trial of methotrexate in steroid-dependent asthma. *Lancet*, **336**, 137–40.

Siersted HC, Hansen HS, Hansen N-CG, Hyldebrandt N, Mostgaard G, Oxho H. (1994) Evaluation of peak expiratory flow variability in an adolescent population sample. The Odense schoolchild study. *Am J Respir Crit Care Med*, **149**, 598–603.

Skinner MH. (1990) Adverse reactions and interactions with theophylline. *Drug Safe*, **5**(4), 275–85.

Smith LJ. (1998) The prospects for long-term intervention in asthma with antileukotrienes. *Clin Exp Allergy*, **28** (Suppl 5), 154–63; 171–3.

Sont JK, Willems LN, Bel EH, van Krieken JH, Vandenbroucke JP, Sterk PJ. (1999) Clinical control and histopathologic outcome of asthma when using airway hyperresponsiveness as an additional guide to long-term treatment. The AMPUL Study Group. *Am J Respir Crit Care Med*, **159**(4 Pt 1), 1043–51.

Spector SL, Smith LJ, Glass M. (1994) Effects of 6 weeks of therapy with oral doses of ICI 204, 219, a leukotriene D4 receptor antagonist, in subjects with bronchial asthma. ACCOLATE Asthma Trialists Group. *Am J Respir Crit Care Med*, **150**(3), 618–23.

Sporik R, Holgate ST, Platts-Mills TAE, Cogswell JJ. (1990) Exposure to house-dust mite allergen (Der p I) and the development of asthma in childhood. A prospective study. *N Engl J Med*, **323**, 502–7.

Stewart GE, Diaz JD, Lockey RF, Seleznick MJ, Trudeau WL, Ledford DK. (1994) Comparison of oral pulse methotrexate with placebo in the treatment of severe glucocorticosteroid-dependent asthma. *J Allergy Clin Immunol*, **94**, 482–9.

Storr J, Barrell E, Barry W, Lenney W, Hatcher G. (1987) Effect of a single oral dose of prednisolone in acute childhood asthma. *Lancet*, **1**, 879–82.

Svendsen UG, Frolund L, Madsen F, Nielsen NH. (1989) A comparison of the effects of nedocromil sodium and beclomethasone diproprionate on pulmonary function, symptoms, and bronchial responsiveness in patients with asthma. *J Allergy Clin Immunol*, **84**(2), 224–31.

Svenonius E, Kautto R, Abborelius MJ. (1983) Improvement after training of children with exercise-induced asthma. *Acta Paediatr Scand*, **72**, 23–30.

Toogood JH, Baskerville J, Jennings B, Lefcoe NM, Johansson SA. (1984) Use of spacers to facilitate inhaled corticosteroid treatment of asthma. *Am Rev Respir Dis*, **129**, 723–9.

Toogood JH, Jennings B, Baskerville J, Newhouse M. (1981) Assessment of a device for reducing oropharyngeal complications during beclomethasone treatment of asthma. *Am Rev Respir Dis*, **123**, 113.

Toogood JH, Jennings B, Greenway RW, Chuang L. (1980) Candidiasis and dysphonia complicating beclomethasone treatment of asthma. *J Allergy Clin Immunol*, **65**, 145–53.

Toogood JH. (1998) Side-effects of inhaled corticosteroids. *J Allergy Clin Immunol*, **102**(5), 705–13.

Twentyman OP, Finnerty JP, Harris A, Palmer J, Holgate ST. (1990) Protection against allergen-induced asthma by salmeterol. *Lancet*, **336**, 1338–42.

Ullman A, Hedner J, Svedmyr N. (1990) Inhaled salmeterol and salbutamol in asthmatic patients. An evaluation of asthma symptoms and the possible development of tachyphylaxis. *Am Rev Respir Dis*, **142**, 571–5.

US Department of Health and Human Services. (1991) Executive summary: guidelines for the diagnosis and management of asthma. National Asthma Education Program Expert Panel Report.

US Department of Health and Human Services. (1991) Guidelines for the diagnosis and management of asthma.

van der Molen T, Meyboom-de Jong B, Mulder HH, Postma DS. (1998) Starting with a higher dose of inhaled corticosteroids in primary care asthma treatment. *Am J Respir Crit Care Med*, **158**(1), 121–5.

Wallaert B, Brun P, Ostinelli J, *et al*. (1999) A comparison of two long-acting B-agonists, oral bambuterol and inhaled salmeterol, in the treatment of moderate to severe asthmatic patients with nocturnal symptoms. *Respir Med*, **93**, 33–8.

Wechsler M, Drazen JM. (1999) Churg–Strauss syndrome [letter]. *Lancet*, **353**(9168), 1970–1.

Wenzel SE. (1998) Should antileukotriene therapies be used instead of inhaled corticosteroids in asthma? No. *Am J Respir Crit Care Med*, **158**(6), 1699–701.

Wilding P, Clark M, Coon JT, *et al*. (1997) Effect of long term treatment with salmeterol on asthma control: a double blind, randomised crossover study. *BMJ*, **314**, 1441–6.

Wilson SR, Scamagas P, German DF, *et al*. (1993) A controlled trial of two forms of self-management education for adults with asthma. *Am J Med*, **94**, 564–76.

Wong CS, Pavord ID, Williams J, Britton JR, Tattersfield AE. (1990) Bronchodilator, cardiovascular, and hypokalaemic effects of fenoterol, salbutamol, and terbutaline in asthma. *Lancet*, **336**: 1396–9.

Woolcock AJ, Jenkins CR. (1991) Clinical responses to corticosteroids. In: Kaliner MA, Barnes PJ, Persson CGA, eds. *Asthma, its pathology and treatment. Lung Biology in health and disease, Vol.* 49. New York: Marcel Dekker, 633–65.

Woolcock AJ, Rubinfeld AR, Seale JP, *et al*. (1989) Asthma management plan, 1989. *Med J Aust*, **151**, 650–3.

Woolley M, Anderson SD, Quigley BM. (1990) Duration of protective effect of terbutaline sulfate and cromolyn sodium alone and in combination on exercise-induced asthma. *Chest*, **97**, 39–45.

Childhood asthma

S. GODFREY

INTRODUCTION

Asthma is by far the commonest of all chronic diseases of childhood and the importance of asthma in children both to the individual child, the family and the community cannot be overemphasized. In most developed societies asthma is a very common cause of chronic ill health. In one study in young children it was found that some two-thirds of all drugs prescribed were for the treatment of wheezing and 7% of all children had missed school (for a median period of 7 days in a year) because of wheezing (Hill *et al.*, 1989). While in almost all paediatric diseases there has been a reduction in the time children spend in hospital, this has not been true for hospital admission for asthma, which steadily increased from the mid-1970s at least up until the start of the 1990s (Burr, 1987; Henderson *et al.*, 1992; Lung and Asthma Information Agency, 1996). In a survey from Wales, Burr *et al.* found that the rate of hospital discharges for children with a diagnosis of asthma had increased approximately fourfold over the 16 years from 1970 to 1984 and in a population survey they showed that between 1973 and 1988 the incidence of current wheezing had risen from 4 to 9% (Burr, 1987; Burr *et al.*, 1989). An almost identical increase in the incidence of childhood asthma of approximately 6% per year has also been found between 1988 and 1995 (Venn *et al.*, 1998). In the United States, Richards (1989) found that the hospitalization rate for children with status asthmaticus was approximately doubling every 10 years for the period 1966 to 1986. This increase appeared to be genuine and not simply due to a change in diagnostic criteria. Even more worrying was the increase in asthma mortality in children and young people found by surveys in a number of countries (Burney, 1986; Sears *et al.*, 1986; Burr, 1987). In New Zealand, the epidemic of asthma deaths which reached its peak in the late 1970s primarily affected young people. On a more optimistic note, Anderson *et al.* (1994) in a study of Croydon (UK) children aged 7.5 to 8.5 years reported an approximate increase in asthma of about 16% over a 13-year period from 1978 to 1991 but a substantial decrease in morbidity suggesting better management.

The cost of treating children with asthma places a very considerable burden on the health resources in developed countries owing to the cost of medications, hospitalizations and the time spent by parents and other caretakers in looking after the asthmatic child. In a recent survey of the cost of chronic illnesses in over 300 000 children in the Washington State Medicaid healthcare programme, asthma accounted for 12.5% of the total annual health expenditure, and apart from prematurity-related diseases was many times more costly to the programme than all other chronic diseases of childhood (Iryes *et al.*, 1997). Although the cost of caring for the individual asthmatic child was not particularly great, the number of asthmatics was much greater than the number with other diseases and hence the total cost was much higher.

INCIDENCE OF CHILDHOOD ASTHMA

While almost everyone agrees that asthma in childhood is very common its true incidence is quite difficult to determine. Hospital-based surveys are of little use for this purpose as they reflect the incidence of more severe asthma and ignore the majority of children whose asthma is managed in the community. Community-based surveys are also problematical because they often consider the incidence in a specific age range and are usually based on answers to questionnaires filled in by parents. A survey in Scotland by Ninan and Russel (1992a) of 8–13-year-olds showed that 10% reported asthma at some time in their life and 20% reported current wheezing. A similar study in Australia by Peat *et al.* (1994) reported an even higher rate of current wheezing of 23–28% but when they measured bronchial reactivity objectively by histamine inhalation only 9–12% of children were classified as currently asthmatic, by having both current wheezing and bronchial hyperreactivity. In the analysis of the Medicaid claims for the treatment of children aged 0–18 years in the Washington study (Iryes *et al.*, 1997), 4.6% were for asthma, suggesting that at least 4.6% of the childhood population required some medication each year for asthma. This figure may have underestimated the true incidence of asthma in this population, considering some asthmatics do not require treatment and others may well have been misdiagnosed as having 'bronchitis' or 'pneumonia'. Results from the International Study of Asthma and Allergies in Childhood (ISAAC) are now available (ISAAC, 1998) and show major differences in the point prevalence of asthma in 13–14-year-old children. The highest incidence is some 30–35% in the UK, Australia and New Zealand and the lowest incidence is some 2–5% in Russia, China and Greece.

In order to attempt to determine both the lifetime prevalence and the point prevalence of asthma we undertook a total population survey from one area of all Israeli boys aged 17 years who by law must be examined for suitability for military service by physicians at an army recruiting office (Auerbach *et al.*, 1993). We examined over 13 000 boys in 1986 and over 21 000 in 1990. Any boy reporting a symptom at any time up to age 17 which could have been due to asthma was examined again by a trained pulmonary physician, performed spirometry and where there was doubt also undertook a 6 minute treadmill run to detect exercise-induced asthma. We also studied 17-year-old girls in the population but the results were not included in the original publication as about 15% of the population of girls were exempted from military service for religious reasons. Our survey (Fig. 16.1) showed a lifetime incidence of asthma in 1990 of 9.6% in boys and 6.0% in girls and a point incidence of asthma at age 17 of 5.9% in boys and 3.7% in girls. It is important to note that the point prevalence of asthma at age 17 was less than the lifetime prevalence and moreover, many of those still asthmatic at age 17 were very mildly affected, suggesting that children do indeed grow out of asthma. As in previous studies asthma was far commoner in boys than girls.

One of the problems with childhood asthma is that the diagnosis is frequently missed. The reason behind the inadequacy in the diagnosis of asthma in children is not clear but it may stem, in part, from the fact that the young asthmatic child often presents with cough as his primary symptom rather than wheeze. This often leads to the erroneous diagnosis of bronchitis or pneumonia, especially since so many attacks in childhood are precipitated by viral infections (Johnson et al., 1995) and are accompanied by fever. In a survey of North Tyneside (UK) children, Speight et al. (1983) found only a very small proportion of wheezing children had been diagnosed as having asthma and some two-thirds had never been treated with a bronchodilator. Similar results were found by Anderson et al. (1983) from a survey in Croyden while Hill et al. (1989) found that about half of the children in Nottingham (UK) who reported wheezing had been diagnosed as asthmatic but treatment still appeared to be inadequate in many cases. A similar picture was found in a survey comparing the prevalence of asthma in New Zealand and Australia (Asher et al., 1988). However, the more recent study by Anderson et al. (1994) suggests that this trend may be reversing and that better management is reducing morbidity.

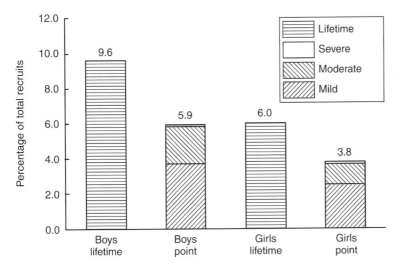

Figure 16.1 *Lifetime prevalence and current severity of asthma in a large population of 17-year-old Israeli recruits for National Service (21 807 boys and 17 985 girls, estimated from corrected 1988 data). Less than half of one percent still required high-dose corticosteroid therapy at age 17 and almost 80% of both boys and girls were symptom-free or virtually so. (Redrawn from the data of Auerbach* et al. *(1993) supplemented with additional data.)*

Death from asthma in childhood is relatively rare but given that the incidence of asthma in children has been rising steadily for many years there might have been an increase in asthma mortality in this age group. Hospital admissions of children for asthma in England and Wales between 1962 and 1993 have been obtained from nationally collected data (Lung and Asthma Information Agency, 1996) and show an increase which was particularly marked from the mid-1970s to mid-1980s where it appeared to have trebled in children aged 0–14 years. Since the start of the 1990s it appears that the admission rate has stopped rising. After the end of the epidemic of asthma deaths in the early 1960s in England and Wales death rates in children derived from the nationally collected data (Lung and Asthma Information Agency, 1992) showed no real change between 1970 and 1990. This, taken with the rising incidence of asthma in the childhood population over this period, suggests that the risk of dying from asthma for an asthmatic child *admitted to hospital* may actually have been falling. Even more important is the finding by Campbell *et al.* (1997) from a study of age-specific mortality from the Office for National Statistics that there has been a real decline in asthma mortality in children of about 6% per annum from 1988 to 1995 at a time when the incidence in the population has been increasing at about 6% per annum (Burr *et al.*, 1989; Venn *et al.*, 1998).

GENERAL FORM OF CHILDHOOD ASTHMA

In the general population about 80% of asthmatic children begin to have symptoms before the age of 4–5 years and only about 10% begin wheezing for the first time in later childhood (Dawson *et al.*, 1969; Blair, 1974; Cserhati *et al.*, 1984). While asthma is commoner in boys than girls, but less common in men than women (Dodge and Burrows, 1980), there does not appear to be any difference in the severity of asthma between boys and girls. The asthmatic child is usually atopic, often first presenting with infantile eczema, which is found in about 60% of hospital attenders in the UK. The eczema usually begins shortly after birth, usually on the cheeks, and may become more generalized before settling into the classical flexural areas of the arms and legs in older children. Although eczema tends to disappear after 2 or 3 years and is gone in almost all asthmatics by 7 or 8 years of age, it does persist in a few children, often the more severe cases (Aberg and Engstrom, 1990). There is a reciprocal relationship in many children between eczema and asthma with one condition alternating with the other in severity. Marked infantile eczema from birth tends to be associated with more troublesome asthma later on (McNicol and Williams, 1973a). Curiously, eczema is much less prominent in warmer climates although children appear to have equally severe asthma. There is often a background of atopic diseases in the family of the asthmatic child. The odds ratio (OR, no increased risk OR = 1.0) for a child having asthma was found to be 2.6 if one first degree relative had asthma and 5.2 if two first degree relatives had asthma (Dold *et al.*, 1992).

The younger asthmatic child is often very troubled by cough, especially at night, rather than frank wheezing and so the diagnosis is often given as 'bronchitis' or 'spastic bronchitis' rather than asthma. There is grave doubt as to whether children even suffer from 'chronic bronchitis' in the adult sense (Taussig *et al.*, 1981). In children with chronic cough but no other lung disease, lung function tests and bronchial provocation challenges by exercise will often produce a typical asthmatic picture (Cloutier and Loughlin, 1981). In a study of children from Australia and New Zealand, no less than 41% of those who reported nocturnal cough were found to have bronchial hyperreactivity to histamine (Asher *et al.*, 1988). This is of practical importance as cough due to asthma should be treated by anti-asthmatic medication and not by 'cough' medicines or antibiotics. On the other hand there are obviously other causes of cough and respiratory symptoms in the young child as discussed below and these must be distinguished by appropriate clinical and laboratory investigations. The cough or 'chesty' episodes in the young child with asthma are typically episodic with symptom-free intervals and are often more common in the winter, presumably related to the increase in viral infections. The older child with asthma typically has episodic attacks of wheezing and breathlessness, usually worse at night or early morning and often accompanied by cough but little or no sputum production. The attacks are separated by symptom-free intervals and the duration of the attack varies from patient to patient. In most children attacks are infrequent but in the more severely affected child symptoms may become more or less continuous. Response to appropriate antiasthmatic medication is usually excellent. Some children, especially the older physically active teenager, may have little or no problem with asthma except in relation to physical exercise (see Chapter 3).

CLASSIFICATION OF ASTHMA SEVERITY

The nature of the attacks of asthma and the pattern of recurrence varies considerably from child to child and this has an important bearing on treatment. In order to develop a rational approach to management it is necessary to have a reasonable and practical method of classification. In recent years a number of national and international committees have prepared guidelines for the management of asthma of which one of the first was a consensus statement for the management of asthma in children (Warner *et al.*, 1989). These guidelines for children have been updated in several subsequent publications but the changes are generally rather small (International Paediatric Asthma Consensus Group, 1992; British Thoracic Society, 1993, 1997; Warner *et al.*, 1998). Apart from addressing the diagnosis and treatment of asthma these guidelines have also attempted to provide a classification of asthma severity in children which is quite similar to that recommended in previous editions of this book and the following represents an edited summary of the various definitions.

The overall severity of asthma may be described in terms of the amount of disturbance the disease causes the child and family without taking into account the severity of the individual attack of asthma which is considered separately. These descriptions mostly relate to the child who has not yet been established on optimal treatment.

Mild asthma

Discrete attacks for no more than 1–2 days occurring no more often than once per month with symptom-free intervals or very brief attacks occurring no more than twice per week. Attacks respond readily to β₂-agonist therapy and do not cause the child to miss more than the occasional day of schooling.

Moderate asthma

Attacks more often than twice weekly with occasional more prolonged exacerbations and requiring frequent or daily medication for relief of symptoms. Such children may well miss occasional days of schooling without adequate treatment.

Severe asthma

Continuous or virtually continuous symptoms with occasional prolonged severe exacerbations and requiring daily medication for relief of symptoms which only respond adequately to corticosteroids. Such children often miss some schooling and are normally unable to keep pace with their peers without adequate treatment.

Mild and moderate asthma may well be seasonal with complete or virtually complete freedom from symptoms once the relevant season (often spring or winter) is over. Severe asthma is rarely seasonal although the severity of symptoms (and need for treatment) may fluctuate from time to time. There are two other forms of asthma which do not fit readily into the above classification and are seen from time to time in children.

Exercise-induced asthma (EIA)

Exercise is a potent stimulus for a short attack of bronchospasm (*see* Chapter 3) and occurs in most asthmatics if they exercise hard enough. Some children, mostly fit, young adolescents have little or no clinical asthma on a day-to-day basis but may be severely handicapped by EIA when they take part in sports. These children can easily be dismissed as neurotic if the condition is not recognized and managed appropriately.

Sudden life-threatening asthma

A few asthmatics suffer from infrequent but devastatingly severe attacks of asthma. Often the onset of an attack is unpredictable, although this form of asthma may occur in the child with marked specific allergy such as from eating nuts. The child may require admission to an intensive care unit and ventilatory support but it is not uncommon for the child to be totally symptom-free in the intervals between attacks. They represent a very high-risk group and their management is problematical.

Whatever the overall pattern of asthma in the child the severity of the individual attacks of asthma varies from time to time. The following represents an edited summary of the various definitions which have been proposed.

Mild/moderate non-life-threatening attack:

- wheezing or coughing without severe distress
- able to talk normally
- little or no tachypnea
- no desaturation (if measured)
- peak flow >70% predicted (if measured)
- excellent response to β_2-agonist therapy

Moderate/severe non-life-threatening attack:

- wheezing or coughing with moderate distress
- unable to talk normally, speaks in phrases
- moderate tachypnea and tachycardia
- saturation 90–95% (if measured)

- peak flow 50–70% predicted (if measured)
- modest response to β_2-agonist therapy

Potentially life-threatening attack:

- severe respiratory distress/retractions
- unable to talk
- exhaustion/confusion
- cyanosis of lips or tongue (in room air)
- silent chest/poor respiratory effort
- marked tachypnea and tachycardia
- saturation <90% (if measured)
- peak flow <33% predicted (if measured)
- no response to β_2-agonist therapy

It is important to note that there is no direct link between the overall severity of the asthma and the severity of the attacks as defined above. It is true that most children with mild asthma suffer from mild attacks but it is not at all rare for such a child to have a moderate or severe attack from time to time and this does not alter the fact that the pattern of attack frequency is still mild. At the other end of the scale, most children with severe asthma have mild or moderate attacks that are nevertheless so frequent as to disturb their everyday activities and only rarely are the attacks both frequent and severe.

CONTRIBUTING FACTORS IN CHILDHOOD ASTHMA

Bronchial hyperreactivity

As with asthma in adults, the basis of asthma in children is bronchial hyperreactivity which means that the intrathoracic airways of the asthmatic child narrow to a far greater degree than those of a normal child in response to various known and unknown stimuli. There has been some confusion in the literature as to the meaning of bronchial reactivity in epidemiological terms and the results of non-specific bronchial provocation tests have sometimes been interpreted to show that quite a large proportion of non-asthmatic children are 'hyperreactive' while some asthmatics are not hyperreactive (Lee et al., 1983; Asher et al., 1988). However, at least some of this confusion is due to the arbitrary choice of a cut-off level to define an abnormal response to methacholine or histamine rather than using a definition based on statistical techniques (see Chapter 3). Given that we define asthma as an unusual degree of reversible airways obstruction, then asthmatics must have, by definition, bronchial hyperreactivity, and whether we measure this clinically or physiologically is immaterial.

   We now know that asthma in children, as in adults, is characterized by an immunological type of inflammation of the airways in which there is damage to the epithelium, basement-membrane thickening and infiltration with lymphocytes, eosinophils and mast cells, amongst others. These pathological changes are associated with bronchial hyperreactivity to non-specific challenges by methacholine or histamine. Foresi et al. (1990) undertook bronchial biopsies in adult asthmatics during remission and found an excellent correlation between bronchial hyperreactivity and both the shedding of epithelial cells into bronchoalveolar lavage fluid and intraepithelial cellularity. These pathological changes in the airway in asthma can be largely or completely reversed by treatment with corticosteroids which is accompanied by a reduction though not complete eradication of bronchial hyperreactivity. The bronchial hyperreactivity in children with asthma differs in an important respect from the bronchial hyperreactivity that can be demonstrated in some children with other types of paediatric chronic obstructive pulmonary diseases (PCOPD), such as cystic fibrosis or primary ciliary dyskinesia. We have shown that non-specific bronchial hyperreactivity to methacholine is present in children with PCOPD, often to the level found in asthma, but hyperreactivity to physical exercise or inhaled adenosine-5'-monophosphate is highly specific and only present in asthmatic children (Avital *et al.*, 1995). The finding of some types of bronchial hyperreactivity in other chronic lung diseases of childhood does not mean that they are asthmatics.

Genetic background

It must be admitted that we do not know why the asthmatic airways are hyperreactive, whether this is from birth or acquired, nor why it seems to disappear during later childhood or puberty in most children as they 'grow out' of their asthma (Balfour-Lynn *et al.*, 1980). A number of years ago we noticed that there was a relatively high incidence of atopy and bronchial hyperreactivity amongst the totally healthy relatives of asthmatic children and wheezy infants (Konig and Godfrey, 1974). We also noticed a much higher concordance for asthma and bronchial hyperreactivity in identical twins (57–71%) as compared with fraternal twins (0–19%) (Konig and Godfrey, 1974). However, concordance was not perfect in the identical twins suggesting that environmental trigger factors may be needed to act on the genetic predisposition to develop asthma. The more recent Finnish studies of twins by Nieminen *et al.* (1991) found a heritability estimate of about 36% for asthma while a Swedish study calculated a heritability index for asthma of 76% in boys and 62% in girls (Lichtenstein and Svartengren, 1997). Over the last few years the hunt has really been on to find where the supposed genes controlling asthma in children are hiding with various studies suggesting links between atopy or bronchial hyperreactivity and certain markers on different chromosomes (Cookson, 1995; Postma *et al.*, 1995; van Herwerden *et al.*, 1995). It now seems very likely that childhood asthma is (a) closely allied to and probably coinherited with atopy and (b) that the gene(s) is permissive in nature since concordance in identical twins is not perfect and therefore some environmental factor(s) is needed to activate them.

Allergy

There is no doubt that inflammation related to allergic processes is of fundamental importance in asthma, especially in childhood asthma. The problem is to determine the importance of specific allergies in the initiation and persistence of the asthma. The large majority of asthmatic children come from an atopic family background (Dold *et al.*, 1992) and positive skin tests to one or more common allergens are found in about 93% of patients (Russell and Jones, 1976). It is interesting that the incidence of positive skin tests increases in older children, just at the time that their asthma is tending to improve. Only some 5–7% of children are skin-test negative 'intrinsic' asthmatics which is considerably less common than in adults. Most children react to a number of allergens, including the house dust mite, moulds and pollens, but reaction to *Aspergillus* is rare, and classical allergic bronchopulmonary aspergillosis is even rarer. The importance of house dust mite allergy is as yet undetermined, but it is tempting to link it to the nocturnal exacerbation of cough or wheeze which is so common in childhood asthma. The role of specific allergies in provoking individual attacks of asthma in children is hotly disputed between those who believe this to be of major importance and those who see little objective evidence to support this concept. Perhaps the most important feature of allergic responses in the asthmatic child is that allergenic stimulation not only produces an immediate and often a late response but also increases airway inflammation and hence the general level of bronchial hyperreactivity for days or even weeks (Cockcroft *et al.*, 1977; Mussaffi *et al.*, 1986). This means that allergic stimulation, even if it only produces mild or insignificant symptoms, may be responsible for the persistence of increased responsiveness to a whole variety of other, non-specific stimuli. It has been well documented that asthmatics with allergic asthma are more likely to develop exercise-induced asthma when the relevant allergen is present in the environment (Karjalainen *et al.*, 1989; Benckhuijsen *et al.*, 1996). It is quite reasonable to consider the possibility that frequent exposure to house dust mites at night in a mite-sensitive child might well be responsible for the sensitivity to exercise and other stimuli.

Smoking and pollution

While there is no evidence that environmental pollution can cause a child to become asthmatic without a familial or genetic predisposition it is now certain that pollution, especially by tobacco smoke, can increase the incidence of lower respiratory tract disease and provoke attacks of asthma. Even passive cigarette smoking in adult asthmatics has been shown to provoke a fall in lung function and increase their level of non-specific bronchial reactivity (Menon *et al.*, 1992). Murray and Morrison (1986) studied a group of asthmatic children and found that those whose mothers smoked had more symptoms and poorer lung function than those whose mothers did not smoke and these symptoms correlated with the number of cigarettes smoked. This increase in incidence of asthma and lower respiratory tract illnesses in children exposed to environmental tobacco smoke in the home or in day care centres has now been demonstrated in several studies (Martinez *et al.*, 1992; Chilmonczyk *et al.*, 1993; Holberg *et al.*, 1993). Bronchial reactivity is also higher in infants of parents who smoke (Young *et al.*, 1991). Of considerable interest is the observation that even smoking during pregnancy can influence lung function and the incidence of asthma in children after birth. Both reduced resting lung function and increased bronchial reactivity have been demonstrated in the infants of mothers who smoked during pregnancy (Tager *et al.*, 1993; Stick *et al.*, 1996). Environmental pollution other than from cigarettes has also been associated with an increased incidence of asthma in children, especially when combined with maternal smoking (Schmitzberger *et al.*, 1993). Exposure to sulphur dioxide interacts with other stimuli, such as exercise, to increase bronchial responsiveness (Sheppard *et al.*, 1981; Roger *et al.*, 1985). Even the long held belief that poor housing conditions are associated with increased incidence of asthma has now been confirmed objectively. Williamson *et al.* (1997) studied asthmatics and controls and found that dampness in the home confirmed by a surveyor was significantly associated with the incidence and severity of asthma. However, some caution is warranted considering the recent European air pollution study (PEACE) failed to show any correlation between pollution levels and the incidence of childhood asthma (Viegi, 1998).

Infection

One of the commonest provoking factors for asthma attacks in young children is viral infection (Horn *et al.*, 1979). The mechanism by which viruses induce asthma attacks is unknown, although the respiratory syncytial virus (RSV) can induce immunological changes in the host (Welliver *et al.*, 1979, 1981). In a controlled prospective follow-up study at age 3 years of children infected with RSV as infants, there was a significantly increased incidence of IgE antibodies to

RSV and asthma as compared with controls (Sigurs *et al.*, 1995). A common pattern seen in young children is for the child to develop an upper respiratory tract infection with a runny nose and low grade fever and by the next day for it to have developed into a full blown asthma attack. In a study of children attending the emergency room for an acute attack of asthma, evidence of viral infection especially with RSV was significantly more common in those under 2 years of age while in older children evidence of rhinovirus infection and allergy to common inhalants was more likely (Duff *et al.*, 1993). In another study it was estimated that viral infections accounted for some 80–85% of exacerbations of asthma in children aged 9–11 years (Johnson *et al.*, 1995). On the other hand it has been hypothesized, based on a lower rate of childhood asthma in less privileged societies, that viral infections in infancy might actually be protective against developing asthma by enhancing Th1 lymphocyte production at the expense of Th2 cells (Martinez, 1994). Clearly, more data are required to determine whether viral infections are more likely to induce or prevent the onset of asthma but it seems certain that they commonly provoke attacks in the child who is already asthmatic. The relationship between viral infection and asthma has recently been the subject of a comprehensive review by Stein *et al.* (1997) in which they point out the possible interaction between viral infection and atopy and the ways in which viruses may damage the airway epithelium and release chemical mediators. They also suggest that some viruses may inhibit the normal antagonistic Th1 type of lymphocyte response to infection and promote the Th2 type of response which is associated with the production of cytokines involved in the asthmatic response. Thus depending upon the virus and the host response, infection could be either protective or enhancing for asthma.

Because cough is a prominent symptom of asthma in the younger child, the combination of fever, cough and breathlessness often leads to the erroneous diagnosis of pneumonia or bronchitis. The situation may be even more difficult as the inflammation and secretions which are an integral part of the asthmatic process may well cause the physician to hear crepitations and not just wheezing, while infiltrates or atelectasis, especially of the right middle lobe, are quite common in asthma attacks. This inevitably leads to the problem of whether or not bacterial infection can induce asthma and whether or not antibiotics should be used to treat attacks. In fact there is no evidence that bacterial infections can initiate an asthma attack but some children may develop secondary bacterial infections. We performed bronchoalveolar lavage in children with asthma who presented with persistent or recurrent infiltrates in their lungs and found that in about half there was a high neutrophil count in the lavage fluid and a pathogenic organism was cultured (Springer *et al.*, 1992). In such patients it seems as if there really is secondary infection and antibiotic therapy is justified in addition to, but not instead of, anti-asthmatic therapy.

Exercise

A number of purely physical stimuli are able to provoke attacks of asthma in the asthmatic child. The commonest problem encountered in paediatric practice is exercise-induced asthma (EIA, *see* Chapter 3) because children are naturally far more active physically than adults and often take part in competitive physical activities. If the exercise is hard enough and persists for long enough the asthmatic child will develop post-exertional bronchospasm unless protected by appropriate medication. The severity of exercise-induced asthma is modified by the climate of the air being breathed and is substantially reduced if the air is warm and humid. It is also influenced by the type of exercise and is far less common after intermittent exercise such as occurs in most team games as compared with continuous running for 6 to 8 minutes. Swimming rarely causes EIA, probably because the air that the child breathes is relatively humid. Closely related to EIA is hyperventilation-induced asthma (HIA) which may be the mechanism by which laughing or crying can induce an asthma attack. In fact, some children are so sensitive to the cooling or drying of the airways induced by deep breathing that even the effort of performing lung function tests may cause an asthma attack.

Diurnal and seasonal factors

As with adults, many children seem to have more trouble with their asthma at night and it is very common for the child to suffer from frequent nocturnal disturbances while being relatively well in the daytime. This feature of asthma has never been well explained and does not appear to be related to such obvious factors as sleep state (Hetzel and Clark, 1979). Asthmatic children are often worse when there are sudden changes in the weather or in the autumn or spring when the general weather pattern is changing. This has also not been explained but may be related to the seasonal variation in aeroallergens or to the natural cycle of airborne viruses or fungal spores. The weather often influences the level of ionization of the atmosphere and this can affect bronchial reactivity under experimental circumstances although the levels of ionization needed to produce changes in laboratory are far higher than those occurring naturally.

Gastro-oesophageal reflux

It has been recognized that gastro-oesophageal reflux can produce an increase in bronchial reactivity (Wilson *et al.*, 1985; Vincent *et al.*, 1997) and may be responsible for the very severe attacks of nocturnal asthma which occur in some children. It appears that this may be due to reflexes from the lower oesophagus since it has been shown that respiratory symptoms are more closely related to lower than upper oesophageal acidity in children with reflux (Cucchiara *et al.*, 1995). How much this is a feature of asthma in the average patient is far from certain and the interpretation of the results of studies is difficult as the selection of patients tends to be biased in favour of those with significant reflux. In some infants anti-reflux treatment has been accompanied by an improvement in lung function (Eid *et al.*, 1994). Given the natural tendency for asthma to improve with time in children and also the fact that reflux and aspiration can cause airways obstruction in patients without asthma, it is difficult to interpret studies which show improvement in symptoms after anti-reflux treatment. In any child with severe asthma, especially those with severe and alarming nocturnal exacerbations, the possibility of reflux should be investigated.

Emotional factors

There is general agreement that emotional factors can provoke or even ameliorate the asthma, but there is no evidence that they can cause asthma to arise *de novo*. It seems that psychological factors can act on the abnormally labile bronchi of the asthmatic child, possibly via the autonomic nervous system (Miller and Wood, 1997). Such an effect may make airways obstruction worse but can also significantly alleviate exercise-induced asthma in some 40% of children (Godfrey and Silverman, 1973; Boner *et al.*, 1988). Most paediatricians treating children with asthma are familiar with the so-called 'typical' dependent asthmatic child and over-protective mother, and in a study of asthmatic adolescents and their families it has been found that a variety of emotional disorders in the family are associated with severe asthma (Wamboldt *et al.*, 1996). However, even here cause and effect are difficult to separate as studies of wheezy infants and their families suggest that if the infant has anxiety-provoking symptoms then a high proportion of families develop or continue to have dysfunctional behavioural patterns (Gustafsson *et al.*, 1994). In a large survey of physical and mental health in children, carried out some years ago on the Isle of Wight (UK), it was found that asthmatic children had an excess of neurotic and antisocial behaviour patterns, but the incidence was exactly the same as that seen in children with other chronic diseases (Rutter *et al.*, 1970). We found even higher scores for neurotic and antisocial behaviour in the children attending a hospital clinic, but of course these were selected from the more troublesome asthmatic children (Norrish *et al.*, 1977). Some children have extremely severe asthma while at home, which vanishes on going to a residential school and it has been shown experimentally that removal of the parents while the child remains at home will improve a proportion of asthmatic children (Purcell *et al.*, 1969). It is important to realize that the asthma is not caused by abnormal emotional reactions in such situations, but rather the other way around, and this can be seen from the frequent improvement in personality which occurs when effective medication is used. In our own study (Norrish *et al.*, 1977) the correlation of deviant behaviour was with the quality of the control of the asthma and not with the severity of the asthma while in a much more recent study by Meijer *et al.* (1995), more structured and interdependent family relationships were associated with better asthma control independent of asthma severity. Greater perceptual accuracy on the part of the child in detecting respiratory symptoms has been shown, as expected, to be associated with better control of asthma and less morbidity (Fritz *et al.*, 1996).

NATURAL HISTORY

For a long time it has generally been assumed that children grow out of their asthma and this may be one of the reasons why so many children were undertreated. The large majority of children (perhaps about 75%) fall into the group classified as mild asthma (McNicol and Williams, 1973) with infrequent attacks not requiring continuous prophylaxis and virtually all of these children become symptom-free before puberty, often in the early years of childhood. From a detailed long-term follow-up of a population of asthmatic children with perennial asthma attending a hospital clinic in London, Balfour-Lynn (1985) showed that about half of those requiring non-steroidal prophylaxis became symptom-free before puberty and almost all of the others during puberty. About 9% of asthmatic children fell into the severe, corticosteroid-dependent group either from the start of their asthma (rare) or after a number of years with mild or moderate asthma. The majority of these severe asthmatics also improved, but at the time of that study this rarely occurred before puberty. An interesting observation in this long-term follow-up study was that puberty was delayed by about 15 months in asthmatics of both sexes (Fig. 16.2) which was quite independent of the treatment they were receiving (Balfour-Lynn, 1986). More recently it has been suggested that the early introduction of effective antiinflammatory treatment improves the prognosis of childhood asthma, although there appear to be very few objective studies to substantiate this policy. In both adults and children it has been shown that the improvement in lung function on starting corticosteroid therapy is greater when they are started earlier in the disease (Agertoft and Pedersen, 1994; Selroos *et al.*, 1995). However, in both of these studies the follow-up was of relative short duration (2 years in adults, 3–6 years in children) and the improvement in lung function during treatment does not necessarily imply a better prognosis in the long term. In one study lasting up to 3 years it was shown that inhaled corticosteroids improved symptoms and reduced bronchial reactivity albeit not to normal levels but did not 'cure' the asthma since many children who appeared to have gone into remission subsequently relapsed (van Essen-

Zandvliet *et al.*, 1994). Clearly more controlled prospective studies are needed in children to determine the validity of the clinical impression that the prognosis of childhood asthma has improved with the earlier use of inhaled corticosteroids.

Every parent of an asthmatic child wants to know if and when the child will 'grow out' of the disease and whether it is possible to alter the course of the disease by treatment. Such questions are very important but to answer them requires studies of the natural history of asthma lasting many years and these are very difficult to perform. A number of community-based studies have followed asthmatic children until they reached 30–40 years of age (Blair, 1977; Jenkins *et al.*, 1994; Oswald *et al.*, 1994; Strachan *et al.*, 1996) and the results are summarized in Table 16.1. These studies suggest that of children who were already asthmatic by the age of 7–12 years, about 65% will be totally symptom-free or only have minimal symptoms as 30–40-year-old adults. Two of the studies suggest that about 20% of children never lose their asthma and continue with the disease throughout adult life. It seems likely

Table 16.1 *Prognosis of childhood asthma*

Reference	Number	Age of children (Y)	Age of adults (Y)	Symptom-free (%)	With symptoms (%)	Never remitted (%)
Blair (1977)	244	<12	30–40	52	27	21
Jenkins *et al.* (1994)	741	<7	29–32	75	25	–
Oswald *et al.* (1994)	249	<8	35	65	35	–
Strachan *et al.* (1996)	539	<8	34–35	58	21	21
Average	–	–	–	65	35	–

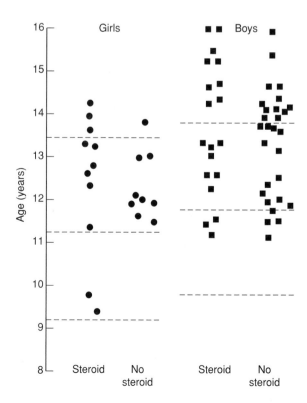

Figure 16.2 *Age of onset of puberty in asthmatic boys and girls classified according to whether or not they received regular inhaled corticosteroid therapy as their main treatment. The horizontal dashed lines represent the mean +2 SD of the age of onset of puberty in healthy British children. Redrawn from the data of Balfour-Lynn (1986).*

that another 15% or so of asthmatic children lose their asthma for a while but relapse before reaching the age of 30–40 years. However, it should be emphasized that these studies were begun some 25–50 years ago when the management of childhood asthma was less effective and before inhaled corticosteroids were available. The prognosis today may be better if indeed it is improved by the earlier use of inhaled corticosteroids. At the present time there does not appear to be any test which can reliably predict the natural history of asthma in any given child other than perhaps the loss of bronchial hyperreactivity which usually coincides with a loss of clinical symptoms (Balfour-Lynn *et al.*, 1980). Inhaled corticosteroids can reduce bronchial hyperreactivity by about two doubling doses which still leaves the child in the hyperreactive range in most cases (van Essen-Zandvliet *et al.*, 1994), but they do reduce the inflammatory changes in the airway and may possibly prevent the development of irreversible changes. There is not the slightest doubt that inadequate treatment is a major factor contributing to the rare but tragic deaths which occur from asthma (Sears *et al.*, 1986).

DIFFERENTIAL DIAGNOSIS

The diagnosis of asthma in children is based on the typical history and clinical finding backed in some cases by laboratory investigations. However, there are a number of other conditions which can produce symptoms similar to those of asthma, especially in the infant and young child, which need to be considered in the differential diagnosis. The cardinal features of asthma are episodes of noisy breathing with cough or wheezing and respiratory distress and similar symptoms may also arise from diseases in any part of the respiratory tract.

Upper airways

- *Adenoid hypertrophy* – very common in infants and preschool children, causing snoring, post-nasal drip and cough especially at night. If very severe and prolonged may cause serious airway obstruction with respiratory failure and cor pulmonale.
- *Congenital laryngeal stridor* – a relatively common group of congenital anomalies (including partial or complete vocal cord paralysis) producing inspiratory stridor and respiratory distress in the newborn and young infant.
- *Laryngo-tracheo-bronchitis (croup)* – usually caused by a viral infection in the infant or young child producing inspiratory stridor, typically worse at night. Some children have repeated attacks which is termed spastic croup and is often confused with asthma.
- *Vocal cord dysfunction* – typically affects adolescents or young adults but can occur in younger children and is usually misdiagnosed as asthma. The condition is due to an emotional disorder (probably hysterical) in which there is vocal cord adduction during inspiration and/or expiration. Unlike asthma, symptoms are not worse at night or while asleep and there is no arterial desaturation during an 'attack'.

Trachea and main bronchi

- *Congenital airway anomalies* – of which the commonest are tracheomalacia or broncho-malacia in which the cartilage rings are not rigid and the airway is unduly floppy resulting in retention of secretions, noisy breathing and a tendency to infection. Tracheo-oesophageal fistula is almost invariably associated with tracheomalacia.
- *Vascular rings* – some of which are entirely innocuous but complete rings surrounding the

trachea, such as those due to a double aortic arch or pulmonary artery sling, are very likely to produce central noisy breathing and airway compression.

- *Aspiration* – gastro-oesophageal reflux is extremely common in otherwise perfectly healthy young infants and rarely causes trouble. Some infants not only reflux but also aspirate gastric contents into the lungs producing recurrent episodes of airway obstruction with generalized wheezing and sometimes with frank pneumonia.
- *Foreign body aspiration* – most common in the 1–3 years age group and especially in boys but usually producing local bronchial obstruction with atelectasis, hyperinflation or pneumonia. Unilateral wheezing should always raise the suspicion of foreign body aspiration.
- *Haemangioma and other tumours* – causing airway obstruction and central airway noisy breathing are extremely rare in childhood. Bronchial adenoma is the commonest airway tumour in children (usually in adolescent girls), but is more likely to cause haemoptysis or pneumonia than noisy breathing.

Small airways

- *Acute viral bronchiolitis* – very common in early infancy occurring in epidemics in the winter and mostly due to infection with the respiratory syncytial virus (RSV). The infant presents with respiratory distress, wheezing and hyperinflation which usually subsides spontaneously over a week or so.
- *Chronic post-bronchiolitic wheezing* – affects up to 40% of infants following acute viral bronchiolitis. The infants have repeated episodes of wheezing which tend to become less severe and less frequent with time and cease after 2–3 years of age unless the child develops classical asthma. The differentiation from asthma may be very difficult and indeed some believe that this is a form of true asthma.
- *Bronchiolitis obliterans* – an uncommon form of paediatric chronic obstructive pulmonary disease with fixed airways obstruction and persistent wheezing which mostly follows severe viral pneumonia, often caused by adenoviral infection. In some cases the disease may affect one lung far more than the other and results in a small, hyperlucent lung, usually termed the Swyer–James syndrome in the paediatric literature or McLeod's syndrome in the adult literature. These children are almost always misdiagnosed as asthmatics until it becomes obvious that their airways obstruction is totally resistant to treatment.
- *Bronchopulmonary dysplasia (BPD)* – a form of generalized chronic obstructive pulmonary disease affecting mainly premature infants who have required intensive care with mechanical ventilation and high levels of inspired oxygen.
- *Primary ciliary dyskinesia* – the 'immotile cilia syndrome' affects a small proportion of children who suffer repeated respiratory infections, otitis media and sinusitis but may present with a relatively mild form of chronic obstructive pulmonary disease that is often mistaken for asthma or cystic fibrosis.
- *Cystic fibrosis* – an autosomal recessive disorder which in most patients causes severe and progressive lung disease and pancreatic insufficiency and results in bronchiectasis. Infants with cystic fibrosis frequently present with a picture of chronic obstructive pulmonary disease which is easily mistaken for bronchiolitis or asthma. Failure to thrive and lung disease in an infant or young child should always raise the possibility of cystic fibrosis.
- *Heart failure* – due to any cause but especially when there is a high pulmonary blood flow often present in infants with variable or persistent wheezing due to obstruction of the small airways. A cardiac abnormality may not be obvious and the problem may be mistaken for asthma or post-bronchiolitic wheezing.

Lung tissue

- *Congenital lobar emphysema* – is one of the less rare developmental anomalies of lung tissue in which usually one lobe and sometimes more is overinflated due to one or other pathological process leading to localized emphysema. The infant not infrequently presents with chronic wheezing.
- α_1-*Anti-trypsin deficiency* – is a rare autosomal recessive inborn error of defence against damage by inflammatory changes, especially those induced by cigarette smoking, which leads to a severe and generalized form of emphysema. The lung disease is extremely rare in infancy and childhood and normally only appears in early or middle adult life.

THE WHEEZY INFANT

The wheezy infant presents one of the commonest and greatest diagnostic and management problems in paediatrics. In countries with well defined seasons there is an epidemic of bronchiolitis in infants each winter which is usually due to infection with the respiratory syncytial virus (RSV). The infection results in wheeze, cough and shortness of breath lasting for a few days and closely resembles an asthma attack clinically, except that the airways obstruction is normally unresponsive to medications effective in children with asthma. There is no doubt that some children with asthma begin to wheeze in the first year or two of life and there is no doubt that many infants with acute viral bronchiolitis have recurrent attacks of wheezing after the initial illness. Of course some infants who wheeze have cystic fibrosis, congenital airway anomalies or other rare conditions, but the real problem is whether it is possible to distinguish the asthmatic from the bronchiolitic as they look so similar clinically. There have been a number of studies which have attempted to determine whether all wheezy infants are really just little asthmatics. One of the most informative was the prospective cohort study of Martinez *et al.* (1995). They found that approximately 40% of infants who wheezed for the first time under the age of 3 years never wheezed again up to the second evaluation at age 6 years and there was some evidence to suggest that the children who wheezed before the age of 3 years and stopped wheezing were different from those who continued to wheeze (Table 16.2). The infants who stopped wheezing early had low values for lung function (forced expiratory flow at resting lung volume, $V_{max}FRC$) at a mean age of 2.4 months which was before they had begun to wheeze. Moreover, while their mothers were likely to be smokers they were unlikely to be asthmatics. The infants who began to wheeze early and continued to wheeze did not have reduced lung function in infancy but did have elevated serum IgE at 9 months of age and were more likely to have mothers who smoked or had asthma and other atopic diseases. Young *et al.* (1995) in Perth (Australia) studied a birth cohort of children to

Table 16.2   *Factors associated with different patterns of wheezing in infants and young children. (From the data of Martinez* et al., *1995)*

	Wheezed only <3 years	Wheezed <3 years and continued
$V_{max}FRC$ <1 year	Reduced	Normal
Mother smokes	Yes	No
Mother with asthma	No	Yes
IgE	Normal	Elevated
Skin tests	Negative	Positive

see whether there were differences between those who wheezed with viral bronchiolitis and those who did not. They also noted a trend for the infants who subsequently developed viral bronchiolitis in the first year of life to have lower values for $V_{max}FRC$ before their first respiratory illness. These bronchiolitics also tended to stop wheezing by the end of the first year (78%) and not to have positive skin tests for allergy. Those who began to wheeze in their second year of life did not have reduced lung function in early infancy but did have an increased incidence of positive skin tests for allergy and a trend for a positive family history of asthma. Similarly, in another birth cohort study, Sporik et al. (1991) found that 24% of infants who first wheezed under two years of age were wheezing at age 11 years compared with 81% who first wheezed after the age of 2 years.

A particularly well conducted long-term controlled study was undertaken some years ago by Pullan and Hey (1982) who followed up 130 infants admitted to hospital at a mean age of 14 weeks with proven RSV bronchiolitis and compared them with matched controls. During the first 4 years of life 38% of the RSV group of infants had repeated episodes of mild wheezing compared with 15% of the controls. However, by the age of 10 years 6.2% of the RSV group and 4.5% of the control group were wheezing but the post-bronchiolitis children had an increased incidence of bronchial hyperreactivity to histamine and exercise but not atopy. These differences suggest that RSV bronchiolitis results in an acute episode of airways obstruction with repeated milder attacks in some infants over the early years of life, does not significantly increase the incidence of true asthma in later childhood but may leave some children with increased bronchial hyperreactivity due to early airway damage. In a similar, albeit uncontrolled, recent study of children aged 10 years who had been admitted with their first episode of wheezing before the age of 2 years, Wennergren et al. (1997) found that 30% of them had asthma that was mild in most cases but the incidence of documented RSV infection in infancy was no more common in those with asthma at age 10 years compared with the symptom-free children. A similar incidence of wheezing in children aged 9–10 years who had suffered from bronchiolitis in infancy was found to be unrelated to a personal or family history of allergy and passive smoking (Noble et al., 1997). In a study of bronchial reactivity and atopy in children aged 11 years with different patterns of wheezing in infancy Stein et al. (1997) were able to define three fairly distinct phenotypes – one which was clearly asthmatic and one which was clearly non-asthmatic bronchiolitis of early infancy (Table 16.3). There were only 6 infants in the intermediate group of Stein et al. (1997) and it is difficult to be certain of its significance. All these studies suggest that some wheezy infants have true (genetically-based) asthma, and some have transient virally-induced wheezing which nevertheless may cause some persistent airway damage.

Clinically and physiologically, the bronchiolitic infant has marked airways obstruction with

Table 16.3   *Findings in later childhood associated with different patterns of wheezing in infants and young children. (From the data of Stein et al., 1997)*

	Wheezed only <3 years	Wheezed aged 3–6 years	Wheezing continued to 11 years
Lung function <1 year	Reduced	Normal	Normal
Lung function in later childhood	Reduced	Normal	Reduced
Hyperreactivity to methacholine in later childhood	No	No	Yes
PEF variability in later childhood	No	Yes	Yes
Skin tests in later childhood	Negative	Negative	Positive
Elevated IgE in later childhood	No	No	Elevated

ventilation–perfusion mismatching and hypoxia. The chest X-ray may well be normal although non-specific infiltrates are not uncommon. Occasionally the infant may be very ill with marked hypoxia and may develop respiratory failure, but this is quite unusual. Quite apart from the problem as to whether or not it is possible to distinguish between the infant with bronchiolitis and asthma there is the very practical question as to whether or not the wheezy infant responds to the medications used to treat wheezing in older children and adults. For many years there has been uncertainty as to whether bronchodilator drugs are effective in the wheezy infant less than 2 years of age. Clinical observations often suggested that infants improved with bronchodilators while objective measurements of lung function mostly failed to show any improvement (Lenney and Milner, 1978). After the development of the thoracic compression (squeeze) technique for measuring forced expiratory flows in infants (Taussig *et al.*, 1982; Godfrey *et al.*, 1983) there was renewed interest in the possibility that bronchodilators might affect small airway function. However, measurements of forced expiratory flow at functional residual capacity ($V_{max}FRC$) also failed to show convincing evidence of improvement with bronchodilator with some studies showing a small improvement and others even showing deterioration (Sly *et al.*, 1991; Tepper *et al.*, 1994; Henderson *et al.*, 1995). The efficacy of inhaled or even oral corticosteroids in the treatment of the wheezy infant is also uncertain. We and others have shown that corticosteroids usually fail to show clinical benefit or shorten the course of the illness in acute viral bronchiolitis (Dabbous *et al.*, 1966; Leer *et al.*, 1969; Webb *et al.*, 1986; Springer *et al.*, 1990). The use of inhaled corticosteroids for the chronically wheezy infant has been investigated objectively in a few studies and the evidence of benefit from such treatment is far from certain. Based on clinical evaluation Carlsen *et al.* (1988) showed improvement with nebulized inhaled beclomethasone dipropionate (BDP) while we were able to show some modest improvement in lung function in chronically wheezy infants when taking nebulized BDP (Maayen *et al.*, 1986). However Stick *et al.* (1995) did not find any improvement in $V_{max}FRC$ in infants taking BDP from a metered dose inhaler and spacer although there was some evidence that BDP prevented the increase in bronchial reactivity seen in the control group. Some clinical studies with budesonide (BUD) given either by metered dose inhaler and a spacer or by nebulizer have shown a modest response (Noble *et al.*, 1992; Reijonen *et al.*, 1996) but objective data on lung function with BUD are lacking. Recently, Richter *et al.* (1998) failed to show any benefit in either lung function or the incidence of later wheezing in infants treated with nebulized budesonide for 6 weeks after acute bronchiolitis. Thus it appears that the airways obstruction in the wheezy infant is usually resistant to drugs normally effective in childhood asthma although there are exceptions and every clinician is aware of the very dramatic response that can be seen in even very young infants.

CLINICAL INVESTIGATION OF THE ASTHMATIC CHILD

History-taking

As with all medicine, history-taking forms the basis of the investigation of childhood asthma, but it is proportionately much more important. In addition, the history must usually be taken from a third party (normally the mother) and this complicates the problem, either because she is unaware of important details or she interprets her observations consciously or unconsciously and presents an 'edited' version. When trying to decide if the child has asthma, attention should be given to the episodic nature of symptoms with clear intervals, at least initially, and the fact that attacks can be provoked in various ways such as by upper respiratory tract infections and exertion. Most asthmatic children are worse during the night and first thing in the morning, and improve during the day. Attention should be paid to the mode of onset and progression of the disease and particularly to the amount of disability it is causing to both the child and the family, including the amount of schooling that is being missed and the number of days of invalidism during which the child cannot undertake normal activities.

The history should pay attention to factors which might be responsible for provoking attacks or making them worse. Care is needed when dealing with the possible role of allergy as this features so highly in popular beliefs about the aetiology of asthma. The vast majority of children with asthma are atopic and react to a number of allergens on skin testing. Parents are often convinced (sometimes by their doctors) that this means that the asthma is simply due to exposure to these allergens. This is of course quite incorrect in most cases and it is necessary to take a careful allergic history to determine which substances (if any) will regularly and invariably provoke an attack when the child is exposed to them. Asthma induced by food is rare in children and should only be accepted after a positive response to a double-blind food challenge (May, 1976; Cant, 1986). Parents are often led to believe that the child is allergic to milk or eggs but questioning reveals that cakes containing these substances are eaten without trouble. No history about asthma would be complete without an enquiry about associated atopic disease such as eczema, hayfever and urticaria in the child and close relatives. Finally, a general medical and paediatric history should be taken because asthmatic children are not immune to other diseases. The physician must always be on guard so as not to miss one of the alternative diagnoses discussed above in the child initially thought to have asthma. In such cases, the physician often finds it frustrating because of the inability to get a clear asthmatic history from the mother – it just does not 'sound right' for asthma and this should alert one to the possibility that one is dealing with something else.

A most important aspect of history-taking concerns the previous treatment that the child has received. It is not only necessary to enquire about what drugs or other types of treatment have been tried, but also how they were taken, for how long and with what effect. It is not at all uncommon for parents (or even their doctors) to misunderstand the use of drugs and to believe that the drug has not worked when in fact it was never taken adequately. If the child is receiving drugs by inhalation it is most important to enquire about the type of inhaler being used, the manner in which it is being used and, in the case of nebulizers, about the output performance of the device.

Physical examination

Conventional physical examination is not particularly helpful in most children with asthma because the presence or absence of wheezing on any particular occasion is no guide to the overall severity of the disease. One of the most useful signs of chronicity is given by the height and weight of the child which should be recorded at every visit. These should be plotted on a centile chart in order to standardize for age and sex. Ideally they should also be standardized for parental height as well, but this is not very important unless the parents are unusual. Asthma is a disease which slows growth and delays puberty quite apart from the effect of any drugs (Hauspie et al., 1977; Balfour-Lynn, 1984), with eventual catch-up growth. But experience suggests that inadequate treatment may exaggerate this phenomenon and, of course, injudicial use of systemic corticosteroids may slow the growth in height and increase weight.

Examination of the chest should pay particular attention to signs of airways obstruction of long standing which can result in the pigeon chest deformity and Harrison's sulcus. These signs are only present in the more severe type of chronic perennial asthmatic and usually indicate previous inadequate treatment. Signs related to the degree of airways obstruction at the time of examination are subject to considerable observer error but the simple criteria discussed above may provide a clue to the severity of an acute attack. No examination of the chest is complete without inspection for cyanosis which is rare, even in status asthmaticus, although some degree of desaturation which can be detected by pulse oximetry is normal in symptomatic asthma. Clubbing of the nails is not a feature of asthma and if present would suggest an alternative diagnosis. Every child should have a general physical examination on the first visit and as often as indicated during follow-up. Attention should be paid to the skin, upper respiratory tract and ears. This is of particular importance in any child whose illness does not fit with the usual pattern of asthma as infections in other sites, particularly the ears and sinuses, could suggest immunodeficiency or primary ciliary dyskinesia, and cystic fibrosis is always a possible diagnosis in a child with chronic obstructive lung disease.

An integral part of the physical examination of the child with asthma who uses any type of device for inhaling medications is to observe exactly how the device is being used either by the child or the parents if they usually administer the medication. The device itself should be inspected to ensure that it is working correctly and that any one-way valves are not sticking while the child breathes through the facemask or mouthpiece. This inspection should be repeated periodically as devices deteriorate with time and patients forget how to use them correctly. Failure to use an inhalation device correctly is a very common cause of treatment failure in children.

Special investigations

At the time of the initial visit or shortly afterwards a number of investigations should be carried out in every asthmatic child, some of which may need to be repeated at intervals.

LUNG FUNCTION TESTING

Tests of lung function are undoubtedly a most useful guide to management and simple lung function tests should be carried out on every child at every attendance at the clinic provided that the child is able to undertake the test reliably. The most useful tests are almost always the simplest and most children over about 6 years can undertake spirometry. Younger children may be able to use a peak flow meter which may be helpful in some cases but the peak flow rate may well be normal or nearly normal in a child with quite considerable obstruction in the smaller airways. Simple tests are useful because they provide objective evidence of the severity of obstruction at the time of the examination which can be compared with the opinion of the mother and the doctor. By repeating the tests at every visit a better idea can be obtained of the pattern of the asthma, i.e. whether the child is always below par or whether he can actually reach his expected value so that this is the ideal to aim for during treatment. Occasionally it is useful to have a more detailed evaluation of lung function if there is some doubt about the validity of the results of peak flow, FEV_1 or flow–volume measurements. This can happen when there is doubt about the reliability of effort-dependent tests of lung function, and in such a situation whole body plethysmography may confirm or refute the presence of lung disease. Whole body plethysmography and measurements of forced expiratory flow are also possible in infants but at present this is confined to highly specialized centres where such tests may help in the differential diagnosis of the very problematic wheezy infant (Beardsmore et al., 1986).

BRONCHIAL REACTIVITY TESTING

Tests of bronchial reactivity can be of major importance in making the diagnosis and evaluating the severity of the asthma. Not all children need to undergo tests of bronchial reactivity. If the diagnosis is clinically obvious and the response to treatment is as expected, tests of bronchial reactivity are probably superfluous for clinical management. They are most useful when the diagnosis is uncertain or when the severity of the asthma is in doubt. There are various ways of measuring non-specific (i.e. non-allergic) bronchial reactivity in children of which the simplest is by physical exercise. A positive response to exercise (a greater than 13% fall in FEV_1 after 6 minutes of strenuous exercise) can be expected in only about 63% of asthmatic children but the specificity of this test is 94%. The inhalation of hyper- or hypotonic fog or isocapnic hyperventilation mimic exercise-induced asthma to some degree but on the whole require more complicated equipment and a greater degree of patient understanding and co-operation.

Bronchial provocation by inhalation has now been widely performed in children using either methacholine or histamine as the challenge. More recently the inhalation of adenosine 5′-monophosphate has been used since it appears to be a highly sensitive and specific challenge for asthma (Avital et al., 1995). The simplest method of performing a challenge is the tidal breathing method (Cockcroft et al., 1977). The agent is nebulized using a simple jet-type nebulizer and delivered to a mouthpiece fitted with a one-way valve through which the child breathes continuously for 2 minutes. An initial control inhalation of phosphate buffer is performed followed by doubling concentrations of challenge agent. Lung function is measured for 3 minutes after each inhalation and the end point of the test (PC_{20}) is the concentration reached when there has been a 20% fall in FEV_1 from the baseline, post-buffer value. The optimal dose of methacholine or histamine for distinguishing the asthmatic from the normal response is a cumulative dose of 6.6 μmol (equivalent to a methacholine step concentration of 3.2 mg/mL). This test has a sensitivity of 92% and a specificity of 89% (Godfrey et al., 1999). In children too young to perform lung function tests the methacholine or adenosine can be delivered to an open facemask rather than to a mouthpiece. We have shown that the end point of the challenge can be judged by the appearance of wheezing heard with a stethoscope, mild desaturation determined by pulse oximetry, tachycardia or tachypnoea (Avital et al., 1988; Noviski et al., 1991). This end point, which we termed the provocation concentration for wheezing (PCW) correlates very well with the PC_{20} in those children old enough to perform both types of test and is about half of one doubling concentration greater than that causing a 20% fall in FEV_1.

Children with asthma generally respond abnormally to exercise, methacholine and adenosine 5′-monophosphate (AMP) challenges while those with other types of chronic lung disease often respond abnormally to methacholine but not to exercise or AMP (Avital et al., 1995). This may be helpful in the differential diagnosis of the child with chronic airways obstruction. In general, children with more active asthma are more reactive to the various challenges but unfortunately there is no close correlation between asthma severity and the degree of bronchial hyperreactivity. Perhaps newer techniques such as the measurement of nitric oxide levels in exhaled air may prove to be useful in this respect (Lundberg et al., 1996; Nelson et al., 1997).

CHEST RADIOGRAPH

Every asthmatic child should have a chest radiograph on the first visit unless one is available from within the previous 6 months. Although there may be radiological changes associated with asthma the main reason for this investigation is to exclude other pulmonary pathology. The chest radiograph should only be repeated for clinical indications such as suspected pneumonia or atelectasis ('middle lobe syndrome'). If a child presents with acute severe asthma, a chest radiograph should always be taken because complications such as pneumothorax or mediastinal emphysema are not all that uncommon (Eggleston et al., 1974).

Infiltrations and localized atelectasis in an asthmatic do not necessarily mean that there is bacterial infection and other corroborative evidence should be sought before instituting antibiotic therapy in addition to the anti-asthmatic treatment. One particular problem that is sometimes encountered in children with even quite mild asthma, especially in warm, dry climates, is bronchocentric granulomatosis or the mucoid impaction syndrome (Katzenstein *et al.*, 1975; Christensen and Hutchins, 1985). This is probably just a more extreme variant of the common middle lobe syndrome but it results in major plugging of relatively large airways with very tenacious bronchial casts which behave like foreign bodies. There may be complete atelectasis of a lobe, usually the left lower lobe, which is resistant to treatment and this can lead on to infection and bronchiectasis. The diagnosis is normally made at bronchoscopy and by finding the characteristic pathology in the bronchial casts. There is no place for computerized tomography (CT) scanning in the routine management of the child with asthma and this should only be performed if there is a real suspicion of other significant pulmonary pathology (e.g. bronchiectasis) or where there is serious doubt as to the diagnosis, such as in an infant in whom a vascular ring is suspected.

BIOCHEMICAL TESTS

Haematological and biochemical investigations are sometimes helpful, especially when the diagnosis is in doubt given that almost all asthmatic children are atopic and should have an elevation of total IgE and eosinophilia (unless receiving systemic corticosteroids). A sweat test is mandatory if cystic fibrosis is suspected and if there is any doubt then genotyping for the known cystic fibrosis genes should be performed. In those patients in whom recurrent infections suggest the possibility of immunodeficiency as an alternative diagnosis, appropriate immunological investigations should be performed. A proportion of younger asthmatics have IgG subclass deficiency (Loftus *et al.*, 1988), although the relationship of this to their asthma is far from clear.

IMMUNOLOGICAL TESTS

Skin testing or the measurement of specific IgE levels are of limited value in most children with asthma but a total lack of response should cast doubt on the diagnosis as only a small minority of asthmatic children fail to respond to common inhalant allergens. If a strong reaction is obtained to a specific allergen, it is only significant when there is a confirmatory history of wheezing on contact with the allergen. There are a number of commercially available so-called *in vitro* allergy diagnostic tests which claim to identify relevant allergies from tests on the blood of the patient. None of these unconventional tests has been shown to be of any real diagnostic value (Shapiro and Anderson, 1988). Very occasionally, a child does develop allergic bronchopulmonary aspergillosis and this will usually be accompanied by a late skin-test reaction and by precipitating antibody in the blood. These tests should be carried out in children with suspicious radiological changes.

BRONCHOSCOPY

Bronchoscopy is indicated when there is doubt about the diagnosis and there is a suspicion that the problem may be foreign body aspiration. In such a situation a flexible fibreoptic instrument would normally be used (Godfrey *et al.*, 1997) unless it were obvious that a foreign body was present in which case rigid open tube bronchoscopy would be required. Persistent or recurrent atelectasis, usually of the right middle lobe, is an indication for bronchoscopy to determine the anatomy and the presence or absence of a pathogenic organism (Springer *et al.*, 1992). Mucoid impaction usually requires rigid open tube bronchoscopy initially for the removal of plugs and this may need to be repeated from time to time. Bronchoscopy has no place in the routine management of the child with asthma and should only be used when there are clear clinical indications.

DIARY RECORDS

Asthma diaries can be used for the follow-up of symptoms in the child with asthma on a day-to-day basis and can be very important during the initial evaluation and when adjusting treatment. Nearly 30 years ago we developed a simple diary card for this purpose (Connolly and Godfrey, 1970) and such an approach is now widely used clinically and for drug trials. The child or parent is asked to record scores every evening about the child's symptoms over the previous 24 hours, and also to give the number of doses of every kind of medication that has been taken. This diary can be used in a semi-quantitative fashion to document the severity of the asthma and the manner in which the score fluctuates and may be of help in determining the cause of exacerbations such as the failure to take prescribed medication. The scores in the diary are, of course, the subjective impressions of the child or parent. This means that comparisons of scores between children are less reliable than comparisons in the individual child at different times.

PEAK EXPIRATORY FLOW MEASUREMENTS

Diurnal peak expiratory flow (PEF) recording in the home is now commonly recommended for asthmatics because of its practicability and the generally accepted belief that it improves management. Asthmatics also have a much larger diurnal variation of lung function than normals and this diurnal variation is greater in those with more severe bronchial hyper-reactivity (Hetzel and Clark, 1980; Ryan et al., 1982). In the statement from the International Paediatric Asthma Consensus Group (1992) the role of PEF in diagnosis and management is emphasized and the group recommends that 'lung function should be normalised with no excess of diurnal variation in peak expiratory flow rate'. However, other studies have cast doubt on the reliability of PEF measurements as an index of asthma severity and in a very thoughtful review Clark et al. (1992) noted (i) that many studies lacked adequate controls, (ii) that any correlation between PEF and subjective assessments was often very weak and (iii) that the value of PEF recording in improving control or compliance was often marginal.

We undertook a study of home monitoring of PEF in 28 children and young adults with asthma of different severity who recorded their symptoms, drug consumption and PEF twice daily for a mean of 82 days over a 12-week period (Uwyyed et al., 1996). We found that PEF measured twice daily at home correlated well with clinical indices of asthma and rescue bronchodilator consumption in those with more severe disease but poorly in those with mild asthma making such measurements of limited value. In a subgroup of 14 patients who were sick on a mean of 19 days the mean difference in PEF between well and sick days was only 14% of predicted. Diurnal PEF variation correlated poorly with other parameters in all groups. From this study it may be concluded that PEF monitoring adds little to daily recording of symptoms and bronchodilator use in young patients with severe asthma, and is too insensitive to register meaningful changes in those with milder asthma. It should probably be restricted to children with specific management problems and should not be used as a guide to treatment on a routine basis.

TREATMENT OF CHRONIC CHILDHOOD ASTHMA

In previous editions of this book, basic strategies were laid out for the pharmacological and other treatments used in the management of childhood asthma. These were based largely on the severity of asthma as indicated by the amount of disturbance it caused to the everyday life of the child and the family, the response to the treatment prescribed, and the ability of the child and family to administer medications. These principles have now been enshrined in the various national and international guidelines for the management of asthma in children and adults (Warner *et al.*, 1989; International Paediatric Asthma Consensus Group, 1992; British Thoracic Society, 1993, 1997; Warner *et al.*, 1998; National Asthma Education Program Expert Panel Report, 1991; National Heart, Lung and Blood Institute, 1992). The amount of disturbance to the everyday life of the child can be evaluated as follows:

- The number of daytime attacks lasting more than 24 hours and needing extra medication
- The presence of completely symptom-free intervals lasting more than 4 weeks without medication
- The frequency of waking at night because of asthma symptoms
- The amount of absence from school or other child care facility because of asthma
- The ability of the child to keep up with peers in normal physical activity
- The number and type of medications required on a regular daily basis
- The frequency of using extra relief medications on an 'as needed' basis
- The frequency of hospital admissions or attendances at the Accident and Emergency Department
- The frequency of any life-threatening episodes of acute asthma requiring intensive care.

The differences between the adult and paediatric guidelines are fairly trivial and mainly involve the type of device for the inhalation of medications and the recommended doses. The guidelines describe 4 or 5 steps of escalating treatment (the number depending upon which side of the Atlantic they were composed), with the recommendation that the patient be started on the step most appropriate to the severity of the asthma. Most now recommend starting treatment on a step higher than would appear to be necessary and stepping down once control has been obtained. This implies an evaluation of severity which has already been discussed but it must be admitted that this can be difficult because many children are already receiving some type of medication when referred for evaluation. In such a situation a reasonable 'guestimate' must be made of the overall asthma severity and the appropriate treatment step instituted. Follow-up is essential to determine whether the current step is appropriate and whether treatment should be increased to the next step if inadequate, or reduced if it appears to be set too high.

Essential to this process of stepwise management is the evaluation of the adequacy of the control of asthma symptoms – the outcome guidelines.

Adequate control – no change in medication required

- Minimal symptoms but not necessarily totally asymptomatic
- Minimal nocturnal asthma
- No limitation of everyday activities, no loss of schooling
- Occasional need for extra bronchodilator medication
- Able to exercise like peers
- PEF >80% predicted or personal best (if being recorded at home)
- No side-effects from medications.

In the more severe asthmatics these ideals may not be achieved completely and the least possible symptoms and disturbance to everyday function will have to be accepted (steps 4 and 5 in the British system – see below). As an extension of these outcome guidelines it is possible to suggest guidelines as to when treatment should be stepped up because of inadequate control or stepped down to test whether less treatment is required.

Inadequate control – increase medication

- Daily symptoms or frequent nocturnal asthma
- Reduced everyday activities or some loss of schooling
- Daily need for extra bronchodilator medication
- PEF < 80% predicted or personal best (if being recorded at home)
- Side-effects from medications may require change in medication.

Adequate control – try to reduce medication

- No symptoms for at least 1–2 months
- No nocturnal asthma
- No limitation of everyday activities, no loss of schooling
- Able to exercise like peers
- No need for extra bronchodilator medication
- PEF >80% predicted (if being recorded at home).

GUIDELINES TO THE PHARMACOLOGICAL MANAGEMENT OF CHRONIC CHILDHOOD ASTHMA

The mainstay of treatment of asthma is the use of drugs to relieve airways obstruction and reduce the immunological inflammatory processes in the airways which cause bronchial hyperreactivity. The individual groups of drugs are considered more fully in other chapters. A simplified version of the five steps in the guidelines for the pharmacological management of childhood asthma is shown in Fig. 16.3 and amplified below. These apply to children above about two years of age because management of the wheezy infant is far less certain and indeed controversial. The specific problem of the management of the wheezy infant will be considered later. Whatever step is decided upon it may be necessary to begin with a short 5-day course of an oral corticosteroid such as prednisolone or betamethasone (which tastes better) at the start of treatment, if the child is significantly obstructed at the time. A major factor in the management of asthma in children is the ability of the child to take medications, especially inhaled medications, and the ability of the parents to administer them to their child. It is quite useless to prescribe a metered dose inhaler without a spacer for most young children and quite unrealistic to expect parents to administer medications through a nebulizer to a screaming infant who is terrified by the noise of the compressor. The choice of inhalation device must be tailored to each child and its efficient use ensured by education of the child and family (and sometimes even the doctor). The most commonly used inhalation devices are the pressurized metered dose inhaler (pMDI) alone or with some type of spacer holding chamber (pMDI-SP), and the jet nebulizer (NEB). The ultrasonic nebulizer is used much less often for the delivery of asthma medications.

Step 1 – used for mild asthma: inhaled β_2-agonist as required

- Use a short-acting β_2-agonist as required for symptom relief (1–2 puffs by pMDI or pMDI-SP usually)

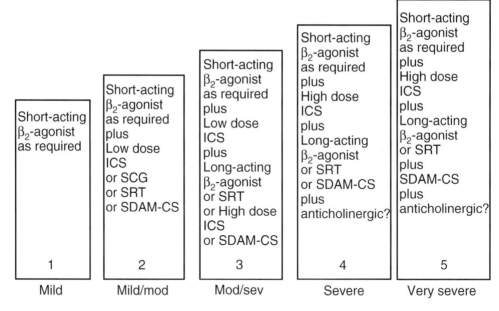

Figure 16.3 *Guideline steps for the management of chronic asthma in children as described in the text. Beneath each step is shown the asthma severity for which the step would be appropriate. ICS, inhaled corticosteroids; SCG, sodium cromoglycate; SRT, slow release theophylline; SDAM-CS, single-dose alternate morning oral corticosteroids; mod, moderate; sev, severe.*

- Oral preparations may be tried in young children but the inhaled route is more effective and much preferred for all children
- If treatment is required more than once daily, move to step 2 after ensuring that the child indeed has a good inhaler technique.

Step 2 – used for mild to moderate asthma: regular inhaled antiinflammatory drugs

- Use a short-acting inhaled β_2-agonist as required for symptom relief
- Add a regular antiinflammatory agent as preventative (prophylactic) medication
- Paediatricians have usually considered that inhaled sodium cromoglycate 3 to 4 times daily is the treatment of choice in children as this drug is entirely without side-effects but is less effective in the very young and less convenient because of dosing frequency than inhaled corticosteroids
- Increasing confidence in the use of inhaled corticosteroids in children means that many now prefer to use these drugs as first line preventative therapy
- Start with a higher dose (400–600 µg twice daily for beclomethasone or budesonide, 200–300 µg for fluticasone) and reduce the dose once control is achieved
- It may be possible to treat these children with oral anti-leukotrienes but this has not yet been adequately investigated
- In young children unable to take inhaled medication, single-dose oral corticosteroids on alternate mornings is used instead.

Step 3 – used for moderate to severe asthma: high dose inhaled corticosteroids or low dose corticosteroid together with a regular bronchodilator

- Use a short-acting inhaled β_2-agonist as required for symptom relief
- Increase inhaled corticosteroids up to 1000 μg daily of beclomethasone or budesonide (and half this amount of fluticasone) for younger children and up to 2000 μg for older children
- Alternatively, a regular twice daily inhaled long-acting β_2-agonist such as salmeterol or formoterol may be used with a lower dose of inhaled corticosteroid
- A relatively low dose of sustained-release oral theophylline to give a blood level of about 10 μg/mL may also be tried as a steroid-sparing strategy
- It may be possible to treat these children by adding oral anti-leukotrienes but this has not yet been adequately investigated
- In young children unable to take inhaled medication, single-dose oral corticosteroids on alternate mornings is used instead.

Step 4 – used for severe asthma: high dose inhaled corticosteroids together with regular bronchodilator

- Use a short-acting inhaled β_2-agonist as required for symptom relief
- Increase inhaled corticosteroids up to 1000 μg daily of beclomethasone or budesonide (and half this amount of fluticasone) for younger children and up to 2000 μg for older children
- Add a regular twice daily inhaled long-acting β_2-agonist such as salmeterol or formoterol
- Alternatively, a relatively low dose of sustained-release oral theophylline, to give a blood level of about 10 μg/mL, may also be tried as a steroid-sparing strategy
- An inhaled anticholinergic such as ipratropium or oxitropium bromide may be combined with the β_2-agonist
- In young children unable to take inhaled medication single-dose oral corticosteroids on alternate mornings is used instead.

Step 5 – used for severe asthma unresponsive to lesser treatment: regular alternate morning oral corticosteroids

- Use a short-acting inhaled β_2-agonist as required for symptom relief
- Inhaled corticosteroids up to 1000 μg daily of beclomethasone or budesonide (and half this amount of fluticasone) for younger children and up to 2000 μg for older children
- Regular twice daily inhaled long-acting β_2-agonist such as salmeterol or formoterol
- Add about 1.0 mg/kg of prednisolone or 0.1 mg/kg of betamethasone (which most children seem to prefer) as a single dose every other morning. It may be possible to reduce the dose of the inhaled corticosteroid.
- Other additional medications should be used as in step 4 as appropriate.

Step-down – used once control has been achieved on a given step

- Treatment should be reviewed every 1–2 months initially and at longer intervals as experienced is gained with the individual child
- Stepwise reduction of treatment may be possible if the patient has been virtually symptom-free and requires little or no rescue additional bronchodilator medication for 1–2 months

- Children with markedly seasonal variations in asthma severity may need to vary their treatment according to the season.

While it is now commonly recommended that treatment with inhaled corticosteroids should be started early in asthma there appear to be very few objective studies to substantiate this policy. More controlled prospective studies are needed in children to determine the validity of the clinical impression that the prognosis of childhood asthma has improved with the earlier use of inhaled corticosteroids.

TREATMENT OF THE WHEEZY INFANT

The management of acute viral bronchiolitis in infancy is basically one of supportive therapy. What is mostly required is to keep the infant well hydrated, fed and oxygenated and await spontaneous recovery, which usually occurs over a few days. As far as medication is concerned it is almost impossible to resist the temptation to treat these infants with inhaled β_2-agonist bronchodilators given by nebulizer even though the evidence that this helps is weak, to say the least. Perhaps more logically a non-selective adrenergic drug that also reduces oedema and is vasoconstrictive should be used, and indeed Kristjansson et al. (1993) have now shown significant improvement in infants treated with racemic adrenaline. Many paediatricians also use systemic corticosteroids for acute bronchiolitis even though controlled trials have shown them to be ineffective in these infants (Dabbous et al., 1966; Leer et al., 1969; Webb et al., 1986; Springer et al., 1990). Other medications such as anticholinergic agents are not more effective and theophylline may actually do more harm than good, considering it makes infants very hyperactive in the neurological sense.

Occasionally, respiratory failure develops and it becomes necessary to ventilate a baby with bronchiolitis, the indications being progressive deterioration in clinical state and in blood gases. For the severely affected infant, especially for those with other complicating factors such as bronchopulmonary dysplasia or congenital heart disease, the use of the antiviral agent ribavirin may be considered although the value of this treatment is the subject of much debate (Milner and Murray, 1989; Kimpen and Schaad, 1997). The drug must be given by inhalation and this is particularly difficult in ventilated infants because it blocks up the respiratory circuit.

The management of the infant with recurrent wheezing less than about two years of age is even more problematical. There is no doubt that a small proportion of such infants do indeed have asthma and respond well to the same medications as do older children. For such infants the guidelines described above are applicable with particular attention to the technique of administration of inhaled medications. However, many infants with recurrent wheezing are not true asthmatics and their disease is probably the result of temporary damage to the small airways following acute viral bronchiolitis. Given that at present the differential diagnosis of non-asthmatic post-bronchiolitic wheezing from infantile asthma is impossible on clinical and physiological grounds, the most logical approach in any chronically wheezy infant is to treat the condition as if it were asthma using the guidelines described above. If there is a good clinical response, then the treatment should be continued as appropriate, but if not, serious consideration should be given to withdrawal of any oral or inhaled corticosteroids that are being used. Most would inevitably continue to receive β_2-agonists but at least these are not likely to be harmful. It is also important to consider alternative diagnoses in the infant who does not respond as discussed above in the differential diagnosis of the infant with noisy breathing. If it is concluded that the infant has post-bronchiolitic wheezing it is most important for the physician to explain the natural history of this condition to the parents so that they will not be unduly surprised or disappointed if the infant has some further wheezing.

ROUTES OF DRUG DELIVERY FOR CHILDREN

The route of drug delivery in asthma is important at all ages but especially in children in whom the ability or willingness to comply with the treatment may assume greater significance. For younger children the oral route would normally be preferred and can be used for β_2-agonists, methylxanthines, corticosteroids and anti-leukotrienes (not yet recommended for children under 6 years of age) but not for cromones. However, a young child may well refuse to swallow the medication, even if it has a good taste, and will almost certainly refuse to take one with a bad taste such as prednisolone.

The inhaled route is now available for all the most important anti-asthmatic medications with the exception of the methylxanthines and anti-leukotrienes and is the preferred route both for adults and children. Pressure-activated metered dose inhalers (pMDI) are currently the cheapest and most widely available devices for inhaling sympathomimetics, anticholinergics and corticosteroids and new formulations are now being produced as the use of CFCs as propellants is being phased out. These pMDIs are very convenient for delivering drugs by inhalation but the technique used by the patient must be perfect. Most children over the age of about 6 or 7 years can be taught to use a pMDI effectively. The age range and applicability of pMDIs can be increased considerably by the use of a spacer between the pMDI and the mouth. The best type for children (and probably adults) is one with both inspiratory and expiratory valves and a volume small enough to make is easily portable. Infants and very young children can be given drugs from pMDIs if a suitable soft facemask is attached to the spacer and held firmly over the mouth and nose. The physician who prescribes the inhaler must take responsibility for ensuring that the child is properly instructed in its use and in our clinic, checking the inhalation technique forms part of the routine examination of the child. An alternative to the pMDI is the dry powder inhaler (DPI) which was introduced originally for sodium cromoglycate, salbutamol and beclomethasone. The original capsule-based devices have been replaced by multidose blister discs or inhalers with powder reservoirs for all the commonly used β_2-agonists, anticholinergics and corticosteroids. These DPIs require much less skill on the part of the patient than the pMDI and are more convenient than the combination of a pMDI and spacer. They are obviously of considerable importance for children and a recent survey in our department has shown that some 3-year-olds, over half the 4-year-olds and virtually every 5-year-old could use the Turbuhaler effectively. The delivery of medications by wet nebulization is particularly useful in children as it requires a minimum of co-operation and can be used at all ages. Sympathomimetics, anticholinergics and an inhaled corticosteroid (budesonide) are available for nebulization. There are many different compressors available and many different nebulizer chambers (*see* Chapter 14). For children it is important to use an efficient system which delivers the recommended dose over about 5–7 minutes because if it takes longer the child may well refuse to co-operate. Since most of the drug is delivered in the first few minutes it is important that the child uses the nebulizer continuously and does not take it off to run about and then return in an intermittent fashion.

ADVERSE EFFECTS OF CORTICOSTEROIDS

A number of studies in children have shown that inhaled corticosteroids, even in reasonable doses, can reduce adrenal function as shown by sensitive and appropriate tests such as the measurement of 24-hour urinary free cortisol (Nassif *et al.*, 1987) or semi-continuous monitoring of plasma cortisol (Law *et al.*, 1986; Phillip *et al.*, 1992). There are differences between drugs and the more modern drugs such as budesonide or fluticasone are less likely to have adverse effects compared to older drugs such as beclomethasone (Pedersen and Fuglsang, 1988). However, clinically evident adrenal insufficiency has not been a problem in children taking reasonable doses of inhaled corticosteroids provided they have not also been receiving oral corticosteroids. Nevertheless, it is wise to keep the dose of inhaled corticosteroid to the lowest that controls symptoms adequately.

Boot *et al.* (1997) studied the possible effect of inhaled corticosteroids on bone density and metabolism in children and although there were some uncorrected differences between the asthmatics and healthy controls, when the data were corrected for size and bone age the differences disappeared. A particular worry in this age group is the possibility of growth suppression. Studies by Wolthers *et al.* (Wolthers and Pedersen, 1991) have demonstrated that even normal doses of inhaled corticosteroids can reduce lower leg growth measured by knemometry in a dose-dependent fashion in the short term. The suppression is much less than that seen with oral corticosteroids (Wolthers and Pedersen, 1990), and the newer drug fluticasone had less effect than beclomethasone (Wolthers and Pedersen, 1993; Wolthers *et al.*, 1997). The studies were undertaken in children with very mild asthma so that any positive effect on growth resulting from the beneficial effect of the inhaled corticosteroid on the asthma would not have been seen. In a long-term study of asthmatic children, Ninan and Russel (1992b) showed that inadequate control of the asthma but not the use of corticosteroids adversely affected growth and Reid *et al.* (1996) showed that very young children treated with high-dose nebulized budesonide grew faster after starting treatment. In a very careful study of growth in asthmatic children who were followed until they had passed through puberty, Balfour-Lynn (1986) showed that the final height of asthmatics after passing through puberty was on average just what was predicted by the height centile at entry to the study (Fig. 16.4) at a mean age of 7.5 years when there was no evidence of growth retardation. A slowing of growth in adolescent asthmatic boys was noted by Merkus *et al.* (1993) and in this study those treated with cortico-steroids actually grew faster. A matched controlled retrospective study of adults who had been asthmatics as children also showed no effect of either the asthma or corticosteroid therapy on growth (Silverstein *et al.*, 1997). A meta-analysis of the effect of oral and inhaled corticosteroids on growth in 810 children (Allen *et al.*, 1994) found a small degree of growth impairment with oral therapy but none with inhaled therapy even with higher doses, longer use or worse asthma.

At present it appears that the use of reasonable doses of inhaled corticosteroids may be associated with some degree of biochemical adrenal suppression but despite short-term growth suppression in mild asthmatics there is no evidence of long-term adverse effects on growth in children with significant asthma.

TREATMENT OF ACUTE SEVERE ASTHMA IN CHILDREN

Any child with asthma of whatever grade can occasionally have an attack of acute severe asthma which may or may not be so severe as to be life-threatening as defined by the clinical features described earlier. When we reviewed our own experience some years ago (McKenzie *et al.*, 1979), we noted that just over 50% of children admitted for acute severe asthma had either never been admitted to hospital before or had not had any serious attacks for at least a year. About 25% of those admitted had received no treatment or quite ineffective treatment before being brought to hospital and the others had been given extra doses of β_2-agonists in addition to their usual medication. Most studies of factors related to death from asthma have found inadequate treatment to be important (British Thoracic Society, 1982; Sears *et al.*, 1986; Asthma Mortality

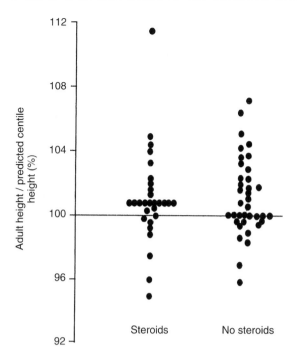

Figure 16.4   *Final post-puberty height as percentage of that predicted from the height centile in 60 asthmatic children (boys and girls) at the onset of asthma classified according to whether or not they received regular inhaled corticosteroid therapy as their main treatment. (Redrawn from the data of Balfour-Lynn, 1986.)*

Task Force, 1987; Martin *et al.*, 1995). Death from asthma is fortunately rare in children but even so it has been estimated that about 40% of asthma deaths could have been avoided (Robertson *et al.*, 1992). In most patients who die from asthma there is a background of chronic undertreatment for various reasons and inadequate management of the final episode, which is due about equally to delay on the part of the patient in seeking help and inadequate treatment by the physician (Carswell, 1985; Fletcher *et al.*, 1990; Robertson *et al.*, 1992; Martin *et al.*, 1995; Tough *et al.*, 1996). In the survey from Australia Robertson *et al.* (1992) noted that about one-third of children who died from asthma were judged to have been mild asthmatics prior to the terminal illness. However, it should be noted that these surveys of the factors surrounding death from asthma were all undertaken some 10 years ago and there does not appear to be any really up-to-date information on this important topic.

The various guidelines that have been prepared for the management of childhood asthma have also addressed the management of acute exacerbations with relatively minor differences in approach. In some there are different recommendations for management at home or in hospital, which is a useful approach. A simplified version of this two-phase approach is shown in Fig. 16.5 and amplified below.

The correct management of acute exacerbations of asthma depends upon:

For ambulatory patients:
- Correct interpretations of warning symptoms at home
- Correct treatment at home
- Recognition of when hospital treatment is needed.

For children coming to hospital:
- Correct evaluation in Accident and Emergency Department
- Correct treatment in Accident and Emergency Department
- Recognition of when transfer to intensive care is needed
- Correct timing of discharge from hospital.

(A)

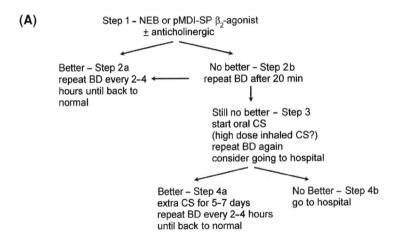

Step 1 - NEB or pMDI-SP β₂-agonist
± anticholinergic

Better – Step 2a
repeat BD every 2-4
hours until back to
normal

No better – Step 2b
repeat BD after 20 min

Still no better – Step 3
start oral CS
(high dose inhaled CS?)
repeat BD again
consider going to hospital

Better – Step 4a
extra CS for 5-7 days
repeat BD every 2-4 hours
until back to normal

No Better – Step 4b
go to hospital

(B)

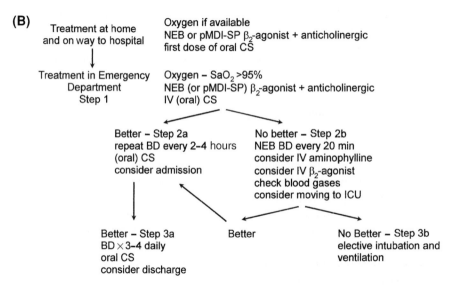

Treatment at home
and on way to hospital

Oxygen if available
NEB or pMDI-SP β₂-agonist + anticholinergic
first dose of oral CS

Treatment in Emergency
Department
Step 1

Oxygen – SaO₂ >95%
NEB (or pMDI-SP) β₂-agonist + anticholinergic
IV (oral) CS

Better – Step 2a
repeat BD every 2-4 hours
(oral) CS
consider admission

No better – Step 2b
NEB BD every 20 min
consider IV aminophylline
consider IV β₂-agonist
check blood gases
consider moving to ICU

Better – Step 3a
BD × 3-4 daily
oral CS
consider discharge

Better

No Better – Step 3b
elective intubation and
ventilation

Figure 16.5 *(A) Algorithm for the management of an acute but not life-threatening attack of asthma on an ambulatory basis. (B) Algorithm for the management of a potentially life-threatening attack of asthma. NEB, nebulizer; pMDI-SP pressurised metered dose inhaler with a spacer; BD, bronchodilator; CS, corticosteroid; SaO₂, oxygen saturation; IV, intravenous; ICU, intensive care unit.*

For all patients:
- Correct follow-up and modification of treatment.

AMBULATORY TREATMENT FOR NON-LIFE-THREATENING ATTACK

Step 1

- Nebulized β₂-agonist bronchodilator if nebulizer available
- pMDI + spacer β₂-agonist is good alternative.

Step 2

- Feeling better – repeat bronchodilator every 2–4 hours until back to usual state
- No better – repeat step 1 after 20 minutes and if still no better, move to next step.

Step 3

- Start oral corticosteroids (beginning of 3–5 day course) and repeat bronchodilator after 20 minutes
- If no better consider going straight to hospital or calling an ambulance
- If better, take extra bronchodilator as needed until back to usual state
- Some would recommend doubling the dose of inhaled corticosteroid if being used as alternative to starting oral corticosteroid provided patient is not deteriorating.

TREATMENT OF POTENTIALLY LIFE-THREATENING ATTACK

Treatment at home and on way to hospital

- Oxygen if available
- Nebulized β_2-agonist combined with anticholinergic if nebulizer available, or pMDI + spacer β_2-agonist and anticholinergic
- First dose of oral prednisolone.

Evaluation in Accident and Emergency Department

- Quick history including medications already taken in past 24 hours
- Quick, relevant physical examination (cyanosis, retractions, air entry)
  - Tachycardia and tachypnea suggests severe asthma
  - Bradycardia, hypotension suggest severe asthma
  - Pulse oximetry – saturation < 90% on room air suggests severe asthma
- Urgent chest radiograph if pneumothorax suspected but don't delay treatment
- Arterial blood gas analysis if asthma thought to be severe.

Treatment in Accident and Emergency Department

STEP 1

- Oxygen by face mask to keep saturation >95%
- Nebulized β_2-agonist combined with anticholinergic
- Oral prednisolone if child relatively well and willing and able to swallow medications otherwise intravenous methylprednisolone or hydrocortisone

If the patient improves, progress to:

STEP 2A

- Oxygen as needed
- Repeat bronchodilator every 2–4 hours

- Oral/intravenous corticosteroids once daily (6-hourly dosing is traditional but unnecessary)
- Monitor heart rate, respiratory rate and saturation.

Continuing improvement, progress to:

STEP 3A

- Stop intravenous therapy
- Regular inhaled bronchodilators
- Oral corticosteroids once daily (twice-daily dosing is traditional but unnecessary)
- Consider discharge and changes in regular medication.

If the patient does not improve after step 1, progress to:

STEP 2B

- Add nebulized anticholinergic if not already being used
- Nebulized bronchodilators every 20 minutes
- Consider intravenous aminophylline (only maintenance dose if patient takes theophylline preparations at home)
- Measure theophylline level if aminophylline is being used
- Consider intravenous β_2-agonist
- Repeat blood gas measurement
- Measure electrolytes and glucose
- Beware of inappropriate antidiuretic hormone secretion – do not overload with fluids
- Consider moving the patient to intensive care if:
  - Becoming tired with weak respiratory effort
  - Becoming comatosed
  - Arterial $PO2 < 60$ mmHg (< 8 kPa) or saturation $< 90\%$ on $>60\%$ inspired O_2
  - Arterial $PCO_2 > 45$ mmHg (> 6 kPa)

Remember that elective intubation and ventilation is always better than an emergency procedure. *Never give sedatives* unless the patient is intubated and ventilated. When the child starts improving with or without a period of ventilation, continue with steps 2a and 3a.

Discharge from hospital after acute attack of asthma

CRITERIA FOR DISCHARGE

- Symptom-free or return to usual ambulatory condition
- Good air entry and wheeze-free on examination
- PEF >75% predicted or personal best if it can be measured
- Saturation >92% breathing room air
- Full understanding by child and/or family of medications to be taken
- Ability to use any prescribed inhaler device correctly
- Discharge medications being taken correctly while still in hospital
- Adequately supportive home conditions.

DISCHARGE MANAGEMENT SHOULD INCLUDE

- Steadily reducing course of oral corticosteroids over about 1 week
- Regular inhaled bronchodilators until completely symptom-free, then as needed

- Increased dose of inhaled corticosteroids for 2–3 weeks if taken before admission
- Consider starting prophylaxis if not used before admission
- Written self-management 'action plan' (revised if necessary)
- Asthma symptom diary if considered necessary.

NON-PHARMACOLOGICAL MANAGEMENT OF CHILDHOOD ASTHMA

Allergic Management

Almost all children with asthma are atopic, and skin testing reveals a positive response to multiple allergens in about 95% of patients (McNicol and Williams, 1973b; Russell and Jones, 1976). There is also not the least doubt that allergenic stimulation is a major cause for the persistence and exacerbation of the increased bronchial reactivity that is the physiological basis of asthma (Cockcroft et al., 1977; Mussaffi et al., 1986). Avoidance of relevant allergens, particularly the house dust mite, can reduce bronchial reactivity and asthma symptoms (Platts-Mills et al., 1982; Murray and Ferguson, 1983) but avoidance of multiple allergens (or even a single allergen) is rarely practical in children. It is often believed that milk allergy is an important cause of wheezing, especially in infants, but controlled observations have shown that food allergy rarely causes asthma (Cant, 1986). Despite the undoubted theoretical importance of allergy in childhood asthma, the evidence that immunotherapy injections are of value to the large majority of asthmatics is still controversial. In adult asthmatics, carefully selected by having symptoms related specifically to ragweed, Creticos et al. (1996) showed that hyposensitization improved morning lung function, reduced skin and bronchial reactivity to ragweed, but the reduction in medication requirements was only evident in the first year of the two-year study. A meta-analysis by Abramson et al. (1995) of 20 randomized placebo-controlled double-blind trials of hyposensitization in adults and children showed significant improvement in symptoms, medication and bronchial hyperreactivity. However, in a recent study by Adkinson et al. (1997) asthmatic children requiring daily medication for control of symptoms were treated by hyposensitization and allergen avoidance in a controlled trial for two years but failed to show any clinical benefit or reduction in bronchial hyperreactivity. Moreover, there was a 34% incidence of adverse systemic reactions to the injections in the treated group compared with 7% in the control group. Even effective mite avoidance cannot be guaranteed to improve asthma in mite-sensitive children. Frederick et al. (1997) used mite impermeable bed coverings to reduce mite exposure for 3 months in asthmatic children and although this reduced the amount of **Der-p-1** allergen retrievable from the bedding there was no clinical effect and no change in bronchial hyperreactivity to histamine.

If careful history-taking, coupled with proper skin testing confirm an important allergic component in provoking or prolonging the asthma, then every reasonable attempt should be made to avoid contact with the allergen. It is possible to undertake simple but effective measures without making the life of the family intolerable. Reduction of exposure to mite antigens can be achieved by the removal of unnecessary dust-collecting fabrics, regular dusting and vacuuming of the room and its contents, and the use of an impermeable mattress cover. If there is real evidence of allergy to household pets then the animal should be removed but perhaps only after first removing the child to a house where there are no pets and noting improvement in the asthma. Because of the supposed importance of food allergens, many children have quite absurd exclusion diets inflicted upon them which make their lives and those of their parents almost intolerable. Fortunately most children have the good sense to ignore the diet whenever possible. Only if there is an absolutely certain and unfailing causal relationship between a food such as peanuts and exacerbations of asthma should the item be rigorously excluded from the diet.

Environmental factors

Air pollution and pollen levels can certainly aggravate asthma and this is sometimes taken to indicate that the family should move to another area. With adequate medications it should rarely if ever be necessary for such a drastic course and almost all children can be managed adequately in their own homes. Of course the asthmatic patient should never smoke and children must be taught this at an early age. Smoking by other members of the family in the home must also be strongly discouraged. Residential treatment for children with asthma has proved to be beneficial in some cases, but these are usually children who have been inadequately treated at home, either because of inadequate medical advice or because of inadequate compliance with treatment.

Gastro-oesophageal reflux

There is no doubt that some children with asthma also have gastro-oesophageal reflux and this may even be the true cause of symptoms in the very young infant. In older asthmatic children and adults it is far from clear which comes first, the asthma or the reflux, and there is also uncertainty as to the efficacy of anti-reflux treatment for such patients (Cucchiara *et al.*, 1995; Vincent *et al.*, 1997). For those children with chronic asthma that is severe and poorly responsive to conventional therapy, the possibility of gastro-oesophageal reflux as a major contributing factor should be considered and if present every effort should be made to treat the child medically before considering surgery.

Psychological management

Children with troublesome asthma sometimes have overt emotional problems and this has been taken as evidence that asthma is a 'psychological' disease. While there is evidence that emotional factors on their own can induce a normal child to become asthmatic there is equally no doubt that they can adversely influence the disease in the genuinely asthmatic child. This is often manifest as inability or failure to comply with management plans due to the inappropriate response of the child or more usually of the family. Adverse social circumstances and poor family bonding are contributing factors to asthma mortality discussed above. Various methods have been tried for the psychological treatment of childhood asthma but education of the child and the family about asthma management is probably the single most useful approach. Ready access to advice and treatment will often prevent the development of the 'problem asthmatic family'. In some situations it may be appropriate to try to modify the reaction of the child and the family to situations which provoke attacks by various forms of behaviour therapy.

Other treatments

There is a belief by some that 'breathing exercises' or physical training can improve or cure asthma, while many asthmatic children are prevented from taking part in sports or normal physical activities because it is supposed to be bad for them. There is no evidence that any kind of breathing exercises are of value in treating asthma except to help remove secretions during the resolution phase of status asthmaticus and to help re-expand an atelectatic middle lobe. Physical exercise is a powerful trigger factor for asthma and many active young asthmatics find this to be very troublesome if they are not given adequate medication to protect them from exercise-induced asthma. Although physical exercise is good for asthmatic children and is to be encouraged there is little evidence to suggest that it has a significant influence on the course of the disease. The various forms of complimentary or alternative medicine such as acupuncture and homeopathy have not been shown to be effective in treating asthma by controlled clinical trials and cannot be recommended for any but those with the very mildest disease. There could be a real danger if the child with significant asthma were taken off effective antiinflammatory treatment because of a belief in alternative medicine unless this be undertaken under very controlled conditions.

LIVING WITH CHILDHOOD ASTHMA

The successful management of asthma depends to a very large degree on providing the child and those with responsibility for his or her care with a good understanding of the nature of asthma and its treatment. The physician must take time to explain this to the child and the parents in terms that they can understand and the message must be reinforced at subsequent visits. There are a number of important points that should be made during the discussion.

1 There is no cure for asthma but there is excellent treatment which can allow virtually all asthmatics to lead normal lives. Almost all children become completely symptom-free or almost so during or by the end of childhood. There is some evidence that good treatment encourages this tendency to grow out of asthma.
2 Asthma is rarely fatal but in those cases where it is, there has almost always been inadequate treatment or failure to comply with medical advice. Children do not need to be over-protected because they have asthma but parents need to appreciate when things are not going well.
3 Far more patients die because they do not get corticosteroid therapy than the reverse. In conventional doses, corticosteroids are not harmful to children (or adults) and they form the mainstay of the treatment of chronic asthma at all ages.
4 Compliance with treatment is essential and the major causes of inadequate control of asthma and consequent suffering are: failure to take prescribed medications regularly; failure to take the prescribed dose; and failure to use inhalers properly.

Given that there are many drugs available to treat asthma and many different devices for the inhalation of medications, it is most important that the child and the family be provided with a written treatment plan which is consistent with the needs of the child and their ability to comply with the plan. The simpler the regimen, the more likely is patient and family compliance and successful control of asthma.

Schooling and the asthmatic child

With proper management asthma should cause little or no interference with schooling in the large majority of asthmatic children. They should be able to take part in all normal activities, including games and competitive sports. However, some children on three-times daily prophylactic medication (usually sodium cromoglycate) will need to take their medication at school and others may need to take their β_2-agonist when needed, especially before physical exercise. Because it is often difficult and sometimes impossible to arrange for children to receive regular medication while at school, a drug regimen which can be given once or twice daily rather than three or four times a day is much preferred. This is perhaps one reason why inhaled corticosteroids are being used more often by paediatricians to treat even mild to moderate chronic childhood asthma. For those children who must take medications at school every attempt should be made to avoid the child becoming embarrassed by having to take the treatment in front of other children.

Teachers and other caretakers should be able to deal with asthmatic children in their care since at least 10–15% of the class are likely to have asthma. This means that they should know which children in their class have asthma, something about the nature of the disease and its treatment. In particular they should appreciate that exercise can be difficult for the asthmatic child who may need to take a β_2-agonist before exercise. They should also be able to recognize deteriorating asthma in a pupil and inform the parents and know how to administer inhaled medications for an acute attack. It is self-evident that teachers and other role models should not smoke and should strongly discourage smoking by children, especially asthmatics.

The best place for an asthmatic child is to live at home and attend a regular school. While special residential homes and schools may have a place in the management of the child whose home circumstances prevent the receiving of adequate treatment, they have no place in the management of the adequately treated child with a normal social and family background. Every attempt must be made to provide adequate treatment and support, with the help of the excellent lay organizations that exist for this purpose where relevant, so that the child is left with healthy lungs and a healthy mind when the asthma subsides.

CONCLUSION

Asthma is a common condition in children and although most are mildly affected the quality of life of many children is seriously disturbed unless adequate treatment is provided. This involves making the diagnosis correctly and excluding other diagnoses, the evaluation of the severity of the asthma in terms of the amount of disturbance to the everyday life of the child, and the prescription of appropriate treatment taking into account the ability of the child and family to comply with the management plan. Tests of lung function and bronchial reactivity are available for children of almost all ages and should be utilized when clinically indicated to assist in management. Guidelines for the management of asthma in children are similar to those for adults with emphasis on antiinflammatory treatment for the child with frequent symptoms. Corticosteroids used sensibly and in reasonable doses do not adversely affect growth in asthmatic children who require them but do cause adrenal suppression, which is not clinically evident. About two-thirds of children with asthma can be expected to 'grow out of' their disease completely and there is some evidence that the early introduction of effective treatment improves the prognosis.

REFERENCES

Aberg N, Engstrom I. (1990) Natural history of allergic diseases in childhood. *Acta Paediatr Scand*, **79**, 206–11.

Abramson MJ, Puy RM, Weiner JM. (1995) Is allergen immunotherapy effective in asthma? A meta-analysis of randomized controlled trials. *Am J Respir Crit Care Med*, **151**, 969–74.

Adkinson NF, Eggleston PA, Eney D, *et al*. (1997) A controlled trial of immunotherapy for asthma in allergic children. *New Engl J Med*, **336**, 324–31.

Agertoft L, Pedersen S. (1994) Effects of longterm treatment with an inhaled corticosteroid on growth and pulmonary function in asthmatic children. *Respir Med*, **88**, 373–81.

Allen DB, Mullen M, Mullen B. (1994) A meta-analysis of the effect of oral and inhaled corticosteroids on growth. *J Allergy Clin Immunol*, **93**, 967–76.

Anderson HR, Bailey PA, Cooper JS, Palmer JC, West S. (1983) Morbidity and school absence caused by asthma and wheezing illness. *Arch Dis Child*, **58**, 777–84.

Anderson HR, Butland BK, Strachan DP. (1994) Trends in prevalence and severity of childhood asthma. *BMJ*, **308**, 1600–4.

Asher MI, Pattemore PK, Harrison AC, *et al.* (1988) International comparison of the prevalence of asthma symptoms and bronchial hyperresponsiveness. *Am Rev Respir Dis*, **138**, 524–9.

Asthma Mortality Task Force. (1987) Recommendations of Asthma Mortality Task Force. *J Allergy Clin Immunol*, **80**, 364–6.

Auerbach I, Springer C, Godfrey S. (1993) Total population survey of the frequency and severity of asthma in 17 year old boys in an urban area in Israel. *Thorax*, **48**, 139–41.

Avital A, Bar-Yishay E, Springer C, Godfrey S. (1988) Bronchial provocation tests in young children using tracheal auscultation. *J Pediatr*, **112**, 591–4.

Avital A, Springer C, Bar-Yishay E, Godfrey S. (1995) Adenosine, methacholine, and exercise challenges in children with asthma or paediatric chronic obstructive pulmonary disease. *Thorax*, **50**, 511–16.

Balfour-Lynn L. (1985) Childhood asthma and puberty. *Arch Dis Child*, **60**, 231–5.

Balfour-Lynn L. (1986) Growth and childhood asthma. *Arch Dis Child*, **61**, 1049–55.

Balfour-Lynn L, Tooley M, Godfrey S. (1980) Relationship of exercise-induced asthma to clinical asthma in childhood. *Arch Dis Child*, **56**, 450–4.

Baraldi E, Azzolin NM, Zanconato S, Dario C, Zacchello F. (1997) Corticosteroids decrease exhaled nitric oxide in children with acute asthma. *J Pediatr*, **131**, 381–5.

Beardsmore CS, Godfrey S, Shani N, Maayan Ch, Bar-Yishay E. (1986) Airway resistance measurements throughout the respiratory cycle in infants. *Respiration*, **49**, 81–93.

Benckhuijsen J, van den Bos J-W, van Velzen E, de Bruin R, Aalbers R. (1996) Differences in the effect of allergen avoidance on bronchial hyperresponsiveness as measured by methacholine, adenosine 5′-monophosphate, and exercise in asthmatic children. *Pediatr Pulmonol*, **22**, 147–53.

Blair H. (1977) Natural history of childhood asthma. 20-year follow up. *Arch Dis Child*, **52**, 613–19.

Blair H. (1974) The incidence of asthma, hay fever and infantile eczema in an East London group practice of 9145 patients. *Clin Allergy*, **4**, 389–99.

Boner AL, Vallone G, Peroni DG, Piacentini GL, Gaburro D. (1988) Efficacy and duration of action of placebo responses in the prevention of exercise-induced asthma in children. *J Asthma*, **25**, 1–5.

Boot AM, de Jongste JC, Verberne AAPH, Pols HAP, de Munick Keizer-Schrama SMPF. (1997) Bone mineral density and bone metabolism of prepubertal children with asthma after long-term treatment with inhaled corticosteroids. *Pediatr Pulmonol*, **24**, 379–84.

British Thoracic Society. (1982) Death from asthma in two regions of England. *BMJ*, **285**, 1251–5.

British Thoracic Society and others. (1997) The British guidelines on asthma management 1995 review and position statement. *Thorax*, **52** (Suppl 1), S1–21.

Burney PGJ. (1986) Asthma mortality in England and Wales: evidence for a further increase, 1974–84. *Lancet*, **2**, 323–6.

Burr ML, Butland BK, King S, Vaughan-Williams E. (1989) Changes in asthma prevalence: two surveys 15 years apart. *Arch Dis Child*, **64**, 1452–6.

Burr ML. (1987) Is asthma increasing? *J Epidemiol Community Health*, **41**, 185–9.

Campbell MJ, Cogman GR, Holgate ST, Johnson SL. (1997) Age specific trends in asthma mortality in England and Wales, 1983–95: results of an observational study. *BMJ*, **314**, 1439–41.

Cant A. (1986) The diagnosis and management of food allergy. *Arch Dis Child*, **61**, 730–1.

Carlsen KH, Leegaard J, Larsen S, Orstavik I. (1988) Nebulised beclomethasone dipropionate in recurrent obstructive episodes after acute bronchiolitis. *Arch Dis Child*, **63**, 1428–33.

Carswell F. (1985) Thirty deaths from asthma. *Arch Dis Child*, **60**, 25–8.

Chilmonczyk BA, Salmun LA, Megathlin KN, *et al*. (1993) Association between exposure to environmental tobacco smoke and exacerbation of asthma in children. *N Engl J Med*, **328**, 1665–9.

Christensen WN, Hutchins GM. (1985) Hypereosinophilic mucoid impaction of bronchi in two children under two years of age. *Pediatr Pulmonol*, **1**, 278–83.

Clark NM, Evans D, Mellins RB. (1992) Patient use of peak flow monitoring. *Am Rev Respir Dis*, **145**, 722–5.

Cloutier MM, Loughlin GM. (1981) Chronic cough in children: a manifestation of airway hyperactivity. *Pediatrics*, **67**, 6–12.

Cockcroft DW, Killian DM, Mellon JJA, Hargreave FE. (1977a) Bronchial reactivity to inhaled histamine: a method and clinical survey. *Clin Allergy*, **7**, 235–43.

Cockcroft DW, Ruffin RE, Dolovich J and Hargreave FE. (1977b) Allergen-induced increase in non-allergic bronchial reactivity. *Clin Allergy*, **7**, 503–13.

Connolly N, Godfrey S. (1970) Assessment of the child with asthma. *J Asthma Res*, **8**, 31–6.

Cookson WO. (1995) 11q high-affinity IgE receptor in asthma and allergy. *Clin Exper Allergy*, **25** (Suppl 2), 71–3.

Creticos PS, Reed CE, Normal PS, *et al*. (1996) Ragweed immunotherapy in adult asthma. *N Engl J Med*, **334**, 501–6.

Cserhati E, Mezei G, Kelemen J. (1984) Late prognosis of bronchial asthma in children. *Respiration*, **46**, 160–5.

Cucchiara S, Santamaria F, Minella R, *et al*. (1995) Simultaneous prolonged recordings of proximal and distal intraesophageal pH in children with gastroesophageal reflux disease and respiratory symptoms. *Am J Gastroenterol*, **90**, 1791–6.

Dabbous IA, Tkachyk JS, Stamm SJ. (1966) A double blind study on the effect of corticosteroids in the treatment of bronchiolitis. *Pediatrics*, **37**, 477–84.

Dawson B, Horrobin G, Illesley R, Mitchell R. (1969) A survey of childhood asthma in Aberdeen. *Lancet*, **1**, 827–30.

Dodge RR, Burrows B. (1980) The prevalence and incidence of asthma and asthma-like symptoms in a general population sample. *Am Rev Respir Dis*, **122**, 567–75.

Dold S, Wjst M, von Mutius E, Reitmeir P, Stiepel E. (1992) Genetic risk for asthma, allergic rhinitis, and atopic dermatitis. *Arch Dis Child*, **67**, 1018–22.

Duff AL, Pomeranz ES, Gelber LE, *et al*. (1993) Risk factors for acute wheezing in infants and children: viruses, passive smoke, and IgE antibodies to inhalant allergies. *Pediatrics*, **92**, 535–40.

Eggleston PA, Ward BH, Pierson WE, Bierman CW. (1974) Radiographic abnormalities in acute asthma in children. *Pediatrics*, **54**, 442–9.

Eid NS, Shepherd RW, Thomson MA. (1994) Persistent wheezing and gastroesophageal reflux in infants. *Pediatr Pulmonol*, **18**, 39–44.

Fletcher HJ, Ibrahim SA, Speight N. (1990) Survey of asthma deaths in the Northern region, 1970–85. *Arch Dis Child*, **65**, 163–7.

Foresi A, Bertorelli G, Pesci A, Oliveri D. (1990) Inflammatory markers in bronchoalveolar lavage and in bronchial biopsy in asthma and during remission. *Chest*, **98**, 528–35.

Frederick JM, Warner JO, Jessop WJ, Enander I, Warner JA. (1997) Effect of a bed covering system in children with asthma and house dust mite hypersensitivity. *Eur Respir J*, **10**, 361–6.

Fritz GK, McQuaid EL, Spirito A, Klein RB. (1996) Symptom perception in pediatric asthma: relationship to functional morbidity and psychological factors. *J Am Acad Child Adolesc Psychiatry*, **35**, 1033–41.

Godfrey S, Avital A, Maayan C, Rotschild M, Springer C. (1997) Yield from flexible bronchoscopy in children. *Pediatr Pulmonol*, **23**, 261–9.

Godfrey S, Bar-Yishay E, Arad I, Landau LI, Taussig LM. (1983) Flow–volume curves in infants with lung disease. *Pediatrics*, **72**, 517–22.

Godfrey S, Silverman M. (1973) Demonstration of placebo response in asthma by means of exercise testing. *J Psychosom Res*, **17**, 293–7.

Godfrey S, Springer C, Bar-Yishay E, Avital A. (1999) Cut-off points defining normal and asthmatic bronchial reactivity to exercise and inhalation challenges in children and young adults. *Eur Respir J*, **14**, 659–68.

Guidelines on the management of asthma. (1993) *Thorax*, **48**, Suppl S1–S24.

Gustafsson PA, Bjorksten B, Kjellman NI. (1994) Family dysfunction in asthma: a prospective study of illness development. *J Pediatr*, **125**, 493–8.

Hauspie R, Susanne C, Alexander F. (1977) Maturational delay and temporal growth retardation in asthmatic boys. *J Allergy Clin Immunol*, **59**, 200–6.

Henderson AJW, Arnott J, Young S, Warshawski T, Landau LI, LeSouef PN. (1995) The effect of inhaled adrenaline on lung function of recurrently wheezy infants less than 18 months old. *Pediatr Pulmonol*, **20**, 9–15.

Henderson J, Goldacre MJ, Fairweather JM, Marcovitch H. (1992) Conditions accounting for substantial time spent in hospital in children aged 1–14 years. *Arch Dis Child*, **67**, 83–6.

Hetzel MR and Clark TJH. (1979) Does sleep cause nocturnal asthma. *Thorax*, **34**, 749–54.

Hetzel MR, Clark TJH. (1980) Comparison of normal and asthmatic circadian rhythms in peak expiratory flow rate. *Thorax*, **35**, 732–8.

Hill RA, Standen PJ, Tattersfield AE. (1989) Asthma, wheezing, and school absence in primary schools. *Arch Dis Child*, **64**, 246–51.

Holberg CJ, Wright AL, Martinez FD, Morgan WJ, Taussig LM. (1993) Child day care, smoking by caregivers, and lower respiratory tract illness in the first 3 years of life. *Pediatrics*, **91**, 885–92.

Horn MEC, Brain EA, Gregg I, Iiglis JM, Yealland SJ, Taylor P. (1979) Respiratory viral infection and wheezy bronchitis in childhood. *Thorax*, **34**, 23–8.

International Paediatric Asthma Consensus Group. (1992) *Arch Dis Child*, **67**, 240–8.

International Study of Asthma and Allergies in Childhood (ISAAC) Steering Committee. (1998) Worldwide variation in prevalence of symptoms of asthma, allergic rhinoconjunctivitis, and atopic eczema: ISAAC. *Lancet*, **351**, 1225–32.

Iryes HT, Anderson GE, Shaffer TJ, Neff JM. (1997) Expenditure for care of children with chronic diseases enrolled in the Washington State Medicaid program, fiscal year 1993. *Pediatrics*, **100**, 197–204.

Jenkins MA, Hopper JL, Bowes G, Carlin JB, Flander LB, Giles GG. (1994) Factors in childhood as predictors of asthma in adult life. *BMJ*, **309**, 90–4.

Johnson SL, Pattemore PK, Sanderson G, *et al.* (1995) Community study of role of viral infections in exacerbations of asthma in 9–11 year old children. *BMJ*, **310**, 1225–9.

Karjalainen J, Lindqvist A, Laitinen LA. (1989) Seasonal variability of exercise-induced asthma especially outdoors. Effect of birch pollen allergy. *Clin Exper Allergy*, **19**, 273–8.

Katzenstein AL, Liebow AA, Friedman PJ. (1975) Bronchocentric granulomatosis, mucoid impaction, and hypersensitivity reactions to fungi. *Am Rev Respir Dis*, **111**, 497–537.

Kimpen JL, Schaad UB. (1997) Treatment of respiratory syncytial virus bronchiolitis: 1995 poll of members of the European Society for Paediatric Infectious Diseases. *Pediatr Infect Dis J*, **16**, 479–81.

Konig P, Godfrey S. (1973) The prevalence of exercise induced bronchial lability in families of children with asthma. *Arch Dis Child*, **48**, 513–18.

Konig P, Godfrey S. (1974) Exercise bronchial lability in monozygotic (identical) and dizygotic (non-identical) twins. *J Allergy Clin Immunol*, **54**(5), 280–7.

Kristjansson S, Carlsen KCL, Wennergren G, Strannegard I-L, Carlsen K-H. (1993) Nebulised recemic adrenlaine in the treatment of acute bronchiolitis in infants and toddlers. *Arch Dis Child*, **69**, 650–4.

Law CM, Marchant JL, Honour JW, Preece MA, Warner JO. (1986) Nocturnal adrenal suppression in asthmatic children taking inhaled beclomethasone dipropionate. *Lancet*, **1**, 942–4.

Lee DA, Winslow NR, Speight AN, Hey EN. (1983) Prevalence and spectrum of asthma in childhood. *BMJ*, **286**, 1256–8.

Leer JA, Bloomfield NJ, Green JL, *et al.* (1969) Corticosteroid treatment in bronchiolitis. A controlled, collaborative study in 297 infants and children. *Am J Dis Child*, **117**, 495–503.

Lenney W, Milner AD. (1978) At what age do bronchodilator drugs work. *Arch Dis Child*, **53**, 532–5.

Lichtenstein P, Svartengren M. (1997) Genes, environment, and sex: factors of importance in atopic diseases in 7–9 year-old Swedish twins. *Allergy*, **52**, 1079–86.

Loftus BG, Price JF, Lobo-Yeo A, Vergani D. (1988) IgG subclass deficiency in asthma. *Arch Dis Child*, **63**, 1434–7.

Lundberg JON, Nordvaal SL, Weitzberg E, Kollberg H, Alving K. (1996) Exhaled nitric oxide in paediatric asthma and cystic fibrosis. *Arch Dis Child*, **75**, 323–6.

Maayan C, Itzhaki T, Bar-Yishay E, Gross S, Tal A, Godfrey S. (1986) The functional response of infants with persistent wheezing to nebulised beclomethasone dipropionate. *Pediatr Pulmonol*, **2**, 9–14.

Martin AJ, Campbell DA, Gluyas PA, *et al*. (1995) Characteristics of near fatal asthma in childhood. *Pediatr Pulmonol*, **20**, 1–8.

Martinez FD, Cline M, Burrows B. (1992) Increased incidence of asthma in children of smoking mothers. *Pediatrics*, **89**, 21–6.

Martinez FD, Wright AL, Taussig LM, Holberg CJ, Halonen M, Morgan WJ, and the Group Health Medical Associates. (1995) Asthma and wheezing in the first six years of life. *N Engl J Med*, **332**, 133–8.

Martinez FD. (1994) Role of viral infections in the inception of asthma and allergies during childhood: could they be protective? *Thorax*, **49**, 1189–91.

May CD. (1976) Objective clinical and laboratory studies of immediate hypersensitivity reaction to foods in asthmatic children. *J Allergy Clin Immunol*, **58**, 500–15.

McKenzie SA, Edmunds AT, Godfrey S. (1979) Status asthmaticus in children. *Arch Dis Child*, **54**, 581–6.

McNicol KN, Williams HE. (1973a) Spectrum of asthma in children – I. clinical and physiological components. *BMJ*, **4**, 7–11.

McNicol KN, Williams HE. (1973b) Spectrum of asthma in children – II, allergic components. *BMJ*, **4**, 12–16.

Meijer AM, Griffioen RW, van Nierop JC, Oppenheimer L. (1995) Intractable or uncontrolled asthma: psychosocial factors. *J Asthma*, **32**, 265–74.

Menon P, Rando RJ, Stankus RP, Salvaggio JE, Lehrer SB. (1992) Passive cigarette smoke – challenge studies: increase in bronchial reactivity. *J Allergy Clin Immunol*, **89**, 560–6.

Merkus PJFM, van Essen-Zandvliet EEM, Duiverman EJ, van Houwelingen HC, Kerrebijn KF, Quanjer PH. (1993) Long-term effect of inhaled corticosteroids on growth rate in adolescents with asthma. *Pediatrics*, **91**, 1121–6.

Miller BD, Wood BL. (1997) Influence of specific emotional states on autonomic reactivity and pulmonary function in asthmatic children. *J Am Acad Child Adolesc Psychiatry*, **36**, 669–77.

Milner AD, Murray M. (1989) Acute bronchiolitis in infancy: treatment and prognosis. *Thorax*, **44**, 1–5.

Murray AB, Ferguson AC. (1983) Dust-free bedrooms in the treatment of asthmatic children with house dust or house dust mite allergy: a controlled trial. *Pediatrics*, **71**, 418–22.

Murray AB, Morrison BJ. (1986) The effect of cigarette smoke from the mother on bronchial responsiveness and severity of symptoms in children with asthma. *J Allergy Clin Immunol*, **77**, 575–81.

Mussaffi H, Springer C, Godfrey S. (1986) Increased bronchial responsiveness to exercise and histamine after allergen challenge in asthmatic children. *J Allergy Clin Immunol*, **77**, 48–52.

Nassif E, Weinberger M, Sherman B, Brown K. (1987) Extrapulmonary effects of maintenance corticoid therapy with alternate-day prednisone and inhaled beclomethasone in children with chronic asthma. *J Allergy Clin Immunol*, **80**, 518–29.

National Asthma Education Program Expert Panel Report. (1991) Guidelines for the diagnosis and management of asthma. Publication No. 9103024. Bethesda, MD: National Institutes of Health.

National Heart, Lung and Blood Institute, National Institutes of Health. (1992) International consensus report on diagnosis and treatment of asthma. *Eur Respir J*, **5**, 601–41.

Nelson BV, Sears S, Woods J, *et al*. (1997) Expired nitric oxide as a marker for childhood asthma. *J Pediatr*, **130**, 423–7.

Nieminen MM, Kaprio J, Koskenvuo M. (1991) A population-based study of bronchial asthma in adult twin pairs. *Chest*, **100**, 70–5.

Ninan TK, Russell G. (1992) Asthma, inhaled corticosteroid treatment and growth. *Arch Dis Child*, **67**, 703–5.

Ninan TK, Russell G. (1992) Respiratory symptoms and atopy in Aberdeen schoolchildren: evidence from two surveys 25 years apart. *BMJ*, **304**, 873–5.

Noble V, Murray M, Webb MSC, Alexander J, Swarbrick AS, Milner AD. (1997) Respiratory status and allergy nine to 10 years after acute bronchiolitis. *Arch Dis Child*, **76**, 315–19.

Noble V, Ruggins NR, Everard ML, Milner AD. (1992) Inhaled budesonide for chronic wheezing under 18 months of age. *Arch Dis Child*, **67**, 285–8.

Norrish M, Tooley M, Godfrey S. (1977) A clinical, physiological and psychological study of asthmatic children attending a hospital clinic. *Arch Dis Child*, **52**, 912–17.

Noviski N, Cohen L, Springer C, Bar-Yishay E, Avital A, Godfrey S. (1991) Bronchial provocation determined by breath sounds compared with lung function. *Arch Dis Child*, **66**, 952–5.

Oswald H, Phelan PD, Lanigan A, Hibbert M, Bowes G, Olinsky A. (1994) Outcome of childhood asthma in mid-adult life. *BMJ*, **309**, 95–6.

Peat JK, van den Berg RH, Green WF, Mellis CM, Leeder SR, Woolcock AJ. (1994) Changing prevalence of asthma in Australian children. *BMJ*, **308**, 1591–6.

Pedersen S, Fuglsang G. (1988) Urine cortisol excretion in children treated with high doses of inhaled corticosteroids: a comparison of budesonide and beclomethasone. *Eur Respir J*, **1**, 433–5.

Phillip M, Aviram M, Leiberman E, *et al.* (1992) Integrated plasma cortisol concentration in children with asthma receiving long-term inhaled corticosteroids. *Pediatr Pulmonol*, **12**, 84–9.

Platts-Mills TAE, Tovey UR, Mitchell EB, Moszoro H, Nock P, Wilkins SR. (1982) Reduction of bronchial hyperreactivity during prolonged allergen avoidance. *Lancet*, **2**, 675–8.

Postma DS, Bleecker ER, Amelung PJ, *et al.* (1995) Genetic susceptibility to asthma – bronchial hyperresponsiveness coinherited with a major gene for atopy. *N Engl J Med*, **333**, 894–900.

Pullan CR, Hey EN. (1982) Wheezing, asthma and pulmonary dysfunction 10 years after infection with respiratory syncytial virus in infancy. *BMJ*, **284**, 1665–9.

Purcell K, Brady K, Chai H, *et al.* (1969) The effect on asthma in children of experimental separation from the family. *Psychosom Med*, **31**, 144–64.

Reid A, Murphy C, Steen HJ, McGovern V, Shields MD. (1996) Linear growth of very young asthmatic children treated with high-dose nebulized budesonide. *Acta Paediatrica Scand*, **85**, 421–4.

Reijonen T, Korppi M, Kuikka L, Remes K. (1996) Anti-inflammatory therapy reduces wheezing after bronchiolitis. *Arch Pediatr Adolesc Med*, **150**, 512–17.

Richards W. (1989) Hospitalization for children with status asthmaticus: A review. *Pediatrics*, **84**, 111–18.

Richter H, Seddon P. (1998) Early nebulized budesonide in the treatment of bronchiolitis and the prevention of postbronchiolitic wheezing. *J Pediatr*, **132**, 849–53.

Robertson CF, Rubinfeld AR, Bowes G. (1992) Pediatric asthma deaths in Victoria: the mild are at risk. *Pediatr Pulmonol*, **13**, 95–100.

Roger LJ, Kehrl HR, Hazucha M, Horstman DH. (1985) Bronchoconstriction in asthmatics exposed to sulphur dioxode during repeated exercise. *J Appl Physiol*, **59**, 784–91.

Russell G, Jones SP. (1976) Selection of skin tests in childhood asthma. *Br J Dis Chest*, **70**, 104–6.

Rutter M, Tizard J, Whitmore K. (1970) *Education, health and behaviour*. London: Longman Group Ltd.

Ryan G, Latimer KM, Dolovich J, Hargreave FE. (1982) Bronchial responsiveness to histamine: relationship to diurnal variation of peak flow rate, improvement after bronchodilator and airway calibre. *Thorax*, **37**, 423–9.

Schmitzberger R, Rhomberg K, Buchele H, *et al.* (1993) Effects of air pollution on the respiratory tract of children. *Pediatr Pulmonol*, **15**, 68–74.

Sears MR, Rea HH, Fenwick J, *et al.* (1986) Deaths from asthma in New Zealand. *Arch Dis Child*, **61**, 6–10.

Selroos O, Pietinalho A, Lofroos AB, Riska H. (1995) Effect of early vs late intervention with inhaled corticosteroids in asthma. *Chest*, **108**, 1228–34.

Shapiro GG, Anderson JA. (1988) Controversial techniques in allergy. *Pediatrics*, **82**, 935–7.

Sheppard D, Saisho A, Nadel JA, Boushey HA. (1981) Exercise increases sulfur dioxide-induced bronchoconstriction in asthmatic subjects. *Am Rev Respir Dis*, **123**, 486–91.

Sigurs N, Bjarnason R, Sigurbergsson F, Kjellman B, Bjorksten B. (1995) Asthma and immunoglobulin E antibodies after respiratory syncytial virus bronchiolitis: a prospective cohort study with matched controls. *Pediatrics*, **95**, 500–5.

Silverstein MD, Yunginger JW, Reed CE, *et al*. (1997) Attained adult height after childhood asthma: effect of glucocorticoid therapy. *J Allergy Clin Immunol*, **99**, 466–74.

Sly PD, Lanteri CJ, Raven JM. (1991) Do wheezy infants recovering from bronchiolitis respond to inhaled salbutamol? *Pediatr Pulmonol*, **10**, 36–9.

Speight ANP, Lee DA, Hey EN. (1983) Underdiagnosis and undertreatment of asthma in childhood. *BMJ*, **286**, 1253–6.

Sporik R, Holgate ST, Cogswell JJ. (1991) Natural history of asthma in childhood – a birth cohort study. *Arch Dis Child*, **66**, 1050–3.

Springer C, Avital A, Noviski N, *et al*. (1992) The role of infection in the right middle lobe syndrome in asthma. *Arch Dis Child*, **67**, 592–4.

Springer C, Bar-Yishay E, Uwyyed K, Avital A, Vilozni D, Godfrey S. (1990) Corticosteroids do not affect the clinical or physiological status of infants with bronchiolitis. *Pediatr Pulmonol*, **9**, 181–5.

Stein RT, Holberg CJ, Morgan WJ, *et al*. (1997) Peak flow variability, methacholine responsiveness and atopy as markers for detecting different wheezing phenotypes in childhood. *Thorax*, **52**, 946–52.

Stick SM, Burton PR, Clough JB, Cox M, LeSouef PN, Sly PD. (1995) The effects of inhaled beclomethasone dipropionate on lung function and histamine responsiveness in recurrently wheezy infants. *Arch Dis Child*, **73**, 327–32.

Stick SM, Burton PR, Gurrin L, Sly PD, LeSouef PN. (1996) Effects of maternal smoking during pregnancy and a family history of asthma on respiratory function in newborn infants. *Lancet*, **348**, 1060–4.

Strachan DP, Griffiths JM, Johnston IDA, Anderson HR. (1996) Ventilatory function in British adults after asthma or wheezing illness at ages 0–35. *Am J Respir Crit Care Med*, **154**, 1629–35.

Tager IB, Hanrahan JP, Tosteson TD, *et al*. (1993) Lung function, pre- and post-natal smoke exposure, and wheezing in the first year of life. *Am Rev Respir Dis*, **147**, 811–17.

Taussig LM, Landau LI, Godfrey S, Arad I. (1982) Determinants of forced expiratory flows in newborn infants. *J Appl Physiol*, **53**, 1220–7.

Taussig LM, Smith SM, Blumenfeld R. (1981) Chronic bronchitis in childhood: what is it? *Pediatrics*, **67**, 1–5.

Tepper RS, Rosenberg D, Eigen H, Reister T. (1994) Bronchodilator responsiveness in infants with bronchiolitis. *Pediatr Pulmonol*, **17**, 81–5.

Tough SC, Green FH, Paul JE, Wigle DT, Butt JC. (1996) Sudden death from asthma in 108 children and young adults. *J Asthma*, **33**, 179–88.

Trends in asthma mortality in the elderly. Factsheet 92/1 Lung and Asthma Information Agency, St. George's Hospital Medical School, London.

Trends in hospital admissions for asthma. Factsheet 96/2 Lung and Asthma Information Agency, St. George's Hospital Medical School, London.

Uwyyed K, Springer C, Avital A, Bar-Yishay E, Godfrey S. (1996) Home recording of PEF in young asthmatics: does it contribute to management? *Eur Respir J*, **9**, 872–9.

van Essen-Zandvliet EE, Hughes MD, Waalkens HJ, Duiverman EJ, Kerrebijn KF, and the Dutch CNSLD study group. (1994) Remission of childhood asthma after long-term treatment with an inhaled corticosteroid (budesonide): can it be achieved? *Eur Respir J*, **7**, 63–8.

van Herwerden L, Harrap SB, Wong ZYH, *et al*. (1995) Linkage of high-affinity IgE receptor gene with bronchial hyperreactivity, even in absence of atopy. *Lancet*, **346**, 1262–5.

Venn A, Lewis S, Cooper M, Hill J, Britton J. (1998) Increasing prevalence of wheeze and asthma in Nottingham primary schoolchildren 1988–1995. *Eur Respir J*, **11**, 1324–8.

Viegi G. (1998) Air pollution epidemiology and the European Respiratory Society: the PEACE project. *Eur Respir Rev*, **8**, Review 52, 1–3.

Vincent D, Cohen-Jonathan AM, Leport J, *et al*. (1997) Gastro-oesophageal reflux prevalence and relationship with bronchial reactivity in asthma. *Eur Respir J*, **10**, 2255–9.

Wamboldt MZ, Weintraub P, Krafchick D, Wamboldt FS. (1996) Psychiatric family history in adolescents with severe asthma. *J Am Acad Child Adolesc Psychiatry*, **35**, 1042–9.

Warner JO, Gotz M, Landau LI, *et al*. (1989) Management of asthma: a consensus statement. *Arch Dis Child*, **64**, 1065–79.

Warner JO, Naspitz CK, Cropp GJA. (1998) Third international pediatric concensus statement on the management of childhood asthma. *Pediatr Pulmonol*, **25**, 1–17.

Webb MSC, Henry RL, Milner AD. (1986) Oral corticosteroids for wheezing attacks under 18 months. *Arch Dis Child*, **61**, 15–19.

Welliver RC, Kaul A, Ogra PL. (1979) Cell-mediated immune response to respiratory syncytial virus infection: relationship to the development of reactive airways disease. *J Pediatr*, **94**, 370–5.

Welliver RC, Wong DT, Sun M, Middleton E, Vaughan RS, Ogra PL. (1981) The development of respiratory syncytial virus – specific IGE and the release of histamine in nasopharyngeal secretions after infection. *N Engl J Med*, **305**, 841–6.

Wennergren G, Amark M, Amark K, Oskarsdottir S, Sten G, Redfors S. (1997) Wheezing bronchitis reinvestigated at the age of 10 years. *Acta Paediatr*, **86**, 351–5.

Williamson IJ, Martin CJ, McGill G, Monie RDH, Fennerty AG. (1997) Damp housing and asthma: a case-controlled study. *Thorax*, **52**, 229–34.

Wilson NM, Charette L, Thomson AH, Silverman M. (1985) Gastro-oesophageal reflux and childhood asthma: the acid test. *Thorax*, **40**, 592–7.

Wolthers OD, Hansen M, Juul A, Nielsen HK, Pedersen S. (1997) Knemometry, urine cortisol excretion, and measures of insulin-like growth factor axis and collagen turnover in children treated with inhaled glucocorticosteroids. *Pediatr Res*, **41**, 44–50.

Wolthers OD, Pedersen S. (1990) Short-term linear growth in asthmatic children during treatment with prednisolone. *BMJ*, **301**, 145–8.

Wolthers OD, Pedersen S. (1991) Growth of asthmatic children during treatment with budesonide: a double blind trial. *BMJ*, **303**, 163–5.

Wolthers OD, Pedersen S. (1993) Short-term growth during treatment with inhaled fluticasone propionate and beclomethasone dipropionate. *Arch Dis Child*, **68**, 673–6.

Young S, LeSouef PN, Geelhoed GC, Stick SM, Turner KJ, Landau LI. (1991) The influence of a family history of asthma and parental smoking on airway responsiveness in early infancy. *N Engl J Med*, **324**, 1168–73.

Young S, O'Keeffe PT, Arnott J, Landau LI. (1995) Lung function, airway responsiveness, and respiratory symptoms before and after bronchiolitis. *Arch Dis Child*, **72**, 16–24.

17

Health professional and patient education

MARTYN R. PARTRIDGE AND GRETA BARNES

INTRODUCTION

The Global Strategy for Asthma Management makes clear that a successful health system for good asthma care is one in which the value of clear communication and education is recognized (National Heart, Lung and Blood Institute, 1995). It is regarded as essential that:

- There are sufficient numbers of well educated health professionals organized in an effective manner
- There is prompt and correct diagnosis of asthma, with accurate assessment of severity and appropriate prescriptions
- There is adequate funding to ensure that the correct treatments are available, and that those with asthma should use treatments correctly.

An essential component of this care delivery involves provision of well educated health professionals who offer treatments to patients in a manner that makes it likely that they are taken to advantage. To aid health professionals in this process most countries now have their own national guidelines on asthma management or have adapted and adopted those produced by others. Guidelines are:

- A useful summary of research for the busy clinician
- Valuable for setting standards
- Essential as a basis for audit
- An excellent common text for the teaching of nurses, doctors, medical students and others
- A starting point for patient education.

Grimshaw and Russell (1993) reviewed 59 papers reporting evaluation of clinical guidelines on a variety of subjects and all but four detected significant improvements in the process of care following the introduction of guidelines. Nine of the 11 papers that assessed the outcome of care reported significant improvement.

However it is clear that there is more to guidelines than their production, and two further steps are essential, namely their dissemination (educational activities designed to enhance knowledge and understanding) and their implementation (changing health professional behaviour). The relative merits of different ways of undertaking each of these steps has also been reviewed (Grimshaw and Russell, 1994) and is summarized in Table 17.1.

There has been less specific evaluation of the production, dissemination and implementation of asthma guidelines. However experience of the production and dissemination (Partridge *et al.*, 1998), acceptability (Hilton, 1991) and deficiencies (McGovern and Crockett, 1996) of the British Asthma Guidelines (British Thoracic Society, 1990a,b; 1993a,b; 1997) have been published, as have background papers justifying any consensus statements contained within the guidelines (Barnes, 1996; Bosley *et al.*, 1996; Bucknall, 1996; Durham, 1996; Holgate, 1996a,b; Neville, 1996). The UK dissemination project was evaluated by a guidelines awareness survey both before and after launch which showed only patchy awareness of some of the key messages (Partridge *et al.*, 1998).

Clearly a dissemination project alone is unlikely to have a major effect on outcomes but it is essential as a substrate for subsequent additional education. This is likely to be best done at a practice level and coupled with a system of prompting the health professional to enquire of certain factors during a consultation, and in the future this may be done by some form of computerized decision support system.

This area has been explored in a study in primary care by Feder and colleagues (Feder *et al.*, 1995). Their study involved the adaptation of guidelines for local use in both asthma and diabetes. The first were based on the British asthma guidelines and the latter on the St Vincent's declaration. Groups of primary care physicians were invited to take part in the study and participatory practices offered either three lunchtime sessions on asthma or three sessions on diabetes. The practitioners were offered a stamp to be used in the notes when reviewing patients with asthma, and a stamp and a booklet for reviewing diabetic patients. That for asthma prompted the practitioners to ask about daytime symptoms, night-time wakening, time off work or school, and use of reliever inhalers and it prompted them to check inhaler technique and to record peak flow. Those practitioners who received the diabetes education also monitored their asthma outcomes and the asthma-educated group also recorded their outcomes for diabetes care. The results showed that the practices educated in diabetes improved their recording of all variables compared with baseline, and the practices educated in asthma significantly improved their recording of inhaler technique, patients' smoking habits and symptoms, compared to baseline. Analysis of post-intervention prescriptions showed an increased rate of prescribing of antiinflammatory therapies in the asthma-educated practices compared with both baseline and the diabetes-educated practices.

Table 17.1   *Likely efficacy of different methods of introducing clinical practice guidelines*

Probability of being effective	Development	Dissemination	Implementation
High	Internal	Specific educational intervention	Patient-specific reminder at consultation
Above average	Intermediate	Continuing medical education	Patient-specific feedback
Below average	External – local	Mailing targeted groups	General feedback
Low	External – national	Publication in a journal	General reminder

Source: From a systematic review of 91 studies: Grimshaw J and Russell I (1994)

Taking educational initiatives regarding guidelines and optimal management down to the place of work of health professionals therefore seems to be a sensible starting point for implementation. Prompting of doctors during consultations to ask specific questions and to make certain observations also appears to be beneficial. This has been shown to be as true in the emergency room management of asthma (Town *et al.*, 1990), as in this primary care study.

In addition to attention being paid to the education and training of health professionals, equal attention needs to be focused on the way in which care for those with asthma is organized, how it is monitored, how a multidisciplinary team approach may be utilized and how we ensure that care is optimal in the interface between primary and secondary care.

ORGANIZATION OF CARE

Current treatments for asthma should be capable of successfully treating most people who have the condition, but many patients are still not receiving the care they deserve, and many hospitalizations, for example, could have been avoided by different prior care. The key to good management lies in organized care with an emphasis on prevention, and this is clearly preferable to crisis management. An optimal approach requires thorough assessment and diagnosis, a logical guidelines-based approach to treatment, and regular follow-up to monitor patients' symptoms and their response to therapy. In addition, emphasis must be placed on providing good, very often simple, patient education, and this needs to include the appropriate amount of information to suit the individual and enable self-management.

The death rate from asthma has fallen in many countries over the last 10 years, suggesting an improvement in the delivery and receiving of care. In England and Wales mortality from asthma dropped from more than 2000 deaths in 1988 to 1500 per annum in 1993 despite an increased prevalence of the condition, and there has been a similar more recent fall in hospital admission rates. There does not appear to be one single reason for this and few studies have looked at the organization of care (Droogan and Bannigan, 1997). It is likely to be due to several factors (Charlton *et al.*, 1991; Jones and Mullee, 1995). These include the introduction of the British Asthma Guidelines in 1990 (British Thoracic Society, 1990a,b; 1993a,b; 1997), which provided a structured framework and could be followed by all health care professionals; the enhanced role of primary care with the introduction in the UK of a Government sponsored Chronic Disease Management Programme in 1993 (Department of Health, 1993), which led to 90% of general practices implementing structured organized asthma care, usually in the form of clinics; and the greater involvement of specially trained nurses who have an extended role and who have played a major role in changing asthma management in general practice in the UK (Neville *et al.*, 1996). Other countries such as Finland have similarly set up National Programmes for organized asthma management with ambitious targets for reducing morbidity and mortality.

At a clinician level, successful management depends largely on good personal and working relationships between patients, their families, and the health professionals. Good communication and consistent messages regarding treatment, management and advice, both within primary care and across the primary/secondary care interface are essential for the provision of a successful asthma service.

METHODS OF DELIVERING CARE

Shared care

Patients with asthma may access health care either in the community (primary care), in an emergency department or within hospital, either as an inpatient or outpatient. During the

1990s shared care was increasingly recognized as an accepted way of management for asthma and other long-term disorders. It may be offered on several levels: between primary and secondary care; within primary care; and within secondary care. The advantage of such shared care, if successful, is that it is able to provide an integrated and co-ordinated approach between all members of a health professional team and their patients.

The first level of shared care, between the primary (general practice) and secondary (hospital) sector, is relevant for about 5–10% of the total asthma population. Approximately 90% of patients should be capably managed exclusively in general practice. In secondary care, good two-way communication is vital and where successful, has been shown to be of value in the long-term follow-up for some groups of patients with more severe or troublesome diseases (Grampian Asthma Study, 1994). These include patients with 'brittle' or difficult-to-control asthma and those on long-term oral steroid therapy. For people with severe asthma it is important that the interface between primary and secondary care is good and that there is efficient transmission of information between doctors and nurses caring for patients in hospital and their colleagues in general practice.

In several countries, shared care within general practice has become the norm. The drive towards a health service led by primary health care has meant that traditional boundaries between medical and nursing professions have become blurred (Campbell, 1997) and many general practitioners have welcomed the extended role of the nurse. Whilst there are potential benefits of shared care for patients and health professionals alike, there are also potential risks. For example, formalized protocols may contain clinical freedom and stifle innovation, and shared care guidelines must be 'quality' focused rather than cost based.

Increasing involvement of nurses in asthma care: examples from the UK

Until the late 1980s the majority of patients with asthma in the UK consulted their doctor only if they required treatment to relieve their symptoms. Only a minority received prophylactic medication, such as sodium cromoglycate or beclomethasone diproprionate, for which a structured approach to therapy was required, and only in a few instances was care delivered via an asthma clinic (Pearson and Barnes, 1985).

By 1993, there had been a dramatic change and 90% of practices in the UK offered supervision of asthma under a Government-initiated Chronic Disease Management Programme as a result of the changes in the National Health Service (Department of Health, 1993). This allowed general practitioners to claim re-imbursement for asthma care. A postal survey of all 14 251 general practices in the UK, undertaken in 1993, found that 3339 (77%) of the responding 4327 practices ran some form of specialist clinic for those with asthma in primary care (Barnes and Partridge, 1994). Activities reported to be undertaken by the majority of those running asthma clinics included checking inhaler technique, education of patients about asthma, explaining about different treatments and teaching recognition of signs of worsening asthma. Nurses were involved in the majority of the asthma clinics with 26% of the sample (866/3339) operated by the nurse alone and 67% (2248/3339) run by a nurse and general practitioner together. Only 175 respondents (5%) reported asthma clinics run by a general practitioner alone.

A more recent survey of 457 practice nurses undertaken in 1997 (Barnes, 1998) showed that in the practices in which they worked, 58% ran an asthma clinic while 36% organized structured care for their asthma patients but not in a dedicated clinic. Only 7% of practices were seeing patients on an ad hoc basis. Whilst some general practitioners choose to look after their own patients who have asthma, the trend in the UK in group practices is towards the team approach with the nurse playing a major role. The extent of involvement of the practice nurses who responded to the 1997 survey showed that more than three-quarters of the practice nurses could be considered to have maximum involvement in asthma care (Barnes, 1998) (Table 17.2).

Delivery of care in hospital

Appropriately, hospital doctors are involved in delivering care to both outpatients (where they may be seen in general respiratory clinics or dedicated asthma clinics) and for patients requiring admission with acute and severe asthma. Patients need to be seen by respiratory specialists where there is uncertainty about diagnosis, if the patient is not responding to standard asthma therapy, or if they have occupational asthma or 'brittle' disease. Two studies have shown that if the inpatient care of patients suffering from acute asthma is carried out by general physicians rather than respiratory specialists, the patient is much more likely to be subsequently re-admitted (Bucknall et al., 1988; Bell et al., 1991).

As in the primary care arena, the role of the hospital-based nurse specialist has developed considerably during the last few years (Wooler, 1993; Dzyngel et al., 1994). In many hospitals nurses see patients who have been admitted with acute asthma prior to their discharge to ensure that they understand the treatment they have been prescribed and have appropriate follow-up arrangements. This may be particularly valuable where patients are admitted under a non-respiratory physician. The respiratory nurse specialist also spends time providing information and education for the patient and family and checks that they understand about their inhaled therapy and how to use their inhaler. Where appropriate, the nurse supervises the hospital nebulizer service and may also provide the link between the hospital and the community, liaising with practice-based nurses regarding those who have been admitted to hospital with severe asthma. Some hospital-based nurses provide a 'drop in' clinic, which offers an informal setting in which to educate patients and their families about asthma (Wooler, 1993, 1998; Dzyngel et al., 1994; Madge et al., 1997). These clinics provide open referral for general practitioner practice nurses, school nurses and health visitors and can provide a valuable link with the community.

Table 17.2 *Areas of asthma care in general practice in which nurses can be involved*

Minimum role for nurse (patient always sees GP)
  Compiling/maintaining an asthma register
  Taking a structured formal history
  Taking peak flows in surgery
  Teaching how to use peak flow at home and keep diary chart
  Demonstrating, instructing, checking inhaler technique

Medium role for nurse (potential for a GP/nurse clinic)
  Carrying out further tests (e.g. reversibility, exercise)
  Improving asthma education
  Providing explanatory literature
  Spotting poor control with referral back to GP
  Establishing regular follow-up procedures

Maximum role for nurse (autonomy/nurse-run clinic with GP availability)
  Carrying out full assessments and regular follow-up
  Formulating structured treatment plan in conjunction with GP and patient
  Preparing prescription for approval by GP
  Giving telephone advice where appropriate
  Seeing patients first in an 'emergency' i.e. presentation with increased symptoms

In addition to nurses based exclusively in hospitals or in primary care, in some areas nurses have a specific additional responsibility for asthma liaison. The role of the asthma liaison nurse is to facilitate a team approach during a patient's admission to hospital and discharge back to the community, and to be helpful in providing advice on asthma management. The value of the asthma liaison nurse is that she is able to work across the boundaries between primary and secondary care, and may play a key role in the education and updating of nurses working in both primary and secondary care.

One area where co-ordination of care may be especially necessary, but which is often sub-optional, is the care of those attending Emergency Departments. Some of these attenders are repetitively seeking care from these departments and bypassing the opportunity of regular supervision in primary or secondary care clinics. In one national survey of Accident and Emergency Departments throughout the UK, 425 of 1292 patients with asthma attending such departments (32.5%) had been admitted to hospital in the previous 12 months and 316 (24.5%) had attended the same Accident and Emergency Department in the previous 3 months (Partridge *et al.*, 1997). Only a quarter had had any contact with their general practitioner (primary care physician) in the preceding 24 hours. In 30% of cases it was at least a month since the patient had had any contact with his or her general practitioner. The repetitive nature of these attendances may result from a variety of factors but it seems logical that unless any one health professional monitors such attacks, severity may be underestimated, and yet in only very few instances are services organized in such a way that primary care is automatically and promptly notified of such attendances. The potential for reducing morbidity by such a process may be considerable. In the National Survey (Partridge *et al.*, 1997) one fifth of the adults attending emergency departments had been kept awake by their asthma for over three nights before attendance and in another study of those hospitalized because of severe asthma, 53% had been waking for five nights before admission (Blainey *et al.*, 1991). The opportunity for educating these patients as to how they could use this time to alter their own treatment to prevent their asthma deteriorating is being missed if shared care across the interface between primary and secondary care is not co-ordinated.

TRAINING OF NURSES AND DOCTORS IN PRIMARY CARE: THE UK EXPERIENCE

The need for special training for general practitioners and practice nurses was recognized in the UK in the mid-1980s. It became evident that the implementation of preventive care for people with asthma (which needed to include patient education and teaching self-management) demanded expertise and time (Tettersell, 1993). The lessons learnt from the setting-up and running of hypertension clinics from the Medical Research Council's Hypertension Trial (Pearson, 1985) and the subsequent extension of the nurse's role were able to be successfully applied to asthma. By 1987 the Asthma Training Centre (now the National Asthma and Respiratory Training Centre, NARTC) was established with charitable status. The Centre provided independent training programmes for general practitioners and nurses with the aim of improving asthma care in the community (Barnes, 1998). Although training was offered to both groups of health professionals (doctors and nurses), it was chiefly taken up by nurses who were supported by their general practitioners.

Since 1990, an accredited Diploma in Asthma Care programme has been in place (Barnes, 1998) (Table 17.3). Participants undertake 6 months distance learning, receive practical experience and are given face-to-face teaching. The programme culminates in a practical and written assessment and successful students are awarded the NARTC Diploma in Asthma Care.

Table 17.3 *National asthma and respiratory training centre (NARTC) diploma in asthma care. The health professional should be able to:*

- Critically analyse at an appropriate level
    What asthma is
    The incidence of asthma
    Predisposing factors
    Diagnosis
    Treatment
    Management
- Conduct appropriate assessment of a patient with asthma
- Identify the signs of deteriorating asthma
- Monitor and evaluate the patient's condition
- Understand and use appropriate referral strategies
- Have a knowledge and understanding of specific therapeutic interventions such as drug therapy, inhaler devices, etc.
- Demonstrate organizational skills in relation to the management of asthma such as a nurse-run asthma clinic
- Evaluate and audit the process of quality assurance for asthma
- Make a major contribution to the health promotion of patients with the education of fellow professionals

Aim: To educate health professionals in the management of asthma in order to improve the care of patients with asthma in the community.
The course consists of a distance learning package, video, and a 2-day intensive course at the NARTC or regional centres. The course requires approximately 200 hours, with approximately 120 hours over 6 months for the distance learning package, 39 hours of contact teaching and 41 hours of practice assignments. For the diploma to be awarded, candidates must reach a satisfactory level in both written and practical assessments.

Approximately 1600 health professionals (mainly nurses but also doctors, physiotherapists, pharmacists and lung function technicians) undertake the programme throughout the UK each year. In addition courses are held regularly in other countries. A variety of basic training programmes can generally be considered suitable for the nurse who wishes to have a minimum or medium role (Table 17.2) in the management of asthma patients. However, successful completion of the accredited higher level course, coupled with practical experience and regular updating, equips the nurse for involvement at the maximum level, with autonomy to run an asthma clinic.

If nurses take on an extended role, standardized training, which includes assessment, must be recognized as essential. The most important factor to emerge from studies looking at nurse involvement in asthma management is adequate training (Droogan and Bannigan, 1997). Studies identifying an impact on asthma management, using as the criteria for involvement the presence in the practice of a nurse with an NARTC Diploma in Asthma Care found correlation with improved outcomes (Patterson, 1997).

Looking specifically at the nurses engaged in asthma care, a survey conducted in 1993 found that 251 of 1131 nurses running an asthma clinic in the UK, (22%) did so without formal assessed training (Barnes and Partridge, 1994).

A study of patient knowledge about asthma and compliance with therapy also identified the need for adequate training and education of the nurses working with these patients (Tettersell, 1993). Nurses without advanced asthma training were shown to be significantly less likely to discuss patient worries and anxieties, provide a written self-management plan for the patient, or to check peak expiratory flow records kept by the patient before a review appointment.

It is important that nurses should successfully complete a recognized course that includes assessment of safety to practice and evidence of keeping up to date. Simply following a training programme is not evidence of achieving a suitable standard. For example, of the 2846 students studying for the NARTC Diploma in Asthma Care between 1995 and 1997, 518 (19%) failed to reach a satisfactory standard and did not receive the qualification. Of these, 254 re-entered the examination and 162 (64%) were successful the second time.

It is clear that in addition to the need for training in the disease, greater responsibility for nurses demands further training in the area of differential diagnosis and appropriate referral. If specialist asthma nurses were to prescribe, then training on drug interactions and pharmacology would be required. Undoubtedly the training of nurses in primary care has had an impact on prescribing. One audit on the effect of nurse-run clinics in a four-partner general practice found there was an increase in the proportion of patients receiving prophylactic medication from 52% before the establishment of the clinic to 71% afterwards (Charlton et al., 1991). Some have concerns that greater nurse involvement in prescribing may increase costs, as nurses may be more willing to prescribe expensive devices or newer products than doctors. However, in order for the treatment to be cost-effective it is necessary to find a treatment and inhaler device that is appropriate for the individual patient. Specially trained nurses who teach and instruct patients are aware that the most 'expensive' device is the one that the patient either cannot, or will not, use.

Many general practitioners consider that their chief role is to diagnose and initiate the management and treatment of asthma. For this group, undoubtedly the most important training tool has been the introduction of national asthma guidelines. However, guidelines do not teach practical skills and many general practitioners need to be trained how to use the large number of different inhaler devices and also how to demonstrate them to patients.

AUDIT

There is clearly a need to measure the effectiveness of different methods of delivering asthma care. Measurement of good care requires clinical assessment and review of case records, followed by repeat assessment and review (Neville, 1998). The principle of ongoing assessment and review underpins the various audit packages such as the Tayside Stamp, and the Jones morbidity index and the GRASSIC audit package (GRASSIC, 1994). The outcome of good care should primarily lead to patients feeling better, and involve appropriate use of preventative therapy and health service resources. There are several factors which influence the success or otherwise of the delivery of care. It has been shown in the UK that larger general practices have lower hospital asthma admission rates than single-handed practices (Griffiths et al., 1997) and such practices are more likely to employ practice nurses, use computers, have practice managers and to undertake audit (Lees and Bosanquet, 1995). The recent undertaking of audit has been shown to be associated with improved asthma outcomes (Neville et al., 1996). Practices running asthma clinics by a specialist asthma-trained nurse had more patients operating self-management plans, fewer patients with symptoms and days lost due to asthma, fewer acute attacks and were more aggressive in giving patients short courses of systemic steroids than other practices (Griffiths et al., 1997). Improved outcomes in terms of prescriptions paralleling the advice contained in guidelines were also shown to occur when patients were reviewed in an asthma clinic largely run by specialist asthma-trained nurses (Dickison et al., 1997).

COMMUNICATION, PATIENT EDUCATION AND SELF-MANAGEMENT

Every person with asthma has a different personality, has had different past life experiences and a different set of fears and concerns. Realization of these factors by health professionals is essential if a satisfactory partnership of care is to be developed. In addition, to the 'within patient' factors, each person with asthma is influenced in both beneficial and potentially adverse ways by factors around them. Support and reassurance may come from friends, family and sources of information but peer pressure, conflicting media stories and misinformation on the Web may conflict with the aims of health professionals.

Good communication within the health professional/patient consultation can mitigate the adverse effects of these influences and build upon the positive supporting factors. Doctors and nurses need to be aware how common it is for those with asthma not to accept the diagnosis. In one qualitative study of 30 patients with doctor-diagnosed asthma who had been on preventive and reliever inhalers for at least a year, the patients were invited by letter to attend for an interview. Approximately one-half of the sample, when interviewed, were keen to impress upon the interviewer that they did not have asthma. Some claimed their name had got on to the wrong list, others claimed it was the first time that they had been told that they had asthma, while others had clearly heard the word 'asthma' applied to them but still did not accept it – 'She said I had bronchial asthma, so it's bronchial I am'. When asked to describe what the term asthma meant to them, many portrayed very negative images of the condition (Adams et al., 1997). Health professionals also need to appreciate the magnitude of the effect that asthma is having on people's lives. One study revealed that 32% of those with asthma felt depressed, 38% were angry at having the condition and 20% felt different from other people (Sibbald, 1989). These feelings might need to be aired, as might those concerning medication. Steroid phobia may be common, and questions about side-effects of medication are a common reason of persons with asthma to ring a telephone helpline (Crone et al., 1993), but the predominant dislike may be that of the need for regular medication of any type (Osman et al., 1993).

Patients and health professionals may also have different expectations of the condition and its treatment and may have markedly differing goals. We may regard a peak flow chart showing wide variations in flows as being indicative of a need for regular antiinflammatory therapy, whereas to a person with asthma the same chart implies the need for treatment when poorly, but no need when well. Even when theoretical goals are shared, human nature may lead to compromise. Whilst the person with asthma may therefore know that night-time waking with asthma reflects poorly controlled disease they feel more comfortable using a relieving bronchodilator at these times rather than doing what they know to be correct and increasing their preventive therapy.

To deliver effective care to those with asthma we therefore need firstly to recognize the absolute importance of good communication and high standard consultation. This can increase a patient's satisfaction (Beckman and Frankel, 1984), improve compliance (Falvo and Tippy, 1988) and enhance the likelihood of accurate diagnosis (Barsky, 1981). Paradoxically, poor communication is more likely to lead to legal action against the physician (Levinson et al., 1997). Summarizing the benefits of an ideal consultation, Fallowfield has proposed the diagram shown in Fig. 17.1 (Fallowfield, 1992).

Within good communication must be the realization that communication involves more than the spoken word:

- A sender, a message and a recipient where the sender, the health professional, also listens
- A realization that much of what is said during a consultation is soon forgotten
- Accepting that repetition and reinforcement of messages are essential

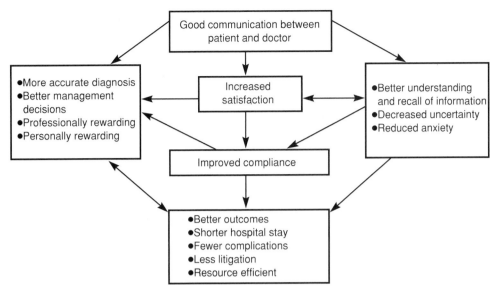

Figure 17.1 *The benefits of an ideal consultation. (Redrawn with the permission of Professor Lesley Fallowfield.)*

- An understanding that each person is an individual with different wants, a differing personality, different fears and concerns and different goals and expectations.

How can we reinforce the spoken word within a consultation and how do patients rate health professionals at the present time? Only 22% of patients in one survey of those with asthma felt that they had had a good discussion with the doctor (Partridge, 1995). Only 27% had had written information about when and how to take their medication and yet simply writing out for the patient a daily regimen can significantly increase correct recall and other outcomes (Sandler *et al.*, 1989; Pedersen, 1992; Raynor *et al.*, 1993). We can also offer patients access to booklets, videos, group support and telephone helplines, and whilst access to such information will not alone improve outcomes it can act as a suitable building block for more personalized information, as summarized in Fig. 17.2.

Whilst compliance with using asthma medication in asthma may be no better or worse than in other long-term conditions it can probably be improved by:

- Patients accepting that asthma can be severe
- Patients accepting that any risk can apply to them
- Patients having had an opportunity to discuss risks versus benefits of treatment
- Patients feeling in control
- There having been good communication between patient and health professional.

The global strategy for asthma management states: 'The aim of patient education, which is a continual process, is to provide the patient with asthma, and the patient's family with suitable information and training so that the patient can keep well and adjust treatment according to a medication plan developed with the health care professional' (National Heart, Lung and Blood Institute, 1995).

The key components are described as:

- The development of a partnership
- Acceptance that this is a continuing process

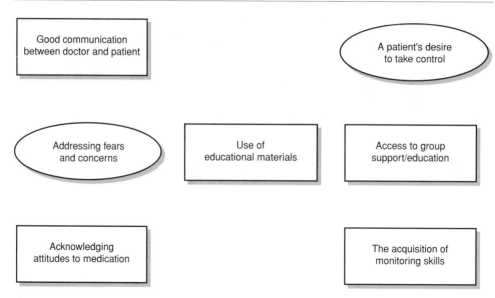

Figure 17.2 *The components of successful patient education and self-management.*

- A sharing of information
- A full discussion of expectation
- Expression of fears and concerns.

The patient then requires information about:

- Diagnosis
- Difference between relievers and preventers
- Training in the use of inhaler devices
- Advice regarding prevention and allergen avoidance
- Signs that suggest asthma is worsening
- Training in monitoring the asthma
- Advice about how and when to seek medical attention.

Following this the person with asthma receives:

- A guided self-management plan
- Regular supervision, revision, reward and reinforcement.

Perhaps most elucidation is required of the term 'self-management'. All patients with asthma self-manage their own condition to some extent, in that they self-treat with reliever inhalers when they perceive a need, and they consult doctors when unwell. In a wider context self-management involves the patient and his or her family, knowing how to adjust the immediate environment to reduce allergen exposure, how to adjust lifestyles (for example, to avoid a smoky atmosphere), and how to self-medicate and to adjust medication to reduce the risks of the asthma slipping from control. The term may have different meaning to others who may regard it as a delegation of care from the health professional to the patient – to guard against that we should perhaps refer to 'guided self-management' to emphasize the ongoing nature of this process within a partnership of care. When talking with doctors and nurses working in different fields we should appreciate that the term self-management may mean different things to others. 'Self-management' may imply mainly lifestyle changes and this may be the case in other longer term conditions such as hypertension, obesity or rheumatoid arthritis, where the self-adjustment by patients may involve diet and exercise for example, more than changes in their prescribed medication. Where self-management involves more lifestyle changes than drug change, teaching of it may be appropriately given by lay people or indeed by fellow patients, and this is a common approach in some arthritis self-management programmes in the UK and USA. In other diseases self-management involves more the patient altering the prescribed medication; at this end of the spectrum this may more accurately be described as 'self-treatment' and sometimes the written advice received by such patients is referred to as an 'action plan'. Where self-management involves a significant component of self-treatment, for example as in diabetes or asthma, the teaching of self-management skills is, of necessity, health professional-rather than lay-led. These concepts are summarized in Fig. 17.3.

An example of an asthma self-treatment (action) plan is shown in Table 17.4. Whilst such plans were promoted in guidelines 9–10 years ago, good evidence in favour of self-treatment has only become available more recently.

Several studies have compared self-monitoring and use of detailed self-treatment (action) plans with usual care in adults and shown improved outcomes in the form of reduced hospitalization rates, emergency doctor visits, time off work, and use of reserve medications. These studies (Ignacio-Garcia and Gonzalez-Santos, 1995; Lahdensuo *et al.*, 1996) were based upon action plans, which advised patients to alter their therapy in response to changes in

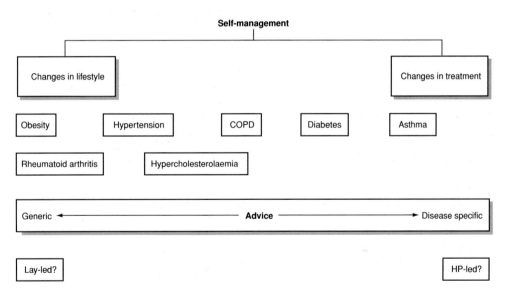

Figure 17.3   *What does self-management mean and involve? This illustration demonstrates how the spectrum of self-management involves both lifestyle changes (e.g. exercise, dieting, allergen avoidance) and self-adjustment of prescribed medication (self-treatment). For some diseases self-management involves predominantly changes in lifestyle (e.g. arthritis, obesity and hypertension), and here generic advice regarding the value of weight reduction and regular instruction may be offered by lay people (or those with the condition) and could even be generic and offered to those with several different conditions at the same time. For other conditions, e.g. diabetes and asthma, lifestyle changes such as diet, exercise and allergen avoidance are equally important, but the main self-motivated intervention is altering prescribed medication to maintain control of the condition and prevent deterioration to a crisis level. Under these circumstances it seems best that self-management (in this case, predominantly self-treatment) is best supervised or guided in a co-management manner with the health professional (HP).*

Table 17.4 *Self-management plan*

ZONE 1

Your asthma is under control if
- it does not disturb your sleep
- it does not restrict your usual activities
  and
- your peak flow readings are above_____

    ACTION
    Your preventer is_____
    You should normally take
    _____puffs/doses
    _____times every day (using a spacer)
    _____even when you are feeling well
    Your reliever is_____
    You should normally only take it when you are
    short of breath, coughing or wheezing, or
    before exercise
    Your other medicines are

ZONE 2
(Your doctor or nurse may decide not to use this zone)
Your asthma is getting worse if
- you are needing to use your

  _____
  (reliever inhaler) more than usual
- you are waking at night with asthma
  symptoms
  and
- your peak flow readings have fallen to
  between_____ and_____

ACTION
Increase your usual medicines
- increase your

  _____
  (preventer inhaler) to

  _____
- Continue to take your

  _____
  (reliever inhaler) to relieve your asthma
  symptoms

ZONE 3

Your asthma is severe if
- you are getting increasingly breathless
- you are needing to use your

  _____
  (reliever/inhaler) every
  _____hours or more often
  and
- your peak flow readings have fallen to
  between_____and_____

ACTION
- Take

  _____prednisolone (steroid) tablets
  (strength_____mg each) and then

  _____

  _____
- Discuss with your doctor how and when to
  stop taking the tablets
- Continue to take your

  _____

  (reliever and preventer inhalers) as prescribed

ZONE 4

It is a medical alert/emergency if
- your symptoms continue to get worse
  and
- your peak flow readings have fallen to below

  _____

Do not be afraid of causing a fuss
Your doctor will want to see you urgently

ACTION
Get help immediately
- Telephone your doctor straightaway on

  _____

  or call an ambulance
- Take
  _____prednisolone (steroid) tablets
  (strength _____ mg each) immediately
- Continue to take your

  _____

  (reliever/inhaler) as needed, or every
  5–10 minutes until the ambulance arrives

symptoms and changes in peak flow. For example, in the study by Lahdensuo and colleagues (1996) patients were advised to double their dose of inhaled steroid for 2 weeks if their peak flow fell below 85% of their optimal personal peak flow, and to start a course of steroid tablets if it fell to below 70% of optimal. Compliance with such changes in treatment was surprisingly good and on 77% of occasions when the patients' condition indicated the need to start a course of steroid tablets, they did so. In this study the self-management group actually had better controlled asthma than the control group but used less steroid tablets overall. This suggests that a feeling of 'being in control' might also enhance compliance with regular therapy, making it less likely that their condition deteriorates to a point where further reserve medication is needed.

The study of Lahdensuo and colleagues (1996) has now been extended by a cost-effectiveness evaluation (Lahdensuo *et al.*, 1998). Whilst the direct health care costs per patient were greater in the self-management group, because of the costs of counselling, the effectiveness of guided self-management reduced indirect costs by such an extent that overall costs were significantly less in the self-managed group.

Whether such action plans used by adults should be based on symptoms or on objective peak flow readings was studied by Turner and colleagues (1998). In this study each patient in a primary care setting was allocated to a nurse-led 6-month asthma education programme and half given action plans based on peak flows (with rather lower thresholds than in Lahdensuo's study) and half given one based on subjective parameters (*see* Table 17.5). Both interventions improved their lung function, symptom scores, quality of life and inhaled steroid dosages compared to baseline, but the only differences between the two groups was that those having peak flow-based action plans made less unscheduled visits to doctors. The additional benefits of peak flow monitoring as part of a self-treatment (action) plan are therefore unproven. It is therefore possibly an issue to discuss with patients as to how they feel about subjective versus objective monitoring and when preferences have been elicited or expressed in studies there is a tendency towards positive comments about objective monitoring (Lloyd and Ali, 1992; D'Souza *et al.*, 1994). One other factor in favour of objective monitoring (which could in time be utilized alongside other methods such as mini hand-held spirometers) is that some patients with asthma may have a diminished ability to perceive a reduction in airway calibre (Kendrick *et al.*, 1993; Kikuchi *et al.*, 1994).

There have been fewer studies of the value of self-management in children. However, in one study all children being admitted to a children's hospital with asthma were allocated to either routine care, or to an educational intervention (Madge *et al.*, 1997). The latter involved a specialist nurse going over with parent and child the circumstances that had led to that

Table 17.5   *A possible symptom-based self-management plan (from Turner et al., 1998)*

1   When you feel normal continue maintenance treatment with:
   (a)   bronchodilators as needed
   (b)   inhaled steroids twice daily
2   If you catch a cold or start to feel tight or awake at night with wheezing or have a persistent cough:
   (a)   double the dose of inhaled steroid until you return to normal
   (b)   Use bronchodilators two puffs every 4 hours as needed
3   If the effect of your bronchodilators lasts only 2 hours and you find doing your normal activities makes you short of breath:
   (a)   Start prednisolone tablets, 40 mg daily
   (b)   Continue this dose for at least 1 week until symptoms have normalized, then reduce prednisolone by 5 mg daily until stopped
4   If the effect of your bronchodilators lasts only 30 minutes or you have difficulty talking:
   (a)   Consult family physician immediately
   (b)   If unavailable call Ambulance (**999 / 911**), or
   (c)   Go directly to hospital emergency department

admission and advising how in future self-management might be used to avoid such an admission. This was reinforced with a written action plan, based where appropriate on subjective and objective (peak flow) monitoring. During a 2–14 month follow-up period there was a significant reduction in readmission rates for the intervention group compared with the traditionally managed group.

A recent systematic review of the effects of self-management education and regular practitioner review in adults with asthma by Gibson and colleagues for the Cochrane Airways Group (Gibson *et al.*, 1999) looked at results from 22 randomized controlled trials of this subject and concluded that when self-management was compared with usual care, there were reductions in hospitalizations, unscheduled visits to the doctor, days off work or school and nocturnal asthma and improvements in peak flow. Educational interventions, which included provision of a written action plan, were associated with better outcomes.

What we need now is a better understanding of who needs what sort of self-management plan, who needs to monitor it objectively and more information about whether the same results of trials in adults can necessarily be applied to children. Finally, we need further information about how to issue such advice most effectively and to determine the relative contributions of doctors, nurses, trained educators, lay educators and group support to the process. Newer interactive methods of offering patients information and self-treatment advice may involve interactive multimedia and more use of telephone consultations.

REFERENCES

Adams S, Pill R, Jones A. (1997) Medication, chronic illness and identity: the perspective of people with asthma. *Soc Sci Med*, **45**, 189–201.

Barnes G. (1998) The nurses's role in asthma management. *Sem Respir Crit Care Med*, **19** (6), 593–601.

Barnes G, Partridge MR. (1994) Community asthma clinics; 1993. Survey of *primary care* by the National Asthma Task Force. *Quality in Health Care*, **3**, 135–6.

Barnes PJ. (1996) Inhaled glucocorticoids: new developments relevant to updating of the asthma management guidelines. *Respir Med*, **90**, 385–90.

Barsky AJ III. (1981) Hidden reasons some patients visit doctors. *Ann Intern Med*, **94**, 492–8.

Beckman HB, Frankel RM. (1984) The effect of physician behaviour on the collection of data. *Ann Intern Med*, **101**, 692–6.

Bell D, Layton AJ, Gabbay J. (1991) Use of a guideline based questionnaire to audit hospital care of acute asthma. *BMJ*, **302**, 1440–3.

Blainey AD, Beale A, Lomas D, Partridge MR. (1991) The cost of acute asthma – how much is preventable? *Health Trends*, **22**, 151–3.

Bosley CM, Corden ZM, Cochrane GM. (1996) Psychosocial factors and asthma. *Respir Med*, **90**, 453–7.

British Thoracic Society and others. (1993a) Guidelines on the management of asthma. *Thorax*, **48**, S1–24.

British Thoracic Society and others. (1993b) Guidelines on the management of asthma. *BMJ*, **306**, 776–82.

British Thoracic Society and others. (1997) British Guidelines on Asthma Management, 1995 review and position statement. *Thorax*, **52**, S1–21.

British Thoracic Society, Research Unit of the Royal College of Physicians of London, King's Fund Centre, National Asthma Campaign. (1990a) Guidelines for management of asthma in adults: I. Chronic persistent asthma. *BMJ*, **301**, 651–3.

British Thoracic Society, Research Unit of the Royal College of Physicians of London, King's Fund Centre, National Asthma Campaign. (1990b) Guidelines for management of asthma in adults: II. Acute severe asthma. *BMJ*, **301**, 767–800.

Bucknall CE. (1996) Definitions of severity and outcome measures. *Respir Med*, **90**, 447–52.

Bucknall CE, Robertson C, Moran F, Stevenson RD. (1988) Management of asthma in hospital: a prospective audit. *BMJ*, **296**, 1637–9.

Campbell S. (1997) Nurse practitioners at the cutting edge of today's NHS. *Primary Care*, **7**, 2–4.

Charlton I, Charlton G, Broomfield J, Mulle MA. (1991) Audit of the effect of a nurse run asthma clinic on workload and patient morbidity in a general practice. *Br J Gen Pract*, **41**, 227–31.

Clough JB. (1996) Recommendations for peak flow monitoring in children. *Respir Med*, **90**, 459–61.

Crone S, Partridge MR, McLean F. (1993) Launching a national helpline. *Health Visitor*, **66**, 94–6.

Department of Health. (1993) On the state of the public health. Annual report of the Chief Medical Officer. London: HMSO.

D'Souza W, Crane J, Burgess C, *et al*. (1994) Community based asthma care: trial of a 'credit card' asthma self management plan. *Eur Respir J*, **7**, 1260–5.

Dickison J, Hutton S, Atkin A. (1997) Implementing the BTS Guidelines. The effect of a nurse-run asthma clinic on prescribed treatment in a North Lincolnshire general practice. *Respir Med*, **91**, 634–40.

Droogan J, Bannigan K. (1997) Organisation of asthma care; what difference does it make? *Nursing Times*, **93**(34), 45–6.

Durham SR. (1996) Allergen avoidance measures. *Respir Med*, **90**, 441–5.

Dzyngel B, Kesten S, Chapman KR. (1994) Assessment of an ambulatory care asthma programme. *J Asthma*, **31**, 291–300.

Fallowfield L. (1992) The ideal consultation. *Br J Hosp Med*, **47**, 364–7.

Falvo D, Tippy P. (1988) Communicating information to patients – patient satisfaction and adherence as associated with resident skill. *J Fam Prac*, **26**, 643–7.

Feder G, Griffiths C, Highton C, Eldridge S, Spence M, Southgate L. (1995) Do clinical guidelines introduced with practice based education improve care of asthmatic and diabetic patients? A randomised controlled trial in general practices in East London. *BMJ*, **311**, 1473–8.

Gibson PG, Coughlan J, Wilson J, *et al*. (1999) Self management education and regular practitioner review for adults with asthma (Cochrane Review). In: *The Cochrane Library*, Issue 1. Oxford: Update Software.

Grampian Asthma Study of integrated care (GRASSIC). (1994) Integrated care for asthma: a clinical, social and economic evaluation. *BMJ*, **308**, 559–64.

Griffiths C, Study P, Naish J, Omar R, Dolan S, Feder G. (1997) Hospital admissions for asthma in East London: associations with characteristics of local general practices, prescribing and population. *BMJ*, **314**, 482–6.

Grimshaw JM, Russell IT. (1993) Effects of clinical guidelines on medical practice: a systematic review of rigorous evaluation. *Lancet*, **342**, 17–22.

Grimshaw JM, Russell IT. (1994) Achieving health gain through clinical guidelines II: Ensuring guidelines change medical practice. *Qual Health Care*, **3**, 45–52.

Hilton S. (1991) Acceptability of Guidelines Recommendations by GPs with an interest in asthma. *Thorax*, **46**, 741.

Holgate ST. (1996a) Inhaled sodium cromoglycate. *Respir Med*, **90**, 393–6.

Holgate ST. (1996b) The efficacy and therapeutic position of nedocromil sodium. *Respir Med*, **90**, 397–400.

Ignacio-Garcia J, Gonzalez-Santos P. (1995) Asthma self management program by home monitoring of peak expiratory flow. *Am J Respir Crit Care Med*, **151**, 353–9.

Jones K, Cleary R, Hyland M. (1999) Predictive value of a simple asthma morbidity index in a general practice population. *Br J Gen Prac*, **49**, 23–6.

Jones KP, Mullee MA. (1995) Proactive nurse-run asthma care in general practice reduces asthma morbidity. Scientific fact or medical assumption? *Br J Gen Pract*, **45**, 497–9.

Kendrick AH, Higgs CMB, Whitfield MJ, Laszio C. (1993) Accuracy of perception of severity of asthma: patients being treated in general practice. *BMJ*, **307**, 422–4.

Kikuchi Y, Okaba S, Tamura G, *et al*. (1994) Chemosensitivity and perception of dyspnoea in patients with a history of near fatal asthma. *N Engl J Med*, **330**, 11329–34.

Lahdensuo A, Haahtela T, Herrala J, *et al*. (1998) A cost effectiveness analysis of guided self managed treatment of asthma in Finland. *BMJ*, **316**(7138), 1138–9.

Lahdensuo A, Haahtela T, Herrala J, *et al*. (1996) Randomised comparison of guided self management and traditional treatments of asthma over one year. *BMJ*, **312**, 748–52.

Lees B, Bosanquet N. (1995) Changes in general practice and its effect on service provision in areas with different socio-economic characteristics. *BMJ*, **311**, 546–50.

Levinson W, Roter DA, Mullody JP. Dull VT, Frankel RM. (1997) Physician–patient communication – the relationship with malpractice claims among *primary care* physicians and surgeons. *JAMA*, **277**, 553–9.

Lloyd BW, Ali MH. (1992) How useful do patients find home peak flow monitoring for children with asthma. *BMJ*, **305**, 1128–9.

Lung and Asthma Information Agency. (1997) Trends in asthma mortality in Great Britain, Fact Sheet 97/3.

Madge P, McColl J, Paton J. (1997) Impact of a nurse-led home management training programme in children admitted to hospital with acute asthma: a randomised controlled study. *Thorax*, **52**, 223–8.

McGovern V, Crockett A. (1996) 1993 BTS Guidelines: impact and short fall. *Asthma J*, **1**, 30–1.

National Heart, Lung and Blood Institute. (1995) Global Initiative for Asthma. Global strategy for asthma management and prevention (NHLBI/WHO Workshop Report). Publication Number 95-3659, Bethesda, MD: National Institutes of Health.

Neville R. (1996) Patient education and guided self management plans – a background paper for the 1995 revision of the 'BTS Guidelines'. *Respir Med*, **90**, 391–2.

Neville R. (1998) Recommended methods and outcomes used to audit asthma care. Ask the experts. London: Class Publishing, 207–8.

Neville RG, Clark RA, Hopkins G, Smith B. (1993) First national audits of acute asthma attacks in general practice. *Thorax*, **48**, 420.

Neville RG, Hoskins G, Smith B, Clark RA. (1996) Observations on the structure, process and clinical outcomes of asthma care in general practice. *Br J Gen Pract*, **46**, 583–7.

Osman L. (1996) The patient perspective. What should a new anti-asthma agent provide? *Drugs*, **52**, (Suppl 6), 29–35.

Osman LM, Russell IT, Friend JA, Legge S, Douglas JG. (1993) Predicting patient attitudes to asthma medication. *Thorax*, **48**, 827–30.

Partridge MR. (1995) Asthma: lessons from patient education. *Patient Educ Counsel*, **25**, 81–6.

Partridge MR, Harrison BDW, Rudolf M, Bellamy D, Silverman M. (1998) The British Asthma Guidelines – their production, dissemination and implementation. *Respir Med*, **92**, 1046–52.

Partridge MR, Latouche D, Trako E, Thurston JGB. (1997) A national census of those attending UK Accident and Emergency Departments with asthma. *J Acc Emerg Med*, **14**, 16–20.

Patterson M. (1997) Inhaled steroids, theophyllines and salmeterol: a comparison of morbidity data from 2375 patients and the prescribing habits of their physicians in primary care. *Am J Resp Crit Care Med*, **155** (4), A891 and poster presented at ATS 1997.

Pearson R, Barnes G. (1985) Asthma clinics in general practice: a practice approach. In: Royal College of General Practitioners manual.

Pedersen S. (1992) Ensuring compliance in children. *Eur Respir J*, **5**, 143–5.

Raynor DK, Booth TG, Blenkinsopp A. (1993) Effect of computer generated reminder charts on patients compliance with drug regimens. *BMJ*, **306**, 1158–61.

Sandler DA, Heaton C, Garner ST, Mitchell JRA. (1989) Patients' and general practitioners' satisfaction with information given on discharge from hospital, audit of new information card. *BMJ*, **299**, 1511–13.

Sibbald B. (1989) Patient self care in acute asthma. *Thorax*, **44**, 97–101.

Tettersell MJ. (1993) Asthma patients knowledge in relation to compliance with drug therapy. *J Adv Nurs*, **18**, 103–13.

Town L, Kwong T, Holst P, Beasley R. (1990) Use of a management plan for treating asthma in an emergency department. *Thorax*, **45**, 702–6.

Turner MO, Taylor D, Bennett R, Fitzgerald JM. (1998) A randomised trial comparing peak expiratory flow and symptom self management plans for patients with asthma attending a *primary care* clinic. *Am J Respir Crit Care Med*, **157**, 540–6.

Wooler E. (1998) The provision of a 'drop-in' clinic for the asthmatic child. *Resp Dis Prac*, **6**, 8–10.

Wooler E. (1993) The role of the asthma nurse specialist. *Paediatr Respir Med*, **1**, 26–8.

18

Allergy and asthma: control and treatment

J. O. WARNER AND J. A. WARNER

INTRODUCTION

The pre-eminent risk factor for the development of asthma in childhood is the presence of allergy and a family history of atopic asthma or eczema. Indeed amongst those children who have had pre-existing atopic eczema, subsequent asthma not only occurs with a very high frequency but is often severe (McNichol and Williams, 1973). Successive studies have highlighted allergy as the one risk factor predicting ongoing asthma amongst infant wheezers (Sporik et al., 1991; van Asperen and Mukhi, 1994). Furthermore, early onset allergy also predicts continuing symptoms and bronchial hyperresponsiveness through adolescence (Peat et al., 1990). These facts, mostly gleaned from epidemiological studies, must focus attention on preventive strategies employing allergen avoidance, immune modulation and even traditional immunotherapy.

ALLERGENS

The pre-eminent allergen associated with asthma worldwide is the house dust mite, *Dermatophagoides pteronyssinus* and/or *Farinae* (Colloff et al., 1992). However, this is clearly not the only allergen that is important in contributing to the allergen load worldwide. In parts of the world where the house dust mite does not exist, other allergens occupy the niche in taking a key role for inducing asthma. Thus, the further north one progresses in Sweden, the less house mites are involved but the animal allergens of cat and dog become the major contributors (Kjellman and Pettersson, 1983). Similarly in the South of France and in Arizona, alternaria mould is of greater importance (Halonen *et al.*, 1997). In addition local pollens, which vary from country to country, also make a significant contribution (Potter and Cadman, 1996). However, it would be true to say that of the ubiquitous and perennial allergens, the house dust mite and cat are associated with the greatest prevalences of disease (Colloff *et al.*, 1992). Indeed in countries where there are a wide range of potential allergens, house dust mite allergy stands out as the key factor predicting ongoing disease.

One additional allergy has recently been highlighted as having a key predictive position in relation to the development of later asthma: egg sensitization in early infancy (Burr *et al.*, 1997). This is the commonest food to induce sensitivity in the young infant and is associated with the development of atopic dermatitis (Rancé *et al.*, 1999). However, successive studies from South Wales (Burr *et al.*, 1997), the multicentre allergy (MAS) study in Germany (Kulig *et al.*, 1998), and ETAC, a multicentre European study (1998) (*see* Table 18.1), have shown that egg sensitization in infancy is extremely strongly predictive of subsequent sensitization to inhalant allergens and to the development of asthma. Indeed from the MAS study, persistent egg sensitivity conferred a 5.5-fold higher risk for the development of asthma (Kulig *et al.*, 1998).

The latter observations raise a key question about the relationship between allergy and asthma. We are well aware that egg is not a common trigger for asthma, though clearly it is a risk factor. Thus, is allergy merely a marker of disease rather than a cause of it? This conundrum is only likely to be unravelled by long-term prospective and controlled intervention studies focusing on allergens. There is no doubt that appropriate aeroallergen avoidance (Woodcock and Custovic, 1998) and even immunotherapy (Bousquet *et al.*, 1990) can improve established allergic asthma. Thus, the role of allergens in aggravating or inciting already existing disease is not in doubt. There are now observations which would suggest that allergens are also playing a key role in actually inducing rather than just inciting disease.

ALLERGY AND HYPERSENSITIVITY

When considering atopic disease, most have a concept of allergy as Gell and Coombs type 1 IgE mediated immediate hypersensitivity. However, allergy and hypersensitivity are defined as the 'altered acquired specific capacity to react'. There are a variety of mechanisms involved, only one of which involves IgE. It is clear that a whole range of cells, cytokines and other molecules are involved in atopic disease.

Primary exposure to an antigen leads to stimulation of innate immune responses and the

Table 18.1 *Associations between egg sensitivity (based on Grade 1 or more RAST) at 1–2 years of age and aeroallergen sensitivity at 2–4 years; and aeroallergen sensitivity at 1–2 years with the risk of asthma by 2–4 years of age. All numbers are percentages of 817 infants.*

Aeroallergen IgE (RAST ≥0.35 i.v./mL)	Egg IgE (<0.35 i.v./mL)	Egg IgE (≥0.35 i.v./mL)	Risk of asthma aged 2–4 years	
			RAST +ve at 1–2 years	RAST −ve at 1–2 years
Cat	10	53	47	33
House dust mite	22	46	51.5	35
Grass pollen	13	46	59	35

RAST, radioallergosorbent test in international units per ML (i.v./mL).
Source: From ETAC Study Group (1998).

engulfment of the antigen by antigen presenting cells. Peptide fragments of antigen are re-presented on the cell surface in association with major histocompatability complex (MHC) molecules which are recognized by T-cell receptors. In association with a range of co-stimulatory molecule interactions and cytokines released by the antigen presenting cell, the T lymphocyte acquires the specific immunological message transmitted by the peptide fragments in the MHC molecule. The T lymphocyte, in turn, expresses a range of cytokines and proliferates, creating a clone of cells that now will recognize the specific antigen.

The T-helper lymphocytes produce a range of cytokines which polarize into two categories. The Th1 cells are associated with stimulation of cell-mediated immunity by the release of interleukin-2 (IL-2) and interferon-gamma (IFN-γ). Th2 cells are associated with allergy and release IL-4, -5, -10 and -13. IL-4 and IL-13 produce a gene deletional switch in B lymphocytes which leads to production of IgE rather than IgM antibodies. IL-5, also released from Th2 cells, attracts and activates eosinophils to the site of exposure. Adhesion molecules in the endothelium are upregulated by many of the above cytokines, which allows eosinophils and also, indeed, neutrophils to adhere to the endothelial surface and migrate out of the vascular space. These leucocytes then release a range of mediators that cause tissue damage, oedema and the airways bronchospasm. All of these latter events can occur in the absence of any IgE-mediated mechanism. Thus it is perhaps not surprising that in some circumstances a Th2-biased response can produce asthma without apparently producing type 1 hypersensitivity. However, in the majority of circumstances, both phenomena co-exist. IL-10, also released by Th2 cells, has a downregulatory effect on Th1 cells, probably by interfering with the production of IL-12 from antigen-presenting cells which would normally stimulate IFN-γ production (Fig. 18.1). Conversely, IFN-γ will downregulate Th2 activities. Thus it is apparent from these mutual inhibitory mechanisms that once a particular pattern of response has been established, it is likely to persist (Holt, 1996).

CONCEPTS OF ALLERGEN AVOIDANCE PROPHYLAXIS

It is generally assumed that the same factors which are involved in the induction of asthma are also likely to incite the disease once established. However, this is not necessarily the case. Thus, strategies of prophylaxis for primary prevention may be very different to those required for the management of established disease. It is, therefore, necessary to distinguish the various steps where modulation of the allergic response or of the environment might be appropriate. Allergen avoidance and so-called immunotherapy or hyposensitization employed in the treatment of atopic asthma might be termed tertiary prophylaxis. Intervention which is

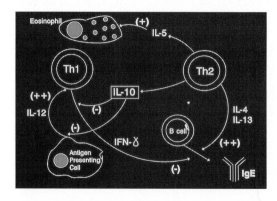

Figure 18.1 *The cytokine 'confusogram' indicating the mutual inhibition of T-helper cell one (Th1) and Th2 activity and its effect on IgE production and eosinophil activation.*

employed in individuals who show signs of allergy but not yet of asthma could be termed secondary prophylaxis, while perhaps the most exciting and speculative of all is primary prophylaxis which would be employed to prevent allergic sensitization in the first place.

The strategies will be discussed in reverse order because most information available is related to tertiary prophylaxis with progressively less associated with secondary and primary interventions. However, the impact of the interventions on the disease are likely to be far greater for primary prophylaxis compared with secondary and tertiary intervention.

TERTIARY PROPHYLAXIS

Lessons from occupational allergic asthma

Sensitization to a range of factors can occur in the work environment. Some are complex proteins such as occur in animal laboratories, and others simple chemicals, probably acting as haptens such as platinum salts and toluene di-isocyanate. Amongst sensitized subjects, some develop asthma and this can become a severe and incapacitating problem. This not uncommon problem provides a unique opportunity to derive lessons in relation to allergen exposure, sensitization and the establishment of asthma in normal domestic environments.

For the majority of occupational allergens, sensitization is more likely to occur in atopic individuals who already have a susceptibility to developing type 1 hypersensitivity. Furthermore, for some of the allergens, co-existent cigarette smoking increases the risk of sensitization and the establishment of asthma. Once asthma has occurred, treatment primarily involves removal from exposure to the offending precipitant. Under such circumstances, many individuals have no further problems. However, a proportion will continue to have asthma despite having no further exposure to the original inducing allergen (Chan-Yeung and Dimich-Ward, 1999).

The key factors (*see* Table 18.2) which discriminate the ongoing asthmatic following occupational allergen exposure are almost certainly highly relevant to atopic asthma in the normal environment. Thus, the ongoing asthmatic has a longer duration of exposure to allergen and a longer duration of symptoms before diagnosis and removal from exposure. As a consequence, such individuals have significantly lower lung function and increased bronchial hyperresponsiveness compared with those who remit. The persistent asthmatics also have a higher sensitivity to the original triggering allergen and are more likely to have an eosinophil-mediated inflammation in the airways (Paggiaro *et al.*, 1994). If such observations are relevant to standard atopic asthma, then the earlier allergen avoidance is instituted after sensitization and the onset of disease, the greater the likelihood of success. Once the disease is well established with 'eosinophilic bronchitis', the less likely allergen avoidance, as a tertiary

Table 18.2   *Influences on outcome after cessation of exposure to allergen*

	Continuing asthma	Asymptomatic
Duration of exposure before onset of symptoms	Prolonged	Short
Duration of symptoms before diagnosis and removal	Prolonged	Short
Lung function at diagnosis	Reduced	Normal or near normal
Sensitivity to allergen on bronchial challenge	High	Low
Eosinophils in bronchial lavage	Increased	Normal

Source: Adapted from a review by Paggiaro *et al.* (1994).

prophylaxis, is likely to have any significant effect. This perhaps accounts for some of the disappointing results from allergen avoidance as tertiary prophylaxis.

House dust mites

As house dust mites are one of the major allergens associated with asthma, strategies to reduce exposure have been extensively investigated as tertiary prophylaxis (Colloff *et al.*, 1992). Unfortunately, the majority of single interventions have failed to achieve a reduction in allergen load sufficient to lead to a clinical improvement. However, in the ideal situation, such as occurs in high altitude/low humidity environments where house dust mites are almost non-existent, very considerable improvement can be achieved. Not only is there a diminution in symptoms and requirement for asthma prophylaxis, but there are also very considerable reductions in bronchial hyperresponsiveness. Indeed, the improvements are far greater than is achieved by conventional asthma prophylaxis. Furthermore, prolonged allergen avoidance in such circumstances also results in a reduction in allergen-induced increases in bronchial hyperresponsiveness (Peroni *et al.*, 1994). Sadly, however, once individuals return to their home environment and further sustained allergen exposure, the problem recurs because once established, immunological memory is very long lasting. Nevertheless, it would seem appropriate to attempt to mimic the environment that exists at high altitude to achieve an improvement in asthma control in the normal domestic situation.

There have been extensive reviews of strategies for house dust mite avoidance (Platts-Mills *et al.*, 1997). The house dust mite most successfully replicates in a condition of relatively high temperature and humidity. Thus, reduction of either will achieve reductions in allergen load. The mite utilizes human dander in association with specific moulds as its primary nutritional source. The bedding, therefore, provides a unique and ideal environment for the mite.

The most successful single strategies for mite reduction and control of disease have involved bed covering systems that separate the mite and its allergen from the asthmatic individual. Provided the mattress, pillow and bed covers are sealed in a mite allergen impermeable encasing, reduction in allergen exposure and asthma can be achieved (Ehnert *et al.*, 1992). However, the clinical effects are relatively modest by comparison with the effects of residence at high altitude.

Attempts have been made to develop sprays that both kill house dust mites and denature the major allergens. While these can be shown to reduce house mite numbers and allergen levels (Warner *et al.*, 1993), the clinical efficacy has been equivocal with many studies showing no effect (Ehnert *et al.*, 1992). High efficiency vacuum cleaners can reduce allergen load but, again, no trials have yet demonstrated that this, as a single intervention, will improve asthma (Hegarty *et al.*, 1995). Effective home ventilation systems have in some countries achieved clinical efficacy (Wichman *et al.*, 1994) while in others, no effects have been demonstrated (Fletcher *et al.*, 1996). The difference would appear to relate to the ambient outdoor humidity. Thus, in Denmark studies have been clinically positive while in the UK, thus far they have been negative. Our own experience is that ventilation systems appreciably reduce allergen load but not sufficiently to reduce symptoms (Warner *et al.*, 2000). Similarly, the use of dehumidifiers in homes has yet to be shown to achieve any effect. These variations in outcome from mite avoidance trials using different forms of interventions have prompted the conclusion from a recently published meta-analysis that this strategy is ineffective (Gotzsche *et al.*, 1998). This sweeping conclusion, which is widely disputed, is unlikely to be correct as it takes little if any account of the degree to which each strategy reduces allergen load.

Our own belief is that single interventions are unlikely to have significant efficacy as all sources of house mite allergen must be tackled. Thus a combination of bed covers with dehumidification and perhaps also further treatment of soft furnishings and carpets are most likely to reduce allergen sufficiently to improve patients clinically. Such combined strategies have yet to be submitted to controlled clinical trial and to cost–benefit analysis. They are urgently required.

Clearly there are a number of interventions which have been shown to have no impact whatsoever, not only on clinical symptoms but also on allergen load. This relates to some forms of anti-mite sprays (Reiser et al., 1990) and ionizers (Warner et al., 1993). Unfortunately advertising regulations that cover domestic products do not have the same rigorous scrutiny that is applied to pharmaceutical interventions. In many countries, therefore, it is possible for manufacturers to intimate that a domestic product will have value in reducing house mites, and thus asthma, in the absence of good controlled clinical trial evidence. This leaves vulnerable asthma families in a highly susceptible position in relation to such advertising. It is incumbent on the physician dealing with such families to be aware of which products have been appropriately investigated.

Cat and dog allergens

Cat and/or dog dander allergy are the next most common associations with atopic asthma after house dust mites. In fact, the major allergens from cat and dog are not the dander itself but are contained in saliva and sebaceous secretions. The particle size is very much smaller than that of house dust mite and, therefore, the allergens are spread much more widely in the environment. Indeed, they can be detected in many locations outside the home (Custovic et al., 1996), which makes avoidance very much more difficult.

Once an asthmatic individual has been shown to be allergic to a particular cat or dog, it would seem entirely appropriate to recommend removal of the animal. However, the allergen persists within the dust in the home for many months and sometimes years. Nevertheless, removal can achieve clinical improvements. One suggested alternative is that regular washing of the animal will remove the major allergens from the dander and thereby reduce allergen load (De Blay et al., 1991). Whilst this can be demonstrated, as yet there have been no controlled clinical trials to demonstrate that this achieves clinical efficacy. Unfortunately, the patient will continue to be exposed to the allergen outside the domestic environment and this may be particularly important in schools where contemporaries who are pet owners themselves, will bring the allergen into the school on their clothes (Lönnkvist et al., 1999).

Other allergens

Clearly there are a number of other domestic pets that have the potential to produce allergic reactions, including birds, rabbits, hamsters, etc. However, the degree of sensitivity to these animals is very much lower than to cats and dogs, probably because of their relatively restricted location within the home.

In North America, it has been shown that cockroach allergens are major contributors to asthma in inner city areas, where this occurs in the socio-economically deprived population. It appears to be much less of a problem in Europe (Rosenstreich et al., 1997).

It is possible to culture moulds from house and bed dust in large quantities. However, the relevance of these moulds to asthma is contentious (Garrett et al., 1998). Mould allergy is very much less common than allergy to house dust mite, animal danders and pollens. Nevertheless, there are occasional examples where indoor moulds may be relevant. Reduced humidity is likely to be a key factor in reducing exposure.

Outdoor allergens can accumulate within the house. It would, therefore, seem prudent to advise pollen-allergic asthmatics to keep their houses and particularly their bedrooms sealed during the day and only open windows at night when the outdoor pollen count is low. Ventilation systems with heat exchangers can be equipped with appropriate filters to avoid drawing pollen allergens into the house.

Foods

In general, food-induced asthma is rare and even when it occurs, food avoidance does not achieve a significant improvement in disease. However, there are occasional cases where food allergens are involved. Recently, it has been identified that this is particularly the case in a small percentage of very brittle asthmatics (Ayres *et al.*, 1998). Thus when all else fails in dealing with the very severe asthmatic, it would seem appropriate to consider dietary manipulations in an attempt to achieve improvement.

Immunotherapy

Immunotherapy involves the administration of ever increasing doses of the allergen which is causing problems in an atopic individual in an attempt to induce some form of tolerance. Normally this is administered by subcutaneous injection and has been shown to be of clinical benefit compared with placebo in relation to insect venom hypersensitivity, seasonal allergic rhinoconjunctivitis and asthma, and even for house dust mite, cat- and dog-sensitive asthmatic children (De Blay *et al.*, 1991). However, the treatment is not without hazards in that during the course of treatment, acute severe allergic reactions including anaphylaxis and death can occur (BSACI Working Party, 1993). Furthermore, there have been too few head-to-head comparisons between immunotherapy and other more conventional approaches to asthma therapy to be able to position it in therapeutic algorithms. Cost–benefit analyses have also not been performed. Thus in the majority of guidelines, immunotherapy is not recommended for the management of atopic asthma. It might have a role in the seasonal asthmatic and can sometimes be effective where a single major allergen is involved.

However, the scientific basis for the use of this therapy has advanced appreciably. It is clear that therapeutic efficacy is linked to the loss of the late allergen-induced reaction observed in many patients after bronchial challenge (Warner *et al.*, 1978). Furthermore, immunotherapy produces a lymphocyte switching from Th2 predominance towards Th1 in terms of the pattern of cytokines released by allergen (Varney *et al.*, 1993). There is also some limited evidence that immunotherapy, unlike pharmacotherapy, will modify the natural history of disease by reducing the development of new allergen sensitivities in mono-sensitized children (Des-Roches *et al.*, 1997), and preventing or delaying onset of asthma in pollen-sensitized, allergic rhinitic children (Jacobsen *et al.*, 1996). Thus immunotherapy may well have a renaissance in asthma management.

SECONDARY PROPHYLAXIS

Allergen avoidance

Much of the earlier efforts in allergen avoidance have been focused on infant feeding and, in particular, on avoidance of early exposure to cow's milk protein and sometimes also egg, fish, nuts, etc. Most of the studies commenced avoidance in the postnatal period and results have been very variable, with no clear cut view emerging. Furthermore, elimination of cow's milk may be a risk for impaired growth in young children (Isolauri *et al.*, 1998). One suggestion has been that allergen exposure continues in relation to the mother's diet. Thus, one or two studies have shown somewhat better outcomes when the mothers have adopted an avoidance diet during lactation (Arshad *et al.*, 1991). Our own observations of this would suggest that postnatal, maternal and infant dieting not only has no effect on the subsequent prevalence of disease but might even increase the severity of the ensuing problems.

There are only two published studies which have combined aeroallergen and food allergen avoidance in infancy. Both showed significant effects on early food allergy and atopic dermatitis but with continuing follow-up, the effects diminished (Matthew *et al.*, 1977; Hide *et al.*, 1996). Indeed in one very large and meticulously conducted study, the final conclusion was that the effort was not justified by the outcome (Zeiger *et al.*, 1992).

Neonatal immunomodulation

As results of postnatal allergen avoidance have proved so disappointing, it has been proposed that an attempt should be made to induce a Th1 immunizing response to allergen in the immediate postnatal period. This might be achieved by high exposure to relevant allergens as distinct from the normal low dose exposure which is likely to occur with inhalants in the respiratory tract during the first months of life (Holt, 1994). Facilitation of a Th1 response might be achieved by utilizing fusion proteins where the allergen is combined with a cytokine such as IL-12 that will induce a Th1 response. This valid and credible proposal has arisen from observations that there appears to be a reciprocal relationship between early exposure to infection and allergy. Thus, allergy and allergic disease is less common in individuals who are tuberculin positive (Shirakawa *et al.*, 1997) or have had measles rather than being immunized against measles (Shaheen *et al.*, 1996). It is probably not even necessary for active infection to induce a Th1 response. The microbial flora of the infant's gut will lead to significant exposures to lipopolysaccharide under perfectly normal circumstances, which will induce a normal immunizing Th1 response. However, in the affluent environment, gut microbial flora of the small baby has changed appreciably and may well have led to the loss of a normal immunizing influence which would prevent the development of allergy (Bjorksten *et al.*, 1999). This would explain much of the distribution of atopic disease in the Western world.

However, the approaches proposed above are at present in the realms of speculation and much more needs to be learned about the mechanisms before embarking on any clinical studies.

Pharmacotherapy

There are some programmes reviewing intervention in children with established allergic disease but without asthma. This would appear to be a very fruitful line of research. One study employing ketotifen, an antihistamine which has very weak, if any, anti-asthma properties, was given to infants with atopic dermatitis, and showed a reduced prevalence of asthma in the active group compared with the placebo group after a year of treatment (Iikura *et al.*, 1992). The effect was observed only in those atopic dermatitis children who also had a raised total IgE level.

There is now another very large multi-national study further investigating the proposition that treating with an antihistamine, cetirizine, which has an effect on eosinophil trafficking, might prevent the development of asthma in individuals with atopic dermatitis (ETAC Study Group, 1998). Over 18 months of treatment those infants with sensitivity to house dust mite and/or grass pollen were significantly less likely to develop asthma than those taking placebo.

PRIMARY PROPHYLAXIS

Mechanisms of fetal sensitization

The main problem with all of the above studies is that the intervention was employed postnatally, and as has been suggested by Martinez and colleagues, it is likely to already be too late to employ preventive strategies when 'the cord has been cut' (Brown *et al.*, 1997). We and many others have now shown that the foetus is far from immunologically naïve. Indeed, we can identify allergen-specific cellular responses as early as 20–22 weeks of gestation (Jones *et al.*, 1996). As pregnancy is Th2 (allergy-biased phenomenon) one component modulating the mother's immune response to foeto/paternal antigens, it is perhaps not surprising that a high percentage of newborn babies are not only sensitized to allergens, to which they have been exposed via the mother, but also have a Th2-biased response (Prescott *et al.*, 1998). Whether this persists and results in allergic disease may be influenced by their microbial exposure in early childhood (Fig. 18.2).

We have recently demonstrated that the amniotic fluid contains significant levels not only of a range of cytokines biased towards the Th2 spectrum but also IgE. Indeed the levels of IgE in the amniotic fluid are proportionate to the maternal levels. It is clear, therefore, that although IgE does not cross the placenta to the foetal circulation, the foetus is exposed to maternal IgE and Th2 cytokines in the amniotic fluid (Jones *et al.*, 1998).

The foetus not only swallows with a highly efficient cycling of proteins through the foetal gut but also makes significant respiratory movement. This, together with the highly permeable skin, means that there is every possibility that the cytokines and the IgE will have an influence on the foetal immune responses. The foetal gut is colonized by HLA-DR expressing antigen-presenting cells even in the first trimester. IgE binding to dendritic cells will increase their capacity to present antigen 100–1000-fold. This, therefore, would be a credible route by which foetal sensitization occurs. Indeed one could propose that this mechanism has evolved to equip the newborn baby to handle its mother's parasites at a time when it would otherwise be extremely susceptible to overwhelming parasitic disease. That this does not occur is well established as being due to efficient generation of Th2 response and IgE generation against parasites in the newborn (Malhotra *et al.*, 1999).

Antenatal intervention

These data set the scene for generating a hypothesis that the critical period for allergen exposure and, therefore, for intervention, is antenatally. Thus future trials of allergen avoidance must commence virtually at conception. Such studies are now running and it remains to be seen whether they will be more successful than later interventions. However, there are one or two additional facts that would support the view that intervention antenatally will be effective. It has been shown that the presence of IgG/anti-IgE antibodies in the newborn, which must have been generated by the mother, are protective against the development of allergy and subsequent allergic disease. We have shown that the levels of IgG antibody downregulate the T-cell response to allergen. Perhaps, therefore, some form of maternal immune modulation will protect the foetus (Warner *et al.*, 1997).

CONCLUSIONS

The allergist's view of asthma control is that a focus on allergens will prove extremely fruitful in the future. However, before we plunge into major community-based strategies, we must

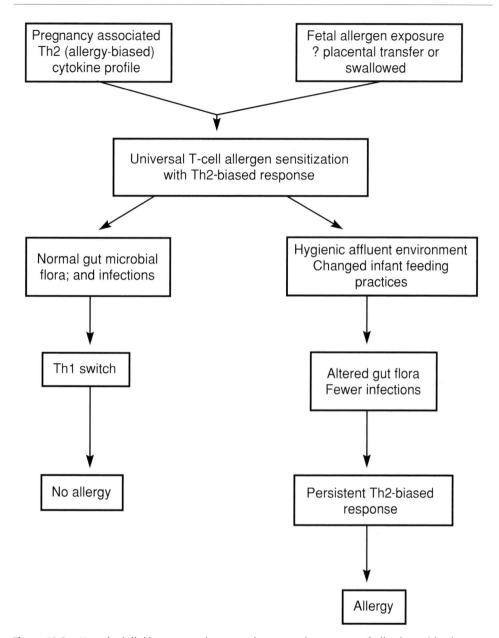

Figure 18.2 *Hypothesis linking ante- and post-natal events to the ontogeny of allergic sensitization.*

elaborate further on the mechanisms and when they are operative. The other prerequisite for establishing such programmes is to identify with high sensitivity and specificity the at-risk population.

REFERENCES

Abramson MJ, Puy RM, Weiner JM. (1995) Is allergen immunotherapy effective in asthma? A meta analysis of randomised controlled trials. *Am J Respir Crit Care Med*, **151**, 969–74.

Arshad SH, Matthews S, Gant C, Hide DW. (1991) Effect of allergen avoidance on development of allergic disorders in infancy. *Lancet*, **339**, 1493–7.

Ayres JG, Miles JF, Barnes PJ. (1998) Brittle asthma. *Thorax*, **53**, 315–21.

Bjorksten B, Naaber P, Sepp E, Mikelsaar M. (1999) The intestinal microflora in allergic Estonian and Swedish two-year old children. *Clin Exp Allergy*, **29**, 342–6.

Bousquet J, Hejjasic A, Michel FB. (1990) Specific immunotherapy in asthma. *J Allergy Clin Immunol*, **86**, 292–305.

Brown MA, Halonen MJ, Martinez FD. (1997) Cutting the cord: is birth already too late for primary prevention of allergy? *Clin Exp Allergy*, **27**, 4–6.

BSACI Working Party Report. (1993) Position paper on allergen immunotherapy. *Clin Exp Allergy*, **23**(Suppl. 3), 1–44.

Burr ML, Merritt TG, Dunstan FD, McGuire MJ. (1997) The development of allergy in high risk children. *Clin Exp Allergy*, **27**, 1247–53.

Chan-Yeung M, Dimich-Ward H. (1999) Natural history of occupational lung diseases. *Europ Respir Monograph 11*, **4**, 46–63.

Colloff MJ, Ayres J, Carswell F, *et al.* (1992) The control of allergens of dust mites and domestic pets: a position paper. *Clin Exp Allergy*, **22**(Suppl. 2), 1–28.

Custovic A, Green R, Taggart SCO, *et al.* (1996) Domestic allergens in public places to dog (Can f 1) and cockroach (Bla g 2) allergens in dust and mite, cat, dog and cockroach allergens in the air in public buildings. *Clin Exp Allergy*, **26**, 1246–52.

Custovic A, Simpson A, Chapman MD, Woodcock A. (1998) Allergen avoidance in the treatment of asthma and atopic disorders. *Thorax*, **53**, 63–72.

De Blay F, Chapman MD, Platts-Mills TNE. (1991) Airborne cat allergen Fel d 1 environmental control with cat *in situ*. *Am Rev Respir Dis*, **143**, 1334–9.

Des-Roches A, Paradis L, Menardo JL, *et al.* (1997) Immunotherapy with a standardised *Dermatophagoides pteronyssinus* extract VI. Specific immunotherapy prevents the onset of new sensitizations in children. *J Allergy Clin Immunol*, **99**, 450–3.

Ehnert B, Lau-Schadendorf S, Weber A, *et al.* (1992) Reducing domestic exposure to dust mite allergen reduces bronchial hyperactivity in sensitive children with asthma. *J Allergy Clin Immunol*, **90**, 135–8.

ETAC Study Group. (1998) Allergic factors associated with the development of asthma and the influence of cetirizine in a double blind randomised placebo controlled trial: first results of ETAC. *Pediatr Allergy Immunol*, **9**, 116–24.

Fletcher AM, Pickering CAC, Custovic A, *et al.* (1996) Reduction in humidity as a method of controlling mites and mite allergens: the use of mechanical ventilation in British domestic dwellings. *Clin Exp Allergy*, **26**, 1051–6.

Garrett MH, Rayment PR, Hooper MA, *et al.* (1998) Indoor airborne fungal spores, home dampness and associations with environmental factors and respiratory health in children. *Clin Exp Allergy*, **28**, 459–67.

Gotzsche PC, Hammarquist C, Burr M. (1998) House dust mite control measures in the management of asthma: meta analysis. *BMJ*, **317**, 1105–10.

Halonen M, Stern D, Wright AL, *et al.* (1997) Alternaria is a major allergen for asthma in children raised in a desert environment. *Am J Respir Crit Care Med*, **155**, 1356–61.

Hegarty JM, Rouhbakhsh S, Warner JA, Warner JO. (1995) A comparison of the effect of conventional and filter vacuum cleaners on airborne house dust mite allergen. *Respir Med*, **89**, 279–84.

Hide DW, Matthews S, Tariq S, Arshad SH. (1996) Allergen avoidance in infancy and allergy at 4 years of age. *Allergy*, **51**, 89–93.

Holt PG. (1994) A potential vaccine strategy for asthma and allied atopic diseases. *Lancet*, **344**, 456–8.

Holt PG. (1996) Primary allergic sensitization to environmental antigens: perinatal T-cell priming as a determinant of responder phenotype in adulthood. *J Exp Med*, **183**, 1297–301.

Iikura Y, Naspitz CK, Mikawa S, *et al.* (1992) Prevention of asthma by ketotifen in infants with atopic dermatitis. *Ann Allergy*, **68**, 233–6.

Isolauri E, Sutas Y, Salo MK, *et al.* (1998) Elimination diet in cow's milk allergy: risk for impaired growth in young children. *J Pediatr*, **132**, 1004–9.

Jacobsen L, Dreborg S, Møller C, *et al.* (1996) Immunotherapy as a preventive treatment. *J Allergy Clin Immunol*, **97**, 232 (Abstract).

Jones AC, Miles EA, Warner JO, *et al.* (1996) Peripheral blood mononuclear cell proliferative responses to mitogenic and allergenic stimulae during gestation. *Pediatr Allergy Immunol*, **7**, 109–16.

Jones CA, Warner JA, Warner JO. (1998) Fetal swallowing of IgE. *Lancet*, **351**, 1859 (Research Letter).

Kjellman B, Pettersson R. (1983) The problem of furred pets in childhood atopic disease. *Allergy*, **38**, 65–73.

Kulig M, Vergmann R, Tacke U, Wahn U, Guggenmoos-Holzmann I, and the MASS Study Group. (1998) Long lasting sensitization to food during the first two years precedes allergic airway disease. *Pediatr Allergy Immunol*, **9**, 61–7.

Lönnkvist K, Hallden G, Dahlen SE, *et al.* (1999) Markers of inflammation and bronchial reactivity in children with asthma exposed to animal dander in school dust. *Pediatr Allergy Immunol*, **10**, 45–52.

Malhotra I, Mungai P, Wamachi A. (1999) Helminth and bacillus Calmette–Guerin-induced immunity in children sensitized *in utero* to filariasis and schistosomiasis. *J Immunol*, **162**, 6843–8.

Matthew DJ, Taylor B, Norman AP, *et al.* (1977) Prevention of eczema. *Lancet*, **1**, 321–4.

McNichol KN, Williams HE. (1973) Spectrum of asthma in children. 2. Allergic components. *BMJ*, **4**, 12–16.

Paggiaro PL, Vagaggini B, Bacci E, *et al.* (1994) Prognosis of occupational asthma. *Eur Respir J*, **7**, 761–7.

Peat JK, Salome CM, Woolcock AJ. (1990) Longitudinal changes in atopy during a 4-year period: relation to bronchial hyperresponsiveness and respiratory symptoms in a population sample of Australian school children. *J Allergy Clin Immunol*, **85**, 65–74.

Peroni DG, Boner AL, Vallone G, *et al.* (1994) Effective allergen avoidance at high altitude reduces allergen induced bronchial hyperresponsiveness. *Am J Respir Crit Care Med*, **149**, 1442–6.

Platts-Mills TAE, Vervloet D, Wayne RT, *et al.* (1997) Indoor allergens and asthma. Report of 3rd International Workshop. *J Allergy Clin Immunol*, **100**, S1–24.

Potter PC, Cadman A. (1996) Pollen allergy in South Africa. *Clin Exp Allergy*, **26**, 1347–54.

Prescott S, Macaubas C, Holt B, *et al.* (1998) Transplacental priming of the human immune system to environmental allergens: universal skewing of initial T-cell responses towards Th-2 cytokine profile. *J Immunol*, **160**, 4730–7.

Rancé F, Kanny G, Dutau G, Moneret-Vautrin DA. (1999) Food hypersensitivity in children: clinical aspects and distribution of allergens. *Pediatr Allergy Immunol*, **10**, 33–8.

Reiser J, Ingram D, Mitchell EB, Warner JO. (1990) House dust mite allergen levels and an anti-mite mattress spray (Natamycin) in the treatment of childhood asthma. *Clin Exp Allergy*, **20**, 561–7.

Rosenstreich DL, Eggleston P, Kattan M, *et al.* (1997) The role of cockroach allergy and exposure to cockroach allergen in causing morbidity amongst inner city children with asthma. *N Engl J Med*, **336**, 1356–63.

Shaheen SO, Abbay P, Hall AJ, *et al.* (1996) Measles and atopy in Guinea Bissau. *Lancet*, **347**, 1792–6.

Shirakawa T, Nomota T, Shimazoo S *et al.* (1997) The inverse association between tuberculin responses and atopic disorders. *Science*, **775**, 77–9.

Sporik R, Holgate ST, Cogswell JJ. (1991) Natural history of asthma in childhood – a birth cohort study. *Arch Dis Child*, **66**, 1050–3.

van Asperen PP, Mukhi A. (1994) Role of atopy in the natural history of wheeze and bronchial hyperresponsiveness in childhood. *Pediatr Allergy Immunol*, **5**, 178–83.

Varney VA, Hamid QA, Gaga M, *et al.* (1993) Influence of grass pollen immunotherapy on cellular infiltration and cytokine mRNA expression during allergen induced late phase cutaneous responses. *J Clin Invest*, **92**, 644–51.

Warner JA, Frederick JM, Bryant TN, *et al.* (2000) Mechanical ventilation and high efficiency vacuum cleaning: a combined strategy of mite and mite allergen reduction in the control of mite sensitive asthma. *J Allergy Clin Immunol*, **105**, 75–82.

Warner JA, Jones CA, Jones AC, *et al.* (1997) Immune responses during pregnancy and the development of allergic disease. *Pediatr Allergy Immunol*, **8** (Suppl. 10), 5–10.

Warner JA, Marchant JL, Warner JO. (1993) A double blind trial of ionisers in house dust mite sensitive asthmatic children. *Thorax*, **48**, 330–3.

Warner JA, Marchant JL, Warner JO. (1993) Allergen avoidance in the homes of allergic asthmatic children: the effect of Allersearch DMS. *Clin Exp Allergy*, **23**, 279–86.

Warner JO, Price JF, Soothill JF, Hey EN. (1978) Controlled trial of hyposensitization to *Dermatophagoides pteronyssinus* in children with asthma. *Lancet*, **2**, 912–15.

Wichman M, Emenius G, Egmar A-C, *et al.* (1994) Reduced mite allergen levels in dwellings with mechanical exhaust and supply ventilation. *Clin Exp Allergy*, **24**, 109–14.

Woodcock A, Custovic A. (1998) Role of the indoor environment in determining the severity of asthma. *Thorax*, **53** (Suppl.2), 47–51.

Zeiger RS, Heller S, Mellon MH, *et al.* (1992) Genetic and environmental factors affecting the development of atopy through age 4 in children of atopic parents: a prospective randomised study of food allergen avoidance. *Pediatr Allergy Immunol*, **3**, 110–27.

Index